Barry B. Halliwell · Henrik E. Poulsen
Editors

Cigarette Smoke and Oxidative Stress

Barry B. Halliwell · Henrik E. Poulsen
Editors

Cigarette Smoke and Oxidative Stress

With 66 Figures, 18 in Color and 8 Tables

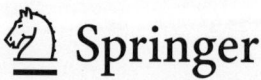
Springer

Barry B. Halliwell
Pharmacology Group
University of London King's College
Manresa Road, London SW3 6LX
UK

Henrik E. Poulsen
Dept. of Clinical Pharmalogy,
Rigshospitalet
University Hospital Copenhagen
Tagensvej 20, 2200 Copenhagen N
Denmark

Library of Congress Control Number: 2006925085

ISBN-10 3-540-31410-5 Springer Berlin Heidelberg New York
ISBN-13 978-3-540-31410-3 Springer Berlin Heidelberg New York

This work is subject to copyright. All rights are reserved, whether the whole or part of the material is concerned, specifically the rights of translation, reprinting, reuse of illustrations, recitation, broadcasting, reproduction on microfilm or in any other way, and storage in data banks. Duplication of this publication or parts therof is permitted only under the provisions of the German Copyright Law of September 9, 1965, in its current version, and permission for use must always be obtained from Springer-Verlag. Violations are liable for prosecution under the German Copyright Law.

Springer is a part of Springer Science + Business Media
springeronline.com
© Springer-Verlag Berlin Heidelberg 2006
Printed in Germany

The use of general descriptive names, registered names, trademarks, etc. in this publication does not imply, even in the absence of a specific statement, that such names are exempt from the relevant protective laws and regulations and therefore free for general use.

Product liability: The publishers cannot guarantee the accuracy of any information about dosage and application contained in this book. In every individual case the user must check such information by consulting the relevant literature.

Editor: Dr. Ute Heilmann
Desk Editor: Meike Stoeck
Production & Typesetting: LE-TeX Jelonek, Schmidt & Vöckler GbR, Leipzig
Cover: Frido Steinen-Broo, Estudio Calamar, Spain

Printed on acid-free paper   21/3100/YL   5 4 3 2 1 0

Preface

From a public health point of view, there is little doubt that one of the most important preventable causes of disease worldwide is tobacco smoking. It is also clear that tobacco smoke contains a vast number of chemicals with important biological effects in disease processes. The gas phase of tobacco smoke is oxidizing, the tar phase is reducing, and whole smoke is roughly neutral, so its effects on oxidative stress may be an "antioxidant paradox."

From a scientific point of view, we found it of interest to make a comprehensive overview of what we presently know about oxidative stress and tobacco smoke, because smoking is presently the best-known common condition associated with oxidative stress, and it may serve as a model for others. To this end, we have asked distinguished researchers from the public and the private sectors to evaluate the present scientific status in their particular area. Authors were selected purely because of their scientific merits.

We do not claim that all the well-described health hazards associated with cigarette smoking stem from oxidative stress, nor should we. However, we ought to be able to find out, and for some of those health hazards, we can already say. We hope this book will stimulate more research to find answers to the remaining questions.

Barry Halliwell and Henrik E. Poulsen

Contents

1. **Oxidative Stress** 1
   Barry B. Halliwell and Henrik E. Poulsen

2. **Tobacco Smoke Constituents Affecting Oxidative Stress** 5
   Jan B. Wooten, Salem Chouchane, and Thomas E. McGrath

3. **Oxidative Modifications of Proteins and Lipids by Cigarette Smoke (CS). A Central Role for Unsaturated Aldehydes in CS-Mediated Airway Inflammation** 47
   Albert van der Vliet

4. **Cigarette Smoke-Induced Redox Signaling and Gene Expression in In Vitro and In Vivo Models** 75
   Thomas Müller and Stephan Gebel

5. **Redox Effects of Cigarette Smoke in Lung Inflammation** 113
   Irfan Rahman

6. **Oxidative Stress in the Pathogenesis of Chronic Obstructive Pulmonary Disease** 165
   Irfan Rahman

7. **Modulation of Cigarette Smoke Effects by Diet and Antioxidants** 199
   Marion Dietrich and Gladys Block

8. **Modulation of Cigarette Smoke Effects by Antioxidants: Oxidative Stress and Degenerative Diseases** 215
   Jari Kaikkonen and Jukka T. Salonen

9. **Smoking Depletes Vitamin C: Should Smokers Be Recommended to Take Supplements?** 237
   Jens Lykkesfeldt

10. **Experimental In Vitro Exposure Methods for Studying the Effects of Inhalable Compounds** 261
    Michaela Aufderheide

11	**Oxidative Stress in Laboratory Animals Exposed to Cigarette Smoke, with Special Reference to Chronic Obstructive Pulmonary Disease**	279
	Chris Coggins	
12	**Pulmonary Effects of Cigarette Smoke in Humans**	293
	Nick H.T. ten Hacken and Dirkje S. Postma	
13	**Smoking and Oxidative Stress: Vascular Damage**	339
	Thomas Münzel, Felix Post, and Ascan Warnholtz	
14	**Nrf2: a Transcription Factor that Modifies Susceptibility to Cigarette Smoke-Induced Pulmonary Oxidative Stress and Emphysema**	365
	Shyam Biswal and Thomas W. Kensler	
15	**Tobacco Smoke and Skin Aging**	379
	Akimichi Morita	
16	**Cigarette Smoke and Oxidative DNA Modification**	387
	Henrik E. Poulsen, Allan Weimann, and Barry B. Halliwell	

Contributors

Michaela Aufderheide
Fraunhofer Institute of Toxicology and Aerosol Research Drug Research and Clinical Inhalation, Nikolai-Fuchs-Strasse 1, 30625 Hannover, Germany

Shyam Biswal
Division of Toxicological Sciences, Department of Environmental Health Sciences, Johns Hopkins Bloomberg School of Public Health, 615 N. Wolfe Street, Baltimore, MD 21205, USA

Gladys Block
Division of Health Policy and Management, School of Public Health, University of California, Berkeley, CA 94720, USA

Salem Chouchane
Philip Morris USA Postgraduate Research Program, USA

Chris Coggins
1266 Carson Watts Road, King,NC 27021-7453, USA

Marion Dietrich
Nutritional Epidemiology, JM USDA HNRCA at Tufts University, 711 Washington Street, Boston, MA 02111, USA

Stephan Gebel
Philip Morris Research Laboratories GmbH, Fuggerstrasse 3, 51149 Cologne, Germany

Nick H.T. ten Hacken
University Medical Center Groningen, Postbox 3001, 9700 RB Groningen, The Netherlands

Barry B. Halliwell
Pharmacology Group, University of London King's College, Manresa Road, London SW3 6LX, UK

Jari Kaikkonen
Oy Jurilab Ltd., Microkatu 1, 70210 Kuopio, Finland

Contributors

Thomas Kensler
Division of Toxicological Sciences, Department of Environmental Health Sciences, Johns Hopkins Bloomberg School of Public Health, 615 N. Wolfe Street, Baltimore, MD 21205, USA

Jens Lykkesfeldt
Section of Biomedicine, Department of Veterinary Pathobiology, Royal Veterinary & Agricultural University, 9 Ridebanevej, 1870 Frederiksberg C, Copenhagen, Denmark

Thomas E. McGrath
Philip Morris USA Research Center, 4201 Commerce Road, Richmond VA 23234, USA
Current address: Philip Morris International, Neuchâtel, Switzerland

Akimichi Morita
Department of Geriatric and Environmental Dermatology, Nogoya City University Graduate School of Medical Sciences, Nagoya 467-8601, Japan

Thomas Müller
Philip Morris Research Laboratories GmbH, Fuggerstrasse 3, 51149 Cologne, Germany

Thomas Münzel
II Medizinische Klinik und Poliklinik Johannes Gutenberg-Universität Mainz, Langenbeckstrasse 1, 55131 Mainz, Germany

Felix Post
II Medizinische Klinik und Poliklinik Johannes Gutenberg-Universität Mainz, Langenbeckstrasse 1, 55131 Mainz, Germany

Dirkje S. Postma
Department of Pulmonology, University Hospital, University of Groningen, Postbus 30001, Hanseplein 1, 9700 RB Groningen, The Netherlands

Henrik F. Poulsen
Dept. of Clinical Pharmacology, Q7642, Rigshospitalet, University Hospital Copenhagen, Tagensvej 20, 2200 Copenhagen N, Denmark

Irfan Rahman
Division of Lung Biology and Disease Program, University of Rochester Medical Center, Rochester, NY 14642, USA

Jukka T. Salonen
Oy Jurilab Ltd., Kuopio, Finland

Albert Van der Vliet
Department of Pathology, University of Vermont, College of Medicine, Burlington, VT 05405, USA

Ascan Warnholtz
II Medizinische Klinik und Poliklinik Johannes Gutenberg-Universität Mainz, Langenbeckstrasse 1, 55131 Mainz, Germany

Jan B. Wooten
Philip Morris USA Research Center, 4201 Commerce Road, Richmond, VA 23234, USA

Allan Weimann
Dept. of Clinical Pharmalogy, Q7642, Rigshospitalet, University Hospital Copenhagen, Tagensvej 20, 2200 Copenhagen N, Denmark

Chapter 1

Oxidative Stress

Barry B. Halliwell and Henrik E. Poulsen

Contents

1.1	What is Oxidative Stress?	2
1.2	Oxidative Stress	2
1.3	Measurement of Oxidative Stress	3
1.4	Biomarkers of Oxidative Stress	3
	References	4

1.1 What is Oxidative Stress?

Oxygen was discovered by the Swedish scientist Carl Wilhelm Scheele and reported in his thesis *Luft und dem Feuer* (Air and Fire) from Uppsala and Leipzig in 1777. Later it was realized that in higher animals, breathing supplies the cells with oxygen and serves to eliminate the carbon dioxide formed from cellular metabolism. The well-known reaction between oxygen and fuel (e.g., carbon in wood) requires high temperatures. However, it was discovered that special proteins in the cells—enzymes—are able to catalyze this combustion at body temperature. The trick is that the enzymes can bind both oxygen and the substrate and bring them into close proximity so that chemical reaction can occur and the liberated energy can be stored as ATP for use elsewhere and later in the cell.

Oxygen was consequently considered a good thing. However, experience from exposure to high-oxygen concentrations in deep-sea divers and premature babies showed that organ damage could be a result of exposure to too much oxygen. As we learned to measure oxidative damage better, we realized that it happens in vivo even at normal atmospheric O_2 levels.

It is now well established that free radical chemistry occurs in biology, and it is also becoming increasingly clear that free radicals not only function in cellular respiration, as damaging species, but also in the signaling systems within cells. As an example of the acceptance of these phenomena, the journal *Nature Medicine* has "oxidative stress" among its limited number of keywords for paper submission.

1.2 Oxidative Stress

Oxidative stress was initially defined by Sies (1985, 1986) as a serious imbalance between oxidation and antioxidants, "a disturbance in the prooxidant–antioxidant balance in favor of the former, leading to potential damage." The definition seems simple; however, it builds on definitions about oxidation, antioxidants, and balance.

The definition of oxidation seems also simple: loss of electrons by a species, gain of oxygen, or loss of hydrogen. However, if something is oxidized, something else must be reduced. The effect depends on the context. As put forward by Buettner (1993), there is a pecking order of oxidants. In biology, substances very high in the pecking order (e.g., the hydroxyl radical) will almost always be an oxidant; other substances (e.g., NO· or H_2O_2, can act as oxidants or reductants, depending on whether they react with substances lower or higher in the pecking order.

An antioxidant is more difficult to define. A popular (but not comprehensive) definition was put forward by Halliwell: An antioxidant is any substance that, when present at low concentrations as compared with those of an oxidizable substrate, significantly delays or prevents the oxidation of that substrate. (Its shortcomings are discussed in an upcoming book, *Free Radicals in Biology and Medicine*, 4th ed., Halliwell and Gutteridge, 2006.) As argued above, the chemical terms are oxidation and reduction, and an antioxidant is clearly different from a reducing agent. A reducing agent may even be a prooxidant if it reduces oxygen to free radicals or converts transition metal ions to lower oxidation states that react more readily with peroxides. Many biological reducing agents are Janus-faced: They can be anti- or prooxidants, depending on the levels of O_2 and transition metal ions around.

Balance or imbalance is poorly defined. Generally, we think of our environment as an oxidative environment, and this presumably is true for outer surfaces of the body. However, our knowledge is limited regarding intracellular conditions. They are generally reducing, but with some subcellular variations (e.g., the endoplasmic reticulum is more oxidized than the mitochondria). Even within the cytosol there might be considerable differences between locations close to the cell membrane and close to the nuclear membrane. It could be that there is a balance between oxidants and antioxidants, but it seems rather unlikely. The cell must rapidly and transiently modulate its redox state to send signals.

1.3 Measurement of Oxidative Stress

The term oxidative stress rests on definitions that are not always sufficiently clear; consequently, oxidative stress is a somewhat vague term, as is oxidative damage. Halliwell and Whiteman (2004) have defined the latter as "the biomolecular damage that can be caused by direct attack of reactive species during oxidative stress."

In very simple noncompartmentalized systems, e.g., an in vitro system with a limited number of oxidants and targets for oxidation, it is often self-evident how oxidative stress is defined and measured: by simply measuring antioxidants, free radicals, and other reactive species (RS) and doing a balance sheet. Care must be taken: What is seen depends on what is measured. RS can be measured directly (e.g., by electron spin resonance or various trapping methods), or indirectly by examining end products of their reaction with biomolecules (oxidative damage).

More-complicated systems need much more careful approaches. A cell is compartmentalized with many different molecular targets for oxidation. Lipids in the outer cell membrane most probably have quite a different oxidative environment as compared with the inner mitochondrial membranes. Nucleic acids also exist in different compartments, and the oxidative environment is quite different between transcribing and nontranscribing DNA in the nucleus, DNA in the mitochondria, and the different types of RNA. Likewise for protein oxidation, plasma proteins and cellular proteins exist in different compartments and thereby in different oxidative environments.

At the next level of complexity, different organs and different parts of the organs may present quite different conditions. For example, the liver receives a mixture of arterial and venous blood and thereby much lower oxygen concentrations than most other organs, and even within the liver, cells in the first part of the sinusoid live in a quite different oxidative environment than those in the end of the sinusoid.

That the structure and organization is complicated should not make researchers refrain from trying to define the system under investigation. Rather, it should in many cases make us more humble in the interpretation of data obtained in complicated systems, and more careful in defining and understanding the limitations of simple methods used to investigate complicated systems.

1.4 Biomarkers of Oxidative Stress

When considering the effect of increased oxidative stress (or decreased for that matter), the issue of target is mandatory. From a general point of view, lipids, proteins, carbohydrates, and DNA are considered important macromolecules. For measurement of the oxidation of these molecules, the biomarker approach is most often used. A biomarker of disease is defined as a molecular indicator of a specific biological property, a biochemical feature or facet that can be used to measure the progress of disease or the effects of treatment. The reader should be aware that there are other forms of biomarkers, e.g., biomarkers of exposure.

Such a biomarker should fulfill certain criteria, as given in Table 1.1.

Table 1.1 Criteria for the ideal biomarker of oxidative stress

No.	Criterion
1	It should be predictive of development of the disease or condition under investigation (example: lipid peroxidation in plasma should predict arteriosclerotic events or cardiovascular death).
2	It should reflect biological event(s) that can be related to the pathogenesis of the disease or condition.
3	It should be stable over short periods (weeks, months) in stable individuals.
4	It should produce identical results when the same sample is measured in different laboratories.
5	The sample from which it is measured should be stable on storage.
6	The biomarker should relate to immediate events within short periods or should reflect integration of events over a well-defined period.
7	Preferentially, the biomarker measurement should be noninvasive or measurable in an easily available biological specimen (example: urine, sputum) or in minimally invasively obtainable biological specimen (example blood or plasma).
8	The cost of sample analysis should be low, and it should be possible to perform a large number of analyses within a reasonable time.

Whereas the methods to measure events that are related to oxidative stress—be it oxidation, free radicals, or antioxidants—are numerous, it should be realized that very few, if any, of them fulfill the criteria in Table 1.1, and hence cannot yet be considered biomarkers of oxidative stress. To our knowledge, there are no publications that in a proper scientific way fulfill criterion 1, namely predictive of development of disease. Nonetheless, recent studies with F_2-isoprostanes and 3-nitrotyrosine look promising in this direction.

References

Buettner GR (1993) The pecking order of free radicals and antioxidants: lipid peroxidation, α-tocopherol, and ascorbate. Arch Biochem Biophys 300:535–543
Halliwell B, Whiteman M (2004) Measuring reactive species and oxidative damage in vivo and in cell culture: how should you do it and what do the results mean? Br J Pharmacol 142:231–255
Sies H (1985) Introductory remarks. In: Sies H (ed) Oxidative stress. Academic, London, pp 1–8
Sies H (1986) Biochemistry of oxidative stress. Angew Chem Int Ed Eng 25:1058–1071

Chapter 2

Tobacco Smoke Constituents Affecting Oxidative Stress

Jan B. Wooten, Salem Chouchane, and Thomas E. McGrath

Contents

2.1	Introduction	6
2.1.1	Pyrolysis and Combustion inside Cigarettes	7
2.1.2	Cigarette Smoke Properties	7
2.2	An Overview of Cigarette Smoke Chemistry and Oxidative Stress	8
2.2.1	Particulate-Phase Constituents	9
2.2.1.1	Free Radicals	9
2.2.1.2	Quinones	10
2.2.1.3	Trace Heavy Metals	11
2.2.2	Gas-Phase Constituents	13
2.2.2.1	Oxidizing Radicals and RNS	13
2.2.2.2	Peroxynitrite	14
2.2.2.3	Glutathione Depleting Substances	14
2.3	Tobacco Leaf Constituents Affecting Smoke Chemistry and Toxicity	16
2.3.1	Phenolic Compounds	16
2.3.1.1	Phenolic Compound Yields in TPM	17
2.3.1.2	Effect of Temperature on Phenolic Compound Yields	19
2.3.1.3	Effect of Water Extraction on Phenolic Compound Yields	20
2.3.1.4	Phenolic Compound Formation from Tobacco Constituents	21
2.3.2	Trace Heavy Metals	24
2.4	Free Radicals, ROS, and RNS	26
2.4.1	Particulate-Phase Free Radicals	27

Contents

2.4.2	Gas-Phase Free Radicals	31
2.4.3	Cytotoxicity of TPM Constituents	31
2.4.4	ROS and RNS in Aqueous Solutions of Cigarette Smoke	36
2.4.4.1	Superoxide and Hydroxyl Radicals	36
2.4.4.2	Hydrogen Peroxide	37
2.4.4.3	NO• and Peroxynitrite	38
2.5	Summary	39
	References	40

2.1 Introduction

Cigarette smoke is a highly complex aerosol composed of several thousand chemical substances distributed between the gas and the particulate phases. A frequently cited estimate for the number of these constituents is ca. 4,700 (Dube and Green 1982). The enormous complexity of cigarette smoke is the result of multiple thermolytic processes that occur in heated tobacco within the confines of the burning cigarette rod. These processes involve distillation, pyrolysis, and combustion, and are influenced by factors including the design of the cigarette (Norman 1999) and the composition of the tobacco (Bokelman and Ryan 1985; Leffingwell 1999). Numerous organic chemical classes are represented in cigarette smoke including saturated and unsaturated hydrocarbons, alcohols, aldehydes, ketones, carboxylic acids, esters, phenols, nitriles, terpenoids, and alkaloids (Baker 1999; Dube and Green 1982; Hoffmann et al. 2001). Whereas the composition of cigarette smoke is complex, certain smoke constituents have received greater analytical scrutiny than have others, either because of their greater relative abundance in smoke (which makes them easy to analyze), their known pharmacological properties (Seeman et al. 2004), and/or because they are believed to be carcinogenic or potentially harmful to smokers (IARC Monographs 1986; USCPSC 1993).

Large numbers of data on the composition of mainstream smoke have been published, and the subject has been reviewed in detail (Baker 1999). The objective of this chapter is to take a more focused look at the chemical constituents in cigarette smoke that relate to oxidative stress. In particular, we examine smoke constituents that are known to (1) increase oxidant burden, (2) decrease antioxidant protection, or (3) result in the generation of reactive oxygen species (ROS) and reactive nitrogen species (RNS). Section 1 provides a brief description of the thermal conditions inside a burning cigarette and some relevant properties of cigarette smoke. Section 2 is an overview of the existing information related to smoke chemistry and oxidative stress. Section 3 explores how certain tobacco leaf constituents affect the delivery of some of the cigarette smoke constituents known to influence oxidative stress. Phenolic compounds originate from the pyrolysis of polyphenols, carbohydrates, and other precursors in tobacco leaves, whereas trace metal ions present initially in the leaves are known to transfer to cigarette smoke. This discussion draws on recent results from our own laboratory and literature reports. Section 4 discusses the important topic of free radicals, ROS, and reactive RNS, their potential involvement in the toxicity of cigarette smoke in general, and the in vitro cytotoxicity of individual smoke constituents in particular. Special emphasis is given to the role of free radicals and the redox chemistry of phenolic compounds, including some current results.

2.1.1 Pyrolysis and Combustion inside Cigarettes

Before discussing cigarette smoke and oxidative stress, we present some basic principles of cigarette smoke formation and properties that may help to convey the complexity of tobacco smoke. An elaborate description of the fluctuating thermal gradients and vapor environment inside a cigarette during smoking has been given by Baker (1999). The chemical complexity of cigarette smoke is strongly dependent on the heating conditions inside the lit cigarette. To summarize briefly, when a smoker lights and draws on a cigarette, the temperature of the ignited tobacco rises rapidly, and a hot coal forms at the lit end of the cigarette that is the center of combustion (the combustion zone). Peak temperatures inside the coal can exceed 900 °C. The high temperature inside the coal during a puff causes an increase in the viscosity of the air flowing through the coal and a concomitant increase in the resistance to the draw of air through the cigarette. This effect forces air to be drawn primarily from the periphery of the coal at the paper burn line rather than through the center of the coal. The depletion of oxygen due to combustion inside the coal and the flux of air around the coal results in the formation of a region immediately behind the coal that is depleted of oxygen, but where the temperatures remain high enough to promote the thermal decomposition of the unburned tobacco. For this reason, this area behind the coal is known as the pyrolysis/distillation zone. Copious amounts of volatile and semivolatile smoke constituents evolve from this zone. These constituents result in part from the pyrolysis of tobacco and in part from distillation of volatile constituents native to tobacco because of the heat of the encroaching coal.

The smoke constituents drawn through the cigarette rod during a puff and delivered to the smoker are termed mainstream smoke. In the interim period between puffs when no air is being drawn through the cigarette, the coal undergoes smoldering combustion driven primarily by diffusion of oxygen into the coal. The smoke escapes from the periphery of the coal to the surrounding air. This smoke is termed sidestream smoke. Typical coal temperatures during smoldering combustion are less than 800 °C. The different thermal conditions and air flow through and around the coal during smoldering combustion, in comparison to combustion during a puff, causes the sidestream and mainstream smoke composition to differ significantly, the primary difference being the relative abundance of the smoke constituents (Baker 1999).

2.1.2 Cigarette Smoke Properties

The smoke emitted from a lit cigarette is a dense aerosol composed of microscopic droplets, known as the particulate phase, dispersed in a vapor of air and other gases derived from the burning tobacco. The particulate phase of cigarette smoke overall acts as a reducing agent, which may play a role in its toxicity (Church and Pryor 1985; Lakritz et al. 1972; Schmeltz et al. 1977). There are some 10^9–10^{10} particles per cubic centimeter in fresh mainstream smoke, and the particle size varies from 0.1 to 1.0 μm in diameter. The standard method for separating the particulate fraction of cigarette smoke from the gas-phase constituents is to pass the cigarette smoke through a fiberglass filter called a Cambridge pad (Baker 1999; Dube and Green 1982). This filter has a trapping efficiency of 99% for particles with an aerodynamic diameter larger than 0.1 μm. Thus, the particulate phase of mainstream smoke is defined operationally by the method employed to trap nonvolatile and semivolatile materials.

The total particulate matter (TPM) includes *all* the material collected on the Cambridge pad (Baker 2002). Tar is the term applied to the smoke particulate fraction collected on the Cambridge pad, minus the content of nicotine and water. A small portion of the mainstream smoke constituents are distributed between the gas and particulate phases. These organic substances are described as semivolatile constituents, and they typically have molecular weights in the range of ca. 60–200 (Baker 1999). The gas phase of cigarette smoke is the component that passes unobstructed through the Cambridge filter pad, which includes the gaseous constituents (oxygen, nitrogen, nitric oxide, carbon dioxide, carbon monoxide, etc.) and the volatile and some semivolatile organic constituents.

The TPM collected on a Cambridge filter pad is mostly soluble in either water or organic solvents (at least 95–99%), and thus differs from respirable particulate matter such as carbon black (e.g., diesel exhaust particles and other forms of soot) that is prevalent in the environment. Such materials have been termed poorly soluble particles (PSP) and have recently attracted the interest of researchers because of potential adverse effects related to the generation of ROS. Primarily surface-driven mechanisms have been invoked to explain ROS generation from PSPs and therefore appear to differ from the ROS generation mechanisms of cigarette smoke (Knaapen et al. 2004). ROS generation in cigarette smoke particulate matter is believed to be based on the redox cycling of quinones derived from TPM constituents (Dellinger et al. 2001).

2.2 An Overview of Cigarette Smoke Chemistry and Oxidative Stress

In this section, we discuss a number of chemical classes of smoke constituents that have been documented to affect oxidative stress. Because of the complexity of cigarette smoke, however, it is impossible to be comprehensive, and much remains unknown. We also do not attempt to address the relative importance of the various chemical classes to induce oxidative stress as there are many complex biological interactions and processes involved. Rather, we focus on the chemistry of the smoke constituents, citing the appropriate literature references that make the connection between the smoke constituents and their biological effects. Among the smoke constituents that we include in our overview are organic compounds or metal ions that act as electrophiles, free radicals, reactive anions or metal ions that act as reducing agents (donate an electron), or free radicals or metal ions that act as oxidizing agents (accept an electron).

ROS and RNS are generated when mainstream cigarette smoke interacts with aqueous media or physiological fluids. Some smoke constituents become involved in oxidative stress only after they are chemically modified by metabolic processes in vivo. For example, benzo[*a*]pyrene can be metabolized to its corresponding quinone, which can generate ROS via a redox cycling mechanism (Briede et al. 2004; Winston et al. 1993).

This quinone and related substances that are not initially present in cigarette smoke are not otherwise included in our discussion. Another distinction can be made between oxidants that form by the direct action of cigarette smoke constituents and secondary oxidants that form in response to inflammation resulting from smoking-related oxidative stress. These topics are addressed in other chapters.

2.2.1 Particulate-Phase Constituents

2.2.1.1 Free Radicals

Free radicals were discovered in cigarette smoke and other charred organic materials soon after the development of electron paramagnetic resonance spectroscopy (EPR) (Lyons et al. 1958). However, it was not until 1983 that Prof. William A. Pryor of Louisiana State University employed EPR to associate cigarette tar radicals with hydroquinone and catechol, and to suggest their possible involvement with smoking-related diseases (Pryor et al. 1983a, c). Subsequently, the Pryor research group conducted many studies to characterize the smoke radicals, and in vitro assays were performed, suggesting that cigarette smoke could cause oxidative stress or oxidative damage to essential biological molecules. For example, Church and Pryor (1985) proposed that the excess superoxide that forms in lung tissue in response to exposure to cigarette smoke might be one possible mechanism responsible for the inactivation of α_1-protease inhibitor, a protein associated with the onset of emphysema in deficient individuals. In the same report, the authors noted that cigarette tar incubated with DNA exhibits an EPR signal in the recovered DNA. Later, it was shown that DNA damage could occur by the attack of hydroxyl radicals generated from the bound tar radicals (Pryor 1992; Pryor et al. 1998). Pryor (1992) noted that such molecular damage is not unique to tobacco smoke, but also occurs from smoke from other sources such as diesel fuel and wood.

Extensive studies were initiated by the Pryor group to characterize the cigarette TPM radicals. Organic extracts of cigarette smoke condensate revealed the presence of as many as five different EPR signals (Church and Pryor 1985). Treating the alcoholic extract of TPM with sodium hydroxide in the presence of air gave an EPR spectrum dominated by the characteristic five-line spectrum of the *p*-benzosemiquinone radical, thus revealing an abundant source of radical precursors (Pryor et al. 1983b). Subsequently, the semiquinone radicals were shown to be concentrated in the aqueous extract of cigarette tar (ACT). The EPR spectrum of fresh ACT in air-saturated pH 10 buffer solutions was found to exhibit the intense resonances of the semiquinone radicals of both hydroquinone and catechol. The pattern of resonances in the ACT spectrum was indistinguishable from the combined spectra of pure hydroquinone and catechol allowed to autooxidize in air-saturated solutions at pH 9, showing that the radicals in ACT derive from the hydroquinone and catechol in cigarette smoke.

The Pryor group (Zang et al. 1995) and "Tanigawa et al. (1994)" also demonstrated by EPR spin-trapping experiments that aqueous dimethyl sulfoxide (DMSO) solutions of ACT, buffered at pH 9 and saturated with air, contain superoxide radical anions, one of the ROS involved in oxidative stress. The mechanism proposed for the formation of superoxide in ACT was the autoxidation of the hydroquinone anion (and related anions) in air to give benzosemiquinone radical and superoxide, as shown in Fig. 2.1 (Brunmark and Cadenas 1989; Zang et al. 1995). Spin-trapped adducts of the hydroxyl radical, another important stress-related ROS, were also identified in ACT. The mechanism put forth for the formation of hydroxyl radicals was the catalytic disproportionation of hydrogen peroxide (H_2O_2) by transition metal ions, the well-known Fenton reaction (Cosgrove et al. 1985).

Hydrogen peroxide is a naturally occurring by-product of oxidative stress. It is formed during normal respiration in living organisms by catalytic disproportionation of superoxide radicals by superoxide dismutase (SOD). Another enzyme, catalase, is highly efficient at converting H_2O_2 to "innocuous products, water, and molecular oxygen." If this cellular defense mechanism is overwhelmed, the excess H_2O_2 can undergo disproportionation via the Fenton reaction to form hydroxyl radicals. The hydroxyl radicals derived from H_2O_2 are highly oxidizing species that are well known to cause oxidative damage to essential biomolecules, including DNA (Halliwell and Gutteridge 1999). H_2O_2 has been found in ACT and in aged unbuffered aqueous solutions of catechol, a smoke constituent abundant in both ACT and TPM. The H_2O_2 concentration in smoke condensate has been shown to increase with age, pH, and temperature (Nakayama et al. 1989; Stone et al. 1995). Exogenous H_2O_2 found in cigarette smoke and H_2O_2 that forms by the physiological response to smoke constituents are presumed to be a source of oxidative stress and/or damage in smokers.

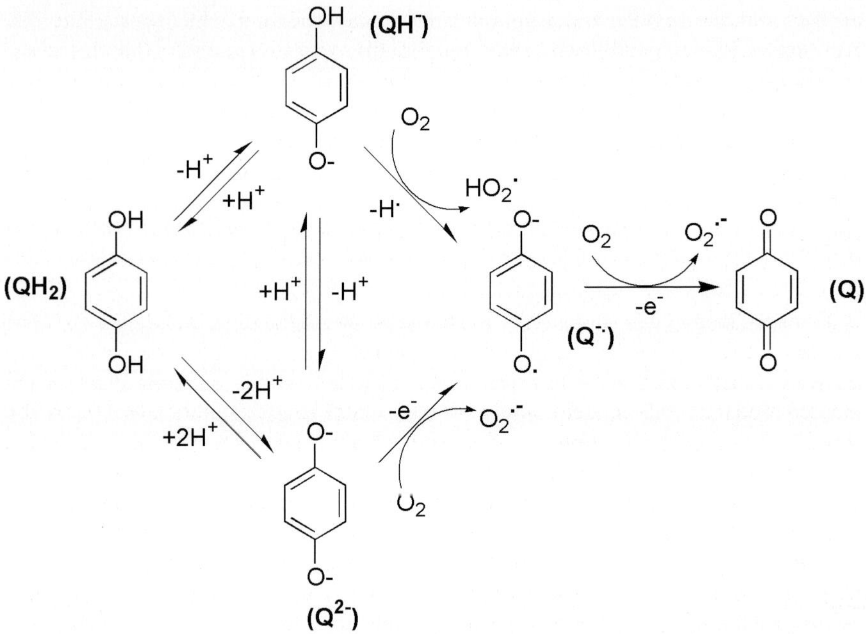

Fig. 2.1 Generation of semiquinone and superoxide radicals by autooxidation of hydroquinone, an abundant dihydroxybenzene found in the particulate phase of cigarette smoke (Zang et al. 1995)

2.2.1.2 Quinones

Quinones are readily formed from cigarette smoke constituents that can undergo autooxidation. Benzoquinone, for example, forms by the autooxidation of hydroquinone in

ACT (Sect. 2.1.1) or by oxidation in vivo in living organisms. The toxicology of quinones has been studied extensively (Bolton et al. 2000; Monks et al. 1992). In general, the toxicity of quinones is believed to occur by two mechanisms, the redox cycling mechanism, which generates excess ROS as byproducts, and the formation of covalent bonds with essential biological molecules (especially molecules containing thiol groups) (Rodriguez et al. 2004; Seung et al. 1998). Both mechanisms can contribute to the onset of oxidative stress. Quinones derived from cigarette smoke constituents undergo redox cycling in living organisms by entering into the NADPH reductase pathway (Bolton et al. 2000; Hirakawa et al. 2002; Squadrito et al. 2001). The reduction of quinones by NADPH or ascorbate regenerates the parent quinols, thereby creating the redox cycle (Roginsky et al. 1999a). Redox cycling of xenobiotic quinones can significantly increase the cellular burden of ROS and deplete their antioxidant defenses.

Whereas redox cycling of quinones is recognized as a significant source of oxidative stress from cigarette smoke, α,β-unsaturated ketones derived from particulate-phase constituents, such as benzoquinone, can also undergo electrophilic substitution in a manner similar to a number of gas-phase constituents such as acrolein (see Sect. 2.2.3). For example, pure benzoquinone in oxygenated aqueous solutions undergoes Michael addition via a semiquinone intermediate to form intensely colored condensation products; the color of the solution changes to a deep purple within minutes of dissolution, an indication of the presence of conjugated Michael addition products. This can occur for various quinones even at physiological pH, depending on the pK of the parent dihydroxybenzene (Pedersen 2002) and the redox potentials of the corresponding semiquinone radicals (Roginsky et al. 1999b). Quinones react readily with cellular nucleophiles, especially glutathione (GSH) and other thiols (Lau et al. 1988).

2.2.1.3 Trace Heavy Metals

Tobacco plants transport metal ions from the soil through the roots into the leaves (Lougon-Moulin et al. 2004; Tso 1990). Trace amounts of heavy metals accumulate in the leaves, and they are known to transfer in trace quantities from the cured and processed tobacco to mainstream cigarette smoke. These metals include cadmium, lead, mercury, arsenic, iron, copper, chromium, nickel, and selenium (Hoffmann et al. 2001; IARC Monographs 1986; Smith et al. 1997; Stohs and Bagchi 1995). The most abundant redox-inactive metals in cigarette smoke generally are cadmium, lead, mercury, and arsenic. The yield of these metals in cigarette smoke is influenced by cigarette design, but the yield generally correlates with tar yields. The most abundant redox-active metals in cigarette smoke are copper and iron, with copper being more abundant than iron, ca. 0.19 versus ca. 0.042 µg per cigarette, respectively (Stohs et al. 1997).

Many investigations have suggested that metal-induced oxidative stress can be partially responsible for the toxicity of these metals (Ercal et al. 2001). Redox-active metals, such as iron, copper, nickel, and chromium, can undergo redox cycling in oxygenated aqueous solutions, with the concomitant formation of ROS, whereas redox-inactive metals such as lead, cadmium, and mercury can deplete cells of thiol-containing antioxidants and reduce the activity of antioxidant enzymes. Heavy metals can exert other molecular effects such as inhibition of DNA repair and activation of cellular signaling (Bal and Kasprzak 2002; Barchowsky and O'Hara 2003; Kasprzak 2002; Waisberg et al. 2003). Thus, both redox-active and redox-inactive metals can potentially cause an increase in ROS in smokers.

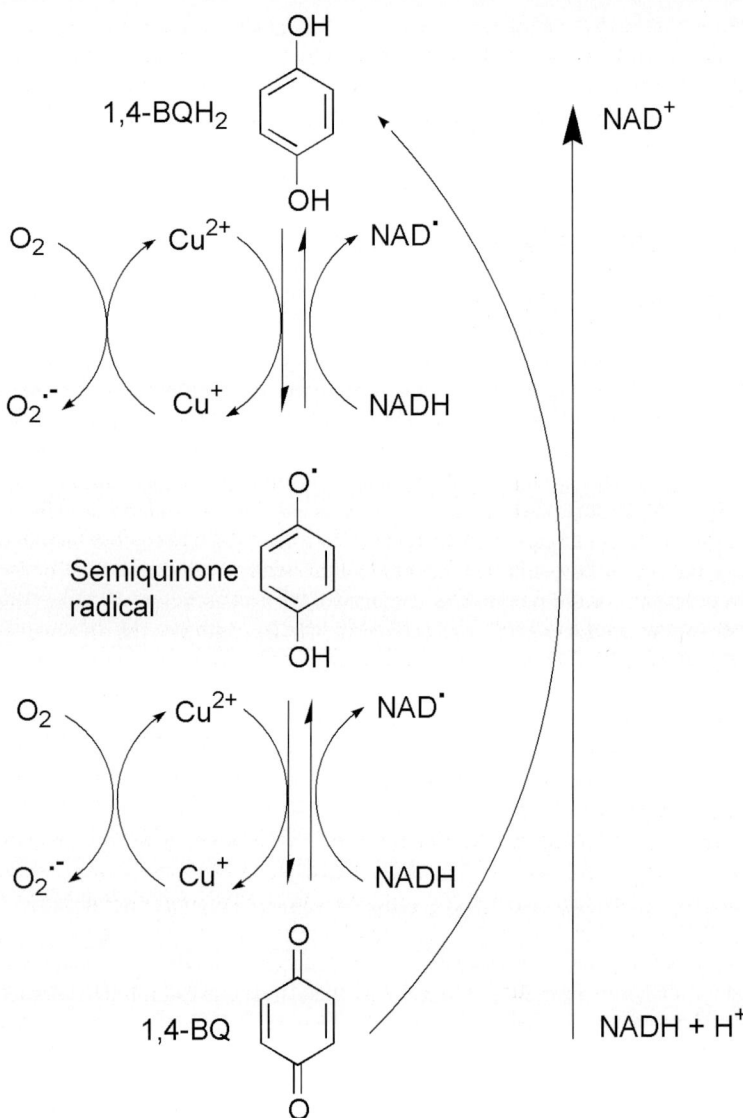

Fig. 2.2 Redox cycling mechanism for the oxidation of quinols to quinones with the formation of reactive oxygen species (Hirakawa et al. 2002)

Transition metals in the tar of cigarette smoke are notable because of their capacity to promote the formation of hydroxyl radicals via the Fenton reaction, both in aqueous extracts of cigarette smoke and in living tissues. In particular, both Fe^{2+} and Cu^{1+} are known to be active in the formation of hydroxyl radicals. These ions can also readily form complexes with many organic molecules, including those that undergo redox cycling (Stohs and Bagchi 1995; Stohs et al. 1997). Cu^{2+} has been shown to oxidize catechol and hydroquinone to their respective quinones. It can enter into a redox cycle involving hydroquinone in the presence of molecular oxygen, forming semiquinone radicals and generating superoxide radical anions, as shown in Fig. 2.2. In contrast, Fe^{3+} does not significantly enhance the rate of oxidation of hydroquinone (Hirakawa et al. 2002; Li and Trush 1993; Li et al. 1995).

2.2.2 Gas-Phase Constituents

2.2.2.1 Oxidizing Radicals and RNS

Cigarette smoke contains abundant oxidizing agents that are found in the gas–vapor phase (Church and Pryor 1985; Pryor 1992). Even though nitric oxide (NO·) is itself a radical, it is neither particularly reactive nor toxic. NO· combines slowly with molecular oxygen in air (over a period of seconds) to form the toxic oxidant and nitrating agent, NO_2·. According to a mechanism proposed by Pryor et al. (1983b), NO_2· reacts rapidly with other smoke constituents such as isoprene and butadiene to form nitroso-carbon-centered radicals. Carbon-centered radicals are generally highly reactive species. The gas-phase carbon-centered radicals in smoke react instantaneously with molecular oxygen to form peroxyl radicals that react with smoke gas-phase NO· to form alkoxyl radicals and NO_2·, thereby creating a continuous cycle. There are two interesting consequences of the above reaction scheme: (1) the oxidizing radicals in cigarette smoke are formed by reactions between the gas-phase constituents, and not primarily by pyrolysis or combustion reactions in the burning tobacco, and (2) the radicals collected inside an enclosed container of gas-phase smoke increase until the supply of NO· is depleted, persisting for several minutes.

Because the radical species that form from reactions of NO· and other gas-phase smoke constituents are all short-lived, spin-trapping methods must be employed to detect them by EPR spectroscopy, as in the case of the reactive oxygen species. The Pryor group employed the spin trap α-phenyl-*N-tert*-butylnitrone (PBN) to detect the oxidizing gas-phase radicals in cigarette smoke. The primary spin adducts found in benzene solutions of PBN bubbled with gas-phase smoke are from alkoxyl radicals, the least reactive, and therefore the longer-lived of the oxidizing radicals. Other researchers developed alternative methods to detect free radicals. For example, Flicker and Green (1998, 2001) developed a chromatographic-based method that is specific for carbon-centered radicals in whole mainstream smoke (including the TPM and the gas phase). The involvement of gas-phase free radicals in oxidative damage is unclear, because it is generally believed that the reactive gas-phase radicals are quenched immediately on contact with surfaces of the respiratory tract (Rahman and MacNee 1996a; 1996b).

NO· itself at physiological concentrations (ca. 0.1–10 n*M*) is relatively unreactive with nonradical molecules (Halliwell and Gutteridge 1999). However, it can react with tyrosyl radical, which is present at the active sites of some enzymes, particularly ribonucleotide reductase (Kwon et al. 1991; Lepoivre et al. 1994). NO· may be converted to a number of more reactive derivatives, known collectively as RNS, such as NO_2·, N_2O_3, and N_2O_4 and $ONOO^-$ (peroxynitrite). DNA damage and nitration of tyrosine in cells exposed to the gas phase of cigarette smoke has been attributed to the action of RNS (Eiserich et al. 1994; Spencer et al. 1995). NO· is reported to enhance the toxicity of phenolic compounds by oxidation to their respective quinones (Urios et al. 2003).

2.2.2.2 Peroxynitrite

Peroxynitrite is an RNS that forms from the reaction of NO· and superoxide. Peroxynitrite is not itself a free radical, being derived from two free radicals, but it is a powerful oxidant that has been shown to induce damage to essential biomolecules in physiological media (Denicola and Radi 2005; Halliwell and Gutterridge 1999). Simultaneous generation of NO· and superoxide favors the production of peroxynitrite anion (Beckman et al. 1990). This peroxynitrite-forming reaction has since been shown to be diffusion controlled (k_{obs} = 6.7×10^9 M^{-1} s^{-1}), indicating that competition between NO· and SOD for superoxide is feasible (Huie and Padmaja 1993), and most of the toxicity of superoxide has been attributed to the formation of peroxynitrite (Koppenol 1998).

It is generally believed that NO· in cigarette smoke reacts with superoxide derived from the reducing constituents in the particulate phase of cigarette smoke, i.e., dihydroxybenzenes such as hydroquinone and catechol, to form peroxynitrite (Müller et al. 1997). Based on kinetic and other considerations, Squadrito and Pryor (1998) proposed that peroxynitrite readily forms in vivo, combining rapidly with abundant intracellular carbon dioxide to form metastable nitrating, nitrosating, and oxidizing intermediates. Apart from carbon dioxide, peroxynitrite is believed to react rapidly only with molecules localized in the cellular vicinity of its formation. Peroxynitrite can react with and inactivate essential proteins including hemoglobin, myeloperoxidase, GSH peroxidase, and others. Because peroxynitrite is short-lived in living tissues and difficult to measure directly, the detection of 3-nitrotyrosine (the nitration product of tyrosine by peroxynitrite) is usually taken as evidence of its existence in vivo (Eiserich et al. 1994; Reiter et al. 2000).

Peroxynitrite has been identified as an oxidative stress-inducing compound of aqueous cigarette smoke fractions (Müller and Gebel 1994, 1998; Müller et al. 1997). After depletion of intracellular GSH content by electrophilic aldehydes, peroxynitrite interferes with specific target molecules, resulting in the activation of stress-related signal transduction and gene expression in cigarette smoke-treated cells in vitro (Müller and Gebel 1994). Furthermore, gene expression profiling in respiratory tract tissues obtained from cigarette smoke-exposed rats revealed a pronounced activation of stress response via upregulation of oxidative stress-related genes, many of which counteract cigarette smoke-induced peroxynitrite stress (Bosio et al. 2002), although other nitration reactions can occur.

2.2.2.3 Glutathione Depleting Substances

Glutathione is abundant in cytoplasm, nuclei, and mitochondria and is the major water-soluble antioxidant in these cell compartments at millimolar concentrations (Ault and Lawrence 2003). High levels of GSH are found in the extracellular lung lining fluid (about 100 μmol/l), but not in blood plasma, where concentrations are very low (<1 μmol/l). Among the intracellular nonprotein thiols such as cysteine, homocysteine, α-lipoic acid, and coenzyme A, GSH accounts for more than 90% of the total thiols. GSH and other thiols react more easily with α,β-unsaturated aldehydes at the β-carbon than at the carbonyl carbon (Meacher and Menzel 1999). Both α,β-unsaturated and saturated aldehydes are direct-acting chemicals, i.e., they require no metabolic activation. The yields of acrolein and crotonaldehyde, two α,β-unsaturated aldehydes in cigarette mainstream smoke, range from 5 to 60 and <1 to 25 μg per cigarette, respectively (Counts et al. 2004).

Modifications of intracellular GSH by electrophiles in the gas phase of cigarette smoke were first reported decades ago (Gaisch and Nyffeler 1976; Leuchtenberger et al. 1974, 1976). As shown in Fig. 2.3, electrophilic cigarette smoke constituents react with thiol-containing proteins. Eiserich (1995) reported that the concentration of protein sulfhydryl groups in blood plasma is about 500 μM. After exposure to cigarette smoke, the concentration of protein sulfhydryl groups was reduced by ca. 60%. Reddy et al. (2002) investigated this effect in more detail. Solutions of GSH in phosphate buffer exposed to gas-phase cigarette smoke resulted in a significant depletion of GSH, attributed primarily to reaction with acrolein, and a concomitant appearance of oxidized GSH (GSSG). The amount of GSSG formed, however, accounted for only 25% of the GSH depletion. NO·, which is abundant in the cigarette smoke gas phase, can react with GSH to form S-nitroso-GSH (GSNO), but Reddy et al. (2002) found that only ca. 1% of the overall reduction in GSH could be attributed to GSNO formation. A more recent investigation by Cahours et al. (2004), using an alternative assay, showed similar amounts of GSSG and GS-aldehyde formation, but the relative percentage of GSNO accounted for more than 30% of the overall GSH depletion.

Hagedorn et al. (2003) developed a GSH depletion assay for gas-phase, particulate-phase, and whole mainstream cigarette smoke. GSH consumption was reported to be two and three times higher for particulate phase and whole smoke, respectively, in comparison to gas-phase smoke. The assay showed that the depletion of GSH in solutions of GSH treated with gas-phase cigarette smoke correlates well with the cytotoxicity of the gas phase, as determined by the neutral red uptake (NRU) and 3-(4,5-dimethylthiazol-2-yl)-5-(3-carboxymethoxyphenyl)-2-(4-sulfophenyl)-2H-tetrazolium, inner salt (MTS)–tetrazolium assays.

The conjugation of cigarette smoke electrophiles with GSH can proceed spontaneously or by catalysis by GSH S-transferases. GSH S-conjugates are catabolized to their

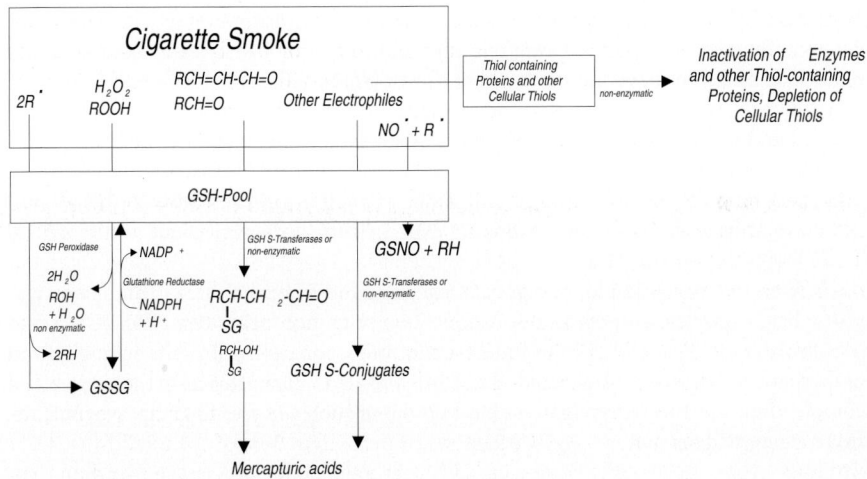

Fig. 2.3 Cigarette smoke-induced depletion of cellular thiols

corresponding mercapturic acids, which are subsequently excreted into the urine. 3-Hydroxypropylmercapturic acid (3-HPMA) is a urinary metabolite of acrolein and can be used as biomarker of cigarette smoke exposure (Mascher et al. 2001). 3-HMPA excretion in smokers as compared with nonsmokers is about three to four times higher (Martin and Tricker 2004).

2.3 Tobacco Leaf Constituents Affecting Smoke Chemistry and Toxicity

2.3.1 Phenolic Compounds

Phenolic compounds are an important class of chemicals that form during the thermal decomposition of biomass (Achladas 1991; Amen-Chen et al. 1997) and tobacco (Schlotzhauer and Chortyk 1987). Their formation, identification and quantification in cigarette smoke has been extensively studied and reviewed (Arrendale et al. 1984; Brunneman et al. 1976; Chen and Moldoveanu 2003; Counts et al. 2005; Crouse et al. 1963; Forehand et al. 2000; Klus and Kuhn 1982; Risner and Cash 1990; Yang and Wender 1962). The most abundant phenolic constituents in tobacco smoke are phenol, dihydroxybenzenes, and their methyl-substituted derivatives. Hydroquinone, catechol, and their methyl-substituted derivatives have been shown by us (see Sect. 4.3) and others (Smith et al. 2002a) to be highly cytotoxic.

Most of the research on phenolic compounds has focused on the formation of catechol and phenol from tobacco, tobacco extracts, and selected tobacco constituents such as polyphenols and lignin (Patterson et al. 1976; Sakuma et al. 1982; Schlotzhauer and Chortyk 1981, 1987; Schlotzhauer et al. 1967, 1982, 1992; Sharma et al. 2000; Spears et al. 1965; Zane and Wender 1963). Despite numerous papers addressing the formation of phenolic compounds from tobacco, there are few data available on their temperature of formation or the contribution of specific tobacco constituents to the yield of phenolic compounds in cigarette smoke TPM (Carmella et al. 1984; Schlotzhauer and Chortyk 1981; Schlotzhauer et al. 1969; Torikaiu et al. 2005). Such information is essential to understand the apportionment of phenolic compounds from tobacco leaf constituents and to develop strategies to reduce the yield of these cytotoxic agents.

We have systematically studied the formation of phenolic compounds from heated tobacco and tobacco leaf constituents in our laboratory. Pyrolysis experiments were carried out in a tube furnace in the heating range from 250 to 600 °C (McGrath et al. 2003). The effect of pyrolysis temperature and water extraction on the formation of phenolic compounds was investigated. Smoking experiments were carried out under Federal Trade Commission smoking conditions (Federal Register 1967, 1980), using cigarettes made from the three individual types of tobacco found in typical American blend cigarettes: bright, burley, and oriental tobaccos. Two reference cigarettes, 2R4F (Chen and Moldoveanu 2003) and IM17 (an industry monitor), containing a representative blend of these tobaccos, were also studied. The 2R4F and IM17 cigarettes have the same blend composition, but the 2R4F cigarette has ventilation holes in the filter tip, whereas the IM17 cigarette does not.

2.3.1.1 Phenolic Compound Yields in TPM

The chemical structures of the ten phenolic compounds in our study (hydroquinone, catechol, resorcinol, 3-methyl catechol, 4-methyl catechol, guaiacol, phenol, o-, m-, and p-cresol) are shown in Fig. 2.4. Quantitative yields of phenolic compounds from smoking and pyrolysis experiments were determined by gas chromatography mass spectrometry (GC/MS) and high-performance liquid chromatography (HPLC). The yield of phenolic compounds was calculated using a calibration curve obtained from the analysis of standard solutions and the yields are reported as the average of three independent measurements. The yields of phenolic compounds in the TPM from the five cigarettes are shown in Fig. 2.5, expressed as micrograms of phenol per milligram of TPM. The TPM yields per cigarette were 7.3±0.7, 14.2±0.2, 16.3±1.0, 8.6±1.3, and 9±1.2 mg, respectively, for the 2R4F, IM17, bright, burley and oriental cigarettes.

Of the ten phenolic compounds measured, hydroquinone and catechol are the most abundant in the TPM of all five cigarettes. The two reference cigarettes gave relatively similar yields of all phenols. Except for the yields of catechol, phenol, and 4-methylcatechol, the yields of phenolic compounds from all three single-component blend cigarettes were quite similar. The 100% bright cigarette gave the highest yield of hydroquinone and 4-methylcatechol. The 100% burley cigarette yielded approximately 47% less catechol as compared with the bright and oriental cigarettes. The trend in the yields of hydroquinone and catechol obtained from the three single-component blend cigarettes followed the order: bright → oriental → burley.

Tobacco polyphenols such as chlorogenic acid and rutin have previously been shown to be precursors of phenolic compounds in cigarette smoke (Carmella et al. 1984; Sakuma et al. 1982; Schlotzhauer et al. 1967, 1982; Sharma et al. 2000; Zane and Wender 1963). The polyphenol content of cigarette tobacco filler ranges from ca. 2.2 mg per cigarette for 100% burley tobacco to ca. 14.22 mg per cigarette for 100% bright tobacco (Table 2.1). Comparison of the polyphenol content of the tobacco filler and the yield of phenolic compounds in the TPM (Fig. 2.5) reveals that the yield of phenolic compounds in the TPM is not directly proportional to the polyphenol content of the tobacco filler. Thus, other tobacco constituents in addition to the polyphenols must contribute to the overall yield of phenolic compounds in cigarette smoke. (see Section 2.3.1.4)

Table 2.1 Polyphenol contents (milligrams per cigarette) for tobacco filler from 2R4F, IM17, and single-tobacco component cigarettes

Cigarette type	Chlorogenic acid	Rutin	Scopoletin	Quinic acid	Caffeic acid	Gentisic acid
2R4F	5.1	1.8	0.01	1.2	0.06	0.01
IM17	6.7	2.2	0.06	1.8	0.13	0.01
Bright	9.7	2.3	0.13	1.9	0.19	0.02
Burley	0.4	0.4	<0.01	1.4	<0.01	<0.01
Oriental	9.0	2.1	<0.01	1.2	0.15	0.01

Polyphenol contents determined from an acetone/water extraction of respective tobacco fillers and quantified by liquid chromatography/mass spectrometry/mass spectrometry

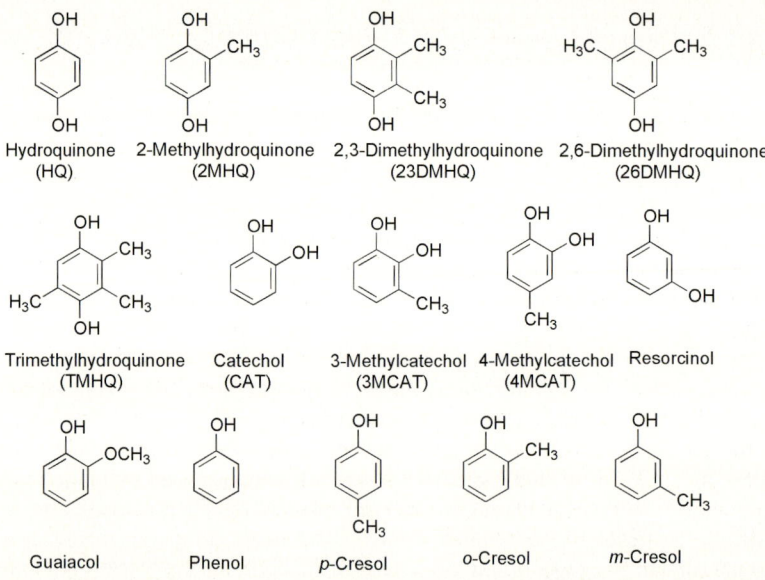

Fig. 2.4 Chemical structures of phenolic compounds found in the total particulate matter (TPM) of mainstream tobacco smoke

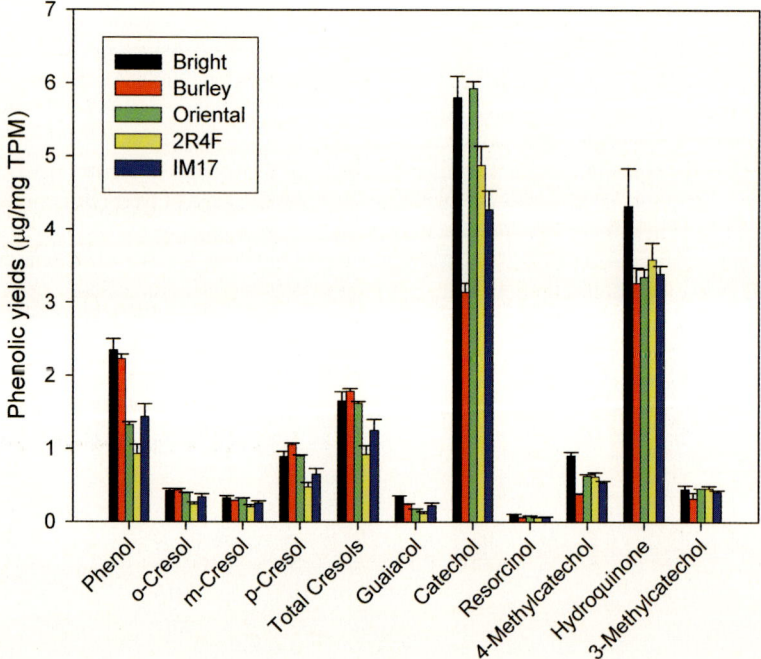

Fig. 2.5 Yields of phenolic compounds in the total particulate matter (*TPM*) of mainstream smoke from several cigarettes smoked under Federal Trade Commission conditions. The cigarettes were three single-component cigarettes containing bright, burley, or oriental tobacco and two reference cigarettes containing the typical American blend of tobaccos (2R4F and IM17)

2.3.1.2 Effect of Temperature on Phenolic Compound Yields

We also investigated the effect of pyrolysis temperature on the formation of phenolic compounds from heated bright tobacco lamina. Samples were first heated at 350 °C for 10 min under helium and the smoke condensate collected and analyzed. The precharred tobacco sample was then heated to 600 °C and held at this temperature for a total of 10 min under helium. The phenolic compounds found in the low-temperature TPM ([LT-TPM] 25–350 °C) and the high-temperature TPM ([HT-TPM] 350–600 °C) were characterized using GC/MS. The constituents of the LT-TPM fraction have previously been described (McGrath et al. 2005). Nicotine is the dominant constituent of the LT-TPM. Furans, furanones, phenols, pyranones, benzenediols, indoles, pyridines, fatty acids, vitamin E, and long-chain hydrocarbons are also present. The HT-TPM fraction was dominated by phenol, mono-, di-, and trimethyl phenols. Indole and methyl indole were also major products, followed by methyl pyridines, substituted pyrroles, methylpyridoindole, stigmasterol, and cholesterol acetates. It is interesting to note that approximately 86% of the total amount of TPM collected by this two-step process forms over the 25–350 °C temperature region.

The relative yields of phenols produced over the two temperature regions of 25–350 °C and 350–600 °C, expressed as a percentage of the total yields formed at 600 °C, are shown in Fig. 2.6. Hydroquinone (96%), catechol (97%), guaiacol (95%), 3-methylcatechol

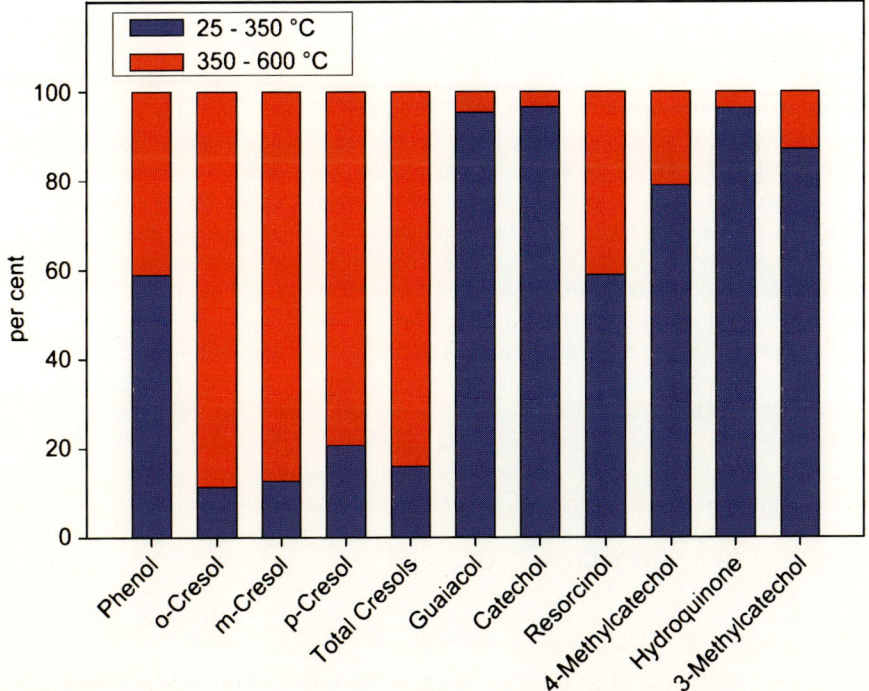

Fig. 2.6 Temperature formation range for phenolic compounds in the total particulate matter (TPM) of bright tobacco heated in a tube furnace under flowing helium for 10 min

(87%) and 4-methylcatechol (79%) are formed predominantly in the LT-TPM fraction, whereas o-cresol (89%), m-cresol (87%), and p-cresol (79%) form predominantly in the HT-TPM fraction. Formation of phenol (59%:41%) and resorcinol (59%:41%) appears to span the two temperature regions. The total yield of the ten phenolic compounds studied accounts for approximately 4% of the total weight of TPM formed.

2.3.1.3 Effect of Water Extraction on Phenolic Compound Yields

To investigate the effect of removing or concentrating potential phenolic precursors from tobacco on the yields of phenolic compounds in cigarette smoke, we extracted samples of bright, burley, and oriental lamina with water. Tobacco polyphenols and brown pigments can be removed and isolated from tobacco by extraction with water, methanol, acetone, and water/methanol solutions (Chortyk et al. 1966; Schlotzhauer and Chortyk 1981; Schlotzhauer et al. 1972, 1969, 1992; Wright et al. 1960, 1964; Zane and Wender 1963). Extraction with water leads to about a 50, 40, and 53% reduction in sample weight of the bright, burley, and oriental lamina, respectively. Water extraction removes the more polar constituents such as inorganic salts, organic salts, polyphenols and alkaloids, while concentrating (on a per-unit weight basis) various carbohydrate, lignin, and lipophilic constituents such as waxes, fatty acids, and high-molecular-weight sterols.

The water-extracted lamina samples were heated at 600 °C under helium, and the yield of phenolic compounds formed were compared with the nonextracted samples. Significant reductions in the yields of hydroquinone (50–60%), catechol (37–41%) and phenol (50–55%) on a per-unit weight basis were observed in the TPM of heated bright and oriental tobacco. A 40% reduction in the yield of hydroquinone was also observed for the TPM of extracted burley tobacco, but, by comparison, there was only a slight reduction in the yield of phenol (21%) and cresols (9%), and there was a significant increase of catechol (85%). When the yields of phenolic compounds from the water-extracted tobacco are normalized to the total amount of material extracted, larger reductions are observed. Decreases of 63–82% for hydroquinone, 53–74% for phenol, and 35–57% for cresols were observed for the burley, oriental, and bright samples, respectively. Whereas the catechol also decreased to around 71% for both bright and oriental tobaccos, the yield of catechol for burley increased slightly by 11%.

Consistent with previous work carried out on the formation of phenol and catechol from extracted tobacco, we found that extraction of tobacco lamina with water removes precursors of hydroquinone, catechol, and phenol from bright and oriental tobacco. Extraction of burley lamina also removes hydroquinone precursors, but significantly concentrates catechol precursors. Because of the longer curing times employed for burley tobacco, precursors to catechol such as chlorogenic acid may be polymerized via enzymatic reactions to water insoluble polymeric precursors (Kameswararo and Gopalachari 1965; Wright et al. 1960, 1964).

2.3.1.4 Phenolic Compound Formation from Tobacco Constituents

To identify possible tobacco precursors of hydroquinone and catechol, we pyrolyzed a number of polyphenolic, carbohydrate, and lignin samples at 600 °C under helium for 10 min and analyzed the collected TPM condensate for hydroquinone, catechol, phenol, and cresols (sum of o-, m-, and p-cresols) by HPLC. The chemical structures of the polyphenols (gentisic, quinic, chlorogenic, and caffeic acids, scopoletin, and rutin) are shown in Fig. 2.7. The yields of hydroquinone, catechol, phenol, and cresols produced from the pyrolysis of these compounds added to bright tobacco under helium gas are shown in Fig. 2.8. The increase in the yield of hydroquinone from the addition of gentisic acid was ca. 6 times higher than that from quinic acid and ca. 17 times higher than from chlorogenic acid on a per-unit weight basis.

The yields of hydroquinone, catechol, phenol, and cresols from the 600 °C pyrolysis of the individual tobacco cell wall constituents are shown in Fig. 2.9. Comparable yields of hydroquinone, catechol, and phenol were formed from cellulose, xylan, glucose, and fructose, with slightly lower amounts of hydroquinone being formed from the pectin sample. The yield of cresols was very similar for cellulose and pectin, with slightly lower yields being formed from glucose and fructose. Although the yield of hydroquinone from the model lignin sample is comparable to the carbohydrates pyrolyzed, the yields of catechol, phenol, and cresols are approximately 9, 11, and 13 times higher, respectively, compared with the cell wall carbohydrates.

Among the 11 tobacco constituents studied, gentisic, quinic, and chlorogenic acids were found to be the most significant precursors of hydroquinone. Caffeic, chlorogenic, and quinic acids are major precursors to catechol, followed by lignin and then the carbohydrates. Lignin yields significantly more catechol compared with the cell wall carbohydrates, (Carmella et al. 1984; Schlotzhauer et al. 1982) but significantly less in comparison to chlorogenic or caffeic acid (ca. 4 and 17 times lower, respectively, on a per-unit weight basis).

To estimate the contribution of each tobacco leaf constituent to the overall yield of the phenolic compounds from the pyrolysis of tobacco, we normalized the yield of phenolic compounds from each of the precursors studied to the amount of each precursor reported in bright tobacco. The estimated level of phenolic compounds from each precursor in bright tobacco leaf lamina is given in Table 2.2. For the normalization step, glucose was used to represent the total reducing sugars, and amounts of cellulose, pectin, hemicellulose, reducing sugars, and lignin were taken from the work of Leffingwell (1999) and Bokelman and Ryan (1985). The amounts of free quinic, caffeic, chlorogenic, and gentisic acids were obtained experimentally from the liquid chromatography mass spectrometry (LC/MS) analysis of an acetone/water extract of bright tobacco.

The carbohydrates and lignin constituents in tobacco were found *not* to be major precursors to hydroquinone. Even though they make up ca. 46% of the weight of tobacco, together they only account for 6–8% of the overall yield of hydroquinone. The polyphenols, which account for less than 2% of the weight of tobacco, account for ca. 17% of the overall hydroquinone yield. Chlorogenic acid and the estimated free quinic acid level account for ca. 11 and 6%, respectively.

From the pyrolysis of the individual tobacco constituents at 600 °C presented in Figs. 2.8 and 2.9, we found that caffeic, chlorogenic, and quinic acids are the major pre-

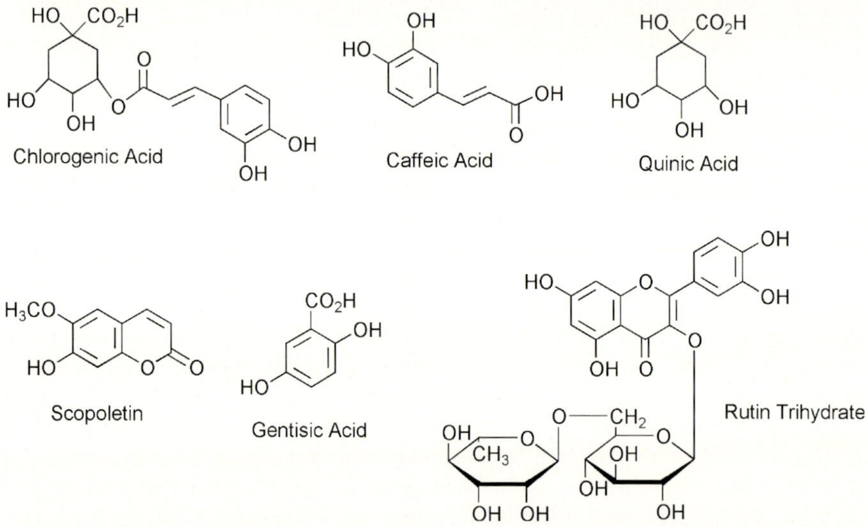

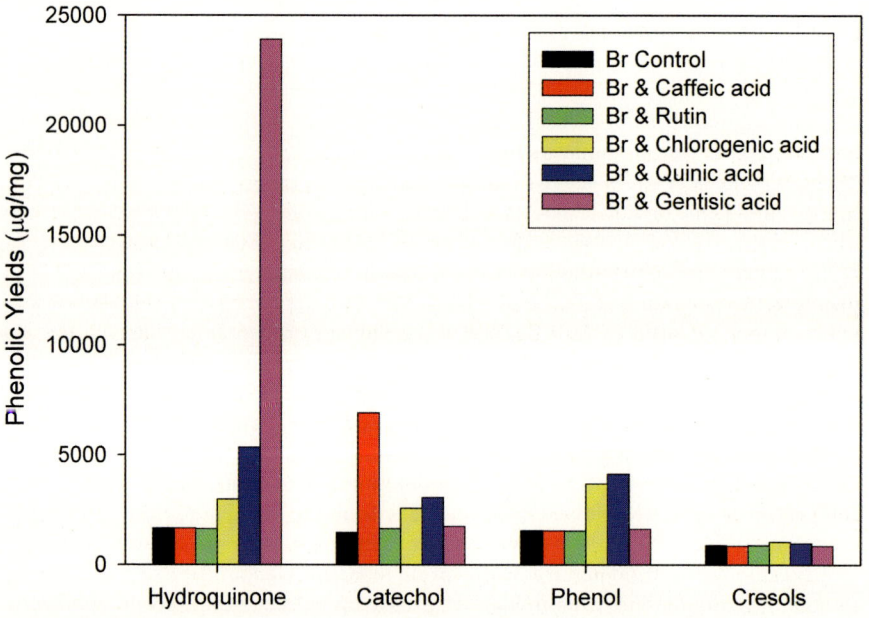

Fig. 2.7 Chemical structures of phenolic precursor compounds found in bright tobacco

Fig. 2.8 Yield of phenolic compounds from 1 g bright tobacco mixed with 60 mg of the indicated phenolic precursors and heated at 600 °C for 10 min under flowing helium in a tube furnace

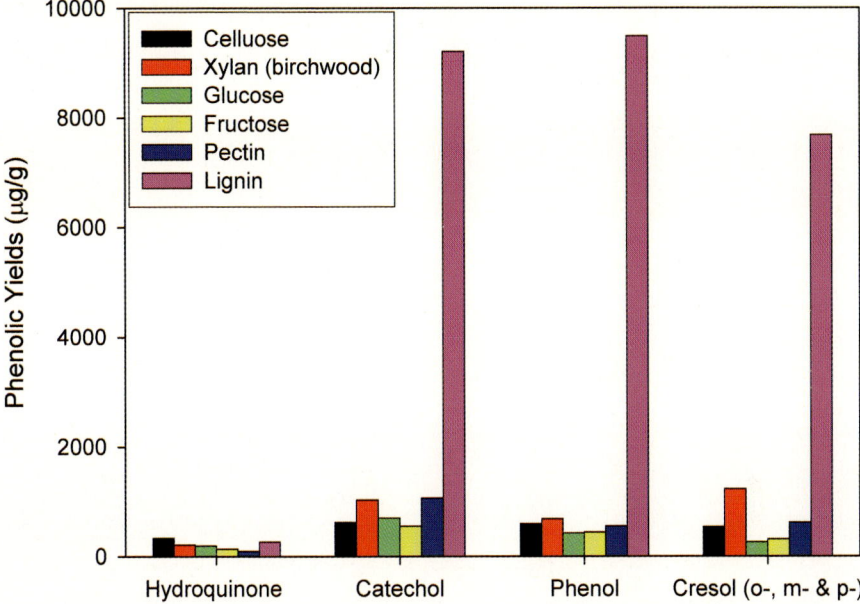

Fig. 2.9 Yield of phenolic compounds from several tobacco leaf constituents heated at 600 °C under flowing helium for 10 min

cursors to catechol, followed by rutin, lignin and, to a lesser extent, the polysaccharides. Upon normalization of the yields, the carbohydrate and lignin together were found to account for approximately one third of the overall catechol yield. Although the carbohydrate content in tobacco is generally approximately five times higher than that of lignin, lignin accounts for 11% of the total yield of catechol, followed by hemicellulose (6.1%), pectin (6.6%), glucose (6%), and cellulose (3.7%). Of the polyphenols, chlorogenic acid (11%), quinic acid (2.7%), caffeic acid (1.2%), and rutin (0.8%) contribute ca. 16% towards the overall yield of catechol. The individual contributions from the pyrolysis for chlorogenic acid, glucose, cellulose, and rutin to the overall yield of catechol reported here are very similar to those previously reported by Carmella et al. (1984).

Based on the assumptions employed for the normalization, we found that ca. 24% of the overall hydroquinone yield and ca. 49% of the overall catechol yield can be accounted for by the 11 tobacco constituents examined. It should be noted that the addition of potassium nitrate and potassium acetate to pure cellulose (1% [w/w] potassium levels) led to a threefold increase in the yields of hydroquinone and catechol. Calcium (in the form of $CaCO_3$) also significantly increases the yield of catechol when added to cellulose. The influence of the two most abundant endogenous inorganic cations (potassium and calcium) can potentially increase the overall contribution of tobacco carbohydrates to catechol yields.

Table 2.2 Estimated source apportionment for hydroquinone and catechol in the TPM of smoke from 100% bright tobacco heated at 600 °C for 10 min under helium

	Wt%	HQ yield[a]	Percentage of total[b]	CAT yield[a]	Percentage of total
Carbohydrates					
Cellulose	10	38	2.4	62	3.7
Glucose	14	34	2.1	100	6.0
Pectin	10	13	0.8	110	6.6
Hemicellulose	10	20	1.2	102	6.1
Lignin	2	5	0.3	184	11.0
Polyphenols					
Chlorogenic acid	0.84	183	11.0	155	10.5
Rutin	0.41	1	0.1	12	0.8
Quinic acid	0.15	92	5.5	39	2.7
Caffeic acid	0.02	0	0.0	18	1.2
Gentisic acid	0.0015	6	0.4	0	0.0

Wt% Estimated weight percentage of each component in bright tobacco lamina (Bokelman and Ryan 1985)

[a]Yields of hydroquinone (*HQ*) and catechol (*CAT*), respectively, for each tobacco constituent normalized to the amount of each constituent found in a methanol/water extract of bright tobacco

[b]Contribution to the total yield

2.3.2 Trace Heavy Metals

The yields reported in the literature of trace metals that transfer from the cigarette tobacco to the mainstream cigarette smoke vary widely. For example, Purkis et al. (2003) reported the yields of several trace metals in the TPM from three different cigarettes (5-, 8-, and 12-mg tar delivery), tested by five independent laboratories under the same smoking regime. For the 8-mg product, the yield (nanograms per cigarette) for cadmium was 20.6–35.3; for lead, 8.8–16.8; for mercury, 0.4–3.5; for arsenic, 1.9–2.2; for chromium, 2–8.7; for nickel, 2–5.3; and for selenium, 0.8–6. Although the Cambridge filter is the most common method of collecting organic compounds from cigarette smoke condensate, it is not suitable for the collection of tar from mainstream cigarette smoke for trace metal analysis because of the trace metal impurities in the pad. Instead, quartz glass filters have been used for collection of inorganic compounds in tobacco smoke, because their background contamination is relatively low. Although cold traps and jet impaction traps have been employed, electrostatic precipitation into quartz tubes has become the preferred technique for collection of cigarette smoke condensate for trace metal analysis. Samples must be handled with meticulous care to avoid potential sources of metal contamination from the laboratory environment (Counts et al. 2004, 2005; Gregg et al. 2004; Roemer et al. 2004). In general, the use of an isolation clean room is required for accurate trace metal analysis.

A variety of analytical techniques has been employed for determining trace metals in mainstream cigarette smoke. In the most recently reported measurements, the two

Table 2.3 Trace metal analysis for 1R4F research cigarettes and three commercial products reported by different labs under different smoking regimes

Reference	Cigarette	Smoking Conditions	Tar (mg/cig.)	Cd (ng/cig.)	Pb (ng/cig.)	Hg (ng/cig.)	As (ng/cig.)	Cr (ng/cig.)	Ni (ng/cig.)	Se (ng/cig.)	Method	No. labs/reps.
Gregg et al. 2004	1R4F	ISO[a]	9	63.2	39.3	4.6	6.1	–[b]	–[b]	–[b]	ICP-MS	2 labs (average)
Torrence et al. 2002	1R4F	FTC[c]	9	64.2±6.3[d]	38.2+/–1.8	–[e]	6.9±0.5	–[e]	–[e]	–[e]	ICP-MS	20 cigarettes
Chang et al. 2002	1R4F	FTC	9	–[e]	–[e]	5±0.4	–[e]	–[e]	–[e]	–[e]	CV-AAS	20 cigarettes
Chen and Moldoveanu 2003	1R4F	ISO	9.38	55.1	42.5	5.4	12.2	57.7	6.4	34.9	Various	1–4 labs
Counts et al. 2004	1R4F	ISO	9.1±0.4	64.4±2.9	36.7±1.5	5.5±0.5	4.7±0.8	–[b]	–[b]	–[b]	GF/CV-AAS	20 cigarettes/replicates
Counts et al. 2004, 2005	1R4F	MDPH[f]	19.1±0.8	143.6	69.5	10	11.2	–[b]	–[b]	–[b]	GF/CV-AAS	20 cigarettes/replicates
	1R4F	HC[g]	26.3±1.4	160.1	89	10.1	11.9	–[b]	–[b]	–[b]	GF/CV-AAS	20 cigarettes/replicates

Cd cadmium, *Pb* lead, *Hg* mercury, *As* arsenic, *Cr* chromium, *Ni* nickel, *Se* selenium, *mg/cig.* milligrams per cigarette, *ng/cig.* nanograms per cigarette, *labs/reps.* laboratories/replicates, *ISO* International Organization for Standardization, *ICP-MS* inductively coupled plasma mass spectrometry, *FTC* Federal Trade Commission, *CV-AAS* cold-vapor atomic absorption spectrometry, *GF/CV-ASS* graphite-furnace atomic absorption spectrometry, *MDPH* Massachusetts Department of Health, *HC* Health Canada

[a]ISO puffing conditions: 35-ml volume, 60-s interval, 2-s duration
[b]Below detection limit or too low to quantify
[c]FTC puffing conditions; 35-ml volume, 60-s interval, 2-s duration
[d]Mean±SD
[e]not measured
[f]MDPH puffing protocol: 45-ml volume, 30-s interval, 2-s duration, 50% filter ventilation blocking
[g]HC puffing protocol: 55-ml volume, 30-s interval, 2-s duration, 100% filter ventilation blocking

most common techniques were either inductively coupled plasma mass spectrometry (ICP-MS), or graphite-furnace (GF-) or cold-vapor atomic absorption spectrometry (CV-AAS). Because of its higher volatility, mercury is usually measured by cold-vapor atomic absorption spectrometry (Chang et al. 2002; McDaniel et al. 2001).

The yields of several trace metals in the mainstream smoke collected under International Organization for Standardization (ISO) smoking machine conditions from 48 commercial brands of filtered cigarettes were reported by Counts et al. (2004). The tar yield in the various brands ranged from 0.9 to 14.4 mg per cigarette. To a very good approximation, the amount of cadmium, lead, mercury, and arsenic in the smoke condensate was found to be proportional to the yield of tar per cigarette. The overall yield of trace metals showed a dependence on the cigarette brand, design, and the smoking machine conditions employed (Counts et al. 2005). For the 48 brands tested, the range of the average yield per cigarette for each metal was cadmium, 1.6–101.1 ng (48 brands); lead, 13.0–31.4 ng (5 brands); mercury, 1.5–4.7 ng (40 brands); and arsenic, 3.9–5.5 ng (3 brands). For the brands not included in this summary, the levels of these metals in the cigarettes were either below the detection limits of the analytical methods, or too low to quantify. A similar survey of cigarette brands sold in the United Kingdom was made by Gregg et al. (2004). In both studies, some of the variation in trace metal yields between cigarettes was likely because of the variation in the trace metal composition of regional cigarette tobaccos. Other reviews of metal ions in cigarette smoke include (Baker 1999; Hoffmann et al. 2001; IARC Monographs 1986; Smith et al. 1997). In some of these reports, single values are given for the yield of particular metals without indicating the cigarette design, TPM yield, or smoking regimen (see examples cited by Baker [1999] and Stohs et al. [1977]). Such reports are not very meaningful in light of the large range in tar yields reported for different commercial products.

The remaining toxic elements that have been assayed in commercial cigarette products are nickel, chromium, and selenium. The yields of these elements in the most recent studies with commercial filtered cigarettes are either below the detection limit of the methods or too low to quantify (<2 ng per cigarette), over a range of cigarette tar yields. (See, for example, the results of Counts et al. [2004, 2005], Gregg et al. [2004], and the summary for 1R4F research cigarettes given in Table 2.3.) In a systematic comparison of the analyses of 1R4F research cigarettes by four different laboratories, Chen and Moldoveanu (2003) reported high values of 57.7, 6.4, and 34.9 ng per cigarette for chromium, nickel, and selenium, respectively (Table 2.3). The authors noted that different analytical limits of quantification between laboratories contributed to uncertainties in several reported yields. Other potential contributors to these analytical variations are the laboratory environmental or apparatus contaminates addressed by Torrence et al. (2002). Thus, appropriate analysis precautions appear necessary to ensure that accurate data are available for health, regulatory, and tobacco science groups.

2.4 Free Radicals, ROS, and RNS

Cigarette smoke contains a large amount of free radicals (Pryor et al. 1983a, c) and constituents that readily produce free radicals (Cosgrove et al. 1985; Pryor et al. 1983a). The free radicals in cigarette smoke can be classified into two categories: (1) free radicals that form during the burning of tobacco and the smoking process and (2) free radicals that are *not* initially present in the smoke, but are generated either when the gas phase or the

TPM constituents are oxidized in the smoke aerosol, or when they dissolve in oxygenated aqueous solutions or biological media. The first category includes the radicals in the TPM and the gas phase, whereas the second category includes semiquinone radicals, ROS, and RNS.

2.4.1 Particulate-Phase Free Radicals

The TPM free radicals from cigarette smoke are known to be stable and last for an indefinitely long period of time (Chouchane et al. 2005; Pryor et al. 1983a, c, 1998; Zang et al. 1995). They can be detected using EPR either directly on the filter used to collect the TPM or in solution by extraction of the TPM. A cellulose filter is employed because the Cambridge pad exhibits a background EPR signal. Figure 2.10 shows the EPR signal of cigarette smoke TPM free radicals detected directly on a cellulose filter (Chouchane et al. 2005). The EPR signal is characterized by a broad singlet with a g-factor equal to 2.0028. The EPR spectrum in Fig. 2.10 is very similar to previously reported spectra (Pryor et al. 1983a; Pryor et al. 1983c). The concentration of these radicals in TPM can be as great as 10^{17} radicals per gram of TPM depending on the tobacco, cigarette type, and the smoking regime. The chemical nature of the radicals in cigarette smoke TPM has never been fully characterized. The accepted view of TPM radicals is that they consist primarily of semiquinone radicals in a polymeric tarry matrix. (Pryor et al. 1983a; Pryor et al. 1983c). Semiquinones undoubtedly account for part of the radicals, but recent findings suggest that the TPM radicals are not simply semiquinone radicals, but can be distinguished as oxygen-centered radicals or carbon-centered radicals (Chouchane et al. 2005).

Using bright tobacco cigarette filler heated in a tube furnace under helium atmosphere, we observed that the free radical yield in TPM increases with the heating temperature, as shown in Fig. 2.11. Maskos et al. (2005) made similar observations and showed that the TPM radicals from bright tobacco filler heated at 200–400 °C exhibit g-factors that vary from 2.0039 to 2.0050, characteristic of oxygen-centered radicals, whereas radicals from tobacco heated at ca. 600 °C exhibit a g-factor equal to 2.0028, characteristic of carbon-centered radicals. Experiments in our laboratory showed that TPM radicals from both cigarette smoke and pyrolyzed tobacco undergo an aging process when exposed to air, exhibiting an increase in the intensity of the EPR signals and a shift in the g-factors after the TPM is aged for more than 24 h, as shown in Fig. 2.12. The results of Maskos et al. (2005) and our own suggest that a significant fraction of the cigarette smoke radicals trapped on the filter is initially carbon-centered radicals that convert to oxygen-centered radicals on exposure to molecular oxygen in air.

In experiments utilizing a smoking machine, we measured the yield of free radicals in the TPM from several cigarettes containing different amounts of polyphenolic compounds in the tobacco filler, as shown in Fig. 2.13 (Chouchane et al. 2005). The cigarettes used in our study were the same cigarettes employed in the phenolic compound analysis (see Sect. 2.3.1). We found that the yield of free radicals generated in the TPM of the smoke from these cigarettes was *not* directly related to the total amount of polyphenolic compounds in the tobacco leaf filler. For example, a cigarette containing 100% bright tobacco, which contains a significantly higher amount of polyphenolic compounds in comparison to burley tobacco (Table 2.1), did not generate the highest amount of free radicals in the TPM. However, with the exception of the bright cigarettes, a slight trend was observed between the TPM radicals and the dihydroxybenzenes in the TPM

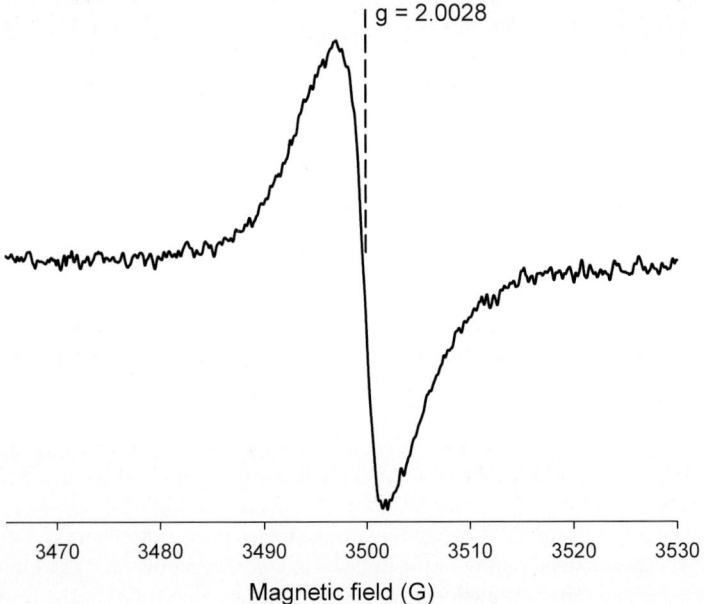

Fig. 2.10 EPR signal of free radicals in the total particulate matter (TPM) of mainstream smoke from a single 2R4F cigarette. The spectrum of the fresh TPM was measured directly on the cellulose collection filter (Chouchane et al. 2005)

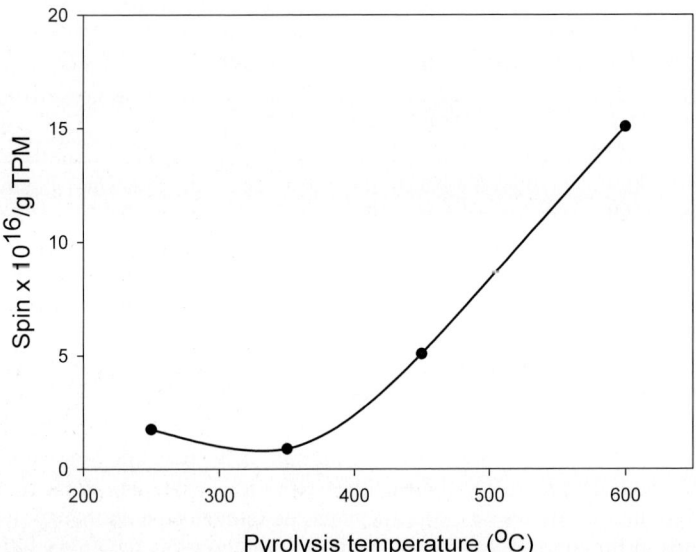

Fig. 2.11 Effect of pyrolysis temperature on the yield of free radicals in the total particulate matter (*TPM*) from bright tobacco. The tobacco was heated for 10 min in a tube furnace at the indicated temperatures under a helium atmosphere

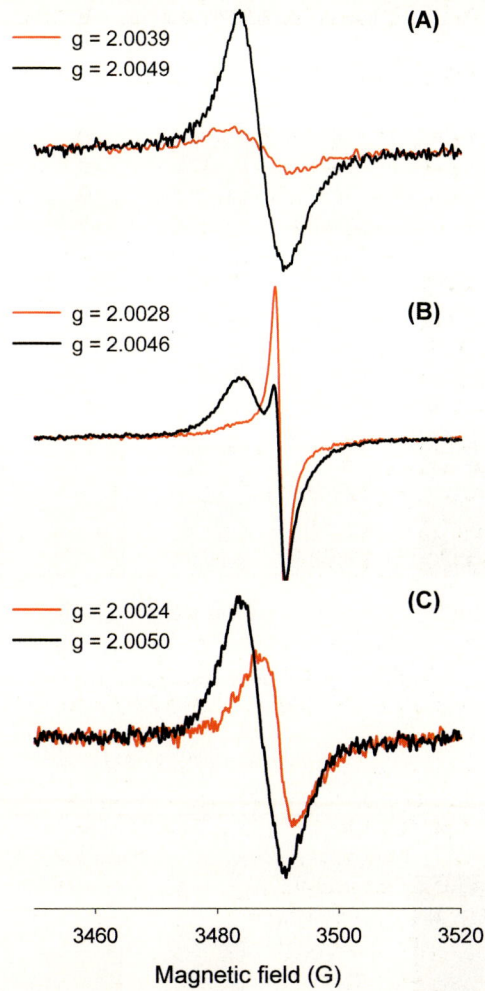

Fig. 2.12 Effect of aging on the free radicals in the total particulate matter (TPM) of smoke from 100% bright tobacco cigarettes or bright tobacco heated under helium in a tube furnace. EPR spectra of free radicals in fresh (·····) and aged (—) TPM for a week from **a** tobacco pyrolyzed in at tube furnace at 450 °C, **b** tobacco pyrolyzed at 600 °C in a tube furnace, and **c** a smoked cigarette

(Fig. 2.14), suggesting that these phenolic compounds do contribute to the formation of the TPM radicals. This result differs, however, from the data previously reported by Blakley et al. (2001) that showed that, there is no relationship between the radicals and the yield of phenolics in the TPM.

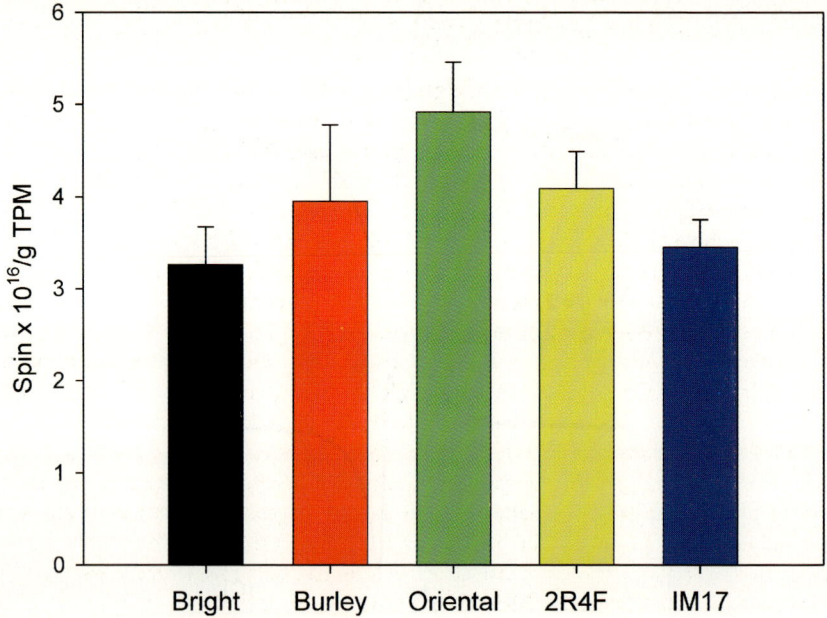

Fig. 2.13 Yield of free radicals in fresh total particulate matter (*TPM*) of mainstream smoke of different cigarettes (Chouchane et al. 2005)

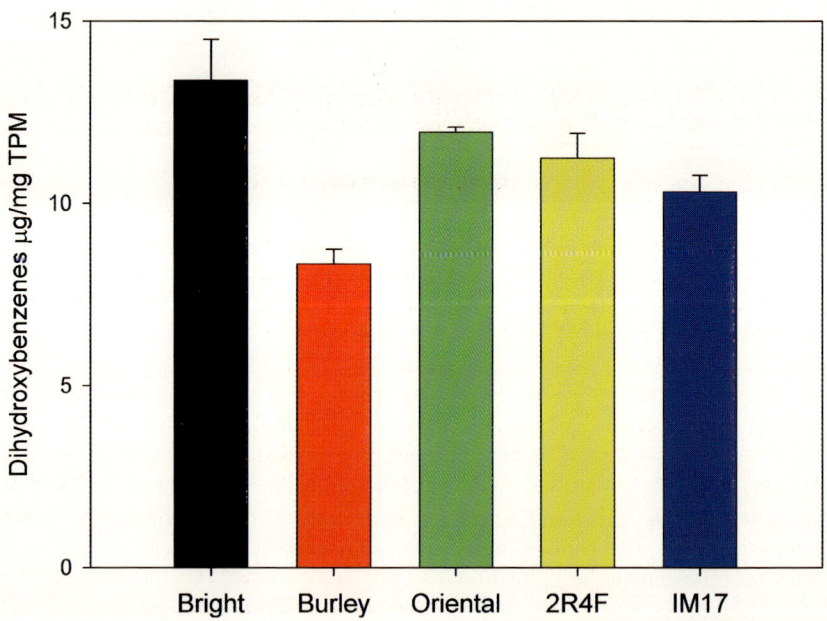

Fig. 2.14 Yield of dihydroxybenzenes in the total particulate matter (*TPM*) of mainstream from different cigarette smoke (Chouchane et al. 2005)

2.4.2 Gas-Phase Free Radicals

The radicals in the gas–vapor phase of cigarette smoke are oxidizing, and they are generally more reactive than are the TPM radicals. EPR spin-trapping techniques are usually used to detect the free radicals in the gas phase of cigarette smoke, typically using the spin trap PBN in benzene solution (Bluhm et al. 1971). Figure 2.15 shows the resulting EPR signal of the gas phase of cigarette smoke, separated from the TPM by a Cambridge filter, and bubbled into a benzene solution of 100 mM PBN (Chouchane et al. 2005). The measured hyperfine coupling constants of the radical adducts (confirmed by spectral simulation) are a_N = 13.9 G and a_H = 2.0 G, and the g-factor is 2.00565. These parameters are in agreement with previously reported hyperfine coupling constants for the PBN adducts of alkoxyl radicals (Pryor et al. 1983a, c). Quantification of the gas-phase radicals from different cigarettes shows that the yield of radicals per cigarette falls in the order: 2R4F > IM17 > burley > oriental > bright (Fig. 2.16) (Chouchane et al. 2005).

NO· is known to be the predominant precursor of other cigarette smoke gas-phase radicals (Sect. 2.2.1). Nitrate, amino acids, ammonium salts, and other nitrogen-containing compounds can potentially produce NO· in the gas phase of cigarette smoke by thermolytic decomposition. Notably, however, gas-phase free radicals can also be produced by heating tobacco leaf constituents that do not contain nitrogen, e.g., cellulose (Pryor et al. 1983a). Im et al. (2003) showed that the evolution of NO· from heated tobacco occurs in two distinct temperature regimes from primarily two sources. Between 275 and 375 °C, under pyrolytic or combustion conditions, the source of NO· was attributed to the decomposition of nitrate. At a higher temperature range (425–525 °C), NO· is produced only in an oxidative environment. In this thermal regime, the NO· was attributed to the oxidation of the char, which contains nitrogen originating from the decomposition of amino acids and protein at lower temperatures.

2.4.3 Cytotoxicity of TPM Constituents

The TPM of cigarette smoke is a very complex mixture that contains numerous substituted phenolic compounds (Smith et al. 2002a). Among these compounds, the dihydroxybenzenes are notable because they can act either as prooxidants or antioxidants. In this section, we present evidence for their possible involvement in the cytotoxicity of cigarette smoke TPM. As discussed in Sect. 3.1.1, the most abundant phenolic compounds found in the TPM from blended or single tobacco cigarettes are phenol, dihydroxybenzenes, and their methyl-substituted derivatives, with hydroquinone and catechol exhibiting the highest yields (see Fig. 2.5). Hydroquinone and catechol are abundant in the smoke of commercial cigarettes (Baker 1999; Counts et al. 2004; Roemer et al. 2004). They are known to generate semiquinone and superoxide radicals via the redox cycling mechanism in aqueous solutions (Samuni et al. 2003; Squadrito et al. 2001), and they have been shown to induce damage in physiological systems (DeCaprio 1999; Deisinger et al. 1996; do Céu Silva et al. 2003; McCue et al. 2003).

We have measured the in vitro cytotoxicity of hydroquinone, catechol, and their methyl-substituted derivatives. The results, given in Table 2.4 (Chouchane et al. 2004), are reported in terms of the 50% effective concentration (EC_{50}), the effective concentration required to kill 50% of mouse embryo BALB/c 3T3 cells in the NRU assay. We found that the methyl-substituted dihydroxybenzenes exhibited a higher cytotoxicity

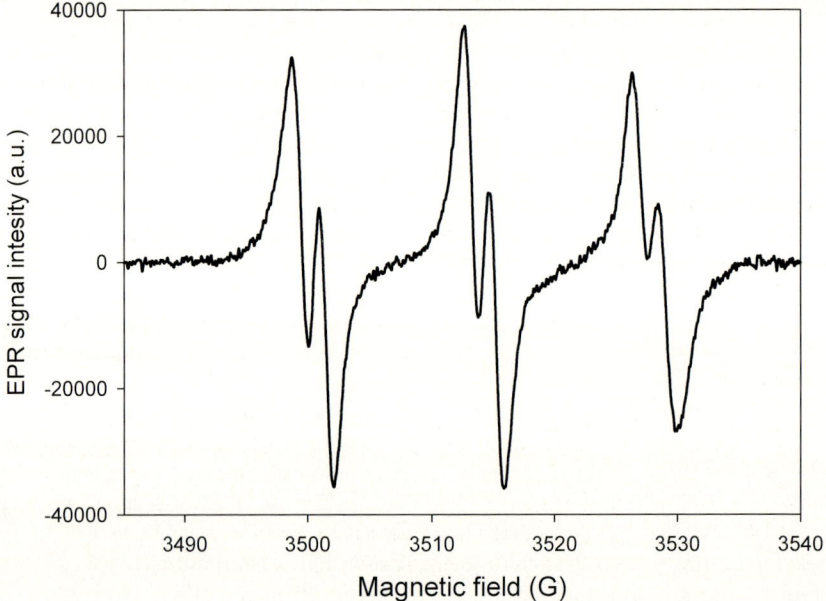

Fig. 2.15 EPR signal of spin adducts of radicals in the gas phase of cigarette smoke. The gas phase was separated from the total particulate matter (TPM) using a Cambridge pad and bubbled into a solution of benzene containing a 100-mM α-phenyl-N-*tert*-butylnitrone (PBN) spin trap. The sample was degassed and analyzed by EPR spectroscopy (Chouchane et al. 2005)

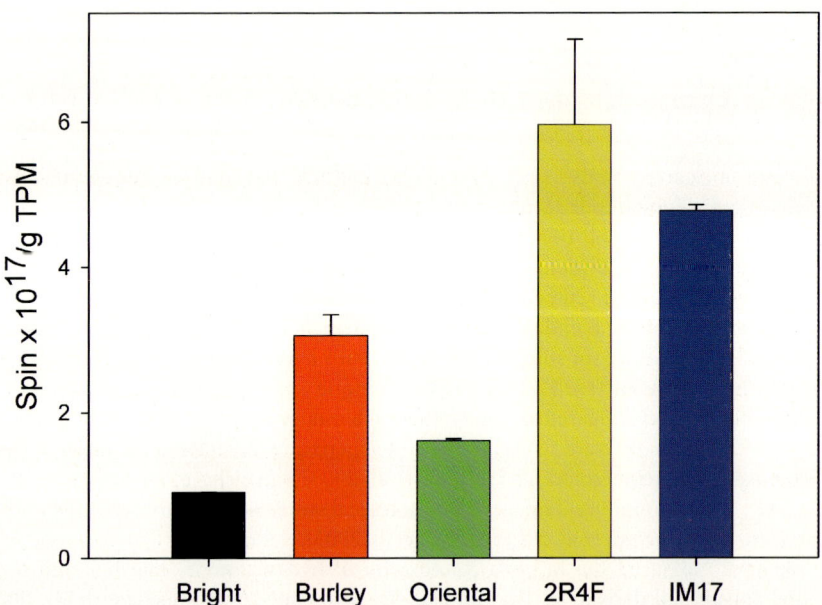

Fig. 2.16 Yield of free radicals found in the gas phase of mainstream smoke from different cigarettes (Chouchane et al. 2005)

than did their unsubstituted parent compounds. Similar results were reported for substituted phenols by Moridani et al. (2003), who attributed the difference in cytotoxicity to their higher lipophilic character and their lower redox potentials. The dihydroxybenzenes shown in Fig. 2.4 are present in the TPM of cigarette smoke, together with many other substances in a complex matrix. The EC_{50} values of the pure compounds, however, do not necessarily reflect the cytotoxicity of such a mixture. The cytotoxicity of the matrix depends on a number of factors such as the structure, concentration, and redox potentials of the individual dihydroxybenzenes. Moreover, molecular interactions between the dihydroxybenzenes (and their oxidation products) and other TPM constituents can affect the cytotoxicity of a mixture of TPM constituents.

Table 2.4 Yield of dihydroxybenzenes in the total particulate matter from 2R4F cigarettes and their specific in vitro cytotoxicity expressed as the 50% effective concentration (EC_{50}) determined by the neutral red uptake assay (Chouchane et al. 2004)

Dihydroxybenzenes	EC_{50} (mM)	Yield (µg/cig.)
Hydroquinone	0.021±0.004	39.3±1.26[a]
2-Methylhydroquinone	0.011±0.001	4.02±0.03[b]
2,3-Dimethylhydroquinone	0.015±0.005	1.37±0.07[b]
2,6-Dimethylhydroquinone	0.016±0.002	0.49±0.04[b]
Trimethylhydroquinone	0.026	1.83±0.03[b]
Catechol	0.33	45.3±0.52[c]
3-Methylcatechol	0.036±0.005	5.3
4-Methylcatechol	0.052±0.013	4.4
Total		102.0

EC_{50} 50% effective concentration, *µg/cig.* micrograms per cigarette
[a] Mean±SD, $n=3$
[b] Mean±SD, $n=4$
[c] Mean±SD, $n=10$

When dissolved in the cell culture medium employed in the cytotoxicity assay (e.g., Dubelcco's Modified Eagle's Medium (DMEM), we found that the dihydroxybenzenes generate significant amounts of the corresponding semiquinone radicals, as represented by their EPR spectra shown in Fig. 2.17. However, the yield of semiquinone radicals depends on the structure of each dihydroxybenzene and its redox potential. Standard one-electron reduction potentials for the redox couple $Q/Q^{-\cdot}$ at 25 °C and pH 7.0 have previously been reported for several dihydroxybenzenes found in TPM including hydroquinone, 78 mV; methylhydroquinone, 23 mV; 2,3-dimethylhydroquinone, −74 mV; 2,6-dimethylhydroquinone, −80 mV; and trimethylhydroquinone, −165 mV (Wardman 1989). The reduction potential decreases with methyl substitution. Among the most abundant dihydroxybenzenes in TPM, hydroquinone is the most potent semiquinone radical generator (Fig. 2.18), and it has a high reduction potential. The reduction potentials of the dihydroxybenzenes increase with their capacity to undergo autoxidation and generate semiquinone radicals, as shown in Fig. 2.19. An association between the cytotoxicity of quinones and their reduction potential has been previously proposed. Nemeikaite-Ceniene et al. (2002), for example, observed that the toxicity of natural hydroxyanthraquinones increases at pH 7 with an increase of their reduction potential, pointing to an oxidative stress mechanism.

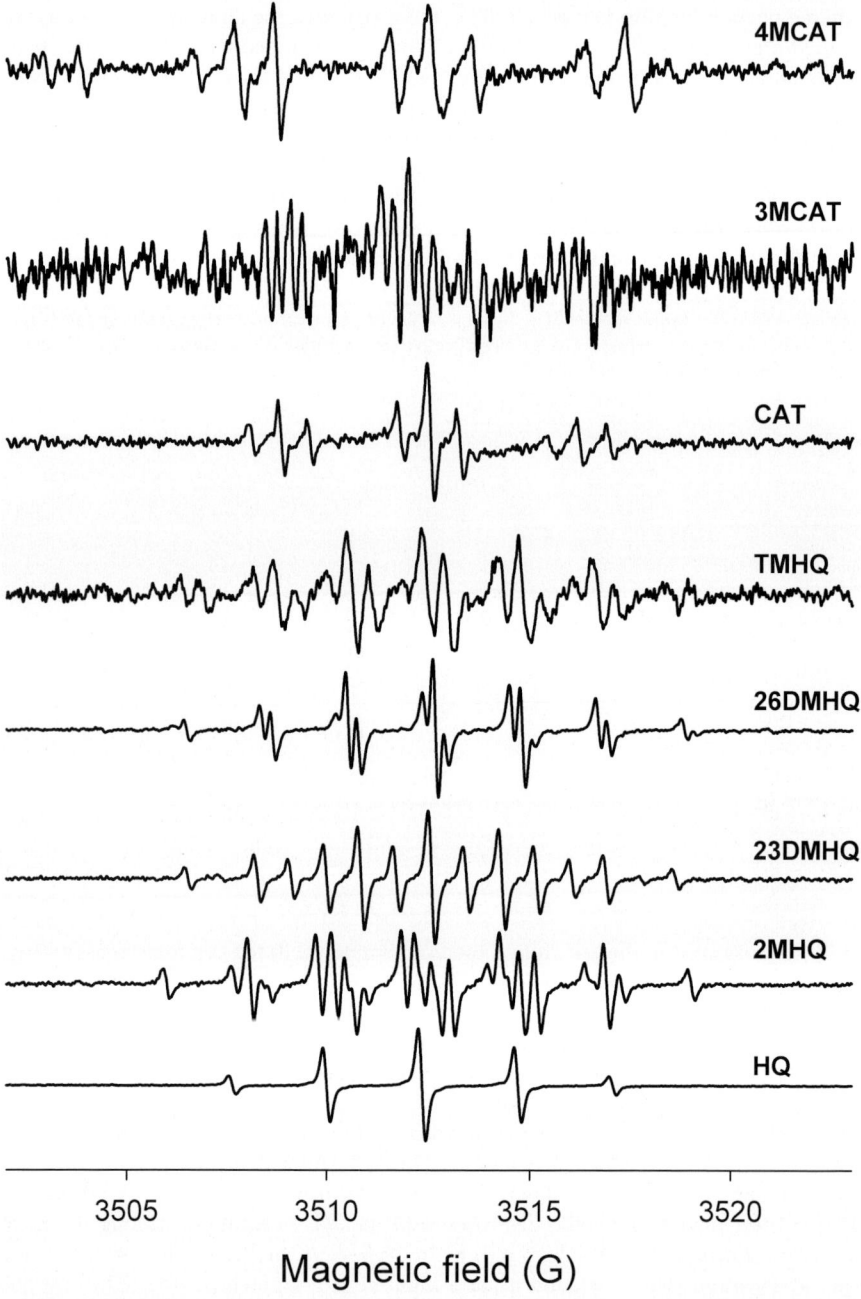

Fig. 2.17 EPR spectra of semiquinone radicals observed in 1-mM solutions of dihydroxybenzenes in DMEM (Chouchane et al. 2004)

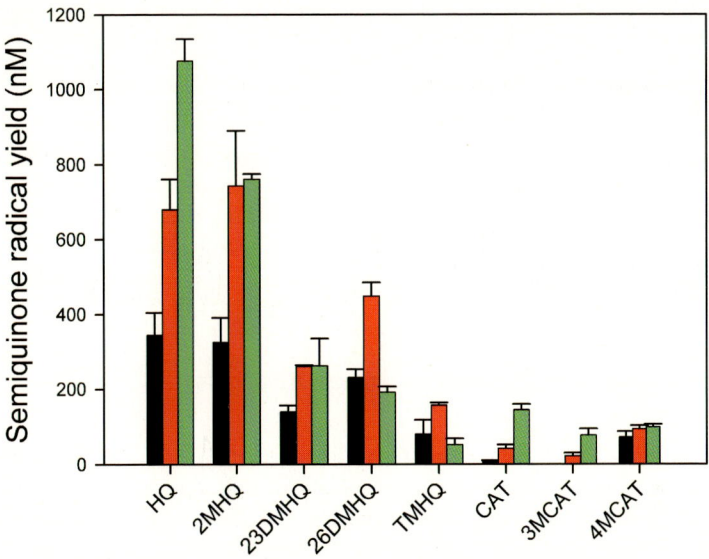

Fig. 2.18 Yield of semiquinone radicals obtained when 1-mM dihydroxybenzenes were dissolved in cell culture medium DMEM (Chouchane et al. 2004)

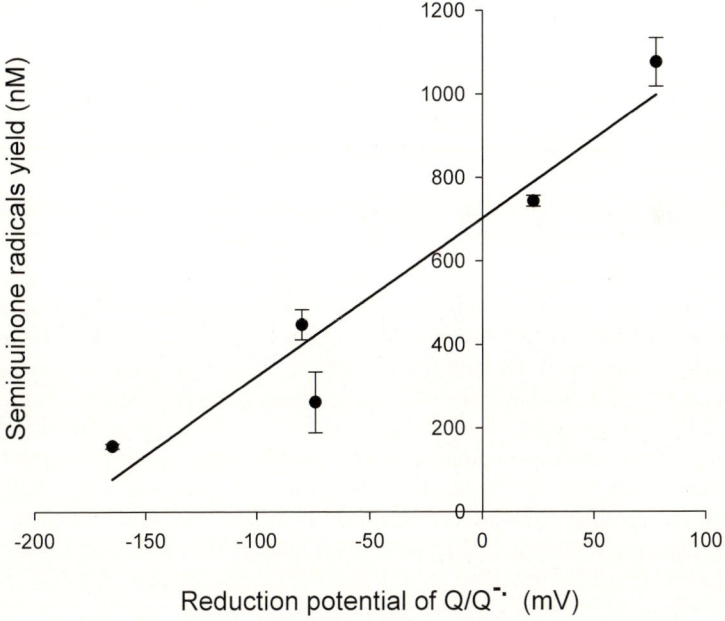

Fig. 2.19 Yield of semiquinone radicals formed in 1-mM solutions of dihydroxybenzenes dissolved in DMEM versus their respective reduction potentials to the semiquinone radical (Q/Q$^{-\cdot}$) (Chouchane et al. 2004)

2.4.4 ROS and RNS in Aqueous Solutions of Cigarette Smoke

The examination of the chemistry of cigarette smoke-bubbled aqueous solutions is important on two counts. First, immediately after a smoker takes a puff, smoke enters an environment of high humidity, and the smoke deposits in the epithelial lining fluid (ELF) of the respiratory tract. Second, reactive species can form in aqueous solutions of cigarette smoke that are not generated inside the burning cigarette, but rather form in solution by reaction between smoke constituents, or by reactions of smoke constituents with dissolved oxygen.

2.4.4.1 Superoxide and Hydroxyl Radicals

Several cigarette smoke constituents have been suggested to be responsible for the generation of reactive oxygen species. Among these constituents, dihydroxybenzenes are good candidates. Oxidation of hydroquinone (QH_2) by molecular oxygen in aqueous solution generates the semiquinone ($Q^-\cdot$) and superoxide radicals following reaction 1:

$$QH_2 + O_2 \rightarrow Q^-\cdot + O_2^-\cdot + 2H^+ \quad (1)$$

Spontaneous disproportionation of the superoxide radical anion, or catalytic disproportionation in vivo by SOD, generates H_2O_2 (reaction 2). In the presence of transition metal ions, H_2O_2 can undergo disproportionation to generate hydroxyl radical, a powerful oxidant (reaction 3).

$$O_2^-\cdot + 2H^+ \rightarrow H_2O_2 \quad (2)$$

$$H_2O_2 + Fe^{2+} \rightarrow \cdot OH + OH^- + Fe^{3+} \quad (3)$$

Superoxide and hydroxyl radicals have been shown to form in aqueous extracts of cigarette smoke (Pryor et al. 1998; Zang et al. 1995). It was also shown that aqueous extracts of TPM produce hydroxyl radicals that can be spin-trapped with 5,5-dimethyl-1-pyrroline-N-oxide (DMPO). The hydroxyl radicals arise from the metal mediated decomposition of H_2O_2, as shown above (Cosgrove et al. 1985; Pryor 1992).

The DMPO–superoxide radical adduct is unstable, with a half-life of 80 s at pH 6 and 35 s at pH 8. The superoxide spin adduct slowly decays to form the DMPO–hydroxyl radical adduct (Buettner and Oberley 1978; Finkelstein et al. 1979, 1980, 1982). The Pryor group observed superoxide radicals in ACT in a high-pH solution, but not hydroxyl radicals. In the same study, superoxide radicals were detected in ACT by employing a much higher concentration of DMPO (ca. 1 M) (Zang et al. 1995). With the development of new spin-trap molecules for reactive oxygen species, particularly superoxide radical, it is possible to overcome some of the problems encountered with the use of DMPO. 5-Diethoxyphosphoryl-5-methyl-1-pyrroline-N-oxide (DEPMPO), for example, can trap both superoxide and hydroxyl radicals. The DEPMPO–superoxide radical adduct has a half-life of 13 min (Frejaville et al. 1995), allowing its detection by EPR within a shorter period in comparison with the DMPO adduct. As shown in

Fig. 2.20, when whole cigarette smoke is passed through a phosphate buffered solution pH 7.4 containing DEPMPO (100 mM), both superoxide radical and hydroxyl radical are trapped. Under the same experimental conditions using DMPO, only superoxide radicals are trapped.

If superoxide is involved in the adverse effects of cigarette smoke, a strategy aimed at the elimination of excess superoxide might minimizes these effects. For example, acute exposure to cigarette smoke is known to induce the infiltration of neutrophils into the airways in guinea pigs, a phenomenon associated with a defensive response to oxidative stress. This response is manifest by activation of the nuclear factor-kappaB (NF-κB) transcription factor and increased expression of interleukin 8 (IL-8) mRNA (Nishikawa et al. 1999). Prior treatment of the guinea pigs with SOD, to reduce the accumulation of superoxide, inhibited neutrophil accumulation and reduced both NF-κB activation and IL-8 mRNA expression. Another example was reported by (Smith et al. 2002b): Intratracheal instillation of a SOD-mimetic (AEOL 10150, a manganese porphyrin) into the airways of rats was shown to provide a marked protective effect against cigarette smoke-induced inflammation and damage.

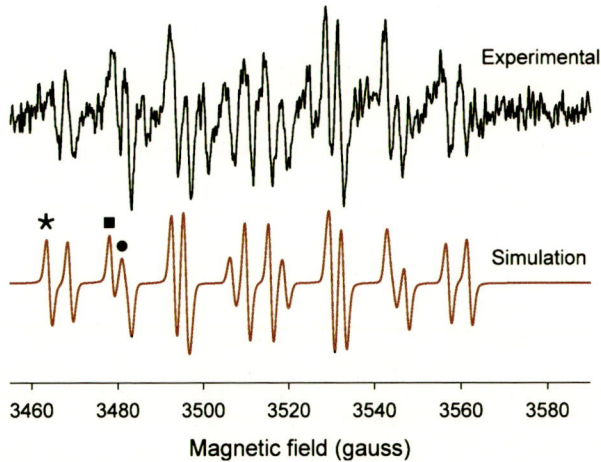

Fig. 2.20 EPR signal of spin adducts of superoxide radicals and hydroxyl radicals trapped in a phosphate buffer pH 7.4 containing 5-diethoxyphosphoryl-5-methyl-1-pyrroline-N-oxide (DEPMPO) 100 mM bubbled with whole mainstream smoke. ■ DEPMPO-superoxide radical adduct, • DEPMPO-hydroxyl radical adduct, * DEPMPO-carboxyl radical adduct

2.4.4.2 Hydrogen Peroxide

There are relatively few reports of H_2O_2 measurements in cigarette smoke under any conditions. One difficulty in analyzing for H_2O_2 is its transient nature, and the established methods of analysis are slow and laborious. Both a polarographic method developed for the analysis of H_2O_2 in TPM (Nakayama et al. 1989) and a previously reported colorimetric method developed to analyze whole smoke (Nakayama et al. 1984) require the removal of the organic phase by chromatography or solvent extraction as a preliminary step in the analysis. Another approach to measure H_2O_2 in cigarette tar is to use an oxygen electrode, but the oxygen electrode is not specific to H_2O_2, and the addition of catalase to the analyte solutions is required to confirm that the oxygen adsorbed species is because of H_2O_2 (Stone et al. 1995).

By application of the polarographic method, Nakayama et al. (1989) found that the aqueous extracts of cigarette tar produce H_2O_2 for prolonged periods up to 24 h and longer. The dihydroxybenzenes in tar, i.e., hydroquinone, catechol, etc., provide an ample reservoir for the formation of semiquinone radicals via autooxidation. The semiquinone radicals generate superoxide radical anions in oxygenated solutions for extended periods, producing H_2O_2 by dismutation. Other pathways of H_2O_2 formation may exist, but they have not been clearly delineated as the semiquinone pathway. The primary source of H_2O_2 in cigarette tar is believed to be superoxide formed by the reduction of atmospheric oxygen by semiquinone radicals in the tar (Tanigawa et al. 1994).

In a series of experiments by Nakayama et al. (1989) on experimental and commercial cigarettes, extracts of TPM in phosphate buffer were bubbled with oxygen for 1 min and incubated in the dark. The yield of H_2O_2 after 4 h ranged from 37 to 123 µM per cigarette. The study included both filtered (with and without ventilation) and nonfiltered cigarettes, and the yield of H_2O_2 varied depending on the cigarette design. In general, nonfiltered cigarettes yielded higher amounts of H_2O_2 than do filtered cigarettes. The results were not normalized to the amount of TPM delivered, but the authors showed that the overall yield of H_2O_2 in most cigarettes is proportional to the yield of TPM

Recently, a fluorometric method was developed that detects the oxidized form of Amplex Red, a fluorescent dye, in the presence of horseradish peroxidase and H_2O_2 (Yan et al. 2005). This method has several advantages over the polarographic method: (1) it only requires a 2-min incubation time and is therefore faster than are previous methods, (2) the H_2O_2 does not have to be separated from the tar matrix, (3) it can be applied to small samples, and (4) the method is readily adapted for automation. Applying their method, Yan et al. (2005) bubbled five puffs of whole smoke from 1R4F or 2R4F research cigarettes into phosphate buffered saline solution (PBS) containing the fluorescent dye, using a smoking machine. Concentrations of 3–8 micromolar H_2O_2 were found in the whole smoke bubbled samples, while there was negligible H_2O_2 formation from gas-phase smoke bubbled samples. Others have developed electrochemical means of detecting hydrogen peroxide. H_2O_2 is an electrochemically active species that will disproportionate at the surface of a metallic electrode. For example, an amperometric detection principle similar to the oxygen detection using the Clark electrode has been utilized. Hydrogen peroxide is selectively detected by an electrode after passing through a H_2O_2 permeable membrane. This method can compliment the flurometric approach with direct quantitative measurement in biological samples in the low nM range.

2.4.4.3 NO· and Peroxynitrite

NO· and peroxynitrites are the major reactive nitrogen species derived from cigarette smoke. The yields of NO· from 49 commercial cigarettes smoked on a smoking machine under ISO conditions were reported to be 78–487 µg per cigarette (Counts et al. 2005). As described in Sect. 2.2.1, NO· forms in the cigarette gas phase from the burning of different tobacco constituents. Im et al. (2003) showed that NO· from heated tobacco is produced in two distinct temperature ranges, a low-temperature range (275–375 °C) in an oxygen-free atmosphere, and a high-temperature range (425–525 °C) that requires an oxygen-containing atmosphere. Nitrates were determined to be the source of NO· formation in the low-temperature ranges, and amino acids and proteins were suggested to be the sources of NO· at the higher-temperature ranges. The individual contribution of these precursors to the overall yield of NO· in cigarette smoke has yet to be determined.

Peroxynitrite forms by the reaction of NO· and superoxide radicals. In smoke-bubbled aqueous solutions, smoke constituents that can reduce molecular oxygen to superoxide, e.g., hydroquinone, continuously generate superoxide, which reacts rapidly with NO· from the gas phase to give peroxynitrite. Alkyl peroxynitrites can also form by reaction of NO· and peroxyl radicals (Halliwell and Gutteridge 1999), which are presumed to form in the gas phase of cigarette smoke (Pryor et al. 1983a, 1984, 1985). Peroxynitrite in cigarette smoke extract has been shown to react with and inactivate the α_1-proteinase inhibitor (Moreno and Pryor 1992). Peroxynitrite has also been identified as an oxidative stress-inducing constituent of aqueous cigarette smoke fractions. After depletion of intracellular GSH by electrophilic aldehydes, peroxynitrite interferes with specific target molecules, resulting in the activation of stress signal transduction and stress gene expression in cigarette smoke-treated cells in vitro (Müller and Gebel 1994, 1998; Müller et al. 1997).

2.5 Summary

Cigarette smoke has considerable potential for inducing oxidative modifications and depletion of antioxidants. In cigarette smoke-exposed aqueous solutions, ROS and RNS form and subsequently act as potent oxidants. Oxidative damage to lipids, proteins, and DNA by cigarette smoke-derived ROS and RNS has been extensively demonstrated both in vitro and in vivo. In many cases, the initially generated reactive intermediates convert cellular constituents into second-generation reactive intermediates (e.g., acrolein, 4-hydroxynonenal) capable of inducing further cytotoxic and genotoxic damage. When free radicals react with nonradicals (e.g., lipids), new radicals can form that may result in a chain reaction of free radicals. Thus, relatively short-lived free radicals may propagate their damaging effects beyond the limits set by their short half-lives and limited diffusion times. ROS and RNS activate numerous redox sensitive signaling pathways that modulate cellular responses, such as inflammation, which may itself result in the formation of endogenous oxidative species. Therefore, the oxidative damage resultant from cigarette smoke exposure is complex and likely mediated by both the oxidative potential of cigarette smoke and indirect biological responses.

Acknowledgements

The authors thank Drs. Matthias Schorp, Susan Plunkett, Mary Ellen Counts, Michael Chang, Kai Lam, and Peter Kuhl for invaluable technical discussions and for their contributions to the text. We are grateful to Dr. Geoffrey Chan and Dr. Peter Lipowicz for their support and encouragement.

References

Achladas GE (1991) Analysis of biomass pyrolysis liquids: separation and characterization of phenols. J Chromatogr A 542:263–275

Amen-Chen C, Pakdel H, Roy C (1997) Separation of phenols from Eucalyptus wood tar. Biomass Bioenergy 13:25–37

Arrendale RF, Severson RF, Chortyk OT (1984) The application of capillary gas chromatography to the analyses of acidic constituents of tobacco leaf and smoke. Beitr Tabak 12:186–197

Ault JG, Lawrence DA (2003) Glutathione distribution in normal and oxidatively stressed cells. Exp Cell Res 285:9–14

Baker RR (1999) Smoke chemistry. In: Davis LD, Nielson MT (eds) Tobacco: production, chemistry and technology. Blackwell, London, pp 308–439

Baker RR (2002) The development and significance of standards for smoking-machine methodology. Beitr Tabak 20:23–41

Bal W, Kasprzak KS (2002) Induction of oxidative DNA damage by carcinogenic metals. Toxicol Lett 127:55–62

Barchowsky A, O'Hara KA (2003) Metal-induced cell signaling and gene activation in lung diseases. Free Radic Biol Med 34:1130–1135

Beckman JS, Beckman TW, Chen J, Marshall PA, Freeman BA (1990) Apparent hydroxyl radical production by peroxynitrite: implications for endothelial injury from nitric oxide and superoxide. Proc Natl Acad Sci USA 87:1620–1624

Blakley RL, Henry DD, Smith CJ (2001) Lack of correlation between cigarette mainstream smoke particulate phase radicals and hydroquinone yield. Food Chem Tox 39:401–406

Bluhm AL, Weinstein J, Sousa JA (1971) Free radicals in tobacco smoke. Nature 229:500

Bokelman GH, Ryan WS Jr (1985) Analysis of bright and burley tobacco laminae and stems. Beitr Tabak Int 13:29–36

Bolton JL, Trush MA, Penning RM, Dryhurst L, Monks TJ (2000) Role of quinones in toxicology. Chem Res Toxicol 13:135–160

Bosio A, Knorr C, Janssen U, Gebel S, Haussmann HJ, Müller T (2002) Kinetics of gene expression profiling in Swiss 3T3 cells exposed to aqueous extracts of cigarette smoke. Carcinogenesis 2002 23:741–748

Briede JJ, Godschalk RWL, Emans MTG, De Kok TMCM, Van Agen E, Van Maanen J, Van Schooten FJ, Kleinjans JCS (2004) In vitro and in vivo studies on oxygen free radical and DNA adduct formation in rat lung and liver during benzo[a]pyrene metabolism. Free Radic Res 38:995–1002

Brunmark A, Cadenas E (1989) Redox and addition chemistry of quinoid compounds and its biological implications. Free Radic Biol Med 7:435–477

Brunneman KD, Lee H, Hoffman D (1976) Chemical studies on tobacco smoke. XLVII. On the quantitative analysis of catechols and their reduction. Anal Lett 9:939–955

Buettner GR, Oberley LW (1978) Considerations in the spin trapping of superoxide and hydroxyl radical in aqueous systems using 5,5-dimethyl-1-pyrroline-1-oxide. Biochem Biophys Res Commun 83:69–74

Cahours X, Renault D, Dubois M, Marchand V, Dumery B (2004) Oxidative effects of cigarette smoke: assessment by fast cell-free method. Presentation at the CORESTA Congress, Kyoto, Japan

Carmella SG, Hecht SS, Tso TC, Hoffman D (1984) Roles of tobacco cellulose, sugars, and chlorogenic acid as precursors to catechol in cigarette smoke. J Agric Food Chem 32:267–273

Chang MJ, McDaniel RL, Nawiral JD, Self DA (2002) A rapid method for the determination of mecury in mainstream cigarette smoke by two-stage amalgamation cold vapor atomic absorption spectroscopy. J Anal Atomic Spec 17:710–715

Chen PX, Moldoveanu SC (2003) Mainstream smoke chemical analyses for 2R4F Kentucky reference cigarette. Beitr Tabak 20:448–458

Chortyk OT, Schlotzhauer SW, Stedman RL (1966) Composition studies on tobacco XXIII-pyrolytic and structural investigations on the polyphenol-amino acid pigments of leaf. Beitr Tabak 3:422–429

Chouchane S, Meruva NK, Brown AP, Wooten JB (2005) Precursors of the free radicals generated in the tar and gas phases of mainstream cigarette smoke. American Chemical Society Division of Fuel Chemistry Preprints 50:419–420

Chouchane S, Müller B, Wittig A, Tewez F, Wooten JB (2004) Involvement of semiquinone radicals generated from dihydroxybenzenes in the in-vitro cytotoxicity of cigarette smoke tar. Free Radic Biol Med 37:S14–S14

Church DF, Pryor WA (1985) Free-radical chemistry of cigarette smoke and its toxicological implications. Environ Health Perspec 64:111–126

Cosgrove JP, Borish ET, Church DF, Pryor WA (1985) The metal-mediated formation of hydroxyl radical by aqueous extracts of cigarette tar. Biochem Biophys Res Commun 132:390–396

Counts ME, Hsu FS, Laffoon SW, Dwyer RW, Cox RH (2004) Mainstream smoke constituent yields and predicting relationships from a worldwide market sample of cigarette brands: ISO smoking conditions. Regul Toxicol Pharmacol 39:111–134

Counts ME, Morton MJ, Laffoon SW, Cox RH, Lipowicz PJ (2005) Smoke composition and predicting relationships for international commercial cigarettes smoked with three machine-smoking conditions. Regul Toxicol Pharmacol 41:185–227

Crouse RH, Garner JW, O'Neill HJ (1963) Determination of phenolic constituents of cigarette smoke by gas chromatograph. J Gas Chromatogr 1:18–22

DeCaprio AP (1999) The toxicology of hydroquinone—relevance to occupational and environmental exposure. Crit Rev Toxicol 29:283–330

Deisinger PJ, Hill TS, English JC (1996) Human exposure to naturally occurring hydroquinone. J Toxicol Environ Health 47:31–46

Dellinger B, Pryor WA, Cueto R, Squadrito GL, Hegde V, Deutsch WA (2001) Role of free radicals in the toxicity of airborne fine particulate matter. Chem Res Toxicol 14:1371–1377

Denicola A, Radi R (2005) Peroxynitrite and drug-dependent toxicity. Toxicology 208:273–288

do Céu Silva M, Gaspar J, Duarte ID, Leão D, Rueff J (2003) Mechanisms of induction of chromosomal aberrations by hydroquinone in V79 cells. Mutagenesis 18:491–496

Dube MFR, Green CR (1982) Methods of collection of smoke for analytical purposes. Rec Adv Tob Sci 8:42–102

Eiserich J, Vossen V, O'Neill CA, Halliwell B, Cross CE, van der Vliet A (1994) Molecular mechanisms of damage by excess nitrogen oxides: nitration of tyrosine by gas-phase cigarette smoke. FEBS Lett 353:53–56

Eiserich JP, van der Vliet A, Handelman GJ, Halliwell B, Cross CE (1995) Dietary antioxidants and cigarette smoke-induced biomolecular damage: a complex interaction. Am J Clin Nutr 62:1490S–1500S

Ercal N, Gurer-Orhan H, Aykin-Burns N (2001) Toxic metals and oxidative stress part I: mechanisms involved in metal-induced oxidative damage. Curr Top Med Chem 1:529–539

Federal Register, August 1, 1967. Cigarettes: testing for tar and nicotine content, vol. 32, no. 147, p. 11178

Federal Register, July 10, 1980. Cigarettes and related matters: carbon monoxide, tar and nicotine content of cigarette smoke; description of new machine and methods to be used in testing, vol. 45, no. 134, pp 46483–46487

Finkelstein E, Rosen GM, Rauckman EJ (1980) Spin trapping of superoxide and hydroxyl radical: practical aspects. Arch Biochem Biophys 200:1–16

Finkelstein E, Rosen GM, Rauckman EJ (1982) Production of hydroxyl radical by decomposition of superoxide spin-trapped adducts. Mol Pharmacol 21:262–265

Finkelstein E, Rosen GM, Rauckman EJ, Paxton J (1979) Spin trapping of superoxide. Mol Pharmacol 16:676–685

Flicker TM, Green SA (1998) Detection and separation of gas-phase carbon-centered radicals from cigarette smoke and diesel exhaust. Anal Chem 70:2008–2012

Flicker TM, Green SA (2001) Comparison of gas-phase free-radical populations in tobacco smoke and model systems by HPLC. Environ Health Perspect 109:765–771

Forehand JB, Dooly GL, Moldoveanu SC (2000) Analysis of polycyclic aromatic hydrocarbons, phenols and aromatic amines in particulate phase cigarette smoke using simultaneous distillation and extraction as a sole sample clean-up step. J Chromatogr A 898:111–124

Frejaville C, Karoui H, Tuccio B, Le Moigne F, Culcasi M, Pietri S, Lauricella R, Tordo P (1995) 5-(Diethoxyphosphoryl)-5-methyl-1-pyrroline-N-oxide: a new efficient phosphorylated nitrone for the in vitro and in vivo spin trapping of oxygen-centered radicals. J Med Chem 38:258–265

Gaisch H, Nyffeler U (1976) The measurement of thiol reactivity in cigarette smoke. Beitr Tabak Int 8:399–403

Gregg E, Hill C, Hollywood M, Kearney M, McAdam K, McLaughlin D, Purkis S, Williams M (2004) The UK smoke constituents testing study. Summary of results and comparison with other studies. Beitr Tabak Int 21:117–138

Hagedorn H-W, Gilch G, Janket D, Scherer G (2003) Mechanistically-based tests for toxicity of tobacco smoke. Presentation at the CORESTA Congress, Freiburg, Germany

Halliwell B, Gutteridge JMC (1999) Free radicals in biology and medicine. Oxford University Press, New York

Hirakawa K, Oikawa S, Hiraku Y, Hirosawa I, Kawanishi S (2002) Catechol and hydroquinone have different redox properties responsible for their differential DNA-damaging ability. Chem Res Toxicol 15:76–82

Hoffmann D, Hoffmann I, El Bayoumy K (2001) The less harmful cigarette: a controversial issue. a tribute to Ernst L. Wynder. Chem Res Toxicol 14:767–790

Huie RE, Padmaja S (1993) The reaction of NO with superoxide. Free Radic Res Commun 18:195–199

IARC Monographs (1986) The evaluation of the carcinogenic risk of chemicals to humans: tobacco smoking, vol. 38, p. 83

Im H, Rasouli F, Hajaligol MR (2003) Formation of nitric oxide during tobacco oxidation. J Agric Food Chem 51:7366–7372

Kameswararo BV, Gopalachari NC (1965) Polyphenolic constituents tobacco—a review. Indian J Appl Chem 28:165–172

Kasprzak KS (2002) Oxidative DNA and protein damage in metal-induced toxicity and carcinogenesis. Free Radic Biol Med 32:958–967

Klus H, Kuhn H (1982) Distribution of various tobacco smoke constituents in main- and sidestream smoke (a review). Beitr Tabak Int 11:229–265

Knaapen AM, Borm PJA, Catrin A, Schins RPF (2004) Inhaled particles and lung cancer. Part A: mechanisms. Int J Cancer 109:799–809

Koppenol WH (1998) The basic chemistry of nitrogen monoxide and peroxynitrite. Free Radic Biol Med 25:385–391

Kwon NS, Stuehr DJ, Nathan CF (1991) Inhibition of tumor cell ribonucleotide reductase by macrophage-derived nitric oxide. J Exp Med 174:761–767

Lakritz L, Stanke-Labesque F, Baker MS, Stedman RL (1972) Composition studies on tobacco XLV. Use of cigarette additives to alter the composition and reducing the properties of cigarette smoke. Beitr Tabak 6:120–123

Lau SS, Hill BA, Highet RJ, Monks TJ (1988) Sequential oxidation and glutathione addition to 1,4-benzoquinone: correlation of toxicity with increased glutathione substitution. Mol Pharmacol 34:829–836

Leffingwell JC (1999) Leaf chemistry: basic chemical constituents of tobacco leaf and differences among tobacco types. In: Davis LD, Nielson MT (eds) Tobacco: production, chemistry and technology. Blackwell, London, pp 265–303

Lepoivre M, Flaman JM, Bobe P, Lemaire G, Henry Y (1994) Quenching of the tyrosyl free radical of ribonucleotide reductase by nitric oxide. Relationship to cytostasis induced in tumor cells by cytotoxic macrophages. J Biol Chem 269:21891–21897

Leuchtenberger C, Leuchtenberger R, Zbinden I (1974) Gas vapour phase constituents and SH reactivity of cigarette smoke influence lung cultures. Nature 247:565–567

Leuchtenberger C, Leuchtenberger R, Zbinden I, Schleh E (1976) SH Reactivity of cigarette smoke and its correlation with carcinogenic effects on hamster lung cultures. Soz Praventivmed 21:47–50

Li YB, Trush MA (1993) Oxidation of hydroquinone by copper: chemical mechanism and biological effects. Arch Biochem Biophys 300:346–355

Li Y, Kuppusamy P, Zweier JL, Trush MA (1995) ESR evidence for the generation of reactive oxygen species from the copper-mediated oxidation of the benzene metabolite, hydroquinone: role in DNA damage. Chem Biol Interact 94:101–120

Lougon-Moulin N, Zhang M, Gadani F, Rossi L, Koller D, Kauss M, Wagner GJ (2004) Critical review of the science and options for reducing cadmium in tobacco (*Nicotiana Tabacum* L.) and other plants. In: Sparks D (ed) Advances in agronomy. Academic, New York, pp 111–180

Lyons MJ, Gibson JF, Ingram DJ (1958) Free-radicals produced in cigarette smoke. Nature 181:1003–1004

Martin LC, Tricker AR (2004) Biological monitoring of urinary metabolites of acrolein, benzene, and 1,3-butadiene in smokers and non-smokers. Presentation at Sixth International Symposium on Biological Monitoring in Occupational and Environmental Health. Heidleburg September 6–8 2004

Mascher DG, Mascher HJ, Scherer G, Schmid ER (2001) High-performance liquid chromatographic-tandem mass spectrometric determination of 3-hydroxypropylmercapturic acid in human urine. J Chromatogr B 750:163–169

Maskos S, Khachatryan L, Cueto R, Pryor WA, Dellinger B (2005) Radicals from the pyrolysis of tobacco. Energy Fuels 19:791–799

McCue JM, Lazis S, Cohen JJ, Modiano JF, Freed BM (2003) Hydroquinone and catechol interfere with T cell cycle entry and progression through the G(1) phase. Mol Immunol 39:995–1001

McDaniel RL, Torrence KM, Self DA, Chang MJ (2001) Determination of mercury in mainstream cigarette smoke by conventional and amalgamation of vapor atomic absorption spectroscopy. Beitr Tabak 39:995–1001

McGrath TE, Chan WG, Hajaligol MR (2003) Low temperature mechanism for the formation of polycyclic aromatic hydrocarbons from the pyrolysis of cellulose. J Anal Appl Pyrolysis 66:51–70

McGrath TE, Wooden JB, Chan WG, Hajaligol MR (2005) Formation of polycyclic aromatic hydrocarbons (PAHs) from tobacco: the link between low temperature residual solid and PAH formation. Food and Chemical Toxicology (submitted).

Meacher DM, Menzel DB (1999) Glutathione depletion in lung cells by low-molecular-weight aldehydes. Cell Biol Toxicol 15:163–171

Monks TJ, Hanzlik RP, Cohen GM, Ross D, Graham DG (1992) Quinone chemistry and toxicity. Toxicol Appl Pharmacol 112:2–16

Moreno JJ, Pryor WA (1992) Inactivation of alpha 1-proteinase inhibitor by peroxynitrite. Chem Res Toxicol 5:425–431

Moridani MY, Siraki A, O'Brien PJ (2003) Quantitative structure toxicity relationships for phenols in isolated rat hepatocytes. Chem Biol Interact 145:213–223

Müller T, Gebel S (1994) Heme oxygenase expression in Swiss 3T3 cells following exposure to aqueous cigarette smoke fractions. Carcinogenesis 15:67–72

Müller T, Gebel S (1998) The cellular stress response induced by aqueous extracts of cigarette smoke is critically dependent on the intracellular glutathione concentration. Carcinogenesis 19:797–801

Müller T, Haussmann HJ, Schepers G (1997) Evidence for peroxynitrite as an oxidative stress-inducing compound of aqueous cigarette smoke fractions. Carcinogenesis 18:295–301

Nakayama T, Church DF, Pryor WA (1989) Quantitative analysis of the hydrogen peroxide formed in aqueous cigarette tar extracts. Free Radic Biol Med 7:9–15

Nakayama T, Kodama M, Nagata C (1984) Generation of hydrogen peroxide and superoxide anion radical from cigarette smoke. Gann 75:95–98

Nemeikaite-Ceniene A, Sergediene E, Nivinskas H, Cenas N (2002) Cytotoxicity of natural hydroxyanthraquinones: role of oxidative stress. Z Naturforsch C 57:822–827

Nishikawa M, Kakemizu N, Ito T, Kudo M, Kaneko T, Suzuki M, Udaka N, Ikeda H, Okubo T (1999) Superoxide mediates cigarette smoke-induced infiltration of neutrophils into the airways through nuclear factor-kappaB activation and IL-8 mRNA expression in guinea pigs in vivo. Am J Respir Cell Mol Biol 20:189–198

Norman A (1999) Cigarette design and materials. In: Davis DL, Nielson MT (eds) Tobacco production, chemistry and technology. Blackwell, London, pp 353–97

Patterson JM, Haider NF, Chen SP, Smith WT (1976) An investigation of some factors affecting phenol production in tobacco pyrolysis. Tob Sci 20:114–116

Pedersen JA (2002) On the application of electron paramagnetic resonance in the study of naturally occurring quinones and quinols. Spectrochim Acta A 58:1257–1270

Pryor WA (1992) Biological effects of cigarette smoke, wood smoke, and the smoke from plastics: the use of electron spin resonance. Free Radic Biol Med 13:659–676

Pryor WA, Dooley MM, Church DF (1984) Inactivation of human alpha-1-proteinase inhibitor by gas-phase cigarette smoke. Biochem Biophys Res Commun 122:676–681

Pryor WA, Hales BJ, Premovic PI, Church DF (1983a) The radicals in cigarette tar: their nature and suggested physiological implications. Science 220:425–427

Pryor WA, Prier DG, Church DF (1983b) Electron-spin resonance study of mainstream and sidestream cigarette smoke: nature of the free radicals in gas-phase cigarette smoke and in cigarette tar. Environ Health Perspect 47:345–355

Pryor WA, Tamura M, Dooley MM, Premovic P, Hales BJ, Church DF (1983c) Reactive oxy-radicals from cigarette smoke and their physiological effects. In: Greenwald R, Cohen G (eds) Oxy-radicals and their scavenger systems: cellular and medical aspects. Elsevier, New York, pp 185–192

Pryor WA, Dooley MM, Church DF (1985) Mechanisms of cigarette smoke toxicity: the inactivation of human alpha-1-proteinase inhibitor by nitric oxide/isoprene mixtures in air. Chem Biol Interact 54:171–183

Pryor WA, Stone K, Zang LY, Bermudez E (1998) Fractionation of aqueous cigarette tar extracts: fractions that contain the tar radical cause DNA damage. Chem Res Toxicol 11:441–448

Purkis SW, Hill CA, Bailey IA (2003) Current measurement reliability of selected smoke analytes. Beitr Tabak Int 20:314–324

Rahman I, MacNee W (1996a) Oxidant/antioxidant imbalance in smokers and chronic obstructive pulmonary disease. Thorax 51:348–350

Rahman I, MacNee W (1996b) Role of oxidants/antioxidants in smoking-induced lung diseases. Free Radic Biol Med 21:669–681

Reddy S, Finkelstein EI, Wong PS, Phung A, Cross CE, van der Vliet A (2002) Identification of glutathione modifications by cigarette smoke. Free Radic Biol Med 33:1490–1498

Reiter CD, Teng RJ, Beckman JS (2000) Superoxide reacts with nitric oxide to nitrate tyrosine at physiological pH via peroxynitrite. J Biol Chem 275:32460–32466

Risner CH, Cash SL (1990) A high-performance liquid chromatographic determination of major phenolic compounds in tobacco smoke. J Chromatogr Sci 28:239–244

Rodriguez CE, Shinyashiki M, Froines J, Yu RC, Fukuto JM, Cho AK (2004) An examination of quinone toxicity using the yeast *Saccharomyces cerevisiae* model system. Toxicology 201:185–196

Roemer E, Stabbert R, Rustemeier K, Veltel DJ, Meisgen TJ, Reininghaus W, Carchman RA, Gaworski CL, Podraza KF (2004) Chemical composition, cytotoxicity and mutagenicity of smoke from US commercial and reference cigarettes smoked under two sets of machine smoking conditions. Toxicology 195:31–52

Roginsky VA, Barsukova TK, Stegmann HB (1999a) Kinetics of redox interaction between substituted quinones and ascorbate under aerobic conditions. Chem Biol Interact 121:177–197

Roginsky VA, Pitz M, Bors W, Michel C (1999b) The kinetics and thermodynamics of quinone-semiquinone-hydroquinone systems under physiological conditions. J Chem Soc Perkin Trans 24:871–876

Sakuma H, Matsushima S, Munakata S, Sugawara S (1982) Pyrolysis of chlorogenic acid and rutin. Agric Biol Chem 46:1311–1317

Samuni AM, Chuang EY, Krishna MC, Stein W, DeGraff W, Russo A, Mitchell JB (2003) Semiquinone radical intermediate in catecholic estrogen-mediated cytotoxicity and mutagenesis: chemoprevention strategies with antioxidants. Proc Natl Acad Sci 100:5390–5395

Schlotzhauer WS, Chortyk OT (1981) Pyrolytic studies on the origin of phenolic compounds in tobacco smoke. Tob Sci 25:6–10

Schlotzhauer WS, Chortyk OT (1987) Recent advances in studies on the pyrosynthesis of cigarette smoke constituents. J Anal Appl Pyrolysis 12:193–222

Schlotzhauer WS, Schmeltz I, Hickey LC (1967) Pyrolytic formation of phenols from some high-molecular-weight tobacco leaf constituents and related non-tobacco materials. Tob Sci 11:31–34

Schlotzhauer WS, Chortyk OT, Higman HC, Schmeltz I (1969) Pyrolytic studies on fractions sequentially extracted from tobacco. Tob Sci 13:153–155

Schlotzhauer WS, Higman EB, Schmeltz I (1972) The chemistry of tobacco and tobacco smoke. Plenum, New York

Schlotzhauer WS, Martin RM, Snook ME, Williamson RE (1982) Pyrolytic studies on the contribution of tobacco leaf constituents to the formation of smoke catechols. J Agric Food Chem 30:372–374

Schlotzhauer WS, Snook ME, Chortyk OT, Wilson RL (1992) Pyrolytic evaluation of low chlorogenic acid tobaccos in the formation of the tobacco smoke co-carcinogen catechol. J Anal Appl Pyrolysis 22:231–238

Schmeltz I, Tosk J, Jacobs G, Hoffmann D (1977) Redox potential and quinone content of cigarette smoke. Anal Chem 49:1924–1929

Seeman JI, Lipowicz PJ, Piade JJ, Poget L, Sanders EB, Snyder JP, Trowbridge CG (2004) On the deposition of volatiles and semivolatiles from cigarette smoke aerosols: relative rates of transfer of nicotine and ammonia from particles to the gas phase. Chem Res Toxicol 17:1020–1037

Seung SA, Lee JY, Lee MY, Park JS, Chung JH (1998) The relative importance of oxidative stress versus arylation in the mechanism of quinone-induced cytotoxicity to platelets. Chem Biol Interact 113:133–144

Sharma RK, Hajaligol MR, Martoglio-Smith PA, Wooten JB, Baliga VL (2000) Characterization of char from pyrolysis of chlorogenic acid. Energy Fuel 14:1083–1093

Smith CJ, Livingston SD, Doolittle DJ (1997) An international literature survey of "IARC Group I carcinogens" reported in mainstream cigarette smoke. Food Chem Toxicol 35:1107–1130

Smith CJ, Perfetti TA, Morton MJ, Rodgman A, Garg R, Selassie CD, Hansch C (2002a) The relative toxicity of substituted phenols reported in cigarette mainstream smoke. Toxicol Sci 69:265–278

Smith KR, Uyeminami DL, Kodavanti UP, Crapo JD, Chang LY, Pinkerton KE (2002b) Inhibition of tobacco smoke-induced lung inflammation by a catalytic antioxidant. Free Radic Biol Med 33:1106–1114

Spears AW, Bell JH, Saunders AO (1965) The contribution of tobacco constituents to phenol yield of cigarettes. Tob Sci 19:19–19

Spencer JP, Jenner A, Chimel K, Aruoma OI, Cross CE, Wu R, Halliwell B (1995) DNA damage in human respiratory tract epithelial cells: damage by gas phase cigarette smoke apparently involves attack by reactive nitrogen species in addition to oxygen radicals. FEBS Lett 375:179–182

Squadrito GL, Cueto R, Dellinger B, Pryor WA (2001) Quinoid redox cycling as a mechanism for sustained free radical generation by inhaled airborne particulate matter. Free Radic Biol Med 31:1132–1138

Squadrito GL, Pryor WA (1998) Oxidative chemistry of nitric oxide: the roles of superoxide, peroxynitrite, and carbon dioxide. Free Radic Biol Med 25:392–403

Stohs SJ, Bagchi D (1995) Oxidative mechanisms in the toxicity of metal ions. Free Radic Biol Med 18:321–336

Stohs SJ, Bagchi D, Bagchi M (1997) Toxicity of trace elements in tobacco smoke. Inhal Toxicol 9:867–890

Stone K, Bermudez E, Zang LY, Carter KM, Queenan KE, Pryor WA (1995) The ESR properties, DNA nicking, and DNA association of aged solutions of catechol versus aqueous extracts of tar from cigarette smoke. Arch Biochem Biophys 319:196–203

Tanigawa T, Yoshikawa T, Takahashi S, Naito Y, Kondo M (1994) Spin trapping of superoxide in aqueous solutions of fresh and aged cigarette smoke. Free Radic Biol Med 17:361–365

Torikaiu K, Uwano Y, Nakamori T, Tarora W, Takahashi H (2005) Study on tobacco components involved in the pyrolytic generation of selected smoke constituents. Food Chem Toxicol 43:559–568

Torrence KM, McDaniel RL, Self DA, Chang MJ (2002) Slurry sampling for the determination of arsenic, cadmium, and lead in mainstream cigarette smoke condensate by graphite furnace-atomic absorption spectrometry and inductively coupled plasma-mass spectrometry. Anal Bioanal Chem 372:72373

Tso TC (1990) Production, physiology and biochemistry of tobacco plants. Ideal, Beltsville, MD

Urios A, Lopez-Gresa MP, Gonzalez MC, Primo J, Martinez A, Herrera G, Escudero JC, O'Connor JE, Blanco M (2003) Nitric oxide promotes strong cytotoxicity of phenolic compounds against *Escherichia coli*: the influence of antioxidant defenses. Free Radic Biol Med 35:1373–1381

USCPSC (1993) U.S. Consumer Product Safety Commission in consultation with the U.S. Department of Health and Human Services. Toxicity testing plan 5

Waisberg M, Joseph P, Hale B, Beyersmann D (2003) Molecular and cellular mechanisms of cadmium carcinogenesis. Toxicology 192:95–117

Wardman P (1989) Reduction potentials of one-electron couples involving free radicals in aqueous solution. J Phys Chem Ref Data 18:1637–1755

Winston GW, Church DF, Cueto R, Pryor WA (1993) Oxygen consumption and oxyradical production from microsomal reduction of aqueous extracts of cigarette tar. Arch Biochem Biophys 304:371–378

Wright HE, Burton WW, Berry RC (1960) Soluble browning reaction pigments of aged Burley tobacco. I. The nondialyzable fraction. Arch Biochem Biophys 86:94–101

Wright HE, Burton WW, Berry RC (1964) Soluble browning reaction pigments of aged Burley tobacco. II. The dialysable fraction. Phytochemistry 3:525–533

Yan F, Williams S, Griffin GD, Jagannathan R, Plunkett SE, VoDinh H (2005) Near-real-time determination of hydrogen peroxide generated from cigarette smoke. J Environ Monitor 7:681–687

Yang CH, Wender SH (1962) Free phenolic acids in cigarette smoke and tobacco. Paper chromatography: separation and identification. J Chromatogr A 8:82–89

Zane A, Wender SH (1963) Pyrolysis products of rutin, quercetin, and chlorogenic acid. Tob Sci 7:21–23

Zang LY, Stone K, Pryor WA (1995) Detection of free radicals in aqueous extracts of cigarette tar by electron spin resonance. Free Radic Biol Med 19:161–167

Chapter 3

Oxidative Modifications of Proteins and Lipids by Cigarette Smoke (CS). A Central Role for Unsaturated Aldehydes in CS-Mediated Airway Inflammation

Albert van der Vliet

Contents

3.1	Introduction	48
3.2	Cigarette Smoking and Airway Inflammation	49
3.2.1	Evidence from Epidemiology and Animal Studies	49
3.2.2	The Chemical Composition of Cigarette Smoke—Particulate Phase versus Gas Phase	50
3.2.3	The Oxidative Capacity of CS—Oxidation of Proteins and Lipids	52
3.3	Cellular Effects of CS	54
3.3.1	CS and Cellular Redox Changes—Seminal Studies	54
3.3.2	Effects on Cell Signaling Pathways and Gene Expression—a Role for α,β-Unsaturated Aldehydes	56
3.4	Unsaturated Aldehydes and Mediators of CS Effects	57
3.4.1	Biological Sources—Environmental Pollutants or Products of Lipid Oxidation?	57
3.4.2	Cellular Defenses against α,β-Unsaturated Aldehydes	58
3.4.3	Effects on Inflammatory–Immune Regulation—Recent Studies	60
3.5	Future Perspectives	63
3.5.1	Strategies to Detect Biological Targets for Unsaturated Aldehydes	63
3.6	Concluding Remarks	66
	References	67

3.1 Introduction

Voluntary and involuntary cigarette smoking remains a major health concern, smoking not only being the main cause of lung cancer, but also being a major causative factor in cardiovascular diseases and chronic lung inflammatory diseases such as emphysema and asthma (Eisner et al. 1998; Schwartz et al. 2000). Although tobacco smoking is a preventable habit, exposure to tobacco smoke may have more long-lasting effects, and its consequences may be manifest long after exposure. In this regard, several clinical and epidemiological studies have indicated that prenatal tobacco smoke exposure or exposures early in life may have a significant affect on lung function, susceptibility to respiratory infection, and asthma risk (DiFranza et al. 2004; Gilliland et al. 2002; Kabesch et al. 2004). Hence, despite necessary efforts to reduce the smoking habit, the more delayed health effects of involuntary smoking can be expected to be a major and growing health issue over the next few decades. Thus, despite continued success in reducing smoking habits in most Western countries, continued research is needed to understand further the mechanistic basis underlying both acute and more chronic and protracted health effects. In particular, the long-term effects of pre- or postnatal smoke exposure require additional investigation, which may lead to improved diagnosis and management of tobacco-related health effects later in life. Determining how tobacco smoke contributes to disease and what components of tobacco smoke are primarily responsible for the adverse health effects of smoking will lead to improved mechanistic understanding of tobacco-related diseases and perhaps open new avenues for therapeutic management of patients with tobacco-related disease.

Although cigarette smoke contains thousands of toxic chemicals including many carcinogens, a wealth of evidence supports the notion that a major part of the toxicity associated with cigarette smoking is related to oxidative stress, caused by reactive oxidants and radical species in tobacco smoke itself or by secondary oxidative events that are initiated by inflammatory–immune processes that are activated by smoke exposure. It is the main purpose of the present chapter to briefly overview the oxidant chemistry of tobacco smoke and to outline the major oxidative modifications in biological targets that are induced by tobacco smoke, with special focus on interactions with biological lipids and proteins. As will be clarified in the next several sections, a large body of evidence supports the notion that a major part of the "oxidative stress" that is induced by cigarette smoke is because of the presence of unsaturated aldehyde species, rather than free radicals, within cigarette smoke. In particular, α,β-unsaturated aldehydes such as acrolein and crotonaldehyde are abundant components of cigarette smoke, and possess high reactivity toward many biological targets. Because similar aldehydes are also produced during the oxidation of biological lipids, e.g., as a result of activated inflammatory–immune processes or initiated by cigarette smoke-derived radicals, this class of molecules may contribute importantly to many of the cellular effects of cigarette smoke. For this reason, the majority of this chapter will be devoted to the biochemistry and cellular effects of this class of molecules as well as cellular defenses against these agents. Finally, some recent efforts and strategies to identify critical cellular targets for these aldehydes will be discussed, as these approaches will be instrumental in future studies aimed at determining the precise role of these agents in cellular and biological effects of cigarette smoke.

3.2 Cigarette Smoking and Airway Inflammation

3.2.1 Evidence from Epidemiology and Animal Studies

In addition to being a major cause of lung cancer (which will be discussed in other chapters in this volume, and hence not further discussed here), cigarette smoking is known to cause activation of inflammatory processes within the central airways, peripheral airways, and the lung parenchyma, even in smokers with normal lung function. Moreover, tobacco smoke exposure also results in increased or altered inflammation in patients with chronic obstructive pulmonary disease (COPD) and is a well-known contributing factor in emphysema or other forms of COPD (Rahman and MacNee 1996; Saetta 1999). Similarly, cigarette smoking is also known to contribute to allergic airway diseases such as asthma, and appears to contribute to increased inflammation with neutrophilia, which is generally associated with increased disease severity (Chalmers et al. 2001; Floreani and Rennard 1999; Rahman and MacNee 1996; Saetta 1999). The ability of environmental tobacco smoke (ETS) to promote airway inflammation has been investigated in several animal studies (Witschi et al. 1997), and ETS exposure was generally found to augment inflammatory responses that were initiated by other stimuli (other environmental pollutants or pathogens), illustrating the ability of tobacco smoke to alter inflammatory–immune processes. An example of such studies is shown in Fig. 3.1, which illustrates the occurrence of airway neutrophilia in mice on exposure to lipopolysaccharide (LPS) from *Escherichia coli*, a response that was augmented when mice were simultaneously exposed to ETS. As shown, ETS exposure markedly augmented the airway neutrophilia as well as epithelial injury (as determined by protein leak, not shown), when combined with LPS challenge, although such ETS exposure alone did not cause significant neutrophilic inflammation. These findings indicate that tobacco smoke can alter ongoing inflammatory–immune processes, which may be a contributing factor in the airway inflammation and decreased lung function in subjects with asthma or COPD.

Clearly, many factors are involved in the contributing effects of tobacco smoking to chronic airway disease, and it is well appreciated that genetic factors contribute importantly to susceptibility to allergic airway diseases such as asthma (Wills-Karp and Ewart 2004) and to the incidence of COPD in smokers, because only 15% of smokers develop COPD (Saetta 1999). Hence, the contributing effects of cigarette smoking to these disorders most likely result from a combination of the various chemical effects of smoke exposure and genetic variability in inflammatory–immune regulation and/or susceptibility to such tobacco smoke-mediated effects. Despite such complexities, it has become increasingly appreciated that the presence of elevated oxidative stress is one common denominator in the relationship between smoking and lung inflammation, asthma, and COPD (Rahman and MacNee 1996). Such oxidative stress is the result of the many reactive oxidizing components within tobacco smoke components as well as the activation of inflammatory–immune processes, and the relative contribution of these events may be difficult to dissect. Furthermore, as outlined above, cigarette smoking contributes importantly to chronic inflammation, and efforts to outline the molecular mechanisms involved in such tobacco smoke-induced inflammation have pointed to various changes in cell function, including apoptotic or necrotic cell death, altered repair following injury, and alterations in pro- or anti-inflammatory cytokine production, by either epithelial cells or by resident or recruited inflammatory–immune cells. In addition, cigarette smoke exposure is known to affect phagocytic clearance of inhaled pathogens or of apoptotic or necrotic neutrophils, and can thereby contribute to more chronic inflammation and impaired host defense. For example, it was recently demonstrated in mice that cigarette smoke exposure suppresses the ability to clear *Pseudomonas aeruginosa* infections, which results in augmented inflammation and clinical presentation (Drannik et al. 2004). As will be discussed in the following sections, many such cellular effects appear to be associated with oxidative stress, which may form the basis of the molecular mechanisms by which cigarette smoke causes such alterations.

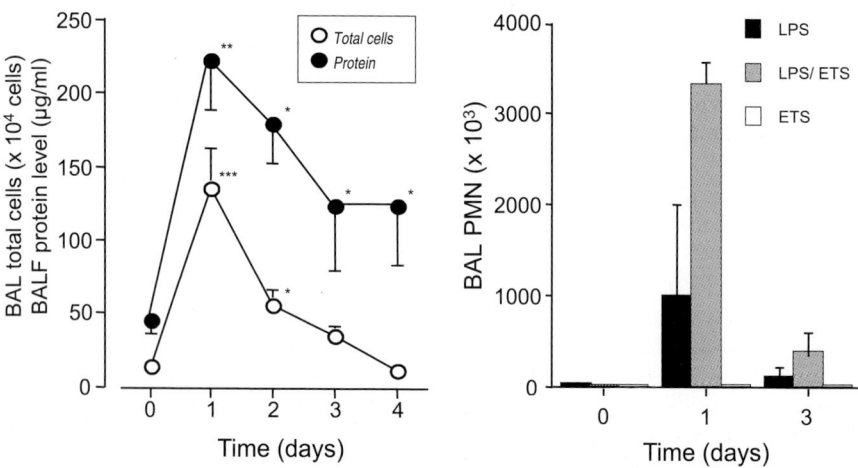

Fig. 3.1 Exposure to environmental tobacco smoke (*ETS*) promotes lipopolysaccharide (*LPS*)-induced airways neutrophilia in mice. **a** Intranasal LPS instillation induces transient airways neutrophilia. LPS (serotype 055:B5; 300 μg/kg) was instilled intranasally into C57Bl6 mice, and lungs were lavaged after 1, 2, 3, or 4 days for total cell count and protein analysis. **b** Effect of ETS on LPS induced airway inflammation. Mice were challenged with LPS as in **a**, and subsequently exposed to ETS for 6 h/day (at the Institute for Toxicology and Environmental Health at the University of California, Davis) starting 18 h after LPS challenge. ETS exposure was monitored and kept at 160 ppm CO, 10 mg/m^3 nicotine, and 50 mg/m^3 total particulate matter, and acrolein concentrations were measured using 2,4-dinitrophenylhydrazine-coated cartridges (SKC, Eighty Four, PA), and found to be 2.1 mg/m^3 (0.9 ppm). Lung lavage was performed immediately after ETS exposure on days 1 and 3 for analysis of total cell count or protein levels.

3.2.2 The Chemical Composition of Cigarette Smoke—Particulate Phase versus Gas Phase

Perhaps the main reason why our understanding of tobacco-related disease is still rather limited is the extremely complex chemical composition of cigarette smoke, which varies depending on smoking habits, the type of tobacco used, and differences between mainstream and sidestream smoke. Moreover, because many components in cigarette smoke (CS) are short-lived and undergo complex chemical reactions, the chemical composition changes substantially during aging within the ambient environment. Physically, CS can be divided into a particulate tar phase (approximately 10^{12} particles per cigarette) and a gas (or vapor) phase, which comprises all components that can pass through a glass-fiber filter that removes >99% of particles greater than 0.1 μm in diameter (Church and

Pryor 1985; see also Chapter 2). The tar phase of CS contains primarily hydrophilic and nonvolatile components, including water, alkaloids (nicotine), phenols, and traces of various aromatic hydrocarbons, nitrogenous aromatics, nitrosamines, etc. The tar phase can be collected on a filter that traps particulate matter or by low-temperature condensation to produce cigarette smoke condensate (CSC). Studies using electron spin resonance (ESR) have demonstrated that the tar phase contains several relatively stable radicals that can form an active redox system capable of reducing O_2 to generate superoxide ($O_2^-\cdot$), hydrogen peroxide (H_2O_2), and other reactive oxygen species (Church and Pryor 1985; Zang et al. 1995). The gas phase of CS contains high concentrations of inorganic gases (O_2, N_2, CO, NO, HCN, H_2S, NH_3) as well as various alkanes, alkenes, alcohols, and saturated and unsaturated aldehydes, as volatile products of organic combustion. Usually, the lower homologs of these different classes of products predominate in abundance. In addition, gas-phase CS represents a source of organic and oxygen free radicals, which are most likely generated by autooxidation of the high levels of nitric oxide (NO·) within CS to the much more oxidizing nitrogen dioxide ($NO_2\cdot$) (Cueto and Pryor 1994; Norman and Keith 1965). Hence, both CS tar-phase components as well as the gas phase may be an important source of oxidative stress associated with smoke exposure.

It is clear from the above that CS contains many oxidizing components, in either the gas phase or the particulate (tar) phase. Elucidating the contribution of such oxidizing components within CS to its various biological or cellular effects has been significantly complicated by the various experimental approaches that have been used to study CS-related effects. Whereas some investigators use fresh whole or filtered CS in their studies, it has been a more common practice to expose cultured cells to extracts of CS, obtained after bubbling smoke through an aqueous solution, or to CSC (see above). Such approaches have obvious practical advantages, as they allow more accurate dose-response studies and increase reproducibility. In addition, these approaches could also be rationalized as reflecting the CS components that may dissolve or condense at the respiratory tract surface (i.e., in lung lining fluids) and are capable of directly targeting airway epithelial cells. A main problem with such approaches, however, is the fact that they are poorly standardized, which has made comparisons between different studies using CS extracts or CSC difficult. In addition, and perhaps more importantly, many volatile CS components are lost during the collection of CS extracts and/or CSC, leading to underappreciation of the potential role(s) of such volatile components in the cellular effects of CS. Even though many of the carcinogenic components of CS (e.g., those causing DNA nicking and mutations) may be successfully collected in CSC, it has been appreciated for many years that volatile components within CS may be primarily responsible for CS-induced alterations in lung cell function (Leuchtenberger et al. 1974). Overall, it should be stressed that any model of exposing cultured cells or laboratory animals to CS is associated with some trade-offs (Rennard 2004). However, a growing number of studies demonstrated the important contributions of volatile constituents of CS in cellular dysfunction or oxidative stress, some of which may be successfully collected when fresh CS extracts are prepared (even though a significant fraction is most likely lost). As will be outlined in the next several sections, gas-phase CS components (such as the α,β-unsaturated aldehydes acrolein and crotonaldehyde) play an important role in the oxidative stress that is induced by cigarette smoke exposure. Hence, the remainder of this chapter will be primarily centered on the role of gas-phase constituents (with special emphasis on unsaturated aldehydes) in CS toxicity, although it is important not to trivialize the contribution of other CS constituents in the carcinogenic or mutagenic properties of CS.

3.2.3 The Oxidative Capacity of CS— Oxidation of Proteins and Lipids

The respiratory tract surface and the epithelial lining fluids represent the first biological targets of inhaled CS. Therefore, in an attempt to characterize the oxidative modifications that may occur within lung surface fluids as well as the local antioxidant defenses within such fluids, several studies have been performed in which blood plasma was exposed to CS, as a model biological fluid with comparable composition. These studies have indicated that exposure of gas-phase (filtered) CS readily depletes plasma levels of antioxidant micronutrients (primarily ascorbate) and that products of lipid peroxidation (lipid hydroperoxides, conjugated dienes) can be detected as soon as ascorbate pools are depleted (Frei 1991). Supplementation of ascorbate was furthermore capable of delaying lipid oxidation by CS, indicating the involvement of oxidizing free radicals. Although many CS-derived radicals could potentially be responsible for the oxidation of ascorbate and initiation of lipid oxidation, subsequent studies have illustrated that the major factor involved in such oxidation is the formation of $NO_2\cdot$ by autooxidation of $NO\cdot$, based on similar rates of ascorbate depletion by comparable concentrations of $NO\cdot$, and a critical dependence on the presence of molecular O_2 (Eiserich et al. 1997). Indeed, several studies indicated that $NO_2\cdot$ is a strong oxidant capable of initiating lipid oxidation (Eiserich et al. 1997). The associations between CS, lipid oxidation, and antioxidant (ascorbate) status have also been confirmed in measurements in smokers, which are found to contain elevated plasma levels of stable lipid oxidation products such as F_2-isoprostanes (Morrow et al. 1995) as well as reduced plasma ascorbate levels (Lykkesfeldt et al. 2000), compared with nonsmoking subjects. Moreover, supplementation with ascorbate appeared to decrease the plasma levels of F_2-isoprostanes in passive smokers (Dietrich et al. 2003).

Using similar studies with isolated blood plasma or with buffered solutions of purified proteins, exposure to CS was also found to cause oxidative modifications in proteins, as illustrated by decreases in protein reduced thiol (-SH) levels, and increased markers of protein oxidation, including protein carbonyls and the tyrosine oxidation products dityrosine and 3-nitrotyrosine (Eiserich et al. 1994; Reznick et al. 1992). The formation of tyrosine oxidation and nitration products by CS most likely involves the intermediate formation of $NO_2\cdot$ (Eiserich et al. 1994), and could be prevented by supplementation with ascorbate. In contrast, thiol depletion and protein carbonyl formation were not altered by supplementation with ascorbate or metal chelators (in an attempt to prevent radical-mediated oxidation), illustrating that these modifications are not because of radical-mediated oxidation, but rather caused by nonradical constituents in CS. As illustrated in Table 3.1, gas-phase CS contains high concentrations of reactive nonradical components, including unsaturated aldehydes such as acrolein and crotonaldehyde, that could conceivably react with nucleophilic targets such as thiols. Indeed, as will be discussed in more detail in subsequent sections, these aldehydes readily react with nucleophilic amino acid residues (including cysteine thiols) by Michael addition, resulting in protein carbonyl adducts, and comparative studies indicated that the depletion of protein-thiol and the formation of protein carbonyls by CS could be accounted for by the major reactive aldehydes within CS (Eiserich et al. 1995; Reznick et al. 1992).

Despite these rather convincing studies, some controversies still remain. First, although protein carbonyl adduct formation by gas-phase CS may be largely independent of radical chemistry and is caused by alkylation by unsaturated aldehydes (Reznick et

Table 3.1 Major Components of Gas-Phase Cigarette Smoke

Component	μmol/cigarette
Inorganic gases	
Carbon dioxide (CO_2)	1,500
Carbon monoxide (CO)	570
Nitric oxide (NO·)	12
Hydrogen cyanide (HCN)	10
Ammonia (NH_3)	6
Nitrogen dioxide (NO_2·)	1
Alkanes, alkenes, etc.	
Methane	50
Isoprene	6
Methanol	6
Acetonitrile	3
Toluene	0.9
Aldehydes	
Acetaldehyde	20
Formaldehyde	2
Acetone	6
Acrolein	0.8
Crotonaldehyde	0.2
Organic radicals	
Alkyl, alkoxyl, peroxyl	0.02

Data from Eiserich et al. (1997) and Norman (1977) and references therein

al. 1992), more recent studies have also described protein carbonyl formation by CS tar-phase components that was preventable by ascorbate (Panda et al. 2001), pointing to differences in oxidative mechanisms between gas-phase and tar-phase CS. Secondly, the relative importance of oxidizing free radicals within gas-phase CS has been questioned, based on a lack of success in detecting oxidizing radicals within fresh CS using ESR (Maranzana and Mehlhorn 1998). Furthermore, studies with erythrocytes demonstrated that exposure to gas-phase CS depleted cell glutahione (GSH) levels more rapidly than ascorbate, and that depletion of GSH diminished the ability of erythrocytes to recycle oxidized ascorbate (Maranzana and Mehlhorn 1998). Thus, direct thiol modifications by CS may be kinetically favored and therefore more important than are free radical-mediated oxidations. This notion is supported by studies towards oxidation of plasma constituents: Whereas CS-mediated oxidation of ascorbate or tyrosine occurred rather slowly over several minutes, as they required NO_2· formation by autooxidative reactions (Cueto and Pryor 1994; Eiserich et al. 1997; Eiserich et al. 1994), thiol depletion by unsaturated aldehydes in CS occurs much more rapidly (Eiserich et al. 1995; Esterbauer et al. 1991).

The chemical modifications of GSH by gas-phase CS were recently investigated using high-performance liquid chromatography (HPLC) and mass spectrometry (MS) approaches, which confirmed that (radical-mediated) oxidation to oxidized GSH (GSSG) occurred to a relatively minor extent, whereas the majority of GSH depletion could be accounted for by alkylation by the major CS-derived unsaturated aldehydes, acrolein and crotonaldehyde (Reddy et al. 2002). In fact, about 50% of the GSH that was depleted by CS could be accounted for its addition to one single aldehyde, acrolein (Reddy et al. 2002). Studies in which various isolated cells were exposed to CS are consistent with this: CS-mediated depletion of GSH occurs largely by alkylation and not by oxidation to GGSG or mixed disulfides (Rahman and MacNee 1996; Reddy et al. 2002), and formation of protein carbonyls is largely the result of Michael addition of aldehydes (Nguyen et al. 2001). Increased carbonyl levels have also been detected in various circulating proteins in smokers as compared with nonsmokers (Lee et al. 1998; Pignatelli et al. 2001), possibly as a result of similar Michael addition. However, markers of free radical-mediated protein oxidation, such as 3-nitrotyrosine, were also found to be increased in smokers (Petruzzelli et al. 1997), illustrating that radical-mediated processes also contribute to increased protein oxidation in smokers. Determination of chemical mechanisms involved in such protein modifications in vivo is more difficult, because they may have been due to indirect oxidative events caused by increased activation of inflammatory processes, rather than direct CS-mediated oxidation. Similarly, the increased presence of lipid oxidation products in smokers (Dietrich et al. 2003; Morrow et al. 1995) may be because of both direct CS-mediated effects and by oxidative processes because of activation of inflammatory/immune cells (Zhang et al. 2002a, b). Conversely, the process of lipid oxidation results in the formation of a range of α,β-unsaturated aldehydes that can alkylate thiols and modify proteins in a manner similar to CS-derived aldehydes. Figure 3.2 illustrates the structural similarities between acrolein and crotonaldehyde (major α,β-unsaturated aldehydes in CS) and malondialdehyde and 4-hydroxy-nonenal (major products of lipid peroxidation). Importantly, acrolein and crotonaldehyde have recently been identified as additional products of lipid oxidation (Uchida 1999).

In summary, alkylations of biological thiols (GSH, protein cysteine residues) by aldehydes appear to be major "oxidative" effects of gas-phase CS. Similarly, as will be discussed in the next paragraph, cellular effects of CS appear to be related to alterations in cellular redox status because of the action of CS-derived unsaturated aldehydes rather than free radicals, most likely because these aldehydes are readily diffusible and capable of entering cells and reacting with many cell targets. Therefore, the biological effects of CS are expected to be because of modifications of critical cell components by unsaturated aldehydes, and by alterations in cellular defenses against these aldehydes, which will be the subject of subsequent sections.

3.3 Cellular Effects of CS

3.3.1 CS and Cellular Redox Changes—Seminal Studies

In seminal observations over 30 years ago, Green (Green 1968) and Leuchtenberger et al. (Leuchtenberger et al. 1974) discovered that adverse effects of CS on alveolar macrophage function or on lung cell alterations could be prevented by reducing agents such as GSH or cysteine, and that volatile CS constituents were primarily responsible for such

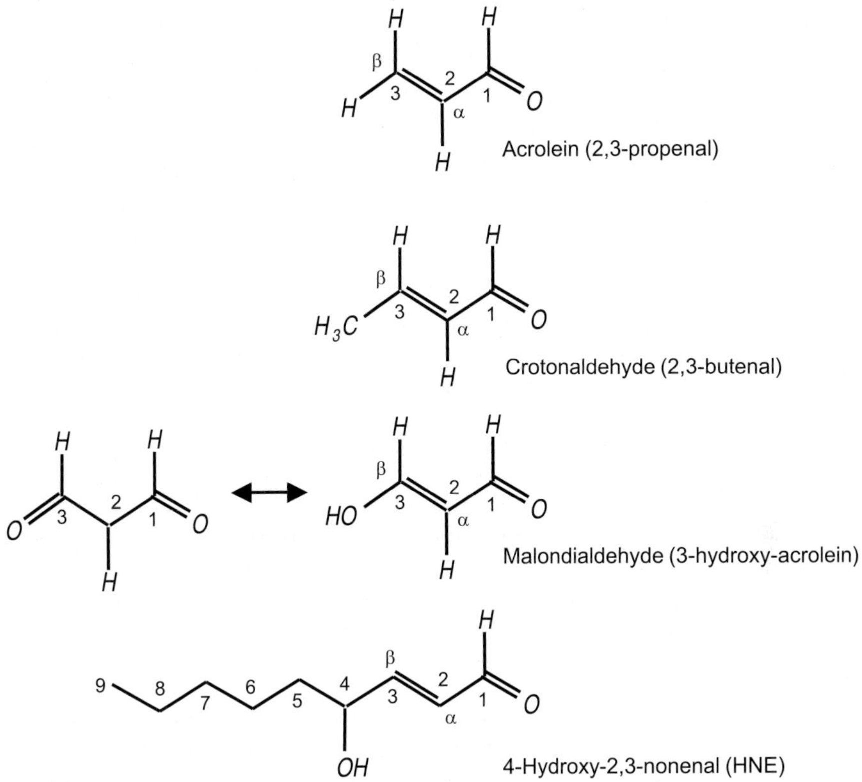

Fig. 3.2 Structures of α,β-unsaturated aldehydes that are present in cigarette smoke (CS) or are formed during lipid peroxidation

effects. In subsequent years, many studies have reported that CS is capable of inducing growth arrest or apoptotic or necrotic cell death (Carnevali et al. 2003; Hoshino et al. 2001; Kim et al. 2004; Rahman and MacNee 1999; Tsuji et al. 2004; Wickenden et al. 2003), or impairing epithelial or phagocytic cell function (Kirkham et al. 2004; Martey et al. 2004; Mio et al. 1997; Nguyen et al. 2001; Wang et al. 2001). In most of these cases, CS effects were related to depletion of cellular GSH and could be countered by reducing agents such as GSH or N-acetylcysteine, leading to the general conclusion that oxidative stress generated by CS exposure is responsible for these effects. Several more recent studies have addressed the ability of CS to alter gene expression, in cultured airway epithelial cells or in lung biopsies from current or ex-smokers, and such studies have revealed reversible upregulation of genes that are involved in oxidative stress, GSH metabolism, xenobiotic metabolism, as well as more persistent changes in several putative oncogenes or tumor suppressor genes (Hackett et al. 2003; Spira et al. 2004; Yoneda et al. 2001). Changes in drug metabolizing and antioxidant genes largely involved genes involved in GSH metabolism (GSH peroxidases, glutamate–cysteine ligase, GSSG reductase, GSH S-transferases), redox balance (alcohol dehydrogenases, aldo-keto reductases, thioredoxin-related genes) or pentose phosphate cycle, suggesting that many of the cellular effects may be related to alterations in cellular redox status or changes in GSH-dependent drug metabolism (Hackett et al. 2003).

3.3.2 Effects on Cell Signaling Pathways and Gene Expression—a Role for α,β-Unsaturated Aldehydes

As discussed in the previous section, the major thiol reactive agents within gas-phase CS are α,β-unsaturated aldehydes, of which acrolein and crotonaldehyde are the main members. Hence, these aldehydes can be expected to contribute greatly to the cellular effects of CS, either by altering cellular redox balance by depleting GSH pools or by direct reaction with redox-sensitive targets in proteins or DNA. Indeed, an increasing number of studies have addressed the cellular effects of such aldehydes (as well as similar aldehydes that are generated during lipid oxidation, such as 4-hydroxynonenal) (Esterbauer et al. 1991; Kehrer and Biswal 2000; Leonarduzzi et al. 2000; Li and Holian 1998), and several such studies have documented that these aldehydes can largely mimic the various cellular effects of CS (Hoshino et al. 2001; Mio et al. 1997; Nguyen et al. 2001; Wang et al. 2001). CSCs or extracts have been found to be capable of activating stress responses in cells, resulting in the activation of extracellular regulated kinase-1/2 (ERK) or p38 mitogen-activated protein kinase (MAPK), and of the transcription factor nuclear factor-kappaB (NF-κB), and these responses are associated with induction of stress response genes (*fos*, heme oxygenase) and inflammatory genes such as interleukin (IL)-8, cyclooxygenase-2 or matrix metalloproteinase-1 (Anto et al. 2002; Martey et al. 2004; Mercer et al. 2004; Muller and Gebel 1998). Again, these effects were found to be largely related to GSH depletion and could in part be attributed to CS-derived aldehydes (Finkelstein et al. 2001; Kehrer and Biswal 2000; Mio et al. 1997; Muller and Gebel 1998). In addition to depleting cellular GSH, acrolein readily inactivates thioredoxin and thioredoxin reductase (Park et al. 2005; Yang et al. 2004), thus potentially affecting cell signaling pathways that are controlled by this redox system. We have demonstrated that CS and acrolein are able to induce tyrosine phosphorylation and p38 MAPK activation in neutrophils, and that p38 MAPK activation is related to functional outcomes such as IL-8 production (Finkelstein et al. 2001). It is important to note that acrolein does not always fully replicate the effects of CS, consistent with some studies that suggest that CS aldehydes may synergize with other CS components (including oxidants) to induce their overall effects (Muller and Gebel 1998). Despite rather consistent reports on the ability of CS to activate MAP kinases, the effects on NF-κB are more controversial, because some studies also demonstrated inhibition of (cytokine-mediated) NF-κB activation by CS (Gebel and Muller 2001; Moodie et al. 2004). These apparent discrepancies may be because of variations between CS preparations used, which may have resulted in variable outcomes because of opposing effects of different CS components. Indeed, whereas certain CS components within CS extracts may activate NF-κB, the volatile component acrolein was found to inhibit NF-κB activation, either by upregulation of the inhibitor IκB or by direct chemical modifications of redox-sensitive proteins involved in NF-κB activation (Kehrer and Biswal 2000; Valacchi et al. 2005) (see next paragraph).

Studies with cultured cells or lung biopsies from smokers have shown that CS exposure induces many changes in gene expression, largely involving those encoding oxidative stress-responsive and phase II drug-metabolizing enzymes (Gebel et al. 2004; Hackett et al. 2003; Spira et al. 2004), which are all (at least in part) transcriptionally regulated by the nuclear factor Nrf2 (NF-E2-related factor) (Gebel et al. 2004). Indeed, acrolein and other unsaturated aldehydes are known activators of Nrf2, presumably by direct chemical modification of the Kelch-like ECH-associating protein 1 (Keap1) sensor, which represses Nrf2 activity (Itoh et al. 2004; Kwak et al. 2003; Levonen et al. 2004; Tirumalai et al. 2002; Wakabayashi et al. 2004). Recently, genetic ablation of Nrf2 in mice was found to enhance susceptibility to cigarette smoke-induced emphysema (Rangasamy et al. 2004), consistent with an important role for oxidative stress, and perhaps aldehyde stress, in the development of this CS-related disorder. One specific consequence of CS exposure to airway epithelial cells is the overproduction of mucin through activation of epidermal growth factor receptors (EGFR) (Shao et al. 2004; Takeyama et al. 2001), and this may contribute to the prominent feature of goblet cell hyperplasia and mucus hypersecretion that is seen in COPD. More-recent studies have suggested that CS-derived aldehydes may be involved in this response, as acrolein has been shown to be able to activate EGFR and to induce expression of mucin genes (Borchers et al. 1999; Deshmukh et al. 2005; Takeuchi et al. 2001). Moreover, such acrolein-induced effects appear to occur in the absence of major cellular redox changes, and appear to be mediated largely by cell surface events such as the activation of cellular metalloproteinases (Deshmukh et al. 2005; Shao et al. 2004). Collectively, these various observations clearly point to an important role for unsaturated aldehydes in overall cellular effects by CS that are thought to contribute to the etiology of CS-related diseases. Therefore, the remainder of this chapter will focus specifically on the biochemistry of these aldehydes.

3.4 Unsaturated Aldehydes and Mediators of CS Effects

3.4.1 Biological Sources—Environmental Pollutants or Products of Lipid Oxidation?

Although the previous section strongly supports a contributing role for unsaturated aldehydes in many of the cellular effects of CS, it is difficult to elucidate their role in vivo without better knowledge regarding the actual doses or concentrations of these aldehydes that reach target cells. Indeed, studies in vitro have shown a wide range of cellular effects of these aldehydes, depending on concentrations that were used, but it is unclear which experimental conditions most accurately resemble in vivo conditions of aldehyde exposure or production. For instance, whereas concentrations of acrolein in mainstream or environmental tobacco smoke can be measured relatively easily, it is much more difficult to determine concentrations that will be encountered within the airways of smokers or of subjects exposed to environmental tobacco smoke. Such determinations are compromised by complications in sampling of specific lung areas, and the reactivity of acrolein with various biological targets, that would result in dramatically underestimating the overall acrolein burden in the lung when based on measurements of unreacted acrolein. Some recent studies documented concentrations of major CS aldehydes (acetaldehyde, acrolein, etc.) in saliva specimens or in exhaled breath condensates (EBC) from nonsmokers and smokers, using chemical derivatization and capillary electrophoresis and/or LC-MS procedures (Andreoli et al. 2003; Annovazzi et al. 2004). These recent findings suggest that acrolein, the main reactive unsaturated aldehyde, can be found in micromolar concentrations in saliva and nanomolar levels in EBC (which, based on dilution associated with EBC collection, corresponds to micromolar levels in lung surface fluids), and were typically several-fold higher in smokers (Andreoli et al. 2003; Annovazzi et al. 2004). As will be discussed in more detail in the next section, such concentrations of these aldehydes can profoundly affect cell function. More intriguingly, increases in acrolein within EBC of smokers were associated with similar increases in 4-hydroxynonenal and malondialdehyde, well-known end products of lipid oxidation (see Fig. 3.2). Because acrolein and crotonaldehyde are not only major components of CS, but can also be produced during oxidation of various lipids (Uchida 1999), these measurements in EBC suggest that the increased acrolein in smokers may originate from increased lipid peroxidation rather than reflect inhaled acrolein from CS itself. Indeed, recent analysis of various lipid oxidation products in exhaled breath condensates and induced sputum from subjects with COPD or asthma revealed comparable increases in lipid oxidation products including acrolein (Corradi et al. 2004). Because the majority of subjects in this latter study were nonsmokers or ex-smokers, the increased acrolein most likely originated from lipid oxidation rather than inhalation of CS.

The above considerations point to another level of complexity with regard to CS-related disease. First, it is apparent that the biological effects of CS may be mediated not only by the abundant reactive aldehydes within CS, but also by the same aldehydes that are generated on lipid peroxidation, because of the activation of inflammatory–immune processes. Moreover, oxidation of unsaturated fatty acids results in the formation of a variety of similar unsaturated aldehydes, of which 4-hydroxynonenal has received the most attention as a major lipid oxidation product with potential functions as a second messenger molecule (Petersen and Doorn 2004). The similarities in reactivity between the various α,β-unsaturated aldehydes suggest that their cellular effects may in fact represent more general responses to a larger family of aldehydes, although their cellular effects may differ and be more specific because of differences in carbon chain length and other functional groups, that may contribute to specificity in target interactions. For reasons of simplicity, and because it represents the major and most reactive α,β-unsaturated aldehyde in CS, the following paragraphs will deal primarily with acrolein, although many aspects may also apply to other α,β-unsaturated aldehyde family members.

3.4.2 Cellular Defenses against α,β-Unsaturated Aldehydes

As discussed in the previous sections, α,β-unsaturated aldehydes are among the main components within CS that may be responsible for its effects on cellular function and are also produced during lipid oxidation, a process that is commonly observed in smokers and may involve reactive components of CS itself, as well as the activation of oxidative pathways as a result of inflammatory–immune processes. For these reasons, many studies have addressed the ability of members of this aldehyde family to activate cell signaling pathways, alter gene expression, and/or cell function (Finkelstein et al. 2001; Kehrer and Biswal 2000; Li and Holian 1998; Petersen and Doorn 2004). The α,β-unsaturated aldehydes comprise a family of compounds that are reactive towards many classes of biomolecules, and both the aldehyde group as well as the unsaturated bond, which gives these compounds their strong electrophilic character, are involved in their reactivity. Hence, various metabolic pathways exist to minimize cell exposure to such aldehydes, and/or their unwanted reaction with critical cell targets (Petersen and Doorn 2004). Figure 3.3 illustrates the several metabolic pathways involved in detoxification of α,β-unsaturated aldehydes such as acrolein. A first class of metabolic enzymes that detoxify aldehydes are the aldehyde dehydrogenases (ALDH), a large family of enzymes that catalyze the pyridine nucleotide-dependent oxidation of aldehydes to the corresponding acids (Sladek 2003). Conversely, aldehydes can also be detoxified by enzymatic reduction of the aldehyde to the corresponding alcohol, by members of the aldo-keto reductase family (AKR), aldose reductase (AR) and/or alcohol dehydrogenase (ADH) (Niknahad et al. 2003; Sanli et al. 2003; Srivastava et al. 1999). Intriguingly, whereas short-chain aldehydes such as acrolein are relatively poor substrates for reduction by AR, its adduct with GSH, formed by spontaneous or glutathione S-transferase (GST) catalyzed conjugation with GSH (see below), is reduced with much higher efficiency by AR (Srivastava et al. 1999), and induction of AR activity has been found to enhance cellular resistance to acrolein (Keightley et al. 2004).

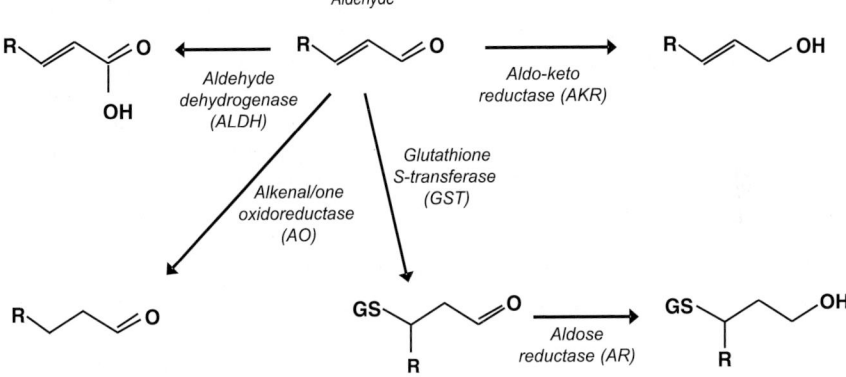

Fig. 3.3 Schematic representation of metabolic pathways in cellular detoxification of α,β-unsaturated aldehydes

Because the unsaturated bond is considered the most reactive moiety within α,β-unsaturated aldehydes, the main detoxification route presumably involves their reduction or conjugation with GSH, the latter catalyzed by a family of GSH S-transferases (Berhane et al. 1994; Hubatsch et al. 1998; Pal et al. 2000). Whereas GST P1-1 is most effective against propenals, including acrolein, GST A1-1 and GST M1-1 are more active against hydroxyalkenals, which are produced during lipid peroxidation (Berhane et al. 1994; Pal et al. 2000). GST A4-4, a member of the alpha class GST family, was found to have particularly high activity against 4-hydroxynonenal and other similar lipid oxidation products (Hubatsch et al. 1998). Inhibition of GST activity increases acrolein toxicity, whereas GST induction can protect cells from acrolein toxicity, illustrating the significance of GST-mediated aldehyde detoxification (Cao et al. 2003; He et al. 1998). Recently, an additional enzyme was identified in the detoxification of α,β-unsaturated aldehydes, known as NAD(P)H-dependent alkenal/one oxidoreductase (Dick and Kensler 2004; Dick et al. 2001). This enzyme was initially discovered as a dithiolthione-inducible gene (*DIG-1*), a homolog of an inactivator of leukotriene B$_4$, and a recently identified enzyme in pig lung that reduces the 13,14 double bond of 15-oxoprostaglandins was found to be virtually identical (Dick et al. 2001; Ensor et al. 1998). Kinetic analysis revealed that this alkenal/one oxidoreductase (AO) may contribute importantly to the detoxification of α,β-unsaturated aldehydes such as acrolein and hydroxynonenal, and that overexpression of AO reduces hydroxynonenal-induced cell toxicity and Michael addition to proteins (Dick et al. 2001).

Although GSTs appear to be most important in detoxifying unsaturated aldehydes, the significance of aldehyde reduction by AR (Keightley et al. 2004) or elimination of their GSH adducts by multidrug resistance protein (Renes et al. 2000), indicates that addition of GSH to these aldehydes does not fully eliminate their toxicity (Ramu et al. 1996). The importance of GSTs in tobacco-related diseases has been illustrated by several reports of increased disease incidence or decreased lung function associated with genetic GST variants (He et al. 2004). Several GST polymorphisms have been identified, including a *GST M1* null allele, which results in a complete lack of GST M1 activity. A similar null allele also exists for *GST T1*. Several studies have indicated that *GST M1*-null or *GST T1*-null children have increased risk for asthma in relation to environmental tobacco smoke or maternal smoking (Gilliland et al. 2002; Kabesch et al. 2004). Moreover, the *GST M1*-null genotype has also been associated with emphysema (Harrison et al. 1997). Finally, a polymorphism in *GST P1* leads to a 105Ile/Val substitution, which affects catalytic activity against substrates including acrolein (Pal et al. 2000), and has been associated with chronic obstructive pulmonary disease in a Japanese population (Ishii et al. 1999). Collectively, these associations with genetic GST variants may further underscore the potential contribution of unsaturated aldehydes to CS-related disorders.

3.4.3 Effects on Inflammatory–Immune Regulation—Recent Studies

Although many CS constituents are capable of reaching the circulation and thereby contribute to more systemic effects, inhaled (environmental) tobacco smoke will primarily interact with cells at the respiratory surface, which include largely airway and alveolar epithelial cells, as well as alveolar macrophages and extravasated inflammatory–immune cells such as neutrophils, during active episodes of acute or chronic inflammation. Based on geometric considerations, the airway epithelium is the major target for inhaled pollutants such as CS, as it covers the entire surface area of the lung, which in adults resembles the size of a tennis court. Recent studies have clearly established that the airway epithelium may be a main effector in mounting inflammatory responses to inhaled pathogens or allergens (Poynter et al. 2003; Sadikot et al. 2003). Similarly, the epithelium is also thought to be involved in the proinflammatory effects of CS exposure, as reflected by increased neutrophilia and enhanced production of the major neutrophil chemoattractant IL-8, a member of the CXC chemokine family (Chalmers et al. 2001; Mio et al. 1997). Indeed, exposure of cultured respiratory tract epithelial cells to CS extracts was found to cause increased production of IL-8, and increased IL-8 production was also observed on epithelial cell exposure to major aldehyde components in CS, acetaldehyde and acrolein (Mio et al. 1997). Epithelial IL-8 expression is regulated by both transcriptional and posttranscriptional mechanisms (Li et al. 2002), involving the activation of MAP kinases and the transcription factor NF-κB, a main regulator of epithelial cytokine and chemokine expression (Poynter et al. 2003). Recent studies have, however, also shown that α,β-unsaturated aldehydes are capable of inhibiting NF-κB activation, and we recently demonstrated that acrolein at low-micromolar concentrations can inhibit epithelial IL-8 expression by inhibiting NF-κB activation (Valacchi et al. 2005). Similarly, acrolein was also found to inhibit NF-κB activation in macrophages (Li et al. 1999). In this regard, the action of acrolein on NF-κB signaling is analogous to those of structurally analogous α,β-unsaturated carbonyl compounds, such as 4-hydroxynonenal or cyclopentenone prostaglandins (Ji et al. 2001b; Valacchi et al. 2005).

Although the involvement of unsaturated aldehydes on CS-induced proinflammatory signaling is not straightforward, several lines of evidence suggest that they may represent major causative factors in inducing epithelial oxidative injury and apoptotic or necrotic cell death (Hoshino et al. 2001; Rahman and MacNee 1999; Wickenden et al. 2003). Investigations of acrolein-mediated cell death in cultured bronchial epithelial cells revealed the activation of a process reminiscent of apoptosis, as illustrated by DNA fragmentation and phosphatidylserine externalization (Nardini et al. 2002), although this mode of cell death was not accompanied by caspase activation (not shown). Moreover, whereas cell death by acrolein was closely associated with transient GSH depletion, cell supplementation with either ascorbate or α-tocopherol appeared to prevent acrolein-induced cell death and promote restoration of cellular GSH pools, even though initial GSH depletion could not be prevented (Nardini et al. 2002). Accordingly, increases in cellular oxidant production could be observed following acrolein exposure, illustrating secondary oxidative stress that may be responsible for epithelial cell death. Despite the absence of NF-κB activation and proinflammatory cytokine production under these conditions (Valacchi et al. 2005), such acrolein-induced cell death could conceivably release "danger" signals that can activate antigen-presenting cells and thereby contribute to the initiation of immune responses (Gallucci et al. 1999; Shi et al. 2003). Whether acrolein indeed contributes to increase risk of allergic airway diseases, as has been demonstrated in relation to pre- or postnatal CS exposure, still remains to be established.

From the above, it is clear that the proinflammatory effects of tobacco smoke cannot be easily explained by individual activities of bioactive components on individual cell types, as they most likely involve a combination of effects of its many diverse components on various lung cell types. The studies illustrated in Fig. 3.1 indicate that ETS exposure augments neutrophilia induced by other stimuli, even though it did not induce significant inflammation by itself. Such stimulatory effects on preexisting inflammation suggest that inhaled tobacco smoke may act in part by altering the biological properties of extravasated inflammatory cells such as neutrophils. We and others have studied the effects of CS and/or acrolein on various critical neutrophil activities, such as respiratory burst activation, cytokine production, and apoptotic cell death, the latter being a critical factor in the resolution of inflammation (Fadok et al. 1998; Savill 1997). Initial studies of neutrophil respiratory burst activation indicated that CS (and acrolein) dramatically inhibit this important neutrophil activity in host defense (Nguyen et al. 2001), which suggest a causative mechanism by which CS exposure may diminish host defense and contribute to enhanced respiratory childhood infections (DiFranza et al. 2004; Li and Holian 1998). Also, a decreased ability to clear respiratory infection will contribute to increased and more chronic proinflammatory conditions. Further studies in our laboratory have indicated that neutrophil exposure to acrolein results in increased production of IL-8, by a mechanism involving p38 MAPK activation (Finkelstein et al. 2001). Thus, the observed increases in respiratory tract levels of IL-8 in smokers (Chalmers et al. 2001; Mio et al. 1997) may originate (at least in part) from increased production by extravasated neutrophils.

Although much emphasis has been given to cellular mechanisms by which CS may affect processes that result in the activation of inflammation and inflammatory cell recruitment, it is increasingly recognized that the process of inflammation is also critically regulated by mechanisms that control inflammatory cell clearance in order to terminate inflammatory processes. The overall state of inflammation can, in fact, be envisioned as a balance between activating mechanisms that recruit inflammatory cells and processes that eliminate inflammatory cells. Apoptotic cell death, regulated by constitutively expressed pathways and by pro- and anti-inflammatory cytokines, is a critical step in terminating the inflammatory response and removing inflammatory cells from the inflamed site. The molecular events that are involved in neutrophil apoptosis and clearance mechanisms of apoptotic cells have been actively studied in recent years and have been comprehensively reviewed (Haslett 1999; Lauber et al. 2004; Maderna and Godson 2003). Many studies have attempted to address the involvement of CS components such as aldehydes in apoptotic or necrotic cell death in various cell types (Haynes et al. 2001; Ji et al. 2001a; Li et al. 1997; Nardini et al. 2002), and concluded that acrolein and other unsaturated aldehydes induce apoptotic cell death. Studies with freshly isolated neutrophils, however, showed the surprising finding that exposure to micromolar concentrations of acrolein actually blocks the constitutive apoptotic pathway in neutrophils and appears to extend their lifespan (Finkelstein et al. 2001). Further mechanistic studies indicated that these effects are closely associated with dramatic changes in cellular GSH status, which were found to correspond with decreased activation of caspases-3, -8, and -9, critical mediators of both intrinsic and extrinsic apoptotic pathways (Finkelstein et al. 2005). Preliminary studies indicate that such inhibition of neutrophil apoptosis also results in reduced phagocytosis by monocyte-derived macrophages (Finkelstein and van der Vliet, unpublished observations). The significance of such inhibitory effects on neutrophil apoptosis for overall CS-related inflammation is still unclear, but may be profound based on recent studies indicating anti-inflammatory signals that are produced as a result of phagocytic clearance of apoptotic cells (Huynh et al. 2002). Conversely, failure to clear apoptotic or necrotic neutrophils can be expected to result in increased deposition of toxic granule proteins that are released from disintegrating cells, which would contribute to proinflammatory conditions (Haslett 1999). In addition to altering neutrophil apoptosis and potentially interfering with their removal, CS and acrolein have also been demonstrated to decrease the phagocytic capacity of alveolar macrophages (Green 1968; Kirkham et al. 2004), resulting not only in reduced antimicrobial activity, but also in diminished clearance of apoptotic neutrophils, which would collectively promote inflammation.

In summary, it is evident from the previous sections that there are a number of mechanisms by which CS exposure can contribute to chronic airway inflammation and to increasingly common diseases such as asthma and COPD. Furthermore, many of these proinflammatory events can be accounted for by acrolein (and other similarly reactive aldehydes in CS), which affects cell function either by direct modification of critical cell constituents, or indirectly by alteration of the cellular redox status and increasing cellular oxidative stress. Figure 3.4 illustrates the several major mechanisms by which acrolein can promote inflammatory–immune processes in the lung.

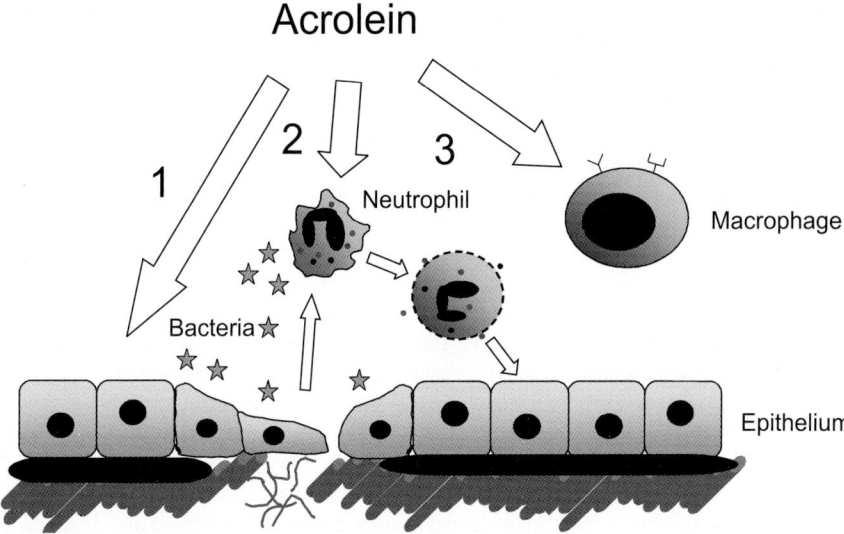

Fig. 3.4 Schematic illustration of the several mechanisms by which acrolein can contribute to airway inflammation. 1. The action of acrolein on airway epithelial cells may cause cell activation and/or injury (Nardini et al. 2002). Such injury, and diminished capacity for repair (Wang et al. 2001), will promote influx of inflammatory cells such as neutrophils. 2. Acrolein can affect neutrophil function by inhibiting oxidative bacterial killing (Nguyen et al. 2001), increasing proinflammatory cytokine production, and interfering with neutrophil apoptosis and promoting necrotic cell death (Finkelstein et al. 2001). Released products from necrotic cells can further promote inflammation by activating or injuring airway epithelial cells. 3. Interaction of acrolein with alveolar macrophages or extracellular proteins results in alterations in macrophage cytokine production (Li and Holian 1998) and in decreased phagocytic activity (Kirkham et al. 2004), further diminishing neutrophil clearance and antimicrobial activity, leading to increased infection and inflammation

3.5 Future Perspectives

3.5.1 Strategies to Detect Biological Targets for Unsaturated Aldehydes

It is evident from the previous paragraphs that acrolein may play a major role in the pro-inflammatory activities of cigarette smoking and/or exposure to environmental tobacco smoke, and that a variety of cellular and chemical mechanisms may be involved in this. The mechanisms by which acrolein could alter cell function involve either direct interaction with critical cell targets, or indirectly by disturbing cellular homeostasis and redox status (Kehrer and Biswal 2000). Delineating the specific mechanisms by which acrolein affects cell function and what are the specific cellular targets for acrolein (or structurally related aldehydes) has been the subject of considerable recent research effort. In the following, some recent strategies that have been used in these endeavors will be discussed, as well as some limitations and remaining challenges.

In order to clarify further mechanisms by which unsaturated aldehydes affect the cell biology of, e.g., airway epithelial cells, alveolar macrophages, or neutrophils, it is imperative to identify the major cellular targets for these aldehydes and to link modifications of such targets to functional alterations. Based on the known reactivity of α,β-unsaturated aldehydes, the major modifications in proteins are likely through Michael addition with the main nucleophilic targets, cysteine, histidine, and lysine residues (Fig. 3.5). In this regard, the ability of acrolein (and other aldehydes) to modify cysteine residues has received the most attention, as such residues are often involved in structural or functional protein alterations induced by oxidative or nitrosative events. However, the relative importance of modification of cysteine residues and other amino acid modifications may vary, depending on the protein of interest and the relative abundance and reactivity of these amino acid residues. Several recent studies have implicated reaction with protein cysteine residues by acrolein as a mechanism by which enzyme function is altered. For example, we have recently determined that formation of Michael adducts in cytoplasmic NADPH oxidase subunits may be responsible for the lack of NADPH oxidase activation in neutrophils (Nguyen et al. 2001). Similarly, the central protein kinase that is involved in the activation of NF-κB, I-κB kinase (IKK), has been shown to be subject to redox regulation (Ji et al. 2001b; Reynaert et al. 2004), and was recently identified as a target for alkylation by 4-hydroxynonenal (Ji et al. 2001b), and by acrolein in airway epithelial cells (Valacchi et al. 2005). Although this was not always demonstrated directly, such inactivation most likely occurred by alkylation of the redox-sensitive cysteine residue in the transactivation loop of IKK, providing a direct mechanism involved in the inhibitory effects of unsaturated aldehydes on NF-κB activation. By analogy, preliminary evidence also suggests that acrolein is capable of inactivating caspase-3 (Finkelstein et al. 2001) by alkylation of a cysteine residue that is also subject to redox regulation (Fadeel et al. 1998; Hampton et al. 2002; Mannick et al. 1999).

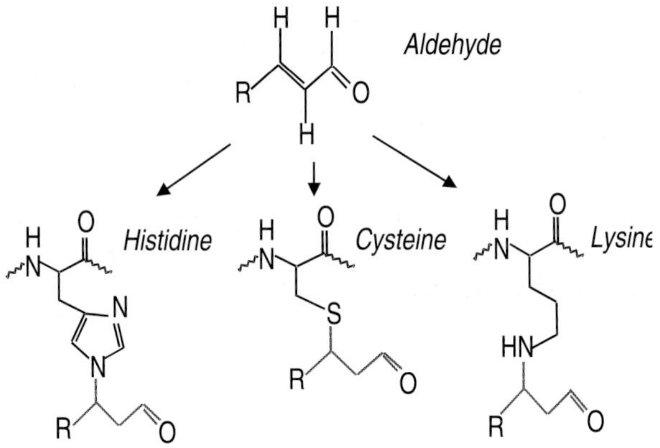

Fig. 3.5 Reaction of α,β-unsaturated aldehydes with protein histidine, lysine, or cysteine residues to form Michael adducts

Despite such examples, identification of the critical protein targets that are modified by acrolein or by other α,β-unsaturated aldehydes is still incomplete, and the exact consequence of such specific modifications to changes in protein interactions or enzymatic function is still largely unknown. One obvious reason for this is the complexity of such chemistry and the diversity of cellular targets. In order to address this issue, advanced proteomic approaches will be needed to identify the exact protein targets, and the precise modification product(s). Several approaches are currently being used in an attempt to identify direct modifications in protein targets by α,β-unsaturated aldehydes, based largely on their ability to form Michael adducts with several amino acid residues (primarily cysteine, lysine, and histidine residues) (Esterbauer et al. 1991; Parola et al. 1998). Such adducts still contain the aldehyde moiety, which can be employed in strategies to detect them directly. Common approaches to detect protein-bound carbonyl adducts involve derivatization with hydrazides such as dinitrophenylhydrazide (DNPH) or biotin-hydrazide, after which these adducts can be separated using two-dimensional gel electrophoresis approaches, or selectively collected with avidin chromatography for identification by LC-MS or matrix-assisted laser desorption ionization (MALDI)-MS approaches (Conrad et al. 2001; Yoo and Regnier 2004). Although such hydrazide derivatization approaches have been well established and would allow detection of a broad range of Michael adducts of unsaturated aldehydes with various amino acid residues, one major limitation of this approach is that protein carbonyls can also be generated by several other oxidative mechanisms (Levine et al. 1994). Hence, such an approach could yield a high number of false positives, although MS/MS approaches could be used to distinguish alkylation by unsaturated aldehydes and other amino acid oxidation products. Another limitation with such an approach is the fact that the aldehyde moiety is still able to react with biological targets (e.g., Schiff base formation with lysine residues), and such reactions can occur secondary to Michael addition with neighboring amino acid residues, depending on protein structure (Esterbauer et al. 1991; Furuhata et al. 2002).

Alternative approaches to identify protein targets for unsaturated aldehydes have been made possible by the development of specific antibodies against protein adducts of, e.g., acrolein or hydroxynonenal (HNE). In fact, these antibodies have been used in several studies to demonstrate the formation of protein–aldehyde adducts in vivo or to detect adduct formation in specific proteins (Levonen et al. 2004; Parola et al. 1998; Uchida 1999). Although such immunochemical approaches may be more selective, the downside of such approaches is that such antibodies recognize only one specific protein adduct as the main epitope and do not cover the full spectrum of aldehyde reactivity with proteins. For instance, commonly used antibodies to detect protein–HNE adducts specifically recognize a Michael adduct with histidine (Levonen et al. 2004; Parola et al. 1998), and most likely do not detect Michael adducts with other amino acid residues such as cysteine residues. In this regard, such approaches could fail to recognize the potentially important reactions with redox-sensitive cysteine residues in various proteins. Furthermore, aldehyde adducts in which the aldehyde moiety has undergone secondary reactions with other targets (by, e.g., Schiff base formation) would also be left undetected. Similarly, an antibody raised against protein–acrolein adducts (Uchida 1999) is known to recognizes a specific epitope formed by Michael addition to lysine residues, Nε-(3-formyl-3,4-dehydropiperidino)-lysine (FDP-lysine), and will similarly not detect Michael adducts with other amino acid residues. Although this antibody has been used successfully to detect protein–acrolein adducts in inflamed tissues (Uchida 1999) and in CS-exposed cells (Nguyen et al. 2001), many potentially important protein modifications (e.g., with cysteine residues) would not be detected.

Whereas endeavors to detect direct cellular targets for unsaturated aldehydes are critical in order to understand the mechanisms by which these agents affect cell function, it has become clear that some redox-sensitive cellular pathways may also be affected indirectly by increased cellular production of oxidants. As such, 4-hydroxynonenal (Uchida et al. 1999), cyclopentenone prostaglandins (Kondo et al. 2001), and acrolein (van der Vliet et al., unpublished observations) have all been shown to rapidly increase cellular oxidant production, presumably related to changes in mitochondrial function. Moreover, recent proteomic analysis of cysteine-containing proteins revealed cysteine oxidation/modification on a number of cellular proteins following exposure to cyclopentenone prostaglandins, which could be reversed by dithiothreitol, thus reflecting reversible oxidation/thiolation rather than irreversible alkylation (Ishii and Uchida 2004). Thus, although redox-sensitive protein cysteine residues may be susceptible targets for direct modification by unsaturated aldehydes, it is important to follow up analysis of protein cysteine status by additional strategies (reduction or secondary MS approaches) in order to distinguish between direct or indirect modifications. This complexity further illustrates the challenges that can be expected in studies aimed at identifying cellular mechanisms by which unsaturated aldehydes affect cell signaling pathways and function.

3.6 Concluding Remarks

In summary, it is apparent that the spectrum of reactions of α,β-unsaturated aldehydes with biological systems is complex and will not be fully characterized by analysis of one single reaction product in proteins. Hence, successful determination of cellular targets for specific α,β-unsaturated aldehydes will most likely require a combination of various approaches, using both more general derivatization strategies as well as more specific immunochemical approaches. Overall, further analysis by MS/MS techniques will be needed to obtain more-specific identification of aldehyde-induced modifications in target proteins. Although this might be a challenging endeavor, such approaches will be important in identifying the major cellular targets for biologically important aldehydes and may lead to critical discoveries of biological targets that are involved in the proposed roles of α,β-unsaturated aldehydes as potential signaling molecules. The realization that acrolein and other common CS aldehydes are not only products of air pollution, but may also be produced endogenously as potential mediators of lipid oxidation has increased the general scope and significance of such studies toward the biological actions of these aldehydes. Continued efforts to identify cellular mechanisms of acrolein (and related aldehydes) and identification of critical targets will not only be instrumental in further understanding the (bio)chemical mechanisms involved in tobacco-related diseases, but also yield further insights into the more general biochemistry of α,β-unsaturated aldehydes that are receiving increasing attention as more general mediators of conditions associated with oxidative stress and inflammation. As such, important continued research into molecular mechanisms of tobacco-related diseases could not only lead to improved diagnosis and therapeutic management of such cases, but also have the added advantage of having much wider implications for a broader range of pathophysiologic conditions.

Acknowledgements

I would like to thank Drs. Erik Finkelstein, Giuseppe Valacchi, Hung Nguyen, and Mirella Nardini for their contribution to some of the studies that were described here, and Kent Pinkerton at ITEH for his assistance in the ETS mouse exposures. Finally, I thank NIH (HL068865) and the University of California Tobacco-Related Disease Research Program (TRDRP) for research support.

References

Andreoli R, Manini P, Corradi M, Mutti A, Niessen WM (2003) Determination of patterns of biologically relevant aldehydes in exhaled breath condensate of healthy subjects by liquid chromatography/atmospheric chemical ionization tandem mass spectrometry. Rapid Commun Mass Spectrom 17:637–45

Annovazzi L, Cattaneo V, Viglio S, Perani E, Zanone C, Rota C, Pecora F, Cetta G, Silvestri M, Iadarola P (2004) High-performance liquid chromatography and capillary electrophoresis: methodological challenges for the determination of biologically relevant low-aliphatic aldehydes in human saliva. Electrophoresis 25:1255–1263

Anto RJ, Mukhopadhyay A, Shishodia S, Gairola CG, Aggarwal BB (2002) Cigarette smoke condensate activates nuclear transcription factor-kappaB through phosphorylation and degradation of IkappaB(alpha): correlation with induction of cyclooxygenase-2. Carcinogenesis 23:1511–1518

Berhane K, Widersten M, Engstrom A, Kozarich JW, Mannervik B (1994) Detoxication of base propenals and other alpha, beta-unsaturated aldehyde products of radical reactions and lipid peroxidation by human glutathione transferases. Proc Natl Acad Sci U S A 91:1480–1484

Borchers MT, Wesselkamper S, Wert SE, Shapiro SD, Leikauf GD (1999) Monocyte inflammation augments acrolein-induced Muc5ac expression in mouse lung. Am J Physiol 277:L489–L497

Cao Z, Hardej D, Trombetta LD, Trush MA, Li Y (2003) Induction of cellular glutathione and glutathione S-transferase by 3H-1,2-dithiole-3-thione in rat aortic smooth muscle A10 cells: protection against acrolein-induced toxicity. Atherosclerosis 166:291–301

Carnevali S, Petruzzelli S, Longoni B, Vanacore R, Barale R, Cipollini M, Scatena F, Paggiaro P, Celi A, Giuntini C (2003) Cigarette smoke extract induces oxidative stress and apoptosis in human lung fibroblasts. Am J Physiol 284:L955–L963

Chalmers GW, MacLeod KJ, Thomson L, Little SA, McSharry C, Thomson NC (2001) Smoking and airway inflammation in patients with mild asthma. Chest 120:1917–1922

Church DF, Pryor WA (1985) Free-radical chemistry of cigarette smoke and its toxicological implications. Environ Health Perspect 64:111–126

Conrad CC, Choi J, Malakowsky CA, Talent JM, Dai R, Marshall P, Gracy RW (2001) Identification of protein carbonyls after two-dimensional electrophoresis. Proteomics 1:829–834

Corradi M, Pignatti P, Manini P, Andreoli R, Goldoni M, Poppa M, Moscato G, Balbi B, Mutti A (2004) Comparison between exhaled and sputum oxidative stress biomarkers in chronic airway inflammation. Eur Respir J 24:1011–1017

Cueto R, Pryor WA (1994) Cigarette smoke chemistry: conversion of nitric oxide to nitrogen dioxide and reactions of nitrogen oxides with other smoke components as studied by Fourier transform infrared spectroscopy. Vib Spectrosc 7:97–111

Deshmukh HS, Case LM, Wesselkamper SC, Borchers MT, Martin LD, Shertzer HG, Nadel JA, Leikauf GD (2005) Metalloproteinases mediate mucin 5AC expression by epidermal growth factor receptor activation. Am J Respir Crit Care Med 171:305–314

Dick RA, Kensler TW (2004) The catalytic and kinetic mechanisms of NADPH-dependent alkenal/one oxidoreductase. J Biol Chem 279:17269–17277

Dick RA, Kwak MK, Sutter TR, Kensler TW (2001) Antioxidative function and substrate specificity of NAD(P)H-dependent alkenal/one oxidoreductase. A new role for leukotriene B4 12-hydroxydehydrogenase/15-oxoprostaglandin 13-reductase. J Biol Chem 276:40803–40810

Dietrich M, Block G, Benowitz NL, Morrow JD, Hudes M, Jacob P III, Norkus EP, Packer L (2003) Vitamin C supplementation decreases oxidative stress biomarker F_2-isoprostanes in plasma of nonsmokers exposed to environmental tobacco smoke. Nutr Cancer 45:176–184

DiFranza JR, Aligne CA, Weitzman M (2004) Prenatal and postnatal environmental tobacco smoke exposure and children's health. Pediatrics 113:1007–1015

Drannik AG, Pouladi MA, Robbins CS, Goncharova SI, Kianpour S, Stampfli MR (2004) Impact of cigarette smoke on clearance and inflammation after *Pseudomonas aeruginosa* infection. Am J Respir Crit Care Med 170:1164–1171

Eiserich JP, Cross CE, van der Vliet A (1997) Nitrogen oxides are important contributors to cigarette smoke-induced ascorbate oxidation. In: Packer L, Fuchs J (eds) Vitamin C in health and disease. Dekker, New York, pp 399–412

Eiserich JP, van der Vliet A, Handelman GJ, Halliwell B, Cross CE (1995) Dietary antioxidants and cigarette smoke-induced biomolecular damage: a complex interaction. Am J Clin Nutr 62: S1490–S1500

Eiserich JP, Vossen V, O'Neill CA, Halliwell B, Cross CE, van der Vliet A (1994) Molecular mechanisms of damage by excess nitrogen oxides: nitration of tyrosine by gas-phase cigarette smoke. FEBS Lett 353:53–56

Eisner MD, Yelin EH, Henke J, Shiboski SC, Blanc PD (1998) Environmental tobacco smoke and adult asthma. The impact of changing exposure status on health outcomes. Am J Respir Crit Care Med 158:170–175

Ensor CM, Zhang H, Tai HH (1998) Purification, cDNA cloning and expression of 15-oxoprostaglandin 13-reductase from pig lung. Biochem J 330(Pt 1):103–108

Esterbauer H, Schaur RJ, Zollner H (1991) Chemistry and biochemistry of 4-hydroxynonenal, malonaldehyde and related aldehydes. Free Radic Biol Med 11:81–128

Fadeel B, Ahlin A, Henter JI, Orrenius S, Hampton MB (1998) Involvement of caspases in neutrophil apoptosis: regulation by reactive oxygen species. Blood 92:4808–4818

Fadok VA, Bratton DL, Konowal A, Freed PW, Westcott JY, Henson PM (1998) Macrophages that have ingested apoptotic cells in vitro inhibit proinflammatory cytokine production through autocrine/paracrine mechanisms involving TGF-beta, PGE2, and PAF. J Clin Invest 101:890–898

Finkelstein EI, Nardini M, van der Vliet A (2001) Inhibition of neutrophil apoptosis by acrolein: a mechanism of tobacco-related lung disease? Am J Physiol 281:L732–L739

Finkelstein EI, Ruben J, Koot CW, Hristova M, van der Vliet A (2005) Regulation of constitutive neutrophil apoptosis by the α,β-unsaturated aldehydes acrolein and 4-hydroxynonenal. Am J Physiol 289:L1019–L1028

Floreani AA, Rennard SI (1999) The role of cigarette smoke in the pathogenesis of asthma and as a trigger for acute symptoms. Curr Opin Pulm Med 5:38–46

Frei B (1991) Ascorbic acid protects lipids in human plasma and low-density lipoprotein against oxidative damage. Am J Clin Nutr 54:1113S–1118S

Furuhata A, Nakamura M, Osawa T, Uchida K (2002) Thiolation of protein-bound carcinogenic aldehyde. An electrophilic acrolein-lysine adduct that covalently binds to thiols. J Biol Chem 277:27919–27926

Gallucci S, Lolkema M, Matzinger P (1999) Natural adjuvants: endogenous activators of dendritic cells. Nat Med 5:1249–1255

Gebel S, Gerstmayer B, Bosio A, Haussmann HJ, Van Miert E, Muller T (2004) Gene expression profiling in respiratory tissues from rats exposed to mainstream cigarette smoke. Carcinogenesis 25:169–178

Gebel S, Muller T (2001) The activity of NF-kappaB in Swiss 3T3 cells exposed to aqueous extracts of cigarette smoke is dependent on thioredoxin. Toxicol Sci 59:75–81

Gilliland FD, Li YF, Dubeau L, Berhane K, Avol E, McConnell R, Gauderman WJ, Peters JM (2002) Effects of glutathione S-transferase M1, maternal smoking during pregnancy, and environmental tobacco smoke on asthma and wheezing in children. Am J Respir Crit Care Med 166:457–463

Green GM (1968) Cigarette smoke: protection of alveolar macrophages by glutathione and cysteine. Science 162:810–811

Hackett NR, Heguy A, Harvey BG, O'Connor TP, Luettich K, Flieder DB, Kaplan R, Crystal RG (2003) Variability of antioxidant-related gene expression in the airway epithelium of cigarette smokers. Am J Respir Cell Mol Biol 29:331–343

Hampton MB, Stamenkovic I, Winterbourn CC (2002) Interaction with substrate sensitises caspase-3 to inactivation by hydrogen peroxide. FEBS Lett 517:229–232

Harrison DJ, Cantlay AM, Rae F, Lamb D, Smith CA (1997) Frequency of glutathione S-transferase M1 deletion in smokers with emphysema and lung cancer. Hum Exp Toxicol 16:356–360

Haslett C (1999) Granulocyte apoptosis and its role in the resolution and control of lung inflammation. Am J Respir Crit Care Med 160:S5–S11

Haynes RL, Brune B, Townsend AJ (2001) Apoptosis in RAW 264.7 cells exposed to 4-hydroxy-2-nonenal: dependence on cytochrome C release but not p53 accumulation. Free Radic Biol Med 30:884–894

He JQ, Connett JE, Anthonisen NR, Pare PD, Sandford AJ (2004) Glutathione S-transferase variants and their interaction with smoking on lung function. Am J Respir Crit Care Med 170:388–394

He NG, Awasthi S, Singhal SS, Trent MB, Boor PJ (1998) The role of glutathione S-transferases as a defense against reactive electrophiles in the blood vessel wall. Toxicol Appl Pharmacol 152:83–89

Hoshino Y, Mio T, Nagai S, Miki H, Ito I, Izumi T (2001) Cytotoxic effects of cigarette smoke extract on an alveolar type II cell-derived cell line. Am J Physiol 281:L509–L516

Hubatsch I, Ridderstrom M, Mannervik B (1998) Human glutathione transferase A4-4: an alpha class enzyme with high catalytic efficiency in the conjugation of 4-hydroxynonenal and other genotoxic products of lipid peroxidation. Biochem J 330(Pt 1):175–179

Huynh ML, Fadok VA, Henson PM (2002) Phosphatidylserine-dependent ingestion of apoptotic cells promotes TGF-beta1 secretion and the resolution of inflammation. J Clin Invest 109:41–50

Ishii T, Matsuse T, Teramoto S, Matsui H, Miyao M, Hosoi T, Takahashi H, Fukuchi Y, Ouchi Y (1999) Glutathione S-transferase P1 (GSTP1) polymorphism in patients with chronic obstructive pulmonary disease. Thorax 54:693–696

Ishii T, Uchida K (2004) Induction of reversible cysteine-targeted protein oxidation by an endogenous electrophile 15-deoxy-delta12,14-prostaglandin J2. Chem Res Toxicol 17:1313–1322

Itoh K, Tong KI, Yamamoto M (2004) Molecular mechanism activating Nrf2-Keap1 pathway in regulation of adaptive response to electrophiles. Free Radic Biol Med 36:1208–1213

Ji C, Amarnath V, Pietenpol JA, Marnett LJ (2001a) 4-hydroxynonenal induces apoptosis via caspase-3 activation and cytochrome c release. Chem Res Toxicol 14:1090–1096

Ji C, Kozak KR, Marnett LJ (2001b) IkappaB kinase, a molecular target for inhibition by 4-hydroxy-2-nonenal. J Biol Chem 276:18223–18228

Kabesch M, Hoefler C, Carr D, Leupold W, Weiland SK, von Mutius E (2004) Glutathione S-transferase deficiency and passive smoking increase childhood asthma. Thorax 59:569–573

Kehrer JP, Biswal SS (2000) The molecular effects of acrolein. Toxicol Sci 57:6–15

Keightley JA, Shang L, Kinter M (2004) Proteomic analysis of oxidative stress-resistant cells: a specific role for aldose reductase overexpression in cytoprotection. Mol Cell Proteomics 3:167–175

Kim H, Liu X, Kobayashi T, Conner H, Kohyama T, Wen FQ, Fang Q, Abe S, Bitterman P, Rennard SI (2004) Reversible cigarette smoke extract-induced DNA damage in human lung fibroblasts. Am J Respir Cell Mol Biol 31:483–490

Kirkham PA, Spooner G, Rahman I, Rossi AG (2004) Macrophage phagocytosis of apoptotic neutrophils is compromised by matrix proteins modified by cigarette smoke and lipid peroxidation products. Biochem Biophys Res Commun 318:32–37

Kondo M, Oya-Ito T, Kumagai T, Osawa T, Uchida K (2001) Cyclopentenone prostaglandins as potential inducers of intracellular oxidative stress. J Biol Chem 276:12076–12083

Kwak MK, Kensler TW, Casero RA Jr (2003) Induction of phase 2 enzymes by serum oxidized polyamines through activation of Nrf2: effect of the polyamine metabolite acrolein. Biochem Biophys Res Commun 305:662–670

Lauber K, Blumenthal SG, Waibel M, Wesselborg S (2004) Clearance of apoptotic cells: getting rid of the corpses. Mol Cell 14:277–287

Lee BM, Lee SK, Kim HS (1998) Inhibition of oxidative DNA damage, 8-OHdG, and carbonyl contents in smokers treated with antioxidants (vitamin E, vitamin C, beta-carotene and red ginseng). Cancer Lett 132:219–227

Leonarduzzi G, Arkan MC, Basaga H, Chiarpotto E, Sevanian A, Poli G (2000) Lipid oxidation products in cell signaling. Free Radic Biol Med 28:1370–1378

Leuchtenberger C, Leuchtenberger R, Zbinden I (1974) Gas vapour phase constituents and SH reactivity of cigarette smoke influence lung cultures. Nature 247:565–567

Levine RL, Williams JA, Stadtman ER, Shacter E (1994) Carbonyl assays for determination of oxidatively modified proteins. Methods Enzymol 233:346–357

Levonen AL, Landar A, Ramachandran A, Ceaser EK, Dickinson DA, Zanoni G, Morrow JD, Darley-Usmar VM (2004) Cellular mechanisms of redox cell signalling: role of cysteine modification in controlling antioxidant defences in response to electrophilic lipid oxidation products. Biochem J 378:373–382

Li J, Kartha S, Iasvovskaia S, Tan A, Bhat RK, Manaligod JM, Page K, Brasier AR, Hershenson MB (2002) Regulation of human airway epithelial cell IL-8 expression by MAP kinases. Am J Physiol 283:L690–L699

Li L, Hamilton RF Jr, Holian A (1999) Effect of acrolein on human alveolar macrophage NF-kappaB activity. Am J Physiol 277:L550–L557

Li L, Hamilton RF Jr, Taylor DE, Holian A (1997) Acrolein-induced cell death in human alveolar macrophages. Toxicol Appl Pharmacol 145:331–339

Li L, Holian A (1998) Acrolein: a respiratory toxin that suppresses pulmonary host defense. Rev Environ Health 13:99–108

Lykkesfeldt J, Christen S, Wallock LM, Chang HH, Jacob RA, Ames BN (2000) Ascorbate is depleted by smoking and repleted by moderate supplementation: a study in male smokers and nonsmokers with matched dietary antioxidant intakes. Am J Clin Nutr 71:530–536

Maderna P, Godson C (2003) Phagocytosis of apoptotic cells and the resolution of inflammation. Biochim Biophys Acta 1639:141–151

Mannick JB, Hausladen A, Liu L, Hess DT, Zeng M, Miao QX, Kane LS, Gow AJ, Stamler JS (1999) Fas-induced caspase denitrosylation. Science 284:651–654

Maranzana A, Mehlhorn RJ (1998) Loss of glutathione, ascorbate recycling, and free radical scavenging in human erythrocytes exposed to filtered cigarette smoke. Arch Biochem Biophys 350:169–182

Martey CA, Pollock SJ, Turner CK, O'Reilly KM, Baglole CJ, Phipps RP, Sime PJ (2004) Cigarette smoke induces cyclooxygenase-2 and microsomal prostaglandin E2 synthase in human lung fibroblasts: implications for lung inflammation and cancer. Am J Physiol 287:L981–L991

Mercer BA, Kolesnikova N, Sonett J, D'Armiento J (2004) Extracellular regulated kinase/mitogen activated protein kinase is up-regulated in pulmonary emphysema and mediates matrix metalloproteinase-1 induction by cigarette smoke. J Biol Chem 279:17690–17696

Mio T, Romberger DJ, Thompson AB, Robbins RA, Heires A, Rennard SI (1997) Cigarette smoke induces interleukin-8 release from human bronchial epithelial cells. Am J Respir Crit Care Med 155:1770–1776

Moodie FM, Marwick JA, Anderson CS, Szulakowski P, Biswas SK, Bauter MR, Kilty I, Rahman I (2004) Oxidative stress and cigarette smoke alter chromatin remodeling but differentially regulate NF-kappaB activation and proinflammatory cytokine release in alveolar epithelial cells. FASEB J 18:1897–1899

Morrow JD, Frei B, Longmire AW, Gaziano JM, Lynch SM, Shyr Y, Strauss WE, Oates JA, Roberts LJ II (1995) Increase in circulating products of lipid peroxidation (F_2-isoprostanes) in smokers. Smoking as a cause of oxidative damage. N Engl J Med 332:1198–1203

Muller T, Gebel S (1998) The cellular stress response induced by aqueous extracts of cigarette smoke is critically dependent on the intracellular glutathione concentration. Carcinogenesis 19:797–801

Nardini M, Finkelstein EI, Reddy S, Valacchi G, Traber M, Cross CE, van der Vliet A (2002) Acrolein-induced cytotoxicity in cultured human bronchial epithelial cells. Modulation by alpha-tocopherol and ascorbic acid. Toxicology 170:173–185

Nguyen H, Finkelstein E, Reznick A, Cross C, van der Vliet A (2001) Cigarette smoke impairs neutrophil respiratory burst activation by aldehyde-induced thiol modifications. Toxicology 160:207–217

Niknahad H, Siraki AG, Shuhendler A, Khan S, Teng S, Galati G, Easson E, Poon R, O'Brien PJ (2003) Modulating carbonyl cytotoxicity in intact rat hepatocytes by inhibiting carbonyl-metabolizing enzymes. I. Aliphatic alkenals. Chem Biol Interact 143–144:107–117

Norman V (1977) An overview of the vapor phase, semivolatile, and non-volatile components of cigarette smoke. In: Tobacco smoke: its formation and composition, vol. 3. Tennessee Eastman, Kingsport, TN, p 28

Norman V, Keith CH (1965) Nitrogen oxides in tobacco smoke. Nature 205:915–916

Pal A, Hu X, Zimniak P, Singh SV (2000) Catalytic efficiencies of allelic variants of human glutathione S-transferase Pi in the glutathione conjugation of alpha,beta-unsaturated aldehydes. Cancer Lett 154:39–43

Panda K, Chattopadhyay R, Chattopadhyay D, Chatterjee IB (2001) Cigarette smoke-induced protein oxidation and proteolysis is exclusively caused by its tar phase: prevention by vitamin C. Toxicol Lett 123:21–32

Park YS, Misonou Y, Fujiwara N, Takahashi M, Miyamoto Y, Koh YH, Suzuki K, Taniguchi N (2005) Induction of thioredoxin reductase as an adaptive response to acrolein in human umbilical vein endothelial cells. Biochem Biophys Res Commun 327:1058–1065

Parola M, Robino G, Marra F, Pinzani M, Bellomo G, Leonarduzzi G, Chiarugi P, Camandola S, Poli G, Waeg G, Gentilini P, Dianzani MU (1998) HNE interacts directly with JNK isoforms in human hepatic stellate cells. J Clin Invest 102:1942–1950

Petersen DR, Doorn JA (2004) Reactions of 4-hydroxynonenal with proteins and cellular targets. Free Radic Biol Med 37:937–45

Petruzzelli S, Puntoni R, Mimotti P, Pulera N, Baliva F, Fornai E, Giuntini C (1997) Plasma 3-nitrotyrosine in cigarette smokers. Am J Respir Crit Care Med 156:1902–1907

Pignatelli B, Li CQ, Boffetta P, Chen Q, Ahrens W, Nyberg F, Mukeria A, Bruske-Hohlfeld I, Fortes C, Constantinescu V, Ischiropoulos H, Ohshima H (2001) Nitrated and oxidized plasma proteins in smokers and lung cancer patients. Cancer Res 61:778–784

Poynter ME, Irvin CG, Janssen-Heininger YM (2003) A prominent role for airway epithelial NF-kappa B activation in lipopolysaccharide-induced airway inflammation. J Immunol 170:6257–6265

Rahman I, MacNee W (1996) Oxidant/antioxidant imbalance in smokers and chronic obstructive pulmonary disease. Thorax 51:348–50

Rahman I, MacNee W (1999) Lung glutathione and oxidative stress: implications in cigarette smoke-induced airway disease. Am J Physiol 277:L1067–L1088

Ramu K, Perry CS, Ahmed T, Pakenham G, Kehrer JP (1996) Studies on the basis for the toxicity of acrolein mercapturates. Toxicol Appl Pharmacol 140:487–498

Rangasamy T, Cho CY, Thimmulappa RK, Zhen L, Srisuma SS, Kensler TW, Yamamoto M, Petrache I, Tuder RM, Biswal S (2004) Genetic ablation of Nrf2 enhances susceptibility to cigarette smoke-induced emphysema in mice. J Clin Invest 114:1248–1259

Reddy S, Finkelstein EI, Wong PS, Phung A, Cross CE, van der Vliet A (2002) Identification of glutathione modifications by cigarette smoke. Free Radic Biol Med 33:1490–1498

Renes J, de Vries EE, Hooiveld GJ, Krikken I, Jansen PL, Muller M (2000) Multidrug resistance protein MRP1 protects against the toxicity of the major lipid peroxidation product 4-hydroxynonenal. Biochem J 350(Pt 2):555–561

Rennard SI (2004) Cigarette smoke in research. Am J Respir Cell Mol Biol 31:479–480

Reynaert NL, Ckless K, Korn SH, Vos N, Guala AS, Wouters EF, van der Vliet A, Janssen-Heininger YM (2004) Nitric oxide represses inhibitory kappaB kinase through S-nitrosylation. Proc Natl Acad Sci U S A 101:8945–8950

Reznick AZ, Cross CE, Hu ML, Suzuki YJ, Khwaja S, Safadi A, Motchnik PA, Packer L, Halliwell B (1992) Modification of plasma proteins by cigarette smoke as measured by protein carbonyl formation. Biochem J 286(Pt 2):607–611

Sadikot RT, Han W, Everhart MB, Zoia O, Peebles RS, Jansen ED, Yull FE, Christman JW, Blackwell TS (2003) Selective I kappa B kinase expression in airway epithelium generates neutrophilic lung inflammation. J Immunol 170:1091–1098

Saetta M (1999) Airway inflammation in chronic obstructive pulmonary disease. Am J Respir Crit Care Med 160:S17–S20

Sanli G, Dudley JI, Blaber M (2003) Structural biology of the aldo-keto reductase family of enzymes: catalysis and cofactor binding. Cell Biochem Biophys 38:79–101

Savill J (1997) Recognition and phagocytosis of cells undergoing apoptosis. Br Med Bull 53:491–508

Schwartz J, Timonen KL, Pekkanen J (2000) Respiratory effects of environmental tobacco smoke in a panel study of asthmatic and symptomatic children. Am J Respir Crit Care Med 161:802–806

Shao MX, Nakanaga T, Nadel JA (2004) Cigarette smoke induces MUC5AC mucin overproduction via tumor necrosis factor-alpha-converting enzyme in human airway epithelial (NCI-H292) cells. Am J Physiol 287:L420–L427

Shi Y, Evans JE, Rock KL (2003) Molecular identification of a danger signal that alerts the immune system to dying cells. Nature 425:516–521

Sladek NE (2003) Human aldehyde dehydrogenases: potential pathological, pharmacological, and toxicological impact. J Biochem Mol Toxicol 17:7–23

Spira A, Beane J, Shah V, Liu G, Schembri F, Yang X, Palma J, Brody JS (2004) Effects of cigarette smoke on the human airway epithelial cell transcriptome. Proc Natl Acad Sci U S A 101:10143–10148

Srivastava S, Watowich SJ, Petrash JM, Srivastava SK, Bhatnagar A (1999) Structural and kinetic determinants of aldehyde reduction by aldose reductase. Biochemistry 38:42–54

Takeuchi K, Kato M, Suzuki H, Akhand AA, Wu J, Hossain K, Miyata T, Matsumoto Y, Nimura Y, Nakashima I (2001) Acrolein induces activation of the epidermal growth factor receptor of human keratinocytes for cell death. J Cell Biochem 81:679–688

Takeyama K, Jung B, Shim JJ, Burgel PR, Dao-Pick T, Ueki IF, Protin U, Kroschel P, Nadel JA (2001) Activation of epidermal growth factor receptors is responsible for mucin synthesis induced by cigarette smoke. Am J Physiol 280:L165–L172

Tirumalai R, Rajesh Kumar T, Mai KH, Biswal S (2002) Acrolein causes transcriptional induction of phase II genes by activation of Nrf2 in human lung type II epithelial (A549) cells. Toxicol Lett 132:27–36

Tsuji T, Aoshiba K, Nagai A (2004) Cigarette smoke induces senescence in alveolar epithelial cells. Am J Respir Cell Mol Biol 31:643–649

Uchida K (1999) Current status of acrolein as a lipid peroxidation product. Trends Cardiovasc Med 9:109–113

Uchida K, Shiraishi M, Naito Y, Torii Y, Nakamura Y, Osawa T (1999) Activation of stress signaling pathways by the end product of lipid peroxidation. 4-hydroxy-2-nonenal is a potential inducer of intracellular peroxide production. J Biol Chem 274:2234–2242

Valacchi G, Pagnin E, Phung A, Nardini M, Schock BC, Cross CE, van der Vliet A (2005) Inhibition of NFkB activation and IL-8 expression in human bronchial epithelial cells by acrolein. Antioxid Redox Signal 7:25–31

Wakabayashi N, Dinkova-Kostova AT, Holtzclaw WD, Kang MI, Kobayashi A, Yamamoto M, Kensler TW, Talalay P (2004) Protection against electrophile and oxidant stress by induction of the phase 2 response: fate of cysteines of the Keap1 sensor modified by inducers. Proc Natl Acad Sci U S A 101:2040–2045

Wang H, Liu X, Umino T, Skold CM, Zhu Y, Kohyama T, Spurzem JR, Romberger DJ, Rennard SI (2001) Cigarette smoke inhibits human bronchial epithelial cell repair processes. Am J Respir Cell Mol Biol 25:772–779

Wickenden JA, Clarke MC, Rossi AG, Rahman I, Faux SP, Donaldson K, MacNee W (2003) Cigarette smoke prevents apoptosis through inhibition of caspase activation and induces necrosis. Am J Respir Cell Mol Biol 29:562–570

Wills-Karp M, Ewart SL (2004) Time to draw breath: asthma-susceptibility genes are identified. Nat Rev Genet 5:376–387

Witschi H, Joad JP, Pinkerton KE (1997) The toxicology of environmental tobacco smoke. Annu Rev Pharmacol Toxicol 37:29–52

Yang X, Wu X, Choi YE, Kern JC, Kehrer JP (2004) Effect of acrolein and glutathione depleting agents on thioredoxin. Toxicology 204:209–218

Yoneda K, Peck K, Chang MM, Chmiel K, Sher YP, Chen J, Yang PC, Chen Y, Wu R (2001) Development of high-density DNA microarray membrane for profiling smoke- and hydrogen peroxide-induced genes in a human bronchial epithelial cell line. Am J Respir Crit Care Med 164: S85–S89

Yoo BS, Regnier FE (2004) Proteomic analysis of carbonylated proteins in two-dimensional gel electrophoresis using avidin-fluorescein affinity staining. Electrophoresis 25:1334–1341

Zang LY, Stone K, Pryor WA (1995) Detection of free radicals in aqueous extracts of cigarette tar by electron spin resonance. Free Radic Biol Med 19:161–167

Zhang R, Brennan ML, Shen Z, MacPherson JC, Schmitt D, Molenda CE, Hazen SL (2002a) Myeloperoxidase functions as a major enzymatic catalyst for initiation of lipid peroxidation at sites of inflammation. J Biol Chem 277:46116–46122

Zhang R, Shen Z, Nauseef WM, Hazen SL (2002b) Defects in leukocyte-mediated initiation of lipid peroxidation in plasma as studied in myeloperoxidase-deficient subjects: systematic identification of multiple endogenous diffusible substrates for myeloperoxidase in plasma. Blood 99:1802–1810

Chapter 4

Cigarette Smoke-Induced Redox Signaling and Gene Expression in In Vitro and In Vivo Models

Thomas Müller and Stephan Gebel

Contents

4.1	Introduction	76
4.2	CS-Dependent Redox Effects on Biomolecules Involved in (Oxidative) Stress Sensing and Signal Generation	77
4.2.1	GSH	77
4.4.2	Thioredoxin	79
4.2.3	Lipids and Membrane Constituents	82
4.2.4	Redox-Sensitive Molecules in Signal Transduction	84
4.3	Activation of Signal Transduction Pathways in CS-Exposed Cells	86
4.3.1	Stress Signaling Pathways	87
4.3.2	Cell Growth-Related Signaling Pathways	89
4.3.3	NF-κB	89
4.4	CS-Induced Differential Gene Expression In Vitro and In Vivo	91
4.4.1	CS-Induced Differential Gene Expression of Single (Model) Genes	91
4.4.2	CS-Induced Differential Gene Expression Studied by Gene Chip/Microarray Analysis	96
4.4.2.1	Studies in Rodent Systems	96
4.4.2.2	Studies in Humans	99
4.5	Concluding Remarks	101
	References	102

4.1 Introduction

Cigarette smoke (CS) is causally related to cancer development and severe inflammation-related diseases, such as chronic obstructive pulmonary disease (COPD), a syndrome that comprises respiratory disorders, e.g., chronic bronchitis, emphysema, bronchiolitis, and small airway disease (see Chapters 3 and 6), and cardiovascular disease (CVD), including subclinical atherosclerosis, coronary heart disease, and stroke (Peto et al. 1992; US Department of Health and Human Services 1989a, b). Chronic CS inhalation contributes significantly to the risk of these diseases, some of which develop within a few years, whereas other pathophysiologic effects require decades to become clinically detectable. In general, the individual risk is largely dependant on the chronically inhaled dose as well as on the susceptibility of the individual smoker to any of these diseases (reviewed for tobacco-related cancers in Wu et al. 2004). Because CS is a complex mixture estimated to be composed of up to 5,000 different chemicals, it is likely that the development of any of these disorders is not caused by a single constituent, but instead is the result of a complex interaction of a vast variety of CS-derived constituents reacting either directly or indirectly with target molecules in the aqueous, O_2-containing extra- and intracellular milieu of tissues of the respiratory tract and at other sites in the organism. Moreover, each exposure to CS triggers an acute pattern of cellular responses which is superimposed onto the existing responses to any chronic CS exposure. Altogether, these cellular/tissue responses are aimed at inactivating reactive CS constituents *and* adapting to the new microenvironmental conditions. This includes repair as well as synthesis activities; self-destructing, apoptotic mechanisms are activated when the degree of damage is beyond the cell's repair capacity. If, however, the cell is overwhelmed by an attack of damaging principles that is not manageable by cellular defense mechanisms, including the activation of apoptotic pathways, e.g., resulting in unrepaired and therefore inheritable genotoxic damage (reflected by mutational and epigenetic lesions) or cell death by an uncoordinated (necrotic) pathway, the severity of damage generally requires the sustained activation of upstream repair and clearance activities, which may ultimately result in chronic inflammation and disease development.

Generally, in anticipation of stressing conditions, cells (and tissues) are equipped with a whole plethora of means and tools in order to adequately cope with stressors derived from any chemical or physical source, as reflected, for example, by high local extra- and intracellular concentrations of antioxidant molecules such as glutathione (GSH), which are used as a kind of innate "redox buffer," or by redox-sensitive stress-sensing systems, resulting in the activation of signaling pathways followed by an efficient genetic response to combat stress more specifically. In view of this complex network of defense, the intention of this chapter is to review data describing (1) the interference of CS and CS-derived constituents with redox-sensitive and stress-sensing molecules, (2) the potential of CS and CS-derived constituents to activate signaling pathways, and finally, (3) the consequent changes in the gene expression pattern.

4.2 CS-Dependent Redox Effects on Biomolecules Involved in (Oxidative) Stress Sensing and Signal Generation

4.2.1 GSH

One of the most striking features of CS is its strong sulfhydryl (-SH) reactivity. This phenomenon was described more than 40 years ago independently by several groups using different experimental approaches (Fenner and Braven 1968; Green 1968; Lange 1961; Sato et al. 1962; summarized in Stauffer 1974), with the most detailed biological analysis of this effect provided by Leuchtenberger et al. (1974, 1976). For example, it was demonstrated that the in vitro phagocytic activity of isolated rabbit alveolar macrophages was significantly impaired on exposure to CS, yet the effect was completely inhibited in the presence of micromolar amounts of GSH or cysteine in the cell culture medium (Green 1968). Other publications described an inhibitory activity present in CS on specific -SH-dependent enzyme systems (Lange 1961; Sato et al. 1962). The evidence that an essential part of the adverse biological activity of CS might be exerted by its pronounced propensity to react with thiol residues was confirmed and further substantiated by Leuchtenberger et al. (1974, 1976), who demonstrated that this chemical trait of CS could be directly correlated with cytotoxic and carcinogenic effects in hamster lung cell cultures, as indicated by the inhibition of DNA and protein synthesis, atypical proliferation, and malignant cell transformation (Leuchtenberger et al. 1976). These authors also reported that the CS-dependent -SH reactivity was apparently largely attributable to the gas/vapor phase of smoke (Leuchtenberger et al. 1974). Although these data linked the CS-dependent -SH reactivity to CS-related biological effects, they provided no clue as to the underlying mechanism(s). Most of the discussion was related to compounds in CS contributing to the thiol reactivity, with much of the experimental focus on gas-phase components (Stauffer 1974).

There is now strong evidence that chronic exposure to the -SH reactivity effected by CS affects the development of CS-related diseases, especially COPD (for review, see Rahman and MacNee 1999). GSH is viewed as a prime inter- and intracellular target, and genes encoding enzymes involved in the GSH pathway are supposed to play a crucial role in the susceptibility to carcinogens in CS (Yang et al. 2004). As described elsewhere in this book (see Chapter 5), the -SH group containing tripeptide GSH constitutes a first-defense extra- and intracellular antioxidant, which protects cells against endogenous and exogenous oxidative stress (Meister 1991, 1994). The conclusion that this nonprotein thiol is a preferred target of an evidently huge number of different and chemically unrelated CS constituents is documented in numerous publications. These publications report, both in vitro and in vivo, the overall effect of GSH depletion by cigarette whole smoke (Bilimoria and Ecobichon 1992; Müller and Gebel 1998); by various CS fractions, including those derived from both the gas phase and the particulate phase (Müller and Gebel 1998; Rahman et al. 1995); and by single compounds present in CS, e.g., the metal carcinogen cadmium (summarized in Waisberg et al. 2003), and the tobacco-related aldehydes, such as acrolein, formaldehyde, and acetaldehyde (Grafström 1994; Horton et al. 1999; Kehrer and Biswal 2000; Müller and Gebel 1998). -SH-reactive compounds in CS are also represented by the CS particulate phase-associated compound benzoquinone (Abdelmohsen et al. 2003) and by nicotine (Yildiz et al. 1998), and are also indirectly formed from CS-derived precursors in an aqueous O_2-containing environment (Müller et al. 1997). In this context, it is important to note that CS exposure in vitro and in vivo generally results in a net loss of GSH, as indicated by decreased levels of reduced GSH, whereas the amount of oxidized glutathione (GSSG) does not significantly increase (Müller and Gebel 1994; Park et al. 1998). This observation can be explained by a direct oxidation of GSH by CS-dependent reactive oxygen species (ROS) to yield GSH sulfenic (R-SOH) or GSH sulfinic acid (R-SO$_2$H); by the reaction of the -SH group with oxides of nitrogen, resulting in the formation of S-nitroso-GSH (GSNO); or by a direct covalent glutathiolation of CS-derived constituents as described for the α,β-unsaturated tobacco-related aldehydes acrolein and crotonaldehyde forming a thiohemiacetal or a thioether (Ohno and Ormstad 1985; Reddy et al. 2002). Moreover, additional routes of GSH consumption are represented by the formation of other conjugates of GSH and CS (yet to be identified), which are produced by the broad spectrum of detoxifying GSH S-transferases (GSTs) (Sellers and Yang 2002; Wu et al. 2004), GSH peroxidases (GPX) and phospholipid-hydroperoxide GSH peroxidases (PHGPx), which inactivate ROS-dependent peroxides and lipid hydroperoxides, respectively, at the expense of GSH (Thomas et al. 1990). Finally, GSH may be consumed in CS-exposed cells by the substantial formation of GSH conjugates with protein thiols, leading to the formation of protein-mixed disulfides (GSSP) catalyzed by the glutaredoxin system (Fernandes and Holmgren 2004). Because this glutathiolation reaction is readily reversible, it has been postulated as an efficient mechanism for protecting crucial protein -SH residues from irreversible damage (Mallis et al. 2002). Hence, in the recovering cell, functional -SH groups in proteins can easily be recovered from corresponding GSSP conjugates through NADPH-dependent electron transfer also mediated by the glutaredoxin system. In fact, significantly elevated GSSP levels were seen in the blood of smokers in a CS dose-dependent manner, suggesting that GSSP is a sensitive biomarker of oxidative stress (Muscat et al. 2004).

Whereas the effect of CS on extra- and intracellular GSH is well-documented, little information is available on how CS-induced GSH depletion provokes inflammatory processes that can enhance the risk of cancer or COPD. Myriad cellular functions, ranging from enzymatic to organelle mechanisms, are based on functional -SH groups presented by critical protein cysteine residues and by GSH itself (Chakravarthi and Bulleid 2004; Hentze et al. 2002; Molteni et al. 2004; Morito et al. 2003), and which are all protected by high local (millimolar) concentrations of GSH. Accordingly, by compromising cellular GSH homeostasis, cells become increasingly vulnerable to oxidative damage and cell death (D'Alessio et al. 2004), and it can be assumed that it is, among other effects, the sum of CS-dependent cellular lesions induced by -SH modification that contribute to the development of CS-dependent adverse effects. The protective function of GSH becomes clearer when we see that GSH concentrations are significantly elevated in bronchial epithelial cells from smokers (Rusznak et al. 2000) as well as in the extracellular lining fluid of chronic smokers, whereas significantly decreased GSH concentrations are found in the extracellular lining fluid of acute smokers (Barnes 2004; Rahman and MacNee 1999). In this context, it is worth noting that kinetic studies in vivo using rat and guinea pig smoking models revealed that exposure to CS acutely decreased pulmonary and renal GSH levels in a dose-dependent manner, particularly in the rat (Bilimoria and Ecobichon 1992). However, diminished GSH pools were found to be replenished after 3 h of exposure (Bilimoria and Ecobichon 1992), a time frame that was also observed in vitro (Gebel and Müller 2001). The conclusion that CS interferes with -SH functions is corroborated by the finding that N-acetyl cysteine (NAC), a precursor of GSH synthesis, has a dramatic chemoprotective effect, both in vitro and in vivo, on CS-induced lesions, such as DNA damage, gene expression, cell survival, and apoptosis (summarized in De Flora et al. 2001).

According to its crucial role as an -SH-residue-protecting agent, the intracellular GSH concentration represents a sensitive stress sensor and, consequently, exhibits signaling potential. This is the overall conclusion from in vitro and in vivo experiments performed in the presence of L-buthionine-[S,R]-sulfoximine (BSO), a selective inhibitor of γ-glutamylcysteine synthetase (γGST), the rate-limiting enzyme in GSH synthesis (Meister 1995). In fact, a direct effect of lowered GSH levels on stress signal transduction and gene activation has been shown by demonstrating increased DNA-binding activity of the transcription factor activated protein-1 (AP-1) and induced reporter gene transcription (Bergelson et al. 1994) as well as for the expression of the antioxidant gene heme oxygenase-1 (*hmox1*) in cells treated with BSO (Maines 1992 and refs. cited therein). However, most of the data based on BSO treatment show that diminished GSH levels strongly intensify the stress signaling activities of compounds that react directly or indirectly with -SH, such as phorone (Oguro 1996), peroxynitrite (Oh-Hashi et al. 2001), arsenite (Shimizu et al. 1998), and asbestos (Janssen 1995), as well as of CS, both in vitro (Müller and Gebel 1998) and in vivo (Park et al. 1998), whereas, if tested, NAC generally decreased the sensitivity towards these toxic compounds. In addition to activating defense mechanisms as represented by the expression of phase II and antioxidant genes, such as γ*gst*, NAD(P)H:quinone oxidoreductase 1 (*nqo1*) and *hmox1*, stress signals, including those emerging from GSH depletion, also address the expression of inflammation-related genes, such as those encoding growth factors, cytokines, and chemokines, partly via activation of the transcription factor nuclear factor-κB (NF-κB) (Adler et al. 1999; Flohé et al. 1997; Wilhelm et al. 1997) (see below). It can therefore be assumed that in chronic smokers, continually compromised GSH levels per se represent a proinflammatory scenario that may ultimately favor cellular and tissue damage.

4.4.2 Thioredoxin

The other major cellular parameter responsible for keeping the cell's redox potential low and consequently the concentration of free -SH residues high is thioredoxin, also known as adult T-cell leukemia-derived factor (for review, see Arnér and Holmgren 2000; Powis and Montfort 2001). Beyond its crucial involvement in ribonucleotide metabolism (Holmgren 1989), another main function of this low-molecular-weight protein (M_r ~12 kDa) is to reduce oxidized -SH residues of functional proteins by means of its dithiol/disulfide (Cys-X-X-Cys) active site, which is fueled by NADPH-released electrons and catalyzed by thioredoxin reductase activity (for review, see Powis and Montfort 2001). In this function, the thioredoxin/thioredoxin reductase system partly overlaps the disulfide reductase activity exerted by the NADPH-dependent GSH/glutaredoxin system, which, however, is uniquely responsible for the protection of critical -SH residues by the formation of GSSP conjugates (Arnér and Holmgren 2000; Aslund and Beckwith 1999; Fernandes and Holmgren 2004). Accordingly, thioredoxin and glutaredoxin, which both belong to the thioredoxin superfamily of disulfide reductases, execute overlapping (i.e., back-up) as well as different disulfide reductase activities, thus further highlighting the biological significance of intracellular reduced thiol residues.

A major important feature of thioredoxin is its ability to interfere with signal transduction pathways by controlling the redox state of certain cysteine residues required by transcription factors to bind to DNA (reviewed in Sun and Oberley 1996). Although the list of transcription factors that rely on the thiol reducing activity of thioredoxin for efficient DNA binding is still growing, it includes such crucial players as NF-κB (Hayashi et al. 1993; Matthews et al. 1992; Okamoto et al. 1992), as well as p53, AP-1, and hypoxia inducible factor-1α (HIF-1α), the latter three via the redox factor Ref-1 (Gaiddon et al. 1999; Hirota et al. 1997; Lando et al. 2000). According to the fundamental impact on the signaling pathways addressing these transcription factors on the cellular response to changed microenvironmental conditions, and based on its ability to sense alterations of the redox potential, the thioredoxin/thioredoxin reductase system should be a central intracellular stress sensor (Aslund and Beckwith 1999). This hypothesis is supported by data demonstrating that thioredoxin also strongly influences decisions on life and death in the cell, as indicated by its potential to inhibit apoptosis signaling kinase-1 (ASK1) (Fiers et al. 1999; Liu et al. 2000; Saitoh et al. 1998), a mitogen-activated protein kinase (MAPK) that relays signals received via the tumor necrosis factor (TNF) receptor/TNF receptor-associated factor 2 (TRAF2) route to c-Jun N-terminal kinase (JNK) and p38 MAPK. In fact, the strong antiapoptotic effect associated with the overexpression of the thioredoxin/thioredoxin reductase system appears to be instrumental in the development of tumors, as indicated by increased levels of thioredoxin in many human tumors, which is associated with tumor aggressiveness (Powis and Montfort 2001). In mechanistic terms, at least part of the antiapoptotic nature harbored by thioredoxin may be related to its strong NF-κB-activating qualities (Harper et al. 2001).

Although the thioredoxin/thioredoxin reductase system is obviously of fundamental biological significance, there is, in contrast to the numerous effects described for GSH, a surprisingly small number of studies dealing with the effects of CS on thioredoxin or the thioredoxin/thioredoxin reductase system. However, using aqueous extracts of CS, no stimulating effect of this type of CS fraction was detectable on the expression of thioredoxin in in vitro-cultured 3T3 cells as observed by Western blotting (Gebel and Müller 2001). This result was recently confirmed at the transcriptional level for the in vivo situation by two independent rat inhalation studies during which the CS-dependent alteration of the gene expression pattern was studied using DNA microarray technology (Gebel et al. 2004; Gebel et al. in preparation). Although the thioredoxin gene was found to be slightly (~2-fold) induced in the airway epithelium of chronic smokers (Spira et al. 2004b), its low or lack of induction in CS-exposed cells and tissues (beyond a homeostatic [background] expression level) is somewhat surprising because recent data indicate that the thioredoxin gene is controlled by the transcription factor nuclear factor erythroid 2-related factor 2 (Nrf2) (Kim et al. 2003), which represents a major target for activation by CS, both in vitro and in vivo (see below). Although the expression of thioredoxin is obviously not a major target of CS exposure, there is still strong, though indirect, evidence for the oxidation of its critical cysteine -SH residues by CS. This was deduced from experiments showing, in the first 2–4 h of exposure in CS-treated 3T3 cells, an almost complete failure of thioredoxin to coprecipitate with the p50 subunit of NF-κB, which was paralleled by a significantly decreased efficiency of NF-κB to bind to DNA (Gebel and Müller 2001). Because NF-κB DNA binding is strictly dependent on

Fig. 4.1 Examples of cellular signal transduction pathways triggered by cigarette smoke (CS) or CS-related components. Transcription factors are depicted in *yellow*, protein kinases in *blue*, antiapoptotic proteins in *green*, and proapoptotic proteins in *red*. *Hatched boxes* represent transcription factor-binding sites, *dashed lines* represent indirect/unknown mode of action, and *dotted lines* represent transcriptional activation. *P* phosphorylation, *U* ubiquitination. See text for details

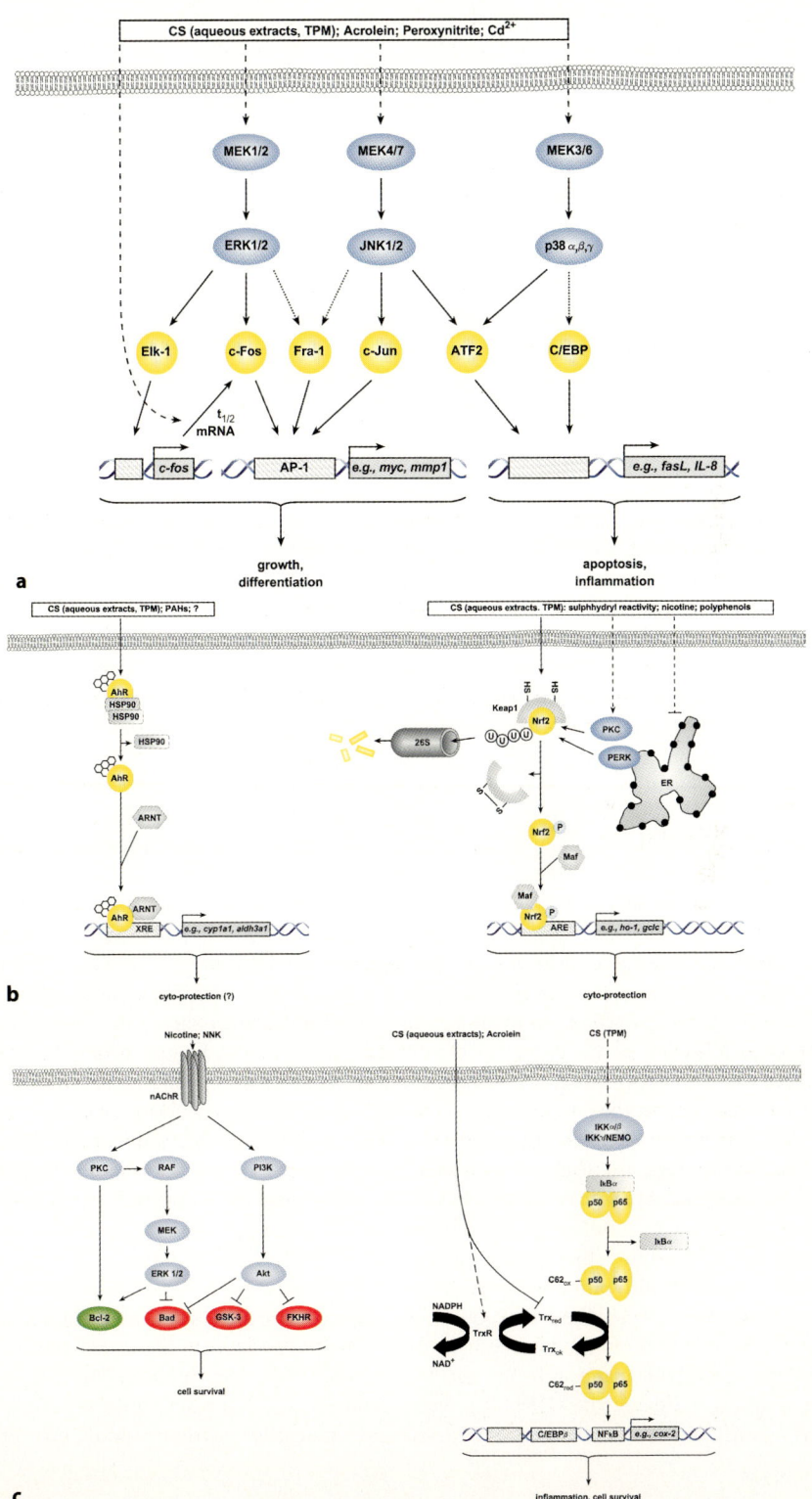

the thiol reductase activity of thioredoxin for DNA binding via its p50 subunit (Hayashi et al. 1993; Matthews et al. 1992; Okamoto et al. 1992) (see Fig. 4.1c), these findings indicate that in the early phase of CS exposure, thioredoxin becomes oxidized. In order to render this oxidized, nonfunctional fraction of thioredoxin protein functional again, it appears that CS-exposed cells and tissues transcriptionally activate the thioredoxin reductase gene as evidenced in vitro by RT-PCR analysis (Gebel and Müller 2001) and in vivo by a reproducible 3- to 5-fold induction of this gene, both in the nasal epithelium and in the lungs of CS-exposed rats (Gebel et al., in preparation). This observation is in accordance with results showing a ~4-fold activation of the thioredoxin reductase gene in the lungs of mice exposed for 3 h to CS (Rangasamy et al. 2004), and with a more than 2-fold induction in the airway epithelium of healthy (chronic) smokers (Hackett et al. 2003; Spira et al. 2004). Because thioredoxin reductases of higher eukaryotes, which are selenium-dependent dimeric flavoproteins, show a broad substrate spectrum, including nondisulfide substrates such as hydroperoxides and vitamin C (Arnér and Holmgren 2000), it appears economically more reasonable to upregulate this more pleiotropic antioxidant tool, rather than its substrate thioredoxin.

Based on its biological significance, there is clearly more experimental work needed to evaluate the role of the thioredoxin/thioredoxin reductase system in CS-related pathobiologic effects. Exploring this role, which appears to be a double-edged sword, as indicated by its potential to act as stress sensor and cellular defense system contrasted with its strong antiapoptotic activities, might also include studies on the chemopreventive potential of selenium, which is currently under debate (Ganther 1999). Finally, the capacity of thioredoxin to release biologically and pharmacologically relevant molecules from their corresponding GSH conjugates, as demonstrated for GSNO (Nikitovic and Holmgren 1996), appears worth investigating in the context of CS exposure.

4.2.3 Lipids and Membrane Constituents

In addition to protein and nonprotein thiols, components of the cellular membrane, such as phospholipids, are targeted by CS-dependent ROS, which may result in the generation of intermediates exhibiting strong proinflammatory signaling character (Niki et al. 1993). Examples of biologically active compounds formed from membrane lipids by CS-induced lipid peroxidation include various oxidized phospholipids that mimic the signaling activities exhibited by platelet-activating factor (PAF), F_2-isoprostanes, and 4-hydroxy-2-nonenal (4-HNE), as well as various other aldehydes, such as acrolein, which are all implicated in the development of CS-related diseases, particularly for COPD (for review, see Barnes 2004) and atherosclerosis (for review, see Stocker and Keaney 2004).

As summarized elsewhere in this book (see Chapter 3), lipid peroxidation reflects the uncontrolled breakdown of polyunsaturated fatty acids by a peroxidation mechanism believed to be induced by free radicals. Radical species involved in these processes either are released directly from CS (Pryor and Stone 1993) or are produced indirectly by their reaction with other biomolecules in the O_2-containing aqueous cellular milieu, leading to the intermediate formation of lipid hydroperoxides (Blair 2001). Hence, the list of CS-derived compounds potentially initiating lipid peroxidation includes hydroxyl radicals ($\cdot$OH), which appear in aqueous solutions of CS via Fenton/Haber-Weiss chemistry, and/or peroxynitrite ($ONOO^-$), which is formed by the reaction of nitric oxide ($NO\cdot$) with superoxide anion ($O_2^-\cdot$) (Pryor and Stone 1993). Other radicals may potentially be formed from the reaction of these compounds with other biomolecules, resulting in the formation of alkoxyl, peroxyl, and nitronium radicals. If not detoxified by PHGPx or GPx1/phospholipase activity (Thomas et al. 1990), such lipid hydroperoxides are further degraded, releasing products with strong proinflammatory signaling activity. For example, oxidation of polyunsaturated fatty acids by this mechanism may produce compounds with PAF-like activities, resulting in the uncontrolled activation of PAF receptors on platelets, monocytes, and leukocytes, which is a powerful trigger of proinflammatory signaling cascades. Eventually, this mechanism favors the formation of atherogenic low-density lipoprotein (LDL) particles as evidenced by the presence of CS-induced breakdown products of polyunsaturated fatty acids exhibiting PAF-like activity in these structures (Marathe et al. 2001).

Other CS-dependent ROS-induced lipid peroxidation products of major biological significance are the F_2-isoprostanes, which arise from uncontrolled arachidonic acid degradation. Because these compounds exhibit thromboxane A_2- and $PGF_{2\alpha}$-like activities and thus induce severe vaso- and bronchoconstriction as well as other lung inflammatory effects, they are supposed to be of key relevance in the development of COPD and CVD (for review, see Cracowski et al. 2002). In fact, increased levels of isoprostanes were identified in the exhaled air of smokers and in COPD patients (Montuschi et al. 2003), implicating a synergistic effect in the pathogenic process. Other end products of lipid peroxidation, i.e., aldehydes (particularly 4-HNE) are highly diffusible thiol-reactive compounds known to exert pleiotropic proinflammatory activities, which may be based, at least in part, on their ability to trigger several growth-related signaling pathways (for review, see Leonarduzzi et al. 2004). For example, it has been demonstrated that 4-HNE binds to, and subsequently activates, the epidermal growth factor (EGF) receptor (Suc et al. 1998) and the platelet-derived growth factor (PDGF) receptor (Escargueil-Blanc et al. 2001), which may catalyze the formation of atherogenic areas induced by oxidized LDL particles. Moreover, 4-HNE has been shown to affect protein kinase C (PKC) activity, especially PKC β_1 and β_2 isozymes (Leonarduzzi et al. 2004), and the stress-related signaling MAPKs JNK and p38MAPK, the latter of which was found to be involved in 4-HNE-induced expression of proinflammatory cyclooxygenase 2 (COX-2) (Kumagai et al. 2000; 2002), the rate-limiting enzyme during prostaglandin and thromboxane synthesis. Although the proinflammatory character of 4-HNE is not under debate, it is surprising that it does not, at least not directly, affect the proinflammatory transcription factor NF-κB, but rather may exert an inhibitory effect on NF-κB (Leonarduzzi et al. 2004). However, this might be explained by the -SH reactivity linked to the aldehyde nature of 4-HNE, because aldehydes have been shown to negatively affect NF-κB activity (Horton et al. 1999), most probably by inactivating the -SH residue of Cys 62 of its p50 subunit, which is required for efficient DNA-binding (Hayashi et al. 1993; Matthews et al. 1992; Okamoto et al. 1992).

Beyond the generation of compounds that cause strong proinflammatory signaling activities by lipid peroxidation, membrane damage itself impairs membrane functions, e.g., by the inactivation or uncontrolled activation of membrane-bound receptors and enzymes. Although no direct data are available for CS or CS-derived fractions, other redox-active chemical and physical treatments have been linked, in mammalian cells for example, with the clustering and internalization of membrane receptors, such as EGF, interleukin 1 (IL-1), and TNF-α coupled with JNK signaling (Rosette and Karin 1996). In addition, environmental stresses such as heat shock, UV irradiation, and oxidative stress caused by H_2O_2 treatment were shown to directly activate membrane-bound acid pH-dependent sphingomyelinase (ASMase), resulting in enhanced levels of the second messenger lipid intermediate ceramide from sphingomyelin. Ceramide generation because of ASMase activation has been correlated with JNK activation and apoptosis in human myeloid leukemia U937 cells (Verheij et al. 1996). In fact, a gradual increase in ceramide levels followed by apoptosis was detected in this cell line on exposure to aqueous extracts of CS (T. Müller, unpublished results). Altogether, these results provide direct and indirect evidence that by interfering with lipid and protein components of biological membranes, CS-derived ROS and reactive nitrogen species (RNS) produce signaling intermediates that may promote the development of a proinflammatory environment.

4.2.4 Redox-Sensitive Molecules in Signal Transduction

Consistent with an apparent biological principle, pathways that transduce signals arising from an impaired redox balance are generally equipped with redox-sensitive components that potentially function as (oxidative) stress sensors. Hence, these pathways are kept silent in the nonstressed cell when facing a sufficiently low redox potential, but in the case of oxidative disturbance become activated through chemical modification(s) of these particular components (for review, see Haddad 2002). Paradigms of signaling pathways that are regulated by such a mechanism are those resulting in the activation of the transcription factors NF-κB, AP-1, and particularly Nrf2 (Fig. 4.1), which mainly orchestrate the cellular stress and antioxidant/phase II-related defensive programs, respectively (Nguyen et al. 2003).

In the unstressed cell, the cap 'n' collar/basic region leucine zipper (CNC/b-Zip) transcription factor Nrf2 is inhibited by a dual mechanism involving its retention in the cytoplasm and its proteolysis through proteasomal degradation. Central to the repression of Nrf2 activity is the actin-binding protein Kelch-like ECH-associating protein 1 (Keap1), which anchors Nrf2 to the cytoplasm via interaction with a specific four amino acid stretch within the Neh2 domain of Nrf2 (for review, see Motohashi and Yamamoto 2004), while the broad complex-tramtrack-bric-a-brac (BTB) and the intervening region (IVR) domains of Keap1 recruit Cullin3, a subunit of the E3 ligase complex, resulting in the ubiquitination and subsequent proteolytic degradation of Nrf2 (Cullinan et al. 2004; Kobayashi et al. 2004; Zhang et al. 2004) (Fig. 4.1b). The efficiency of this regulatory mechanism is reflected by a rapid turnover of Nrf2 in unstressed cells, as expressed by half-lives of less than 20 min. However, if, owing to changes in their microenvironment, cells and tissues are confronted with an imbalanced redox homeostasis arising from electrophiles and oxidants, then this inhibitory mechanism is abruptly abrogated. Because Keap1 is a cysteine-rich molecule, it was hypothesized early on that at least some of these -SH residues might function as sensors for oxidant and electrophile compounds (Dinkova-Kostova et al. 2002). In fact, further investigations revealed direct evidence that -SH-reactive compounds activate Nrf2 through modification (alkylation, oxidation) of essentially two cysteine thiol residues, both located in the IVR domain of Keap1 (Wakabayashi et al. 2004). Mechanistically, modifications of these crucial -SH residues are assumed to induce conformational changes that eventually result in the abrogation of ubiquitin-dependent degradation of Nrf2 and its release from Keap1. Beyond this redox-dependent mechanism, other phosphorylation-dependent activation mechanisms have been reported for Nrf2 (summarized in Motohashi and Yamamoto 2004; Nguyen et al. 2004; see below and Fig. 4.1).

Although the activation of Nrf2 by CS through the Keap1-dependent cysteine thiol-sensitive mechanism outlined above has not been demonstrated directly, there is nevertheless sufficient evidence that the Nrf2/Keap1 system represents a major target for CS-dependent oxidants, as indicated by the finding that $nrf2^{-/-}$ mice are highly susceptible to CS-related inflammatory diseases such as emphysema (Rangasamy et al. 2004), and, more generally, by gene expression studies showing the strong upregulation of the phase II-related gene spectrum in response to CS exposure in vitro (Bosio et al. 2002) and in vivo (Gebel et al. 2004; Spira et al. 2004b). In principle, every CS-dependent -SH-reactive compound (see above) may potentially directly interfere with the specific cysteine thiol sensors provided by Keap1, resulting in the activation of Nrf2, as, for example, has been specifically demonstrated for the CS-dependent metal carcinogen cadmium (Stewart et al. 2003) and the gas-phase component acrolein, which was seen to strongly induce phase II-related genes by a mechanism involving Nrf2 (Tirumalai et al. 2003). Moreover, the interference of electrophilic lipid oxidation products, such as isoprostanes (Levonen et al. 2004), and the end products of lipid peroxidation, such as 4-HNE, with the reactive thiols of Keap1 may represent an indirect mechanism of CS-provoked activation of Nrf2. Finally, in addition to the -SH-sensitive activation mechanism mediated by Keap1, the DNA-binding efficiency of Nrf2 seems, itself, to be dependent on a crucial cysteine thiol, as evidenced by experimentally induced mutagenesis of cysteine to serine in the DNA-binding domain of Nrf2 (Bloom et al. 2002). Considering the strong overall -SH reactivity of CS (see above) together with the paramount relevance of Nrf2 in the cellular defense against oxidative stress, the reactive cysteine thiols of Keap1 represent potential central targets of CS-derived oxidants and electrophiles.

Similar to Nrf2, the other paradigmatic (oxidant) stress responsive transcription factor, i.e., AP-1, is also subject to tight redox regulation (for review, see Dalton et al. 1999; Eferl and Wagner 2003; Karin 1995). However, unlike Nrf2, the redox sensitivity of AP-1 is confined to its DNA-binding activity, which depends on -SH functions provided by critical cysteine residues within the b-Zip proteins potentially forming AP-1, such as proteins of the Jun, Fos, and ATF families. For example, oxidant conditions interfere with the DNA-binding activity of Jun/Fos heterodimers, which led to the identification of Cys-154 in Fos and Cys-272 in Jun as crucial determinants of this parameter (Abate et al. 1990). In this regard, redox regulation of AP-1-related transcription factors is akin to NF-κB, where the -SH function of Cys-62 within the p50 subunit is required for efficient DNA binding (Hayashi et al. 1993; Matthews et al. 1992; Okamoto et al. 1992; see above and Fig. 4.1c). It is therefore not surprising that AP-1 and NF-κB show similar direct effects in response to acute CS exposure, as expressed by significantly reduced DNA-binding capacities, most probably based on the presence of α,β-unsaturated aldehydes such as crotonaldehyde and acrolein (Freed et al. 2003; Gebel and Müller 2001; Kehrer and Biswal 2000; Vayssier et al. 1998b). The apparent paradoxical finding of an increased activity of these transcription factors in CS-related diseases such as COPD may therefore be explained by indirect mechanisms such as chromatin remodeling effects and invasion of proinflammatory cells during chronic CS exposure (Marwick et al. 2004).

In contrast to oxidatively modified -SH functions of Cys-62 within p50 of NF-κB, which are directly dependent on thioredoxin for rereduction, transcription factors of the AP-1 family show an indirect dependence on thioredoxin. In fact, the redox factor Ref-1 was identified as controlling the redox status of cysteine residues relevant for DNA binding in AP-1-related transcription factors, whereas, in turn, oxidized Ref-1 is dependent on thioredoxin for rereduction (Hirota et al. 1997). Notably, in addition to the cysteine-reducing activity, which is not only relevant for AP-1 function but also for p53 and HIF-

1α DNA binding (Gaiddon et al. 1999; Lando et al. 2000), Ref-1 shows the characteristics of a multifunctional protein because it also acts as an apurinic/apyrimidinic endonuclease (Demple et al. 1991). Because this enzyme activity is integral to DNA repair, Ref-1 may represent a central factor in orchestrating/coordinating stress signaling and DNA repair processes. However, despite this obvious functional relevance, no data are available on the direct effects of CS or CS-related components on the activity of Ref-1.

In summary, data gathered over several decades indicate that CS exposure affects the cellular redox potential by mainly interfering with "defensive" nonprotein (i.e., GSH) and critical functional thiol groups of proteins involved in stress sensing and signal generation. The sum of these effects obviously prompts the cell to a comprehensive response at the transcriptional level, resulting in an extensively altered gene expression pattern as described below.

4.3 Activation of Signal Transduction Pathways in CS-Exposed Cells

According to the dimension of alterations seen in the gene expression pattern (see below), strong signaling activities can be expected to occur in CS-exposed cells and tissues. However, somewhat surprisingly, the number of reports in the literature describing the activation of specific signal transduction pathways because of exposure of CS or CS-related compounds is limited and concentrates mainly on the activation of the aryl hydrocarbon (Ah) receptor or on the signaling activities initiated by nicotine and its derivatives.

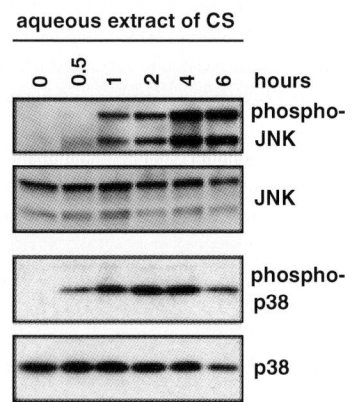

Fig. 4.2 Activation of c-Jun N-terminal kinase (*JNK*) and p38 mitogen-activated protein kinase (MAPK) signaling pathways in Swiss 3T3 cells exposed to aqueous extracts of cigarette smoke. Activation of JNK and p38 MAPK in Swiss 3T3 cells was demonstrated by Western blot analysis using antibodies against activated p38 MAPK (phospho-p38) and JNK (phospho-JNK) and the respective antibodies against the whole proteins

4.3.1 Stress Signaling Pathways

Regarding the induction of stress-related signal transduction pathways, activation of JNK signaling and AP-1 has been observed, for example, in the context of mucin production in the lungs of smokers, which was found to be independent of upstream epidermal growth factor receptor (EGFR) activation (Gensch et al. 2004). Evidence of JNK signaling was also obtained for the CS-induced expression of the AP-1 component *fra-1*, which in this case was dependent on EGFR function based on matrix metalloproteinase (MMP) activation (Zhang et al. 2005), thus confirming that CS-dependent alterations in the extracellular matrix are a trigger of CS-induced cell signaling. There is also evidence for the CS-dependent activation of p38MAPK, which was also demonstrated for the CS-dependent carcinogen cadmium (Alam et al. 2000; Chuang et al. 2000). In fact, our own laboratory observed a sustained activation of both JNK and p38MAPK in Swiss 3T3 cells exposed to aqueous extracts of cigarette smoke (unpublished results; Fig. 4.2). Thus, although data are limited, these results suggest that CS-derived ROS, directly or indirectly (e.g., through lipid peroxidation products such as 4-HNE or by interfering with the extracellular matrix), trigger classical stress-related signal transduction pathways, resulting in the activation of JNK and p38MAPK (Fig. 4.1a).

Beyond JNK and p38MAPK activation, CS and CS-derived compounds have also been reported to activate the other route of MAPK signaling, i.e., the extracellular signal-regulated kinase (ERK) pathway, which, in contrast to JNK and p38MAPK signaling, is mostly involved in transferring cell survival signals (Xia 1995) (Fig. 4.1a). An example of CS as a trigger of ERK signaling has recently been reported by Mercer et al. (2004), who showed that CS-induced expression of the gene encoding matrix metalloproteinase 1 (*MMP1*) was specifically dependent on ERK1/2-activation in human airway epithelial cells in vitro. In vivo experiments supported the assumption that ERK1/2 signaling may be involved in the development of CS-dependent emphysematous symptoms, as expressed by the identification of activated ERK in both airway lining cells and alveolar macrophages of mice exposed to CS as well as in the same cell types in smokers suffering from emphysema (Mercer et al. 2004). In this context it is intriguing to note that the expression of the proinflammatory cytokine IL-8 in alveolar macrophages of smokers was found to be mainly dependent on ERK (and p38MAPK) activation rather than related to the activation of NF-κB (Koch et al. 2004).

In contrast to JNK, p38MAPK, and ERK MAPK signaling, which may enhance inflammatory as well as apoptotic responses, e.g., by activating certain subpopulations of the AP-1 family of transcription factors, activation of the also stress-responsive Nrf2 pathway stimulates cell survival and anti-inflammatory functions. In addition to the mechanism involving the oxidative modification of specific -SH functions of Keap1 as outlined above, phosphorylation by upstream signaling kinases is also believed to be sufficient for activation of Nrf2 as a potent transcription factor of antioxidant and phase II-related genes (reviewed in Motohashi and Yamamoto 2004; Nguyen et al. 2004) (Fig. 4.1b). Accordingly, activation of Nrf2 through phosphorylation of N-terminal serine residues by PKC has been shown in response to oxidative stress and electrophiles (Bloom and Jaiswal 2003; Huang et al. 2000, 2002). Phosphorylation-dependent activation of Nrf2 has also recently been reported to be controlled by PERK, a kinase that becomes induced in response to certain types of stress, resulting in the abrogation of protein synthesis at the endoplasmic reticulum (ER) (Cullinan et al. 2003). Because nicotine (Jin et al. 2004; Mai et al. 2003) and CS-related dihydroxybenzenes such as hydroquinone and catechol (Gopalakrishna et al. 1994) have been described to activate PKC, while at the same time CS acutely interferes with the translational efficiency at the ER (Müller and Gebel 1994), these pathways further represent potential routes for Nrf2 activation by CS. As a consequence of activation, whether via -SH oxidation of specific cysteine residues within Keap1 and/or phosphorylation by upstream signaling kinases such as PKC and PERK, Nrf2 is rapidly released from its negative regulator Keap1 and migrates to the nucleus to initiate, in conjunction with an appropriate dimerization partner (e.g., members of the group of b-Zip small Maf proteins), the antioxidant cellular response at the transcriptional level. In mechanistic terms, this is accomplished by binding of the activated heterodimeric transcription factor to the antioxidant response element (ARE) present in the control region of antioxidant and stress-responsive genes (Motohashi and Yamamoto 2004).

The duality of the cellular defense strategy against environmental stresses is well established. In addition to the expression of antioxidant and phase II genes, which is aimed at inactivating reactive cell damaging species, there is also the activation of phase I-related genes, which code for drug-metabolizing enzymes, such as monooxygenases and dehydrogenases, and help the cell prevent damage from harmful xenobiotics by rendering these compounds accessible to cellular excretion mechanisms (for review, see Nguyen et al. 2003). Typically, the expression of phase I-related genes is orchestrated by cytoplasmic receptors, which, on activation via ligand binding, translocate to the nucleus, where they function as transcription factors in a *cis* element-dependent context. The most prominent representative of this group of transcription factors is the aryl hydrocarbon receptor (AhR) (Denison and Nagy 2003; Nebert et al. 2000, 2004), which is activated by binding to a broad spectrum of xenobiotic ligands, such as polyaromatic hydrocarbons (PAH) and aryl amines. On forming a complex with a particular dimerization partner, i.e., AhR nuclear translocator (ARNT), AhR controls a broad spectrum of genes, including those known to be differentially regulated by CS (see below), by addressing a specific control element known as the xenobiotic responsive element (XRE) (Fig. 4.1b). Interestingly, the efficiency of AhR to function as a transcription factor was recently found to be partly controlled by activated ERK, because ERK activity facilitated ligand-initiated AhR transcriptional activation while targeting the receptor for degradation (Chen et al. 2005).

However, the expression of certain enzymes in response to AhR activation, e.g., cytochrome P450 1A1 (Cyp1A1) (see below), is considered a double-edged sword because there is a risk of reactive (oxygenated) intermediates appearing, which may be harmful to the cell, for example, by forming bulky DNA adducts that may ultimately lead to cancer-initiating mutations (discussed for CS exposure in Bartsch et al. 1992). Thus, inhibition of AhR activity in vivo by 3'-methoxy-4'-nitroflavone, a potent AhR antagonist, completely abolished the DNA genotoxicity induced by CS condensate and benzo[a]pyrene (BaP), a PAH known to be present in CS, in C57Bl/6J mice (Dertinger et al. 2001). This effect was attributed to the abrogated expression of Cyp1A1 in response to AhR inactivation. However, these results should be interpreted with caution because paradoxical effects were reported for murine lines with disrupted *cyp* genes. For example, on exposure to BaP (125 mg/kg/day), *cyp1a1$^{-/-}$* mice exhibited a strict lethal phenotype within 30 d, whereas wild-type mice did not show any lethality within 1 year of treatment. Even more remarkable is the finding that *cyp1a1$^{-/-}$* mice generally harbored much higher amounts of BaP DNA adducts in comparison to their wild-type counterparts (Uno et al. 2004). Hence, these results indicate that the potential detoxification provided by AhR-stimulated Cyp enzymes "is more important than metabolic activation" (Uno et al. 2004).

Clearly, the obvious and important role played by the AhR in cell cycle regulation and apoptosis is only just beginning to emerge (Nebert et al. 2000).

The inducibility of phase I-related genes in the respiratory tract by CS, especially those encoding the cytochrome P450 isozymes, discussed below, was recently described in a detailed review by Ding and Kaminsky (2003).

4.3.2 Cell Growth-Related Signaling Pathways

According to several studies, nicotine is responsible for a strong antiapoptotic cell growth signal delivered by CS. Specifically, nicotine and nicotine-derived compounds, e.g., the tobacco-specific nitrosamine 4-(methylnitrosamino)-1-(3-pyridyl)-1-butanone (NNK), have been reported to activate survival and cell growth signaling pathways, including PKC (Heusch and Maneckjee 1998; Jin et al. 2004; Mai et al. 2003; Maneckjee and Minna 1994) and protein kinase B/Akt (PKB/Akt), most presumably by binding to and activating α_7, α_4, or α_3 variants of nicotinic acetylcholine receptors (nAChR) (Maneckjee and Minna 1994; Schuller et al. 2000; West et al. 2003) (Fig. 4.1c). According to these investigations, nAChRs are not restricted to neuronal cells but, as a result of nicotine exposure, are also expressed in the membranes of cells in other tissues, such as airway epithelial cells and keratinocytes of the oral mucosa, where nicotine specifically interacts with the $\alpha 3\beta 2$ subtype of nAChR, resulting in the activation of survival factors such as Bcl-2, NF-κB, and STAT-1 (Arredondo et al. 2005). Data describing the effects of nicotine-induced activation of PKC support the phosphorylation-dependent induction of antiapoptotic or inactivation of proapoptotic factors controlling the mitochondrion-related intrinsic apoptotic pathway. Accordingly, nicotine-induced PKC has been reported to trigger the activation of the Raf/Erk MAPK pathway, resulting in the phosphorylation-dependent activation of the apoptosis antagonist Bcl2 (Mai et al. 2003) and/or inactivation of the proapoptotic factor Bad (Jin et al. 2004).

Another route of nicotine- and NNK-dependent cell survival signaling affects the activation of PKB/Akt via nAChR binding and phosphatidylinositol 3-kinase (PI3K) activation as described in nonimmortalized human airway epithelial cells in vitro (Fig. 4.1c). This sequence of signaling steps favors the phosphorylation-dependent inactivation of proapoptotic factors, such as glycogen synthase kinase-3 (GSK-3), FKHR, a member of the fork head transcription factor family (West et al. 2003), and Bax (Xin and Deng 2005). As a consequence, nicotine and NNK attenuated the apoptosis induced by model treatments including exposure to etoposide or UV irradiation. Although these in vitro results, which are partially paralleled in vivo by activated PKB/Akt in human lung cancers in smokers (West et al. 2003), point to a growth-stimulating, tumor-promoting potential of nicotine, its role during carcinogenesis remains unclear because nicotine is considered to be neither genotoxic nor carcinogenic (for review, see Hecht 1999).

4.3.3 NF-κB

Regarding the proinflammatory signaling activities of CS, a controversy has emerged on the question of whether CS or CS-derived fractions are capable of *directly* activating the redox-sensitive and proinflammatory transcription factor NF-κB. Several reports describe a direct inhibitory effect of CS on NF-κB in vitro (Favatier and Polla 2001; Freed et al. 2003; Moodie et al. 2004; Vayssier et al. 1998b). As outlined above, this inhibitory effect was attributed mainly to the oxidative modification of Cys 62 of the p50 subunit of NF-κB by α,β-unsaturated aldehydes in CS, such as crotonaldehyde and acrolein, resulting in an impaired DNA-binding activity. In accordance with this concept (Fig. 4.1c), data describing the kinetics of the effect of CS on the DNA-binding activity of NF-κB in Swiss 3T3 fibroblasts in kinetic terms revealed a complex behavior with significantly decreased binding activities seen within the first 2 h of exposure (Gebel and Müller 2001). After 4–6 h of exposure, NF-κB DNA binding recovered, showing binding rates that were slightly elevated over controls (~2-fold). Rebinding of NF-κB was independent of inhibitory protein of κBα (IκBα) degradation but, as described above, correlated with the expression of thioredoxin reductase and the reavailability of reduced thioredoxin (Gebel and Müller 2001), the functional reductase of oxidized Cys 62 within the p50 subunit of NF-κB. Moreover, further studies revealed that aqueous extracts of CS significantly impaired the DNA-binding activities of NF-κB in 3T3 fibroblasts stimulated with tumor necrosis factor α (TNF-α) (Müller and Gebel, unpublished results), a phenomenon that was also described for A549 cells exposed to CS condensate (Moodie et al. 2004). These data clearly indicate that the *direct* response of NF-κB to CS is controlled by redox-dependent mechanisms rather than upstream signaling mechanisms, as has been described for proinflammatory cytokines such as TNF-α. Therefore, chronic inflammation related to CS exposure is, at least according to these data, of an *indirect* nature, e.g., caused by chromatin remodeling effects or cellular damage, resulting in necrosis and the consequent invasion of proinflammatory cells during chronic CS exposure. Finally, even nicotine was shown to interfere with NF-κB activation and cytokine expression in response to lipopolysaccharide (LPS) exposure in monocytic U937 cells, which, as stated by the authors, might explain the immunosuppressive activities observed in the context of CS exposure (Sugano et al. 1998).

The results of a CS-dependent inhibition of NF-κB DNA binding are, however, diametrically opposite to data showing that CS condensate *directly* activates NF-κB in cells of different cell lines (Anto et al. 2002). According to this report, the CS-dependent activation of NF-κB follows the "conventional" route, involving activation of IκB kinase (IKK) followed by degradation of IκBα (Fig. 4.1c). In fact, using various dominant negative mutants of signaling elements known to reside upstream from NF-κB activation, a CS-specific pathway very similar to the pathway of NF-κB stimulation by proinflammatory cytokines such as TNF α was delineated. As evidence of a direct activation of NF-κB by CS condensate, the collinear expression of COX-2 was reported in this study (Anto et al. 2002). Although NF-κB is a key regulator of *cox-2* expression, it is worth noting in this context, that in both the human system and the murine system, the 5'-flanking promoter region of *cox-2* is equipped with several other transcription factor consensus elements in addition to NF-κB-binding sites, including recognition sites for CAAT enhancer-binding protein-β (C/EBPβ) (Caivano et al. 2001; Nie et al. 2003). In fact, the gene coding for C/EBPβ has been shown to become significantly expressed by aqueous extracts of CS in 3T3 cells (Bosio et al. 2002), suggesting that this transcription factor might also be a potential candidate for *cox-2* upregulation seen in CS-exposed cells.

If, as indicated by the results of Anto et al. (2002), CS exposure is a direct inducer of NF-κB, these data would mean that cells and tissues might start a proinflammatory response essentially independent of inflammation-related cytokines released by cells of the immune system. Thus, the question of whether CS is a direct or indirect inducer of an inflammatory response is of fundamental significance, and further efforts should be made to reconcile the conflicting data described above.

4.4 CS-Induced Differential Gene Expression In Vitro and In Vivo

Since entering the post–genome era, with the parallel development of sophisticated tools such as real-time PCR and gene chip/microarray technologies to routinely characterize gene expression on a comprehensive and high throughput basis, the number of publications reporting on the effect of CS on the gene expression profile has steadily increased. As discussed below, in vitro and in vivo investigations making use of these new technologies have not only broadened our understanding of the mechanism of CS-dependent disease formation, but have also raised new questions. Before the scientific and methodological breakthroughs mentioned above, the affect of CS on transcriptional activity in CS-exposed cells and tissues focused mainly on the expression of single (model) genes, which was—and still is—often used as a tool in mode-of-action analysis, i.e., as a molecular reporter aimed at identifying cellular targets as well as CS-dependent compounds involved in the mechanism of gene expression.

4.4.1 CS-Induced Differential Gene Expression of Single (Model) Genes

One of the first genes identified as being strongly induced by CS was *hmox1*. The pronounced sensitivity of this antioxidant gene to CS was deduced from [^{35}S]-methionine protein labeling experiments performed in 3T3 fibroblasts exposed to aqueous extracts of CS (Müller and Gebel 1994). Although CS was found to generally exert a transient inhibitory effect on translation efficiency, the CS-dependent principal expression of a cytoplasmic protein of 32 kDa was observed, which was subsequently identified as HO-1 by Western blotting. These studies also demonstrated that CS-induced HO-1 expression is regulated at the transcriptional level (Müller and Gebel 1994). In fact, almost all studies addressing CS-dependent alteration in the gene expression profile in vitro and in vivo revealed *hmox1* (with some remarkable exceptions, see below) as the most efficiently upregulated gene within the spectrum of antioxidant and phase II-related genes (Table 4.1). In direct agreement with this emerging biological concept, the potential physiological relevance of *hmox1* expression consequent to CS exposure recently became evident when it was found that smokers exhibiting a genetically compromised inducibility of *hmox1* show an increased susceptibility to develop emphysema (Yamada et al. 2000). Based on the paramount antioxidant nature of the enzyme products provided by the HO pathway, i.e., biliverdin and bilirubin (via ubiquitous biliverdin reductase activity), which supply the cell with a kind of SOS redox buffer against an imbalanced redox homeostasis, and apparently because of the release of CO, which has been implicated in the resolution of inflammatory responses (Otterbein et al. 2000), several signaling pathways converge on diverse *cis* regulatory elements identified upstream to the transcriptional start site of *hmox1*. In mechanistic terms, these regulatory elements are part of a complex system consisting of a promoter with a proximal enhancer (E_p) and two distal enhancers (E1 and E2), which, in the murine system, are distributed over more than 10 kb upstream of the transcriptional start site (reviewed in Alam and Cook 2003; Choi and Alam 1996). This ternary system harbors a whole array of *cis* regulatory motifs addressing numerous transcription factors known to be involved in oxidative stress and inflammatory responses, including NF-κB, AP-1, ATF/CREB, Nrf2, and heat

Table 4.1 Selection of genes differentially expressed in connection with cigarette smoke exposure in respiratory tissue samples from animal and human studies, and from one in vitro study

Antioxidant				Xenobiotics metabolism			Inflammation/ emphysema			Miscellaneous		
	I.v.	Animal	Human		Animal	Human		Animal	Human		Animal	Human
hmox1	1	2, 3, 4		cyp1A1	2, 3, 3k, 4	6, 7	gro1/ cxcl1	2		fgfbp1	3	
nqo1		2, 3	7	cyp1B1	2, 3, 3k, 4	6, 7	c3		7↓, 9, 10	fgfr1	4	
gclc		2, 3	6, 7	cyp-2B1/2	2↓		cx3cl1		7↓, 8	gadd45 G	2, 3	
gclm		3	6, 7	cyp1A2	5		cxcl14	3		slc2a1	3	
gsr		3	6	aldh3A1	2, 3, 3k	7	S100A9	3		slc1a4	2, 3	
txnrd1		3	6, 7	adh7	3	6, 7	S100A8	2, 3		cdkn1A (p21)	3, 3k, 5	
txn	1		7				IL1R2	2, 3		IFi204	3k	
prdx1		2, 3	7	ugt1A7	2		IL4Rα	3, 3k		cdc25b	4	
ftl1		3		ugt2B12	2		IL6 st	5		cyclin D1	2↓, 5	
fth1	1	2	7	ugt1A6	2, 3, 4		tnfrsf7	4				
				ugt1A2	4, 5		cd3z	4		cct1	4, 5	
gpx2		3	6, 7	ugt1A10		7	ptgs2	3, 3k		cct3,4,6,8	4	
gpx3			6, 10↓				elf1	4		cct5	5	
				akr1B8	3							
pgd		3	6, 7	akr1C1		7	egr1	3k	8, 9	hspb1	4, 5	
g6pd		2, 3	6	akr1C2		7	fos	2↓, 3k	8, 9	hsf2	5	
				akr1C3		6, 7				dnajb4	5	
sod 2		2, 4		akr1B1		6	lox	3, 3k		dnajc1	5	
sod3		3					eln	3, 3k		dnajb9	5	
cat1		4		gstα4	3		col4a2	3				
				gstα2	3		spi2-2	3		casp7	4	
sqstm1		3, 4		gsto2	3		spi1-2	4↓		casp2	5	
				gstpi2	3		pai1	4		cad	5	
map3k6		3, 3k		gstpi1	2, 4		prtn3	4				
map2k4		4		gstA2		6	spi F1		9	ang2	5	
epas1		3					timp1	2	9	angpt1	5	
mafF		3		esd	3		muc-5AC		7			

Antioxidant			Xenobiotics metabolism			Inflammation/emphysema			Miscellaneous		
	I.v.	Animal	Human		Animal	Human		Animal	Human		Animal	Human
mafG		2	7	aox1	3		cyr61	3k	8	pirin		7
mafK	1			pdk4	3, 3k		ctgf		8	ca12		7
				lpl	3, 3k					ceacam6		7
mt1	1	3, 3k		fmo3	3k		mmp10		7↓			
mt2	1	3, 3k		tst	4		mmp2		9	slit2		7↓
mt1F			7↓	mdr1	4, 5		mmp7		10	slit1		7↓
mt1X			7↓	taldo1		6, 7	ctsB1	4	10	gas6		7↓
mt1G			7↓	tkt		6, 7	ctsK		9	tu3a		7↓

I.v. In vitro, ↓ repressed, *3k* data from nuclear factor erythroid 2-related factor 2 (Nrf2)$^{-/-}$ mice
Genes: **aldh3A1** aldehyde dehydrogenase family 3, subfamily A1; **adh7** alcohol dehydrogenase 7; **akr** aldo-keto reductase; **ang2** angiogenin-related protein; **angpt1** angiopoietin-1; **aox1** aldehyde oxidase 1; **c3** complement 3; **ca12** carbonic anhydrase XII; **cad** caspase-activated DNAse; **casp** caspase; **cat1** catalase 1; **cct** T-complex protein 1; **cd3z** CD3 antigen, zeta polypeptide; **cdc25b** M-phase inducer phosphatase 2; **cdkn1A** cyclin-dependent kinase inhibitor 1A (P21); **ceacam6** carcinoembryonic antigen-related cell adhesion molecule 6; **col4α2** procollagen, type IV, α2; **ctgf** connective tissue growth factor; **cts** cathepsin; **cyp** cytochrome p450; **cyr61** cysteine-rich protein 61; **cx3cl1** chemokine (C-X-3-C motif) ligand 1; **cxcl14** chemokine (C-X-C motif) ligand 14; **dnaj** DNAJ (Hsp40) homolog; **egr1** early growth response protein 1; **elf1** Ets-related transcription factor; **eln** tropoelastin; **epas1** endothelial PAS domain protein 1; **es10** esterase 10; **fgfr1** fibroblast growth factor receptor 1; **fgfbp1** fibroblast growth factor binding protein 1; **fmo3** flavin-containing monooxygenase 3; **fos** c-*fos* oncogene; **fth1** ferritin, heavy chain 1; **ftl1** ferritin, light chain 1; **g6pd** glucose-6-phosphate 1-dehydrogenase; **gadd45G** growth arrest and DNA-damage-inducible 45γ; **gas6** growth arrest-specific 6; **gclc** γ-glutamylcysteine synthetase (catalytic); **gclm** γ-glutamylcysteine synthetase (regulatory); **gpx** glutathione peroxidase; **gro1/cxcl1** chemokine (C-X-C motif) ligand 1; **gsr** glutathione reductase; **gst** glutathione S-transferase; **hmox1** heme oxygenase-1; **hsf2** heat shock transcription factor 2; **hspb1** heat shock 27-kDa protein; **IFi204** interferon-activated gene 204; **IL1R2** interleukin 1 receptor type II; **IL4Rα** interleukin 4 receptor α; **IL6st** interleukin 6 signal transducer; **lox** lysyl oxidase; **lpl** lipoprotein lipase; **maf** transcription factor MAF; **map2k4** mitogen-activated protein kinase kinase 4; **map3k6** mitogen-activated protein kinase kinase kinase 6; **mdr1** multidrug resistance protein 1; **mmp** matrix metalloproteinase; **mt** metallothionein; **muc5AC** mucin 5, subtypes A and C; **nqo1** NAD(P)H quinone oxidoreductase; **pai1** plasminogen activator inhibitor, serpine1; **pdk4** pyruvate dehydrogenase kinase, isoenzyme 4; **pgd** phosphogluconate dehydrogenase; **prdx1** peroxiredoxin 1; **prtn3** trypsin-chymotrypsin-related serine protease; **ptgs2** prostaglandin-endoperoxide synthase 2 (cyclooxygenase-2); **S100A9** S100 calcium-binding potein A9 (MRP-14); **S100A8** S100 calcium-binding protein A8 (MRP-8); **slc** solute carrier family; **slit** slit homolog (Drosophila); **sod2** superoxide dismutase 2 [mn]; **sod3** superoxide dismutase 3 (extracellular); **spi1-2** serine proteinase inhibitor 1-2, serpina1b; **spi2-2** serine proteinase inhibitor 2-2, serpina3n; **spiF1** serine proteinase inhibitor F1, serpinf1; **sqstm1** sequestosome 1; **taldo1** transaldolase 1; **timp1** tissue inhibitor of metalloproteinases 1; **tkt** transketolase; **tnfrsf7** tumor necrosis factor receptor superfamily, member 7, CD27; **tst** thiosulfate sulfurtransferase; **tu3A** tu3A protein; **txn** thioredoxin; **txnrd1** thioredoxin reductase 1; **ugt** UDP glycosyltransferase

References: *1* Bosio et al. (2002), *2* Gebel et al. (2004), *3* Rangasamy et al. (2004), *4* Izzotti et al. (2004a), *5* Izzotti et al. (2004b), *6* Hackett et al. (2003), *7* Spira et al. (2004b), *8* Ning et al. (2004), *9* Spira et al. (2004a), *10* Golpon et al. (2004)

shock factor-1. Current investigations in our laboratory have identified the activation of the transcription factor Nrf2 and its binding to three canonical ARE-like response elements, referred to as stress-responsive elements (StREs), present in both E1 and E2 as major (but not exclusive) contributing mechanism of the CS-induced *hmox1* expression (Knörr-Wittmann et al. 2005). These data correspond directly to recent experiments showing that CS-exposed $nrf2^{-/-}$ mice are prone to emphysema (Rangasamy et al. 2004), which, in turn, confirms the aforementioned observation that smokers harboring a genetic defect in the inducibility of *hmox1* are susceptible to emphysema (Yamada et al. 2000). In summary, these results clearly identify the Nrf2/*hmox1* pathway as a critical defense tool with respect to the development of CS-dependent emphysema and possibly other diseases.

Further characterization of the CS-induced *hmox1* expression in 3T3 fibroblasts (Müller and Gebel 1994) revealed that radicals produced by Fenton/Haber-Weiss chemistry, i.e., hydroxyl radicals, which are potential inducers of *hmox1* (Keyse and Tyrrell 1990) and which were formerly identified as causative principles in CS-mediated DNA strand break formation (Nakayama et al. 1985), could be excluded as a major source of activation. However, increasing the intracellular GSH content by the addition of NAC to the culture medium significantly attenuated the CS-dependent activation of *hmox1*, thus underlining once again the notion that thiol oxidation/modification plays a major role in CS-dependent stress signal initiation and gene expression.

Similar to *hmox1* expression, CS-induced activation of the *c-fos* protooncogene is not affected by inhibitors of hydroxyl radical formation produced by Fenton/Haber-Weiss chemistry but is sensitive to the exogenous addition of NAC (Müller 1995; Müller and Gebel 1998). The *c-fos* gene belongs to the family of stress-, growth-, inflammation-, and differentiation-related genes, whose protein product together with the protein encoded by the *c-jun* protooncogene forms the b-Zip transcription factor AP-1. Expression of *c-fos* represents one of the earliest measurable cellular responses to a variety of chemical and physical stimuli including growth factor treatment, exposure to tumor promoters, and oxidative stress (for review, see Karin 1995). Intriguingly, microarray-based experiments have demonstrated that upregulated expression of *c-fos* has been linked to the pathogenesis of CS-induced COPD (Ning et al. 2004; Spira et al. 2004a).

Studies on the mechanism of *c-fos* expression in 3T3 fibroblasts exposed to aqueous extracts of CS, in comparison to serum (growth factor)-stimulated cells, unraveled a complex regulation characterized by a moderate induction at the transcriptional level and paralleled by a significantly increased half life of the *c-fos* message ($t_{1/2}$ ≥2 h vs <20 min) (Müller 1995). These data suggest that water-soluble compounds delivered by CS interfere with the regulation of (protoonco)gene expression at at least two different regulatory levels, i.e., by promoter activation as a result of upstream stress signaling and, most probably, by interfering with enzymatic systems involved in controlling RNA turnover. For example, some crucial, growth-related mRNA species are subject to rapid turnover via distinct regulatory (AU-rich) elements present in the 3' untranslated region (3' UTR), which promote their deadenylation and eventually rapid degradation (for review, see Shim and Karin 2002).

Further investigations demonstrated that the complex mechanism of CS-dependent *c-fos* expression could be mimicked by exposing the cells to peroxynitrite, a highly reactive nitrogen species (Müller et al. 1997). Peroxynitrite, which is formed in aqueous solution from NO· and O_2^-·, was assumed to be a likely candidate in the *c-fos*-inducing mechanism because of large amounts of NO· delivered by the gas phase of CS and the formation of O_2^-· from quinone/hydroquinone-like redox systems, e.g., provided by dihydroxybenzenes in CS, such as catechol (Pryor and Stone 1993). Evidence for the involvement of peroxynitrite was corroborated by experiments showing that the CS-dependent activation of c-*fos* was sensitive to the presence of specific scavengers of NO· and O_2^{-}·, i.e., oxyhemoglobin and superoxide dismutase (SOD), respectively (Müller et al. 1997). The peroxynitrite concentration calculated as being present in aqueous solutions of CS prepared from the standard reference cigarette used in these investigations proved to be insufficient for inducing c-*fos* on its own. However, the addition of tobacco-related aldehydes, i.e., formaldehyde, acetaldehyde, and acrolein, also at CS-relevant concentrations, reestablished the effects originally seen with aqueous fractions of CS (Müller and Gebel 1998). Further mechanistic studies finally indicated that the presence of tobacco-related aldehydes significantly decreased the intracellular GSH content, which is obviously a prerequisite for peroxynitrite to interfere with crucial target molecules involved in the control of c-*fos* expression (Müller and Gebel 1998). Taken together, these data prove the complexity of the CS-dependent affects on diverse crucial cellular functions, i.e., regulation of transcriptional activity and RNA turnover, even by following the relatively simple experimental approach of exposing cells in culture to aqueous extracts of CS.

Beyond *hmox1* and c-*fos*, several other genes were identified as being induced by CS or CS-related fractions. For example, using cultured human monocytes, it was shown that aqueous extracts of CS upregulate a broad spectrum of genes coding for heat shock proteins (HSPs), including HSP70, HSP90, and HSP110, which, however, did not show any protective effect on CS-induced cytotoxicity (Pinot et al. 1997; Vayssier et al. 1998a). Surprisingly, the CS-dependent expression of *hsp* genes was not sensitive to inhibition by the addition of NAC, indicating that stress signaling pathways upstream to *hsp* expression are activated by CS-related compounds other than those involved in the CS-mediated -SH reactivity. A further interesting observation regarding CS-mediated cytotoxicity made during these investigations is the finding that the expression of the antiapoptotic protein Bcl2 was only seen in cells undergoing necrosis but not in apoptotic cells. In addition, although expression of HSP70 did not show a net effect on CS-mediated cell death, overexpression of HSP70 shifted the mechanism of cell death from necrosis to apoptosis (Vayssier et al. 1998a). However, regarding the ability of CS to induce HSP70, the data reported in these in vitro investigations (Pinot et al. 1997; Vayssier et al. 1998a) are in contrast to a report showing that CS does not induce HSP70 in vivo (Wong et al. 1995).

Finally, the CS-dependent expression of certain inflammation-related genes was also reported before gene expression could be studied on a comprehensive basis using DNA chip technology. For example, the expression and release of the chemoattractant cytokine IL-8 was reported in human bronchial epithelial cells exposed to aqueous extracts of CS in culture and confirmed by increased IL-8 concentrations detected in the bronchoalveolar fluid (BALF) of smokers (Mio et al. 1997). Interestingly, the IL-8 inducing activity of CS was partly attributable to the tobacco-related aldehydes acrolein and acetaldehyde. In the context of CS-induced expression of inflammation-related genes, it should be noted once again that CS is an inducer of the gene encoding the proinflammatory enzyme COX-2, see above.

4.4.2 CS-Induced Differential Gene Expression Studied by Gene Chip/Microarray Analysis

The deciphering of the whole human and several other genomes along with the development of highly sophisticated microarray technologies for routine application has revolutionized many areas of biological sciences, particularly the field of explorative gene expression. As a result, a steadily increasing number of manuscripts have been published reporting on the effect of CS on the human transcriptome and on the transcriptome of rodent model systems, including specific transgenic and knockout models displaying a genotype designed to provide information relevant to the elucidation of the mechanism of CS-dependent disease onset and development at the gene expression level. An attempt to provide an overall summary of the key findings reported in these manuscripts is presented in Table 4.1. However, it should be noted that the comparability of these data is limited by the different experimental approaches used, particularly with regard to the dose and type of CS (mainstream, sidestream, or a mixture of the two) and the study design (e.g., whether the exposure protocols included recovery periods or not) used for exposure, as well as with regard to the diversity of chip technologies applied (whether macroarray, cDNA microarray, or oligonucleotide-based microarray technology).

4.4.2.1 Studies in Rodent Systems

One of the first studies utilizing DNA chip technology to explore differential gene expression induced by CS was performed in murine 3T3 fibroblasts (Bosio et al. 2002). During this kinetic experiment, cells were exposed to subcytotoxic concentrations of aqueous extracts of CS for up to 24 h and profiled for differential gene expression by using a relatively small DNA chip covered with ~500 cDNA probes. As expected, the expression of antioxidant genes, such as *hmox1*, and genes encoding HSP105 and HSP90, was predominant (Bosio et al. 2002), thus confirming the data obtained from investigations on single target genes induced by CS (e.g., Müller and Gebel 1994; Pinot et al. 1997). In kinetic terms, the activation of antioxidant genes was preceded by the upregulation of genes encoding transcription factors implicated in a cellular stress response, such as members of the Jun family of transcription factors, whereas after 24 h, almost all genes returned to normal expression rates. However, the most important finding of this relatively simple approach in vitro was the discovery of an inflammation-related response, which was highlighted by the activation of *kc/gro1* (Bosio et al. 2002), the purported murine homologue of human *Il-8* (Bozic et al. 1994). The CS-dependent expression of this chemoattractant cytokine was subsequently confirmed at the protein level by a gradual increase of KC protein released by CS-exposed cells into the medium (Bosio et al. 2002). From an overall perspective, it appears important to note, that in principle, the CS-dependent signature of differential gene expression in vitro featuring a distinct antioxidant and inflammation-related response was generally observed in almost all microarray studies investigating the CS-induced differential gene expression in vivo.

Recently, in vivo rodent smoking models, including disease-prone transgenic and knockout murine lines, have been used to study the impact of CS (mainstream and sidestream CS) on the differential gene expression in cells of tissues of the respiratory tract. In one of these approaches, Sprague Dawley rats were exposed to relatively low doses of mainstream CS (100 µg TPM/l) following an acute (3 h)- and subchronic (3 h/day, 5 days/week, 3 weeks)-exposure design, with killing of the animals either immediately or after a recovery period of 20 h after (the last) exposure (Gebel et al. 2004). The analysis of differential gene expression induced by CS in the respiratory nasal epithelium (RNE) and in the lungs using a cDNA microarray covered with >2,000 cDNA probes revealed a distinct pattern, which, in general agreement with the results obtained in vitro (Bosio et al. 2002; see above), showed a similar, pronounced antioxidant character, extended by the complexity inherent to an in vivo environment. The antioxidant response was hallmarked by the strong expression of *hmox1*, but also included phase II-related genes such as *nqo1*, *γgcs* (as represented by the catalytic subunits *gclc* and *gclm*), and several genes encoding various isozymes of UDP-glucoronosyltransferases (Table 4.1), which are all, at least in part, transcriptionally regulated by Nrf2 (Nguyen et al. 2003; see above). However, in quantitative terms, there was a striking tissue-dependent difference in the strength of CS-induced antioxidant and phase II-related gene expression, with, in principle, significantly lower expression rates observed in the lungs in comparison to the RNE (Gebel et al. 2004). An obvious explanation for this phenomenon is the deposition gradient of CS-dependent Nrf2/stress gene-inducing compounds from the upper to the lower respiratory tract, whereas tissue-specific differences in the potential inducibility of these genes represent an alternate mechanism to account for this effect.

A further intriguing observation related to the CS-dependent activation of antioxidant and phase II-related genes is the finding that genes in this category demonstrate an adaptive expression behavior during repeated exposures, as indicated by significantly (2- to 5-fold) lower induction rates seen after subchronic versus acute exposure (Gebel et al. 2004). In mechanistic terms, this effect may be explained by a steadily decreasing sensitivity of Nrf2 to become activated by CS-dependent stressors over prolonged exposure periods. Consequently, this effect may gradually compromise the ability of cells of the respiratory tract to adequately respond to CS-dependent (oxidative) stress during chronic exposure, and may therefore be critically involved in CS-dependent diseases such as emphysema (see below). Because, alternatively, the expression activity of this particular subset of genes could also be controlled by the intracellular concentration of the corresponding proteins, quantitative protein analysis and determination of the enzymatic activities are required to clarify this critical issue.

The suggested critical role of the Nrf2-controlled antioxidant and phase II-related gene response as a major defensive cellular tool in CS-dependent disease development was recently elegantly demonstrated by using $nrf2^{-/-}$ mice (Rangasamy et al. 2004). Exposure to an artificial CS sidestream surrogate (89% sidestream smoke and 11% mainstream smoke) for up to 6 months showed that mice with a disrupted *nrf2* gene, in comparison to their wild-type littermates, were significantly more prone to developing emphysema, both with regard to the time of disease onset as well as to the severity of the disease. This was based on a more pronounced bronchoalveolar inflammation, increased levels of oxidant DNA damage, i.e., 8-oxo-7,8-dihydro-2'-deoxyguanosine (8-OH-dG), and an increased number of apoptotic alveolar septal cells in CS-exposed $nrf2^{-/-}$ mice as compared with CS-exposed wild-type mice (Rangasamy et al. 2004). Using microarray analysis, ~50 genes were identified, which remained unaffected in CS-exposed $nrf2^{-/-}$ mice but were relatively strongly induced in CS-treated wild-type littermates, including several phase II-related genes, such as those coding for enzymes involved in GSH metabolism, protective proteins, transcription factors, and, particularly, various antioxidant genes such as *hmox1* and thioredoxin reductase (Table 4.1). Thus, these data directly correspond to the finding that smokers exhibiting a genetically compromised inducibility of *hmox1* show an increased susceptibility to emphysema (Yamada et al. 2000). Scrutinizing the 5' flanking region of the transcriptional start site revealed that the vast majority of the genes presumptively controlled by Nrf2 are equipped with at least one ARE *cis* regulatory consensus sequence site (Rangasamy et al. 2004).

It should be noted, however, that a more thorough analysis of this report (Rangasamy et al. 2004) (including supplementary material) showed that some proinflammatory genes, such as *cox-2*, *cxcl14*, and *IL-1R*, were even more strongly induced in CS-exposed wild-type littermates rather than in smoke-treated $nrf2^{-/-}$ mice, indicating that the inflammation-related phenotype induced by CS in $nrf2^{-/-}$ mice is the result of a complex transcriptional network that is far from being completely understood. Nevertheless, data presented by Rangasamy et al. (2004) represent a major breakthrough in the efforts to link CS-dependent alterations in the gene expression pattern with CS-dependent disease formation, and future chronic studies using this knockout model will demonstrate whether extended exposure might also result in other CS-specific diseases.

In comparison to the distinct expression pattern—in kinetic and quantitative terms—observed for antioxidant and phase II-related genes in CS-exposed rats (Gebel et al. 2004), a completely different expression profile was obtained in the same study for CS-induced genes coding for phase I xenobiotic metabolizing enzymes. The differential expression of these genes was related to *cyp1b1*, *cyp2b1/2*, and, as described for the first time in the context of CS exposure, to the gene coding for aldehyde dehydrogenase type 3 subfamily A1 (ALDH3A1), as well as to *cyp1a1*, which in quantitative terms turned out to be the most strongly CS-dependently induced gene in CS-exposed Sprague Dawley rats, displaying an almost 200-fold induction in lung cells, (Gebel et al. 2004) (Table 4.1). Importantly, in contrast to the various antioxidant and phase II-related genes, the CS-dependent expression pattern of phase I-related genes, which are controlled by cytoplasmic receptors, such as AhR functioning through XRE (see above), does not show any indication of either a deposition gradient or an adaptive response. In this context, it is of note that, in principle, similar results for the expression of phase I-related genes were obtained in CS-exposed $nrf2^{-/-}$ mice, independent of the *nrf2* status (Rangasamy et al. 2004). In view of the paradoxical effects reported for AhR activation and *cyp1A1* expression (see Sect. 4.3.1), it is necessary to identify the role of these genes in the transcriptional network underlying CS-dependent disease onset and development. In this context, the identification of CS-dependent ligands resulting in the activation of, e.g., AhR, as well as the characterization of the CS-induced phenotype in *cyp1a1* knockout and *cyp1a1* overexpressing murine lines might be beneficial.

A further remarkable finding in the respiratory tract of CS-exposed rats (Gebel et al. 2004) was that both antioxidant and phase II- as well as phase I-related genes are controlled in a strict time-dependent manner. This conclusion was based on the fact that the CS-induced transcriptional changes observed immediately after exposure returned almost completely to normal in rats allowed to recover for 20 h, even after 3 weeks of repeated CS exposure. Finally, it should be stressed that subchronic exposure (3 weeks) to relatively low doses of CS is obviously not (yet) sufficient to induce inflammation-related genes. As expressed by a 4-fold upregulation of *gro1*, i.e., the gene encoding the functional rat homologue of *Il-8*, a weak proinflammatory response was only detectable in the lungs after 3 weeks of exposure, which, however, becomes strongly enhanced by the expression of a whole plethora of proinflammatory genes after extended exposure periods (Gebel et al., in preparation).

In two publications, Izzotti et al. (2004 a, b) report on the effect of CS in different specific murine model systems, using the same CS mixture as utilized by Rangasamy et al. (2004) and cDNA macroarray technology for monitoring gene expression. In the first study, SKH-1 hairless mice were exposed for 4 weeks to light and/or CS followed by determination of differential gene expression in the skin and in the lungs. Interestingly, regarding CS exposure, apart from a common phase I response, including the upregulation of *cyp1a1*, clear differences in the pattern of upregulated genes were observed in the two different tissues. In the skin, the expression pattern was characterized by the induction of DNA repair activities aimed at addressing the repair of 8-OH-dG lesions and genes involved in cell cycle regulation, e.g., GADD45 and GADD153, whereas in the lungs, activities aimed at counteracting (oxidative) stress, such as catalase 1 and SOD2 precursor, and at activating the immune response were more prevalent (Izzotti et al. 2004a). In addition, a significant downregulation of the α-1-antitrypsin 1-2 precursor gene was observed in the lungs of CS-exposed mice, which, together with the upregulation of the neutrophil-specific genes cathepsin b (*ctsb*) and proteinase 3 (*prtn3*) (encoding a serine protease), clearly points to an emphysematous response. Although these findings demonstrate tissue-specific effects in the response to cell-stressing microenvironmental changes, it should be noted that statistically significant induction factors were usually between two and three, possibly because of the limited dynamic range provided by cDNA macroarray technology.

In the second study published by Izzotti et al. (2004b), effects of CS on the gene expression in lung tissues are described for F_1 mice produced from crossing lung tumor-prone A/J mice, a proposed surrogate animal model for CS-dependent lung tumor formation (e.g., Witschi et al. 1997), with mice carrying a dominant negative germline *p53* mutation. It was shown that lung tissue cells of the $p53^{+/-}$ offspring, when exposed for 4 weeks to CS, are compromised in upregulating key genes in executing apoptosis, such as caspase-2 precursor, whereas genes coding for growth factors (e.g., vascular endothelial growth factor [VEGF] and PDGF), growth-related transcription factors (various isozymes of PKC), and inflammatory proteins, such as MIP1α, were significantly (2- to 3-fold) induced (Izzotti et al. 2004b). However, the *p53* genotype obviously does not interfere with the CS-triggered transcriptional response of the differential expression of phase I-related genes, as exemplified by the similar high expression rates seen for *cyp1a2* (not seen in CS-exposed rats [Gebel et al. 2004] in mutant [$p53^{+/-}$] and wild-type [$p53^{+/+}$] mice [Izzotti et al. 2004b]). Thus, these results further support the outstanding role of the p53 tumor suppressor in cell cycle regulation and apoptosis induction in stressed cells and tissues in general and for CS-exposed systems in particular, even in a gene dosage-dependent context.

4.4.2.2 Studies in Humans

The first study investigating differential gene expression in smokers and nonsmokers, utilizing microarray technology, focused on differences in the antioxidant gene expression profile in tissues of the upper respiratory tract (Hackett et al. 2003). By analyzing fresh samples of airway epithelium obtained by airway brushing, 44 antioxidant genes were identified to be differentially expressed in phenotypically healthy chronic smokers (>20 pack years) and nonsmokers. Out of these 44 genes, significantly upregulated genes in smokers mainly encode proteins involved in GSH metabolism, such as γGCS, glucose metabolism, such as alcohol dehydrogenase 7 and aldo-keto reductase (also seen in CS-exposed mice [Rangasamy et al. 2004]), and redox homeostasis, including thioredoxin reductase 1 (Hackett et al. 2003) (Table 4.1). Because the gene encoding thioredoxin was not differentially expressed, the latter result corresponds well to data from in vitro and in vivo smoking models (Gebel and Müller 2001; Gebel et al., in preparation; Rangasamy et al. 2004). Surprisingly, there was no mention of the expression of other major CS-related antioxidant target genes identified in rodent smoking models, e.g., *hmox1* and *nqo1*. Finally, a noteworthy finding made during these investigations is the high interindividual variability regarding the magnitude of the response.

The most extensive and thorough study on smoking-related differential gene expression in humans so far has been reported by Spira et al. (2004b). These authors, by also using sample material obtained from bronchoscopy, analyzed the airway transcriptome from current chronic smokers, former smokers, and never smokers, in the context of several variables, such as cumulative exposure, sex, age, and race. Employing DNA microarrays covering ~2,500 transcripts, 97 genes were identified to be significantly differentially regulated in current smokers and nonsmokers, which, according to hierarchical cluster analysis, revealed a specific signature of CS exposure.

A principal finding of this study (Spira et al. 2004b) showed that the spectrum of CS-dependently upregulated genes encoding phase I as well as phase II xenobiotics metabolizing and antioxidant enzymes is consistent with in vitro and in vivo rodent smoking models (Gebel et al. 2004 and references cited therein), thus underlining the suitability of these animal systems for investigating the toxicological effects of CS exposure at the transcriptional level. For example, the antioxidant and phase II-related gene expression in smokers covered, in addition to the several genes implicated in GSH metabolism, the upregulation of *nqo1* and thioredoxin reductase, whereas the phase I response was hallmarked by the strong induction of *cyp1b1* and, most intriguingly, of *aldh3a1* (Table 4.1). Interestingly, *cyp1a1* expression was obviously subject to strong interindividual variability, thus pointing to a high polymorphic variability. However, it is worth noting that, in contrast to the data obtained from rodent smoking models, *hmox1* is missing from the spectrum of differentially expressed genes in human smokers, which, based on the fact that the samples were derived from chronic smokers, might be explained by the adaptation phenomenon seen in rats subchronically exposed to CS (Gebel et al. 2004). Moreover, also in contrast to data from animal studies, thioredoxin was found to be slightly but significantly induced in the airway epithelium of human smokers. Most importantly, however, genes differentially expressed between smokers and never smokers also included several putative oncogenes, which were found to be upregulated in smokers, whereas, conversely, candidate tumor suppressor genes tended to be suppressed, as was also seen for genes supposed to be involved in the regulation of inflammation (Table 4.1). However, the expression of cystatin, which has been shown to correlate with tumor growth and inflammation, significantly correlated with the number of pack years, which renders this gene a potential biomarker of dose and effect.

Apart from these differences between smokers and never smokers, the work by Spira et al. (2004b) uncovered some remarkable characteristics in the gene expression profile of former smokers. For example, cluster analysis of the expression profiles of smokers with a smoking cessation period of more than 2 years were closely related to those of never smokers, whereas profiles of smokers with a smoking cessation period of less than 2 years were closely related to those of current smokers. These results show that most of the CS-specific effects induced at the transcriptional level are reversible, and, therefore, correlate with epidemiological data showing a decreasing relative risk of lung cancer formation in quitters, which is directly proportional to the period after terminating CS exposure (Peto et al. 2000). However, independent of the length of smoking cessation, the relative risk to former smokers of developing lung cancer does not completely return to the level of never smokers (but asymptotically decreases to a relative risk of ~2 [Peto et al. 2000]), which is indicative of at least some irreversible changes induced during chronic CS exposure. Intriguingly, the expression profiles recorded from former smokers uncovered 13 genes that did not return to normal but retained the expression behavior specific for current smokers, even in those individuals who had stopped smoking for 20–30 years (Spira et al. 2004b). Most interestingly, beyond several putative oncogenes and tumor suppressor genes, this particular group of genes also includes three metallothionein genes (four metallothionein isoforms are known so far in humans), which remain decreased in former smokers. The activation of metallothionein genes, which was reported for CS-exposed model systems in vitro (Bosio et al. 2002) and in vivo (Gilks et al. 1998; Rangasamy et al. 2004; Gebel el al. in preparation), has been implicated as a transient response to any form of stress or injury providing cytoprotective action. Based on its unique zinc/cysteine thiolate coordination, which renders the complex oxidoreductive (Maret and Vallee 1998), metallothionein proteins provide antioxidant protection, particularly regarding the binding and detoxification of heavy metal ions such as cadmium. In addition, metallothionein proteins have been shown to be involved not only in cell proliferation and apoptosis, but also in pathophysiologic processes such as chemoresistance and radiotherapy resistance (for review, see Theocharis et al. 2003). Hence, because of the obvious inability to express efficiently these cytoprotective proteins, former smokers may be compromised in adequately responding to any stressing situation, whereas current smokers, lacking metallothionein expression, are at further increased risk of developing CS-related diseases.

In summary, data presented by Spira et al. (2004b) show that CS exposure activates antioxidant, metabolizing, and host defense functions in the airway epithelium of the upper respiratory tract. In general, these findings are consistent with data obtained from rodent smoking models.

Finally, in addition to the reports describing the effects of CS exposure at the transcriptional level in phenotypically healthy smokers, other publications compare the gene expression profile of diseased tissue with healthy or only mildly affected tissues in smokers with regard to emphysema (Golpon et al. 2004; Ning et al. 2004; Spira et al. 2004a) or diseased tissues in smokers and nonsmokers suffering from lung adenocarcinoma (Powell et al. 2003). Accordingly, expression data reported in these publications are mostly confined to the pathophysiologic process of disease formation and do not reflect the *direct* affect of CS or CS constituents on the gene expression profile. For example, gene expression patterns obtained from emphysematous tissues revealed the upregulation of c-*fos* and *egr1* (Ning et al. 2004; Spira et al. 2004a), which was not seen in tissue samples obtained from healthy smokers or CS-exposed wild-type animals. However, most importantly, both genes were significantly increased in emphysematous-prone $nrf2^{-/-}$ mice (Rangasamy et al. 2004), thus impressively corroborating the relevance of the Nrf2 pathway in the cellular defense against CS-induced stress.

4.5 Concluding Remarks

CS harbors a pronounced (oxidative) stress-inducing potential, which, based on its complex composition, affects exposed cells in a pleiotropic way. Hence, CS-caused effects are reported on small biomolecules, proteins, DNA, higher organized complex structures (such as the cytoskeleton and membranes), and organelles (such as mitochondria and the ER), thereby affecting all tissue and cellular compartments from the extracellular matrix to the nucleus. Moreover, CS-specific effects are *direct*, e.g., as reflected by damage inflicted on proteins, membrane lipids, or DNA, as well as *indirect*, e.g., resulting from imbalance of redox homeostasis or signaling activities. It can be assumed that the sum of these effects determines the pathobiologic activity of CS and, according to improved medicinal and extended (molecular) epidemiological research, it is not surprising that the number of diseases linked to CS exposure has considerably increased (US Department of Health and Human Services 2004). However, it is also obvious that because of the chemical complexity inherent in CS, any mode-of-action analysis must be limited. This dilemma is further intensified by the lack of suitable animal model systems, especially with regard to CS-induced lung cancer formation.

Nevertheless, research over the past decades, profiting from immense progress in genome research and the development of sophisticated technical tools, has unraveled some principal mechanisms that provide a first insight into the biological activities of CS at the subcellular level. For example, previous and recent experiments have demonstrated over and over again that the -SH reactivity inherent to CS, which is characteristic to a large extent for components of both the gas phase and the particulate phase, plays a major role in interfering with crucial cellular and tissue functions. In fact, cells are particularly sensitive to this xenobiotic activity, because myriad cellular functions are controlled by functional -SH groups presented by critical protein cysteine residues. Hence, with the development of DNA microarray technologies and by using techniques to selectively knockout or silence specific genes, the Nrf2 pathway, which is controlled via the -SH-sensitive cytosolic inhibitor Keap1, was identified to be a major target of CS exposure (Knörr-Wittmann et al. 2005) and could be directly linked to a CS-related disease phenotype, i.e., emphysema (Rangasamy et al. 2004). Clearly, this experimental approach, which would be even more improved by integrating proteomics research tools, may be paradigmatic for the investigation of other CS-related pathophysiologic effects, for example, to elucidate the yet unsolved issue of how the CS-induced phase I response affects CS-dependent lung tumor formation. Finally, using this paradigmatic approach, we should be able to define specific biomarkers of disease by scrutinizing gene expression profiles using bioinformatics tools.

Acknowledgements

We thank Lynda Conroy for editorial support and Michaela Woiwode for help in preparing the manuscript.

References

Abate C, Patel L, Rauscher FJ, III, Curran T (1990) Redox regulation of fos and jun DNA-binding activity in vitro. Science 249:1157–1161

Abdelmohsen K, Gerber PA, von Montfort C, Sies H, Klotz L-O (2003) Epidermal growth factor receptor is a common mediator of quinone-induced signaling leading to phosphorylation of Connexin-43: role of glutathione and tyrosine phosphatases. J Biol Chem 278:38360–38367

Adler V, Yin Z, Tew KD, Ronai Z (1999) Role of redox potential and reactive oxygen species in stress signaling. Oncogene 18:6104–6111

Alam J, Cook JL (2003) Transcriptional regulation of the heme oxygenase-1 gene via the stress response element pathway. Curr Pharm Des 9:2499–2511

Alam J, Wicks C, Stewart D, Gong PF, Touchard C, Otterbein S, Choi AMK, Burow ME, Tou JS (2000) Mechanism of heme oxygenase-1 gene activation by cadmium in MCF-7 mammary epithelial cells—role of p38 kinase and Nrf2 transcription factor. J Biol Chem 275:27694–27702

Anto RJ, Mukhopadhyay A, Shishodia S, Gairola CG, Aggarwal BB (2002) Cigarette smoke condensate activates nuclear transcription factor-κB through phosphorylation and degradation of IκBα: correlation with induction of cyclooxygenase-2. Carcinogenesis 23:1511–1518

Arnér ESJ, Holmgren A (2000) Physiological functions of thioredoxin and thioredoxin reductase. Eur J Biochem 267:6102–6109

Arredondo J, Chernyavsky AI, Marubio LM, Beaudet AL, Jolkovsky DL, Pinkerton KE, Grando SA (2005) Receptor-mediated tobacco toxicity: regulation of gene expression through α3β2 nicotinic receptor in oral epithelial cells. Am J Pathol 166:597–613

Aslund F, Beckwith J (1999) Bridge over troubled waters: Sensing stress by disulfide bond formation. Cell 96:751–753

Barnes PJ (2004) Mediators of chronic obstructive pulmonary disease. Pharmacol Rev 56:515–548

Bartsch H, Petruzzelli S, De Flora S, Hietanen E, Camus A-M, Castegnaro M, Alexandrov K, Rojas M, Saracci R, Giuntini C (1992) Carcinogen and metabolism in human lung tissues and the effect of tobacco smoking: results from a case-control multicenter study of lung cancer patients. Environ Health Perspect 98:119–124

Bergelson S, Pinkus R, Daniel V (1994) Intracellular glutathione levels regulate Fos/Jun induction and activation of glutathione S-transferase gene expression. Cancer Res 54:36–40

Bilimoria MH, Ecobichon DJ (1992) Protective antioxidant mechanisms in rat and guinea pig tissues by acute exposure to cigarette smoke. Toxicology 72:131–144

Blair IA (2001) Lipid hydroperoxide-mediated DNA damage. Exp Gerontol 36:1473–1481

Bloom D, Dhakshinamoorthy S, Jaiswal AK (2002) Site-directed mutagenesis of cysteine to serine in the DNA binding region of Nrf2 decreases its capacity to upregulate antioxidant response element-mediated expression and antioxidant induction of NAD(P)H:quinone oxidoreductase1 gene. Oncogene 21:2191–2200

Bloom DA, Jaiswal AK (2003) Phosphorylation of Nrf2 at Ser40 by protein kinase C in response to antioxidants leads to the release of Nrf2 from INrf2, but is not required for Nrf2 stabilization/accumulation in the nucleus and transcriptional activation of antioxidant response element-mediated NAD(P)H:quinone oxidoreductase-1 gene expression. J Biol Chem 278:44675–44682

Bosio A, Knörr C, Janssen U, Gebel S, Haussmann HJ, Müller T (2002) Kinetics of gene expression profiling in Swiss 3T3 cells exposed to aqueous extracts of cigarette smoke. Carcinogenesis 23:741–748

Bozic CR, Gerard NP, Uexkull-Guldenband C, Kolakowski LF Jr, Conklyn MJ, Breslow R, Showell HJ, Gerard C (1994) The murine interleukin 8 type B receptor homologue and its ligands. Expression and biological characterization. J Biol Chem 269:29355–29358

Caivano M, Gorgoni B, Cohen P, Poli V (2001) The induction of cyclooxygenase-2 mRNA in macrophages is biphasic and requires both CCAAT enhancer-binding proteinβ (C/EBPβ) and C/EBPδ transcription factors. J Biol Chem 276:48693–48701

Chakravarthi S, Bulleid NJ (2004) Glutathione is required to regulate the formation of native disulfide bonds within proteins entering the secretory pathway. J Biol Chem 279:39872–39879

Chen S, Operana T, Bonzo J, Nguyen N, Tukey RH (2005) ERK kinase inhibition stabilizes the aryl hydrocarbon receptor: implications for transcriptional activation and protein degradation. J Biol Chem 280:4350–4359

Choi AMK, Alam J (1996) Heme oxygenase-1: function, regulation, and implication of a novel stress-inducible protein in oxidant-induced lung injury. Am J Respir Cell Mol Biol 15:9–19

Chuang SM, Wang IC, Yang JL (2000) Roles of JNK, p38 and ERK mitogen-activated protein kinases in the growth inhibition and apoptosis induced by cadmium. Carcinogenesis 21:1423–1432

Cracowski JL, Durand T, Bessard G (2002) Isoprostanes as a biomarker of lipid peroxidation in humans: physiology, pharmacology and clinical implications. Trends Pharmacol Sci 23:360–366

Cullinan SB, Zhang D, Hannink M, Arvisais E, Kaufman RJ, Diehl JA (2003) Nrf2 is a direct PERK substrate and effector of PERK-dependent cell survival. Mol Cell Biol 23:7198–7209

Cullinan SB, Gordan JD, Jin J, Harper JW, Diehl JA (2004) The Keap1-BTB protein is an adaptor that bridges Nrf2 to a Cul3-based E3 Ligase: oxidative stress sensing by a Cul3-Keap1 ligase. Mol Cell Biol 24:8477–8486

D'Alessio M, Cerella C, Amici C, Pesce C, Coppola S, Fanelli C, De Nicola M, Cristofanon S, Clavarino G, Bergamaschi A, Magrini A, Gualandi G, Ghibelli L (2004) Glutathione depletion up-regulates Bcl-2 in BSO-resistant cells. FASEB J 18:1609–1611

Dalton TP, Shertzer HG, Puga A (1999) Regulation of gene expression by reactive oxygen. Annu Rev Pharmacol Toxicol 39:67–101

De Flora S, Izzotti A, D'Agostini F, Balansky RM (2001) Mechanisms of N-acetylcysteine in the prevention of DNA damage and cancer, with special reference to smoking-related end-points. Carcinogenesis 22:999–1013

Demple B, Herman T, Chen DS (1991) Cloning and expression of APE, the cDNA encoding the major human apurinic endonuclease: Definition of family of DNA repair enzymes. Proc Natl Acad Sci U S A 88:11450–11454

Denison MS, Nagy SR (2003) Activation of the aryl hydrocarbon receptor by structurally diverse exogenous and endogenous chemicals. Annu Rev Pharmacol Toxicol 43:309–334

Dertinger SD, Nazarenko DA, Silverstone AE, Gasiewicz TA (2001) Aryl hydrocarbon receptor signaling plays a significant role in mediating benzo[a]pyrene- and cigarette smoke condensate-induced cytogenic damage in vivo. Carcinogenesis 22:171–177

Ding X, Kaminsky LS (2003) Human extrahepatic cytochromes p450: function in xenobiotic metabolism and tissue-selective chemical toxicity in the respiratory and gastrointestinal tracts. Annu Rev Pharmacol Toxicol 43:149–173

Dinkova-Kostova AT, Holtzclaw WD, Cole RN, Itoh K, Wakabayashi N, Katoh Y, Yamamoto M, Talalay P (2002) Direct evidence that sulfhydryl groups of Keap1 are the sensors regulating induction of phase 2 enzymes that protect against carcinogens and oxidants. Proc Natl Acad Sci U S A 99:11908–11913

Eferl R, Wagner EF (2003) AP-1: A double-edged sword in tumorigenesis. Nat Rev Cancer 3:859–868

Escargueil-Blanc I, Salvayre R, Vacaresse N, Jurgens G, Darblade B, Arnal JF, Parthasarathy S, Negre-salvayre A (2001) Mildly oxidized LDL induces activation of platelet-derived growth factor β-receptor pathway. Circulation 104:1814–1821

Favatier F, Polla BS (2001) Tobacco-smoke-inducible human haem oxygenase-1 gene expression: role of distinct transcription factors and reactive oxygen intermediates. Biochem J 353:475–482

Fenner ML, Braven J (1968) The mechanism of carcinogenesis by tobacco smoke. Further experimental evidence and a prediction from the thiol-defence hypothesis. Br J Cancer 22:474–479

Fernandes AP, Holmgren A (2004) Glutaredoxins: glutathione-dependent redox enzymes with functions far beyond a simple thioredoxin backup system. Antioxid Redox Signal 6:63–74

Fiers W, Beyaert R, Declerq W, Vandenabeele P (1999) More than one way to die: apoptosis, necrosis and reactive oxygen damage. Oncogene 18:7719–7730

Flohé L, Brigelius-Flohé R, Saliou C, Traber MG, Packer L (1997) Redox regulation of NF-κB activation. Free Radic Biol Med 22:1115–1126

Freed BM, Ouyang Y, Rosano TG, Mccue J, Zheng J, Yang Y, Pyatt DW, Lazis S, Irons RD (2003) Suppression of inflammatory cytokine production by cigarette smoke is mediated by acrolein. Toxicologist 72:173

Gaiddon C, Moorthy NC, Prives C (1999) Ref-1 regulates the transactivation and pro-apoptotic functions of p53 in vivo. EMBO J 18:5609–5621

Ganther HE (1999) Selenium metabolism, selenoproteins and mechanisms of cancer prevention: complexities with thioredoxin reductase. Carcinogenesis 20:1657–1666

Gebel S, Gerstmayer B, Bosio A, Haussmann HJ, Miert EV, Müller T (2004) Gene expression profiling in respiratory tissues from rats exposed to mainstream cigarette smoke. Carcinogenesis 25:169–178

Gebel S, Müller T (2001) The activity of NF-κB in Swiss 3T3 cells exposed to aqueous extracts of cigarette smoke is dependent on thioredoxin. Toxicol Sci 59:75–81

Gensch E, Gallup M, Sucher A, Li D, Gebremichael A, Lemjabbar H, Mengistab A, Dasari V, Hotchkiss J, Harkema J, Basbaum C (2004) Tobacco smoke control of mucin production in lung cells requires oxygen radicals AP-1 and JNK. J Biol Chem 279:39085–39093

Gilks CB, Price K, Wright JL, Churg A (1998) Antioxidant gene expression in rat lung after exposure to cigarette smoke. Am J Pathol 152:269–278

Golpon HA, Coldren CD, Zamora MR, Cosgrove GP, Moore MD, Tuder RM, Geraci MW, Voelkel NF (2004) Emphysema lung tissue gene expression profiling. Am J Respir Cell Mol Biol 31:595–600

Gopalakrishna R, Chen Z, Gundimeda U (1994) Tobacco smoke tumor promoters, catechol and hydroquinone, induce oxidative regulation of protein kinase C and influence invasion and metastasis of lung carcinoma cells. Proc Natl Acad Sci U S A 91:12233–12237

Grafström RC (1994) Pathobiological effects of acetaldehyde in cultured human epithelial cells and fibroblasts. Carcinogenesis 15:985–990

Green GM (1968) Cigarette smoke: protection of alveolar macrophages by glutathione and cysteine. Science 162:810–811

Hackett NR, Heguy A, Harvey B-G, O'Connor TP, Luettich K, Flieder DB, Kaplan R, Crystal RG (2003) Variability of antioxidant-related gene expression in the airway epithelium of cigarette smokers. Am J Respir Cell Mol Biol 29:331–343

Haddad JJ (2002) Antioxidant and prooxidant mechanisms in the regulation of redox(y)-sensitive transcription factors. Cell Signal 14:879–897

Harper R, Chang MM, Yoneda K, Pan R, Reddy SP, Wu R (2001) Activation of nuclear factor-κB transcriptional activity in airway epithelial cells by thioredoxin but not by N-acetyl-cysteine and glutathione. Am J Respir Cell Mol Biol 25:178–185

Hayashi T, Ueno Y, Okamoto T (1993) Oxidoreductive regulation of nuclear factor κB—involvement of a cellular reducing catalyst thioredoxin. J Biol Chem 268:11380–11388

Hecht SS (1999) Tobacco smoke carcinogens and lung cancer. J Nat Cancer Inst 91:1194–1210

Hentze H, Schmitz I, Latta M, Krueger A, Krammer PH, Wendel A (2002) Glutathione dependence of caspase-8 activation at the death-inducing signaling complex. J Biol Chem 277:5588–5595

Heusch WL, Maneckjee R (1998) Signalling pathways involved in nicotine regulation of apoptosis of human lung cancer cells. Carcinogenesis 19:551–556

Hirota K, Matsui M, Iwata S, Nishiyama A, Mori K, Yodoi J (1997) AP-1 transcriptional activity is regulated by a direct association between thioredoxin and Ref-1. Proc Natl Acad Sci U S A 94:3633–3638

Holmgren A (1989) Thioredoxin and glutaredoxin systems. J Biol Chem 264:13963–13966

Horton ND, Biswal SS, Corrigan LL, Bratta J, Kehrer JP (1999) Acrolein causes inhibitor κB-independent decreases in nuclear factor κB activation in human lung adenocarcinoma (A549) cells. J Biol Chem 274:9200–9206

Huang H-C, Nguyen T, Pickett CB (2000) Regulation of the antioxidant response element by protein kinase C-mediated phosphorylation of NF-E2-related factor 2. Proc Natl Acad Sci U S A 97:12475–12480

Huang H-C, Nguyen T, Pickett CB (2002) Phosphorylation of Nrf2 at Ser-40 by protein kinase C regulates antioxidant response element-mediated transcription. J Biol Chem 277:42769–42774

Izzotti A, Cartiglia C, Longobardi M, Balansky RM, D'Agostini F, Lubet RA, De Flora S (2004a) Alterations of gene expression in skin and lung of mice exposed to light and cigarette smoke. FASEB J 18:1559–1561

Izzotti A, Cartiglia C, Longobardi M, Bagnasco M, Merello A, You M, Lubet RA, De Flora S (2004b) Gene expression in the lung of p53 mutant mice exposed to cigarette smoke. Cancer Res 64:8566–8572

Janssen YMW (1995) Induction of c-*fos* and c-*jun* proto-oncogene expression by asbestos is ameliorated by *N*-acetyl-L-cysteine in mesothelial cells. Cancer Res 55:2085–2089

Jin Z, Gao F, Flagg T, Deng X (2004) Nicotine induces multi-site phosphorylation of Bad in association with suppression of apoptosis. J Biol Chem 279:23837–23844

Karin M (1995) The regulation of AP-1 activity by mitogen-activated protein kinases. J Biol Chem 270:16483–16486

Kehrer JP, Biswal SS (2000) The molecular effects of acrolein. Toxicol Sci 57:6–15

Keyse SM, Tyrrell RM (1990) Induction of the heme oxygenase gene in human skin fibroblasts by hydrogen peroxide and UVA (365 nm) radiation: evidence for the involvement of the hydroxyl radical. Carcinogenesis 11:787–791

Kim YC, Yamaguchi Y, Kondo N, Masutani H, Yodoi J (2003) Thioredoxin-dependent redox regulation of the antioxidant responsive element (ARE) in electrophile response. Oncogene 22:1860–1865

Knörr-Wittmann C, Hengstermann A, Gebel S, Alam J, Müller T (2005) Characterization of Nrf2 activation and heme oxygenase-1 expression in NIH3T3 cells exposed to aqueous extracts of cigarette smoke. Free Radic Biol Med 39:1438–1448

Kobayashi A, Kang MI, Okawa H, Ohtsuji M, Zenke Y, Chiba T, Igarashi K, Yamamoto M (2004) Oxidative stress sensor Keap1 functions as an adaptor for Cul3-based E3 ligase to regulate proteasomal degradation of Nrf2. Mol Cell Biol 24:7130–7139

Koch A, Giembycz M, Stirling RG, Lim S, Adcock I, Wassermann K, Erdmann E, Chung KF (2004) Effect of smoking on MAP kinase-induced modulation of IL-8 in human alveolar macrophages. Eur Respir J 23:805–812

Kumagai T, Kawamoto Y, Nakamura Y, Hatayama I, Satoh K, Osawa T, Uchida K (2000) 4-hydroxy-2-nonenal, the end product of lipid peroxidation, is a specific inducer of cyclooxygenase-2 gene expression. Biochem Biophys Res Commun 273:437–441

Kumagai T, Nakamura Y, Osawa T, Uchida K (2002) Role of p38 mitogen-activated protein kinase in the 4-hydroxy-2-nonenal-induced cyclooxygenase-2 expression. Arch Biochem Biophys 397:240–245

Lando D, Pongratz I, Poellingers L, Whitelaw ML (2000) A redox mechanism controls differential DNA binding activities of hypoxia-inducible factor (HIF) 1α and the HIF-like factor. J Biol Chem 275:4618–4627

Lange R (1961) Inhibiting effect of tobacco smoke on some crystalline enzymes. Science 134:52–53

Leonarduzzi G, Robbesyn F, Poli G (2004) Signaling kinases modulated by 4-hydroxynonenal. Free Radic Biol Med 37:1694–1702

Leuchtenberger C, Leuchtenberger R, Zbinden I (1974) Gas vapour phase constituents and SH reactivity of cigarette smoke influence lung cultures. Nature 247:565–567

Leuchtenberger C, Leuchtenberger R, Zbinden I, Schleh E (1976) SH Reactivity of cigarette smoke and its correlation with carcinogenic effects on hamster lung cultures. Soz Praventivmed 21:47–50

Levonen AL, Landar A, Ramachandran A, Ceaser EK, Dickinson DA, Zanoni G, Morrow JD, Darley-Usmar VM (2004) Cellular mechanisms of redox cell signalling: role of cysteine modification in controlling antioxidant defences in response to electrophilic lipid oxidation products. Biochem J 378:373–382

Liu H, Nishitoh H, Ichijo H, Kyriakis JM (2000) Activation of apoptosis signal-regulating kinase 1 (ASK1) by tumor necrosis factor receptor-associated factor 2 requires prior dissociation of the ASK1 inhibitor thioredoxin. Mol Cell Biol 20:2198–2208

Mai H, May S, Gao F, Jin Z, Deng X (2003) A functional role for nicotine in Bcl2 phosphorylation and suppression of apoptosis. J Biol Chem 278:1886–1891

Maines MD (1992) Heme oxygenase: clinical applications and functions. CRC Press, Boca Raton, FL

Mallis RJ, Hamann MJ, Zhao W, Zhang T, Hendrich S, Thomas JA (2002) Irreversible thiol oxidation in carbonic anhydrase III: protection by S-glutathiolation and detection in aging rats. Biol Chem Hoppe-Seyler 383:649–662

Maneckjee R, Minna JD (1994) Opioids induce while nicotine suppresses apoptosis in human lung cancer cells. Cell Growth Diff 5:1033–1040

Marathe GK, Prescott SM, Zimmerman GA, McIntyre TM (2001) Oxidized LDL contains inflammatory PAF-like phospholipids. Trends Cardiovasc Med 11:139–142

Maret W, Vallee BL (1998) Thiolate ligands in metallothionein confer redox activity on zinc clusters. Proc Natl Acad Sci U S A 95:3478–3482

Marwick JA, Kirkham PA, Stevenson CS, Danahay H, Giddings J, Butler K, Donaldson K, MacNee W, Rahman I (2004) Cigarette smoke alters chromatin remodeling and induces proinflammatory genes in rat lungs. Am J Respir Cell Mol Biol 31:633–642

Matthews JR, Wakasugi N, Virelizier JL, Yodoi J, Hay RT (1992) Thioredoxin regulates the DNA binding activity of NF-κB by reduction of a disulphide bond involving cysteine 62. Nucl Acid Res 20:3821–3830

Meister A (1991) Glutathione deficiency produced by inhibition of its synthesis, and its reversal: applications in research and therapy. Pharmacol Ther 51:155–194

Meister A (1994) Glutathione, ascorbate, and cellular protection. Cancer Res 54:S1969–S1975

Meister A (1995) Glutathione metabolism. Methods Enzymol 251:3–7

Mercer BA, Kolesnikova N, Sonett J, D'Armiento J (2004) Extracellular-regulated kinase/mitogen activated protein kinase is up-regulated in pulmonary emphysema and mediates matrix metalloproteinase-1 induction by cigarette smoke. J Biol Chem 279:17690–17696

Mio T, Romberger DJ, Thompson AB, Robbins RA, Heires A, Rennard SI (1997) Cigarette smoke induces interleukin-8 release from human bronchial epithelial cells. Am J Crit Care Med 155:1770–1776

Molteni SN, Fassio A, Ciriolo MR, Filomeni G, Pasqualetto E, Fagioli C, Sitia R (2004) Glutathione limits Ero1-dependent oxidation in the endoplasmic reticulum. J Biol Chem 279:32667–32673

Montuschi P, Kharitonov SA, Ciabattoni G, Barnes PJ (2003) Exhaled leukotrienes and prostaglandins in COPD. Thorax 58:585–588

Moodie FM, Marwick JA, Anderson CS, Szulakowski P, Biswas SK, Bauter MR, Kilty I, Rahman I (2004) Oxidative stress and cigarette smoke alter chromatin remodeling but differentially regulate NF-κB activation and proinflammatory cytokine release in alveolar epithelial cells. FASEB J 18:1897–1899

Morito N, Yoh K, Itoh K, Hirayama A, Koyama A, Yamamoto M, Takahashi S (2003) Nrf2 regulates the sensitivity of death receptor signals by affecting intracellular glutathione levels. Oncogene 22:9275–9281

Motohashi H, Yamamoto M (2004) Nrf2-Keap1 defines a physiologically important stress response mechanism. Trends Mol Med 10:549–557

Müller T (1995) Expression of c-*fos* in quiescent Swiss 3T3 cells exposed to aqueous cigarette smoke fractions. Cancer Res 55:1927–1932

Müller T, Gebel S (1994) Heme oxygenase expression in Swiss 3T3 cells following exposure to aqueous cigarette smoke fractions. Carcinogenesis 15:67–72

Müller T, Gebel S (1998) The cellular stress response induced by aqueous extracts of cigarette smoke is critically dependent on the intracellular glutathione concentration. Carcinogenesis 19:797–801

Müller T, Haussmann HJ, Schepers G (1997) Evidence for peroxynitrite as an oxidative stress-inducing compound of aqueous cigarette smoke fractions. Carcinogenesis 18:295–301

Muscat JE, Kleinman W, Colosimo S, Muir A, Lazarus P, Park J, Richie JP (2004) Enhanced protein glutathiolation and oxidative stress in cigarette smokers. Free Radic Biol Med 36:464–470

Nakayama T, Kaneko M, Kodama M, Nagata C (1985) Cigarette smoke induces DNA single-strand breaks in human cells. Nature 314:462–464

Nebert DW, Roe AL, Dieter MZ, Solis WA, Yang Y, Dalton TP (2000) Role of the hydrocarbon receptor and [Ah] gene battery in the oxidative stress response, cell cycle control, and apoptosis. Biochem Pharmacol 59:65–85

Nebert DW, Dalton TP, Okey AB, Gonzalez FJ (2004) Role of aryl hydrocarbon receptor-mediated induction of the CYP1 enzymes in environmental toxicity and cancer. J Biol Chem 279:23847–2350

Nguyen T, Sherratt PJ, Pickett CB (2003) Regulatory mechanisms controlling gene expression mediated by the antioxidant response element. Annu Rev Pharmacol Toxicol 43:233–260

Nguyen T, Yang CS, Pickett CB (2004) The pathways and molecular mechanisms regulating Nrf2 activation in response to chemical stress. Free Radic Biol Med 37:433–441

Nie M, Pang L, Inoue H, Knox AJ (2003) Transcriptional regulation of cyclooxygenase 2 by bradykinin and interleukin-1β in human airway smooth muscle cells: involvement of different promoter elements, transcription factors, and histone H4 acetylation. Mol Cell Biol 23:9233–9244

Niki E, Minamisawa S, Oikawa M, Komuro E (1993) Membrane damage from lipid oxidation induced by free radicals and cigarette smoke. Ann N Y Acad Sci U S A 686:29–37

Nikitovic D, Holmgren A (1996) S-nitrosoglutathione is cleaved by the thioredoxin system with liberation of glutathione and redox regulating nitric oxide. J Biol Chem 271:19180–19185

Ning W, Li CJ, Kaminski N, Feghali-Bostwick CA, Alber SM, Di YP, Otterbein SL, Song R, Hayashi S, Zhou Z, Pinsky DJ, Watkins SC, Pilewski JM, Sciurba FC, Peters DG, Hogg JC, Choi AMK (2004) Comprehensive gene expression profiles reveal pathways related to the pathogenesis of chronic obstructive pulmonary disease. Proc Natl Acad Sci U S A 101:14895–14900

Oguro Tea (1996) Heme oxygenase-1 gene expression by a glutathione depletor, phorone, mediated through AP-1 activation in rats. Biochem Biophys Res Comm 221:259–265

Oh-Hashi K, Maruyama W, Isobe K (2001) Peroxynitrite induces GADD34, 45, and 153 VIA p38 MAPK in human neuroblastoma SH-SY5Y cells. Free Radic Biol Med 30:213–221

Ohno Y, Ormstad K (1985) Formation, toxicity and inactivation of acrolein during biotransformation of cyclophosphamide as studied in freshly isolated cells from rat liver and kidney. Arch Toxicol 57:99–103

Okamoto T, Ogiwara H, Hayashi T, Mitsui A, Kawabe T, Yodoi J (1992) Human thioredoxin/adult T cell leukemia-derived factor activates the enhancer binding protein of human immunodeficiency virus type 1 by thiol redox control mechanism. Int Immunol 4:811–819

Otterbein LE, Bach FH, Alam J, Soares M, Tao LH, Wysk M, Davis RJ, Flavell RA, Choi AM (2000) Carbon monoxide has anti-inflammatory effects involving the mitogen-activated protein kinase pathway. Nat Med 6:422–428

Park E-M, Park Y-M, Gwak Y-S (1998) Oxidative damage in tissues of rats exposed to cigarette smoke. Free Radic Biol Med 25:79–86

Peto R, Darby S, Deo H, Silcocks P, Whitley E, Doll R (2000) Smoking, smoking cessation, and lung cancer in the UK since 1950: combination of national statistics with two case-control studies. Br Med J 321:323–329

Peto R, Lopez AD, Boreham J, Thun M, Heath C Jr (1992) Mortality from tobacco in developed countries: indirect estimation from national vital statistics. Lancet 339:1268–1278

Pinot F, El Yaagoubi A, Christie P, Dinh-Xuan AT, Polla BS (1997) Induction of stress proteins by tobacco smoke in human monocytes: modulation by antioxidants. Cell Stress Chap 2:156–161

Powell CA, Spira A, Derti A, DeLisi C, Liu G, Borczuk A, Busch S, Sahasrabudhe S, Chen Y, Sugarbaker D, Bueno R, Richards WG, Brody JS (2003) Gene expression in lung adenocarcinomas of smokers and nonsmokers. Am J Respir Cell Mol Biol 29:157–162

Powis G, Montfort WR (2001) Properties and biological activities of thioredoxins. Annu Rev Pharmacol Toxicol 41:261–295

Pryor WA, Stone K (1993) Oxidants in cigarette smoke; radicals hydrogen peroxide, peroxynitrate and peroxynitrite. Ann N Y Acad Sci U S A 686:12–28

Rahman I, Li XY, Donaldson K, Harrison DJ, MacNee W (1995) Glutathione homeostasis in alveolar epithelial cells in vitro and lung in vivo under oxidative stress. Am J Physiol 269:L285–L292

Rahman I, MacNee W (1999) Lung glutathione and oxidative stress: implications in cigarette smoke-induced airway disease. Am J Physiol 277:L1067–L1088

Rangasamy T, Cho CY, Thimmulappa RK, Zhen L, Srisuma SS, Kensler TW, Yamamoto M, Petrache I, Tuder RM, Biswal S (2004) Genetic ablation of Nrf2 enhances susceptibility to cigarette smoke-induced emphysema in mice. J Clin Invest 114:1248–1259

Reddy S, Finkelstein EI, Wong PS, Phung A, Cross CE, van der Vliet A (2002) Identification of glutathione modifications by cigarette smoke. Free Radic Biol Med 33:1490–1498

Rosette C, Karin M (1996) Ultraviolet light and osmotic stress: Activation of the JNK cascade through multiple growth factor and cytokine receptors. Science 274:1194–1197

Rusznak C, Mills PR, Devalia JL, Sapsford RJ, Davies RJ, Lozewicz S (2000) Effect of cigarette smoke on the permeability and IL-1β and sICAM-1 release from cultured human bronchial epithelial cells of never-smokers, smokers, and patients with chronic obstructive pulmonary disease. Am J Respir Cell Mol Biol 23:530–536

Saitoh M, Nishitoh H, Fujii M, Takeda K, Tobiume K, Sawada Y, Kawabata M, Miyazono K, Ichijo H (1998) Mammalian thioredoxin is a direct inhibitor of apoptosis signal-regulating kinase (ASK) 1. EMBO J 17:2596–2606

Sato T, Suruki T, Fukijama T (1962) Cigarette smoke: mode of adhesion and haemolyzing and SH-inhibiting factors. Br J Cancer 16:7–14

Schuller HM, Jull BA, Sheppard BJ, Plummer HK (2000) Interaction of tobacco-specific toxicants with the neuronal α7 nicotinic acetylcholine receptor and its associated mitogenic signal transduction pathway: potential role in lung carcinogenesis and pediatric lung disorders. Eur J Pharmacol 393:265–277

Sellers TA, Yang P (2002) Familial and genetic influences on risk of lung cancer. In: King RA, Rotter JI, Motulsky AG (eds) The genetic basis of common diseases. Oxford University Press, New York, NY, pp 700–712

Shim J, Karin M (2002) The control of mRNA stability in response to extracellular stimuli. Mol Cells 14:323–331

Shimizu M, Hochadel JF, Fulmer BA, Waalkes MP (1998) Effect of glutathione depletion and metallothionein gene expression on arsenic-induced cytotoxicity and c-*myc* expression in vitro. Toxicol Sci 45:204–211

Spira A, Beane J, Pinto-Plata V, Kadar A, Liu G, Shah V, Celli B, Brody JS (2004a) Gene expression profiling of human lung tissue from smokers with severe emphysema. Am J Respir Cell Mol Biol 31:601–610

Spira A, Beane J, Shah V, Liu G, Schembri F, Yang X, Palma J, Brody JS (2004b) Effects of cigarette smoke on the human airway epithelial cell transcriptome. Proc Natl Acad Sci U S A 101:10143–10148

Stauffer HP (1974) The interaction of cigarette smoke with thiol groups, a model study. Soz Praventivmed 19:55–58

Stewart D, Killeen E, Naquin R, Alam S, Alam J (2003) Degradation of transcription factor Nrf2 via the ubiquitin-proteasome pathway and stabilization by cadmium. J Biol Chem 278:2396–2402

Stocker R, Keaney JF Jr (2004) Role of oxidative modifications in atherosclerosis. Physiol Rev 84:1381–1478

Suc I, Meilhac O, Lajoie-Mazenc I, Vandaele J, Jurgens G, Salvayre R, Negre-salvayre A (1998) Activation of EGF receptor by oxidized LDL. FASEB J 12:665–671

Sugano N, Shimada K, Ito K, Murai S (1998) Nicotine inhibits production of inflammatory mediators in U937 cells through modulation of nuclear factor-κB activation. Biochem Biophys Res Comm 252:25–28

Sun Y, Oberley LW (1996) Redox regulation of transcriptional activators. Free Radic Biol Med 21:335–348

Theocharis SE, Margeli AP, Koutselinis A (2003) Metallothionein: a multifunctional protein from toxicity to cancer. Int J Biol Markers 18:162–169

Thomas JP, Maiorino M, Ursini F, Girotti AW (1990) Protective action of phospholipid hydroperoxide glutathione peroxidase against membrane-damaging lipid peroxidation. In situ reduction of phospholipid and cholesterol hydroperoxides. J Biol Chem 265:454–461

Tirumalai R, Kumar TR, Mai KH, Biswal S (2003) Acrolein causes transcriptional induction of phase II genes by activation of Nrf2 in human lung type II epithelial (A549) cells. Toxicol Lett 132:27–36

Uno S, Dalton TP, Derkenne S, Curran CP, Miller ML, Shertzer HG, Nebert DW (2004) Oral exposure to benzo[a]pyrene in the mouse: detoxication by inducible cytochrome P450 is more important than metabolic activation. Mol Pharmacol 65:1225–1237

US Department of Health and Human Services (1989a) Chronic obstructive pulmonary disease. In: US Department of Health and Human Services (ed) Public Health Service, Centers for Disease Control, Center for Chronic Disease Prevention and Health Promotion Office on Smoking and Health. Rockville, MD, DHHS Publication No. (CDC) 89–8411, pp 66–68

US Department of Health and Human Services (1989b) Coronary heart disease. In: US Department of Health and Human Services (ed) Public Health Service, Centers for Disease Control, Center for Chronic Disease Prevention and Health Promotion Office on Smoking and Health. Rockville, MD, DHHS Publication No. (CDC) 89–8411, pp 58–65

US Department of Health and Human Services (2004) The Health Consequences of Smoking: A Report of the Surgeon General—Executive Summary. U.S. Department of Health and Human Services, Centers for Disease Control and Prevention, National Center for Chronic Disease Prevention and Health Promotion, Office on Smoking and Health, Atlanta, GA

Vayssier M, Banzet N, Francois D, Bellmann K, Polla BS (1998a) Tobacco smoke induces both apoptosis and necrosis in mammalian cells: Differential effects of HSP70. Am J Physiol 19:L771–L779

Vayssier M, Favatier F, Pinot F, Bachelet M, Polla BS (1998b) Tobacco smoke induces coordinate activation of HSF and inhibition of NFκB in human monocytes: effects of TNFα release. Biochem Biophys Res Comm 252:249–256

Verheij M, Bose R, Lin XH, Yao B, Jarvis WD, Grant S, Birrer MJ, Szabo E, Zon LI, Kyriakis JM, Haimovitz-Friedman A, Fuks Z, Kolesnick RN (1996) Requirement for ceramide-initiated SAPK/JNK signalling in stress-induced apoptosis. Nature 380:75–79

Waisberg M, Joseph P, Hale B, Beyersmann D (2003) Molecular and cellular mechanisms of cadmium carcinogenesis. Toxicology 192:95–117

Wakabayashi N, Dinkova-Kostova AT, Holtzclaw WD, Kang MI, Kobayashi A, Yamamoto M, Kensler TW, Talalay P (2004) Protection against electrophile and oxidant stress by induction of the phase 2 response: fate of cysteines of the Keap1 sensor modified by inducers. Proc Natl Acad Sci U S A 101:2040–2045

West KA, Brognard J, Clark AS, Linnoila IR, Yang X, Swain SM, Harris C, Belinsky S, Dennis PA (2003) Rapid Akt activation by nicotine and a tobacco carcinogen modulates the phenotype of normal human airway epithelial cells. J Clin Invest 111:81–90

Wilhelm D, Bender K, Knebel A, Angel P (1997) The level of intracellular glutathione is a key regulator for the induction of stress-activated signal transduction pathways including Jun N-terminal protein kinases and p38 kinase by alkylating agents. Mol Cell Biol 17:4792–4800

Witschi H, Espiritu I, Peake JL, Wu K, Maronpot RR, Pinkerton KE (1997) The carcinogenicity of environmental tobacco smoke. Carcinogenesis 18:575–586

Wong CG, Rasmussen RE, Bonakdar (1995) Lack of elevation of stress-inducible heat-shock protein 70 in the ferret lung after chronic cigarette smoke inhalation. Inhal Toxicol 7:1163–1171

Wu X, Zhao H, Suk R, Christiani DC (2004) Genetic susceptibility to tobacco-related cancer. Oncogene 23:6500–6523

Xin M, Deng X (2005) Nicotine inactivation of the proapoptotic function of Bax through phosphorylation. J Biol Chem 280:10781–10789

Xia Zea (1995) Opposing effects of ERK and JNK-p38 MAP kinases on apoptosis. Science 270:1326–1331

Yamada N, Yamaya M, Okinaga S, Nakayama K, Sekizawa K, Shibahara S, Sasaki H (2000) Microsatellite polymorphism in the heme oxygenase-1 gene promoter is associated with susceptibility to emphysema. Am J Hum Genet 66:187–195

Yang P, Bamlet WR, Ebbert JO, Taylor WR, de Andrade M (2004) Glutathione pathway genes and lung cancer risk in young and old populations. Carcinogenesis 25:1935–1944

Yildiz D, Ercal N, Amstrong DW (1998) Nicotine enantiomers and oxidative stress. Toxicology 130:155–165

Zhang DD, Lo SC, Cross JV, Templeton DJ, Hannink M (2004) Keap1 is a redox-regulated substrate adaptor protein for a Cul3-dependent ubiquitin ligase complex. Mol Cell Biol 24:10941–10953

Zhang Q, Adiseshaiah P, Reddy SP (2005) MMP/EGFR/MAP kinase signaling regulate fra-1 induction by cigarette smoke in lung epithelial cells. Am J Respir Cell Mol Biol 32:72–81

Chapter 5

Redox Effects of Cigarette Smoke in Lung Inflammation

Irfan Rahman

Contents

5.1	Introduction	114
5.2	Cigarette Smoke and Oxidative Stress	115
5.2.1	Composition of Cigarette Smoke	115
5.2.2	Oxidants in the Cigarette Smoke	116
5.3	ROS-Mediated Lipid Peroxidation Products and Their Role in Biochemical Processes	116
5.3.1	Membrane Lipid Peroxidation	116
5.3.1.1	F_2-Isoprostanes	119
5.3.1.2	4-Hydroxy-2-nonenal	119
5.3.1.3	Acrolein	120
5.4	GSH and Cellular Redox Regulation	121
5.4.1	GSH Metabolism	121
5.4.2	GSH and Oxidative Stress	122
5.4.3	Protein-Thiol Alterations: a Novel Redox Signaling Mechanism and Adaptive Stress Response	124
5.4.3.1	Protein-Thiol Oxidation	124
5.4.3.2	Cysteine Sulfoxidation as Protein Function Modulator	125
5.4.3.3	Protein Function Modulation by Disulfide/Mixed Disulfide Formation: Role of Peroxiredoxin, Sulfiredoxin, and Thioredoxin	126
5.4.3.4	Protein-*S*-Glutathiolation and Oxidative Stress	128
5.4.3.5	*S*-Glutathiolation-Dependent Redox—Adaptive and Signaling Mechanisms	128
5.4.3.5.1	Role of *S*-Glutathiolation in Cellular Resistance to Oxidative Stress	128
5.4.3.5.2	*S*-Glutathiolation and Phosphorylation/Dephosphorylation: a Possible Crosstalk	130

Contents

5.4.3.5.3	S-Glutathiolation and the Proteasome Pathway	131
5.4.3.5.4	S-Glutathiolation Modulation of Transcription Factors	131
5.5	Involvement of Cigarette Smoke in Redox Signaling and Gene Transcription	132
5.5.1	Signal Transduction	132
5.5.2	NF-κB and AP-1 Activation	132
5.5.3	Gene Transcription	135
5.5.3.1	Antioxidant Protective and Stress Response Genes	136
5.5.3.2	Pro- and Anti-Inflammatory Genes	137
5.5.3.3	Aldehyde/Lipid Peroxidation Product-Mediated Gene Expression	140
5.5.3.4	Mucin Genes	141
5.5.3.5	DNA Microarray Profile: Cigarette Smoke-Mediated Gene Expression	141
5.6	Role of ROS and Cigarette Smoke-Induced Oxidative Stress in Chromatin Modeling: Role for Histone Acetylation/Deacetylation and DNA Methylation	143
5.6.1	Role of ROS in Chromatin Remodeling and Gene Transcription: Epigenetics	143
5.6.1.1	Chromatin Remodeling (Histone Acetylation and Deacetylation)	143
5.6.1.1.1	Gene Transcription	145
5.6.1.2	Mechanisms of Transcriptional Regulation	145
5.6.1.2.1	MAPK- and NF-κB-Mediated Histone Acetylation and Deacetylation	145
5.6.1.2.2	Glucocorticoids and Chromatin Remodeling	148
5.6.1.2.3	Coactivator Adenoviral E1A and Chromatin Remodeling	149
5.7	Conclusions	150
	References	151

5.1 Introduction

A multitude of lung diseases such as chronic bronchitis, emphysema, bronchiolitis and small airway diseases has been found to be a direct or indirect consequence of cigarette smoking. These are now classified collectively under chronic obstructive pulmonary disease (COPD), characterized by airflow limitation that is not reversible and usually progressive. Cigarette smoking is also associated with impairment in the pulmonary immune function, pulmonary infections, and bronchooncogenesis. Cigarette smoking also initiates such lung inflammatory responses through a wide variety of mechanisms such as the activation of redox-sensitive transcription factors such as nuclear factor-κB (NF-κB) and activator protein 1 (AP-1), signal transduction (activation of mitogen-activated protein kinase [MAPK] pathways, phosphoinositide 3 [PI-3-kinase, PI-3K] and PI-3K-activated serine–threonine kinase, Akt, and chromatin modeling (histone acetylation/deacetylation), leading to gene expression of proinflammatory mediators (Rahman et al. 1998; (Fig. 5.1).

Cigarette smoke is a complex mixture of various noxious gases and condensed tar particles. These components elicit oxidative stress in lungs by continuous generation of reactive oxygen species (ROS) and various other inflammatory mediators (Chapter 1). Cigarette smoke exposure alters redox glutathione status, and causes oxidation of proteins, DNA, and lipids, which may cause direct lung injury or induce a variety of cellular responses through the generation of secondary metabolically reactive species. Cigarette smoke may induce alterations both within and outside the lung cells in the form of remodeling of the extracellular matrix, mucus hypersecretion, plasma exudation/epithelial permeability, cell death, mitochondrial respiration, cell proliferation, maintenance of surfactant and the antiprotease screen, effective alveolar repair response, and immune modulation in the lung (Gutteridge et al. 2000; Rahman et al. 2000; Richer et al. 1995).

This chapter encompasses the redox effects of cigarette smoke-mediated oxidative stress in lung inflammation, the redox molecular mechanisms of gene expression (cell signaling and chromatin remodeling), and pathophysiologic consequences of oxidants and altered redox balance in these conditions.

5.2 Cigarette Smoke and Oxidative Stress

5.2.1 Composition of Cigarette Smoke

Cigarette smoke contains many potent oxidants, carcinogens/mutagens, and chemicals that stand out as major risk factors for the development of COPD and lung cancer (Rahman and MacNee 1996a, 1999). Mainstream cigarette smoke is a complex mixture of over 5,000 chemical compounds, including high concentrations of oxidants (10^{17} per puff) (Church and Pryor 1985; Pryor and Stone 1993). The aqueous phase of the cigarette smoke condensate (CSC) may undergo redox recycling (because of the presence of free iron) for a considerable time in epithelial lining fluid (ELF) of smokers (Nakayama et al. 1989; Zang et al. 1995). The tar phase of cigarette contains a high concentration of radicals (10^{17} spins per gram), which are relatively stable, e.g., semiquinone radical. The tar phase is also an effective metal chelator and can bind iron (released from the activated macrophages) to produce tar semiquinone and tar Fe^{2+}, which can generate millimolar levels of H_2O_2 for at least 24 h (Nakayama et al. 1989; Zang et al. 1995). Sidestream cigarette smoke contains more than 10^{15} reactive organic compounds per puff, and comprises carbon monoxide, ammonia, formaldehyde, N-nitrosamines, benzo[a]pyrene, benzene, isoprene, ethane, pentane, nicotine, acrolein, acetaldehyde, and other genotoxic and carcinogenic organic compounds.

5.2.2 Oxidants in the Cigarette Smoke

Short-lived oxidants, such as superoxide anion ($O_2^-\cdot$) and nitric oxide (NO·), are predominantly found in the gas phase of cigarette smoke. NO· and $O_2^-\cdot$ immediately react to form the highly reactive and toxic peroxynitrite ($ONOO^-$) molecule. The semiquinone radicals in the tar phase of cigarette can reduce oxygen to produce ROS, such as $O_2^-\cdot$, ·OH and H_2O_2 (Pryor and Stone 1993). Oxidants present in cigarette smoke can further augment alveolar macrophage production of ROS and a host of other mediators, some of which are chemotactic and recruit neutrophils and other inflammatory cells into the lungs. Both neutrophils and macrophages, which are known to migrate in increased numbers into the lungs of cigarette smokers, compared with nonsmokers, can generate ROS via the activation of NADPH oxidases (Bosken et. al. 1992; Chan-Yeung 1988; Chan-Yeung and Dybuncio 1984; Muns et. al. 1995; Rahman and MacNee 1996a; Rahman et. al. 1996b, 1997; Richards et. al. 1989; Van Antwerpen et al. 1995).

5.3 ROS-Mediated Lipid Peroxidation Products and Their Role in Biochemical Processes

5.3.1 Membrane Lipid Peroxidation

$O_2^-\cdot$ and ·OH generated and released by activated immune and inflammatory cells are highly cytotoxic and when generated in close proximity to a cell, oxidize membrane phospholipids (lipid peroxidation), which may initiate a chain reaction. A direct result of such a process is the generation of toxic downstream lipid peroxidation products, such as malondialdehyde (MDA), 4-hydroxy-2-nonenal (4-HNE), acrolein, and F_2-isoprostanes (Fig. 5.2). Some of these products, e.g., 4-HNE and F_2-isoprostanes, may be involved in certain signaling processes in a given cell (Uchida et al. 1999). The peroxidative alteration of polyunsaturated fatty acids severely impairs functions of the membrane, membrane-bound receptors, enzymes, and receptor/enzyme translocation. In addition, there is increased tissue permeability because of loss of membrane fluidity, which has been implicated in the etiogenesis of diverse lung injuries (Morrison et al. 1999; Rahman and MacNee 1996a). Endogenous generation of aldehydes because of lipid peroxidation has been found to underlie many of the pathophysiologic events associated with oxidative stress in cells and tissues (Gutteridge 1995). Lipid peroxidation may also have a role in the signaling events in the molecular mechanisms involved in the lung inflammation observed in COPD.

Fig. 5.1 Mechanisms of reactive oxygen species (*ROS*)-mediated lung inflammation in chronic obstructive pulmonary disease (COPD). Inflammatory response is mediated by oxidants either inhaled and/or released by the activated neutrophils, alveolar macrophages, eosinophils, and epithelial cells, leading to production of ROS and membrane lipid peroxidation. Activation of transcription of the proinflammatory cytokine and chemokine genes, upregulation of adhesion molecules, and increased release of proinflammatory mediators are also involved in the inflammatory responses in patients with COPD

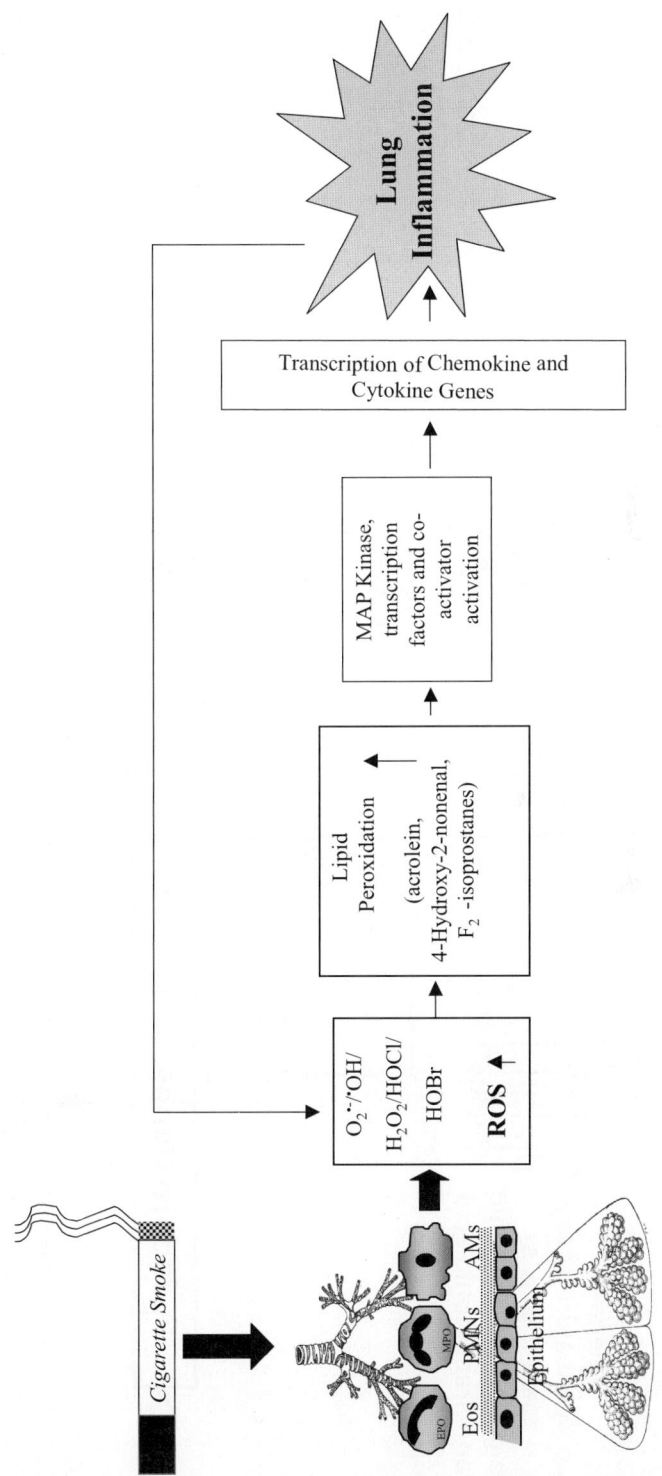

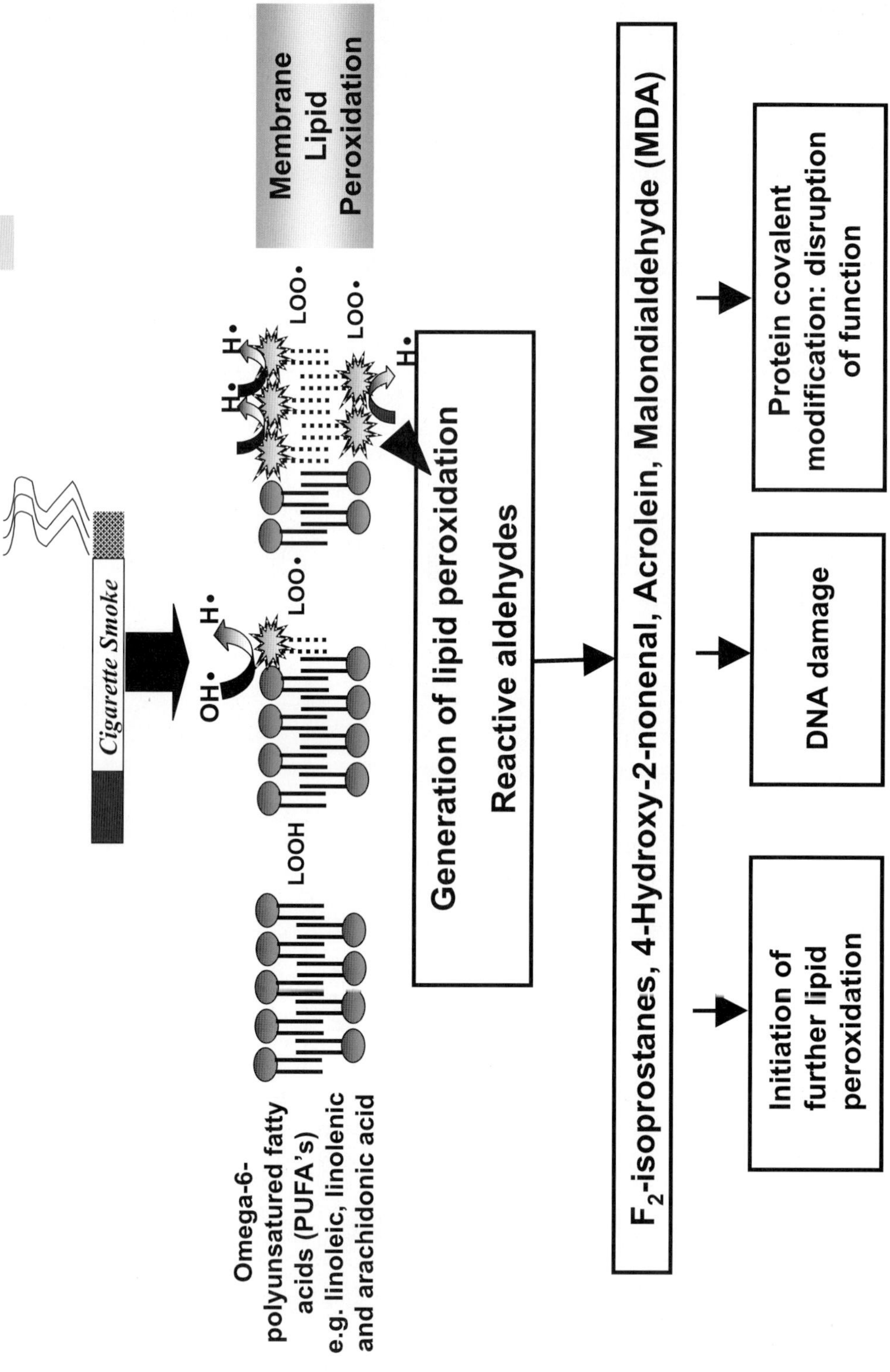
Cigarette Smoke
Omega-6-polyunsatured fatty acids (PUFA's) e.g. linoleic, linolenic and arachidonic acid
LOOH
OH•
H•
LOO•
Membrane Lipid Peroxidation
Generation of lipid peroxidation
Reactive aldehydes
F2-isoprostanes, 4-Hydroxy-2-nonenal, Acrolein, Malondialdehyde (MDA)
Initiation of further lipid peroxidation
DNA damage
Protein covalent modification: disruption of function

Fig 5.2 Mechanism of membrane lipid peroxidation of polyunsaturated fatty acids by cigarette smoke, leading to generation of various reactive aldehydes. The reactive aldehydes triggers several redox signaling events

5.3.1.1 F_2-Isoprostanes

Despite circumstantial data available from in vitro studies suggesting that cigarette smoke may cause oxidative injury, whether this process occurs in vivo has been controversial (Harats et al. 1989). This controversy could largely be attributed to the fact that most methods previously available to assess oxidative stress in humans have been inaccurate and unreliable (Gutteridge and Halliwell 1990). Morrow et al. (1990) then reported a series of bioactive prostaglandin F_2-like compounds (termed F_2-isoprostanes) that are produced as a result of peroxidation of arachidonic acid catalyzed by free radicals and were found to be independent of the cyclooxygenase enzyme in humans. F_2-isoprostanes are initially formed in situ on phospholipids and are subsequently released preformed (Morrow et al. 1992). The level of F_2-isoprostanes is almost two-fold greater in magnitude as compared with cyclooxygenase-derived prostanoids in normal human biological fluids. In addition, a dramatic increase in the levels of F_2-isoprostanes has been observed in the circulation and in association with tissue phospholipids in animal models of oxidant injury.

F_2-isoprostanes are potent smooth muscle constrictors and mitogens. They modulate platelet as well as other cell functions in vitro via membrane receptors (thromboxane A_2) for prostaglandins (Lawson et al. 1999; Morrow and Roberts 1997). The levels of lipid peroxidation end products, such as F_2-isoprostanes and the hydrocarbons ethane and pentane, are increased in exhaled air condensate in smokers and in patients with COPD (Euler et al. 1996; Montuschi et al. 2000; Paredi et al. 2000).

5.3.1.2 4-Hydroxy-2-nonenal

4-HNE is a highly reactive diffusible end product of lipid peroxidation. Increased production of 4-HNE has been associated with several pathological conditions (Grune et al. 1997) and oxidant challenge (Bedossa et al. 1994; Kruman et al. 1997; Mark et al. 1997). In view of an increased 4-HNE production during oxidant challenge, it has been suggested that 4-HNE might act as a mediator in the induction of gene expression by oxidants. A recent screening of oxidized fatty acids in RAW264.7 cells has revealed that 4-HNE might be a major inflammatory mediator in development and progression of atherogenesis (Kumagai et al. 2004). 4-HNE was found to induce the cyclooxygenase 2 (*COX-2*) genes in these cells, thus reflecting the potential role of 4-HNE as perpetrator of inflammation. Cigarette smoke increases phosphorylation of ERK1/2 and nuclear translocation of p50 and p65 subunits of NF-κB, which are important elements involved in COX-2 expression and hence, prostaglandin E2 (PGE2) formation (Martey et al. 2004). Such an inflammatory condition may be an initial step toward epithelial cell transformation. Furthermore, exogenous micromolar 4-HNE increases the expression of several genes, e.g., *HO-1*, collagen a1(I) and aldose reductase, (Basu-Modak et al. 1996; Bedossa et al. 1994; Parola et al. 1993; Spycher et al. 1997). The above results suggest that 4-HNE is involved in the regulation of gene expression even under physiological conditions.

4-HNE also serves as a chemoattractant for neutrophils both in vitro and in vivo (Schaur et al. 1994). In addition, 4-HNE has been reported to have chemotactic, cytotoxic, and immunogenic properties (Steinerova et al. 2001), and these effects were achieved in vitro with 4-HNE concentrations as low as 2.5 μM (Muller et al. 1996). Recent findings from the authors' laboratory indicate increased 4-HNE-modified protein levels in airway and alveolar epithelial cells, endothelial cells, and neutrophils in subjects with airway obstruction, compared with subjects without airway obstruction (Rahman et al. 2002a). This is indicative of not only a definite generation of 4-HNE in COPD subjects, but also corroborates the observation of an increased levels of 4-HNE-modified proteins in lung cells in such subjects. On the physiological front, increased level of 4-HNE-adducts in alveolar epithelium, airway endothelium, and neutrophils was found to be inversely correlated with forced expiratory volume in one second, (FEV_1), further suggesting a role for 4-HNE in the pathogenesis of COPD. 4-HNE is known to induce/regulate various cellular events especially proliferation, apoptosis and activation of signaling pathways (Parola et al. 1999; Uchida et al. 1999). 4-HNE has a high affinity toward cysteine, histidine, and lysine residues; alters protein function; and forms direct protein adducts. An important outcome of 4-HNE generation is its interaction with the important thiol antioxidant glutathione (GSH) (Tjalkens et al. 1999). The conjugation of 4-HNE with GSH might be one of the important mechanisms whereby a cell may lose its antioxidant prowess, leading to oxidative stress. Interestingly, increased formation of 4-HNE has also been reported to induce expression of the glutamate cysteine ligase (*GCL*) gene, which increases synthesis of GSH (Rui-Ming et al. 1998). This might be an important cellular antioxidant adaptation during oxidative stress. Inhibition of lipid peroxidation, specifically the pathways leading to the production of 4-HNE and F_2-isoprostane, may therefore be a target for antioxidant therapy in inflammation and injury in patients with COPD.

ROS-mediated lipid peroxidation has been shown to be involved in epithelial remodeling during lung injury (Gutteridge and Halliwell 2000). The levels of 4-HNE adducts are increased in epithelial cells in patients with COPD, which may be of relevance for the understanding of epithelial changes in this disease. In addition to its ability to increase the expression of proinflammatory mediators, 4-HNE has also been shown to induce apoptosis in T cells (Liu et al. 2000) and cause activation of the epidermal growth factor receptor (EGFR) in human epidermoid carcinoma cells, which results in growth inhibition (Liu et al. 1999). It has recently been shown that 4-HNE also inactivates proteases such as cathepsin B (Crabb et al. 2002), various thiol antioxidant enzymes such as glutathione peroxidase, and key mitochondrial enzymes (Euler et al. 1996; Humphries and Szweda 1998). This may be because of the high affinity of 4-HNE for the sulfhydryl groups present within the active sites of these enzymes.

5.3.1.3 Acrolein

Acrolein (2-propenal) is another thiol reactive, $\alpha,\tilde{\beta}$(beta)-unsaturated aldehyde, which is derived from various environmental sources and combustion of organic systems such as cigarette smoke (Lagrue et al. 1993). Acrolein has a very high affinity for nucleophilic targets, e.g., sulfhydryl groups. Inhalation of acrolein is known to induce changes in rat lung structure and function. Previous studies have shown that acrolein exposure depletes glutathione and inhibits the activity of various glutathione redox system enzymes in the nasal mucosa of rats (Cassee et al. 1996; Lam et al. 1985) and in alveolar A549 epithelial cells in vitro (Kehrer and Biswal 1999). Acrolein inhibits the activity of redox-sensitive transcription factors such as NF-κB and AP-1 by virtue of inducing thiol imbalance as well as covalent modification of cysteine. In a study conducted using alveolar epithelial cells A549, Horton et al. (1999) have demonstrated that acrolein may decrease NF-κB activity by a mechanism independent of I-κB, which normally regulates NF-κB activity.

Exposure of human type II lung epithelial (A549) cells to a nonlethal dose of acrolein (150 fmol/cell for 1 h) depletes 80% of intracellular GSH and increases the transcription of GCL after 6–12 h posttreatment, as an adaptive feedback for replenishing the GSH to normal level. Acrolein exposure of 2 ppm to rats causes bronchioles to be filled with desquamized cells along with isolated peribronchial monocytes (Arumugam et al. 1999). Exposure to acrolein has been shown to reduce ciliary beat frequency in cultured bovine bronchial epithelial cells. In vitro exposure of bovine tracheal epithelial cells to acrolein caused increased release of a series of eicosonoids, such as PGE_2, $PGF_{2\alpha}$, etc. (Cassee et al. 1996; Kehrer and Biswal 1999). Alkylating agents, including acrolein, are versatile mutagens and/or carcinogens because they can react with a variety of nucleophilic sites in DNA, forming adducts with DNA bases (Arumugam et al. 1999). In general, acrolein treatment activates phase II genes transcription as evident by an increase in mRNA for NAD(P)H:quinone oxidoreductase (NQO1). Western blot analysis revealed increased level of the transcription factor nuclear factor erythroid 2-related factor 2 (Nrf2) in the nuclear extract from acrolein-treated cells, and a human NQO1-human antioxidant-response element (ARE) reporter assay has confirmed the involvement of Nrf2 in ARE-mediated transcriptional activation in response to acrolein. Furthermore, increased binding of nuclear proteins to the ARE consensus sequence has been reported in cells treated with acrolein. Enhanced phase II enzyme gene expression by acrolein may form the basis of resistance against cell death and can have implications in cigarette smoke-related lung carcinogenesis. In human lung type II epithelial (A549) cells, acrolein has been shown to induce transcriptional induction of phase II genes by activation of Nrf2. The importance of Nrf2 can be gauged from a recent report by Rangasamy et al. (2004), where they have shown that disruption of the *Nrf2* gene in mice leads to early and more intense emphysema in response to cigarette smoke. In the same study, they have shown that the expression of nearly 50 antioxidant and cytoprotective genes in the lungs may be transcriptionally controlled by Nrf2, and all genes may work in concert to overcome the effects of cigarette smoke. Very recently, Pagnin et al. (2005) have reported that acrolein could inhibit inflammatory responses in the human bronchial epithelial cell line (HBE1) by decreasing interleukin 8 (IL-8) generation via direct or indirect modulation of NF-κB activity.

5.4 GSH and Cellular Redox Regulation

5.4.1 GSH Metabolism

Evidence is rapidly accumulating as to the importance of intracellular redox environment in maintaining proper cellular homeostasis and function. The cells, in particular the lungs, have evolved elaborate mechanisms that ensure proper balance between the prooxidant and antioxidant molecules as defense against constant oxidative challenge. GSH is the most important non–protein sulfhydryl in the cells and plays a key role in the maintenance of the cellular redox status. The redox potential is defined as the ratio of the concentration of oxidizing equivalents to that of reducing equivalents (Forman and Dickinson 2003). Two major redox forms of GSH has been identified in the cells, i.e., reduced GSH (GSH) and oxidized GSH (GSSG) or GSH disulfide. Recently, the two forms were implicated in a range of cellular processes such as cellular signaling, gene expression, and apoptosis (Rahman et al. 2005). GSSG represents a small fraction (1/10th) of the total GSH pool. The normal GSH content of a cell ranges from 1 mM to 10 mM and is a function of the balance between its depletion and synthesis. It is imperative for a cell to maintain this level of GSH for normal functioning. Cells can either excrete GSSG or reduce it back to GSH at the expense of NADPH, the reaction being catalyzed by GSH reductase (GR). However, de novo synthesis of GSH from its amino acid constituents is essential for the elevation of GSH that occurs as an adaptive response to oxidative stress. GSH synthesis involves two enzymatic steps catalyzed by GCL (formerly called as γ-glutamylcysteine synthetase) and glutathione synthetase (Huang et al. 1993). The enzyme GCL is the rate-limiting component of GSH synthesis (Huang et al. 1993). The de novo rate modulation of GSH synthesis is also determined by the cellular levels of the amino acid cysteine. The plasma membrane ectoenzyme γ-glutamyl transpeptidase (γ-GT) plays an important role in the supply of cysteine by hydrolytic release of this amino acid from cysteine-linked sources. γ-GT is the only enzyme that can break the γ-linkage found in GSH and GSH conjugates and release cysteine. It metabolizes the extracellular GSH and preferentially forms γ-glutamylcysteine, which is taken up by cells, bypassing its production by GCL. GCL is composed of a heterodimer containing a 73-kDa heavy catalytic subunit (GCLC) and a 30-kDa light modifying subunit (GCLM) (Huang et al. 1993) (Fig. 5.3). Although the heavy subunit contains all of the catalytic activity, the association of the heavy subunit with the regulatory light subunit can modulate GCL activity. The ratio of the two subunits for physiological function has long been assumed to be 1:1; however, in tissues the ratio varies significantly, and usually GCLC:GCLM is significantly greater than 1:1 (Krzywanski et al. 2004). GCL is regulated by GSH through feedback inhibition. 4-HNE has a high affinity toward cysteine, histidine, and lysine residues; alters protein function; and forms direct protein adducts. As stated earlier, 4-HNE can conjugate with GSH (Tjalkens et al. 1999). The conjugation of 4-HNE with GSH might an important mechanism whereby GSH depletion may occur during oxidative stress. Interestingly, increased formation of 4-HNE has also been reported to induce expression of the *GCL* gene, which increases synthesis of GSH (Rui-Ming et al. 1998) This might be an important cellular antioxidant adaptation during oxidative stress.

5.4.2 GSH and Oxidative Stress

The GSSG/2GSH ratio can serve as a good indicator of the cellular redox state (Park et al. 1998). This ratio in GSH parlance may be determined by the rates of H_2O_2 reduction by glutathione peroxidases (GPx) and GSSG reduction by GSH reductase. Thus, antioxidant enzymes play a critical role in the maintenance of the cellular reductive potential. Several enzymes/proteins involved in the redox system of the cell and their genes such as *MnSOD*, *GCLC*, *GPx*, thioredoxin reductase, and metallothionein are induced by modu-

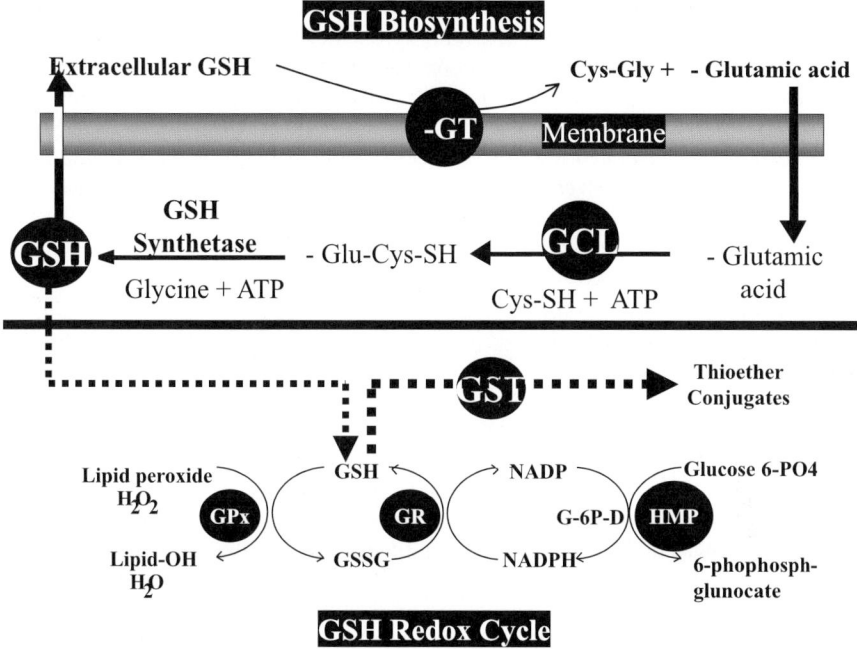

Fig. 5.3 Glutathione (*GSH*) biosynthesis and its redox cycle in lung cells. The steps involved in de novo GSH synthesis and breakdown of extracellular GSH are shown. GSH converts hydrogen and lipid peroxides to nontoxic hydroxy fatty acids and/or water. Glutathione disulfide (GSSG) is subsequently reduced to GSH in the presence of NADPH and glutathione reductase, which are linked with a hexose monophosphate shunt

lation of cellular GSH/GSSG levels in response to various oxidative stresses, including hyperoxia and inflammatory mediators such as tumor necrosis factor-α (TNF-α) and lipopolysaccharide in lung cells (Cotgreave and Gerdes 1998; Das 2001; Das et al. 1995). Intracellular redox status of lung epithelial cells has been shown to be a critical factor in determining cell susceptibility or tolerance to oxidative insults. It has been shown that GSH depletion because of GCL inhibition by buthionine sulfoximine (BSO) sensitizes both A549 and 16-HBE cells to the injurious effects of hyperoxia and H_2O_2, resulting in an increased membrane permeability and activation of NF-κB (Rahman et al. 2001). In contrast, pretreatment of these cell lines with hyperoxia before H_2O_2 exposure protects against the cytotoxic effects of H_2O_2 as well as preventing NF-κB activation. These protective effects were because of an adaptive increase in GSH in response to pretreatment with hyperoxia. Therefore, modulation of intracellular GSH can determine the course of tolerance to subsequent oxidant exposure.

The relationship to redox signaling is provided by the production of GSSG during the enzymatic reduction of hydroperoxides or ONOO⁻ by GSH peroxidases. Normally, GSSG represents less than 1% of the total GSH pool. When H_2O_2 or ONOO⁻ is transiently elevated, an elevation in GSSG, also transient, can occur, providing a possible mechanism for signaling by means of thiol–disulfide exchange. In this scenario, signaling is indirectly dependent on ROS generation. Nonetheless, as this mechanism requires a change in GSSG that is usually only observed during oxidative stress, such signaling is more likely an oxidative stress response rather than physiologic redox signaling. Interesting to note is a recent report wherein it was shown that the sputum levels of GSSG and nitrosothiols are elevated in COPD subjects; the increase was associated with neutrophilic inflammation (Beeh et al. 2004). Therefore, increased GSSG in the sputum may serve as a marker of oxidative stress in lung diseases.

5.4.3 Protein-Thiol Alterations: a Novel Redox Signaling Mechanism and Adaptive Stress Response

5.4.3.1 Protein-Thiol Oxidation

The first evidence that cells may resist oxidative stress via protein thiolation was provided by Dominici and his coworkers (1999). In an elegant study, they showed S-glutathiolation of γ-GT on the surface of U937 lymphoma cells in response to oxidative stress. Initially, an S-glutathiolation-dependent loss of activity was observed for the enzyme wherein the free surface thiols of the enzyme were S-glutathiolated and may be correlated with a concurrent generation of H_2O_2, which is a by-product of γ-GT function. Reversible posttranslational modification of specific amino acid residues on proteins have now been identified as one of the important regulatory mechanism of protein function. Proteins bearing cysteine-thiol (SH) (Cys–SH) residues in the thiolate form (S^-) are considered prone to oxidative modification. Oxidation of protein-Cys-SH (PSH) may interfere with biological functions either as "damage" or in context to oxidant-dependent signal transduction. Although PSH behave like non–protein thiols, their biochemistry is much complicated by their accessibility, steric interference, and charge distribution (Di Simplicio et al. 2003). The response of PSH and their reaction mechanisms vary depending on the source of the PSH, and are influenced by the pK_a, disulfide susceptibility/accessibility to oxidants, and the conformation of the protein at a given time. Oxidative stress can be generated as a result of excessive ROS and or reactive nitrogen species (RNS) production. It is to be noted that NO· may be scavenged with a variety of ROS to form a range of RNS, which may lead to enhanced nitration of protein tyrosine in the lungs and hence, may play a pivotal role in airway inflammation (reviewed in Reynaert et al. 2005). Initially, oxidative thiolation of PSH was recognized as an aftermath of oxidative stress, but recent evidence suggests that such transformations may be of greater biochemical consequence, both as a protective and a signaling mechanism. Therefore, protein S-thiolation and protein S-nitrosation have emerged as a novel area of oxidative biochemistry. A great number of cells have now been recognized to respond to oxidative stress by S-thiolation and S-nitrosation. Although the major mediator of protein thiolation is the thiol antioxidant GSH (which promotes S-glutathiolation), its catabolite-dependent metal reduction has recently been identified to act as a prooxidant capable of modulating redox balance, signal transduction pathways, and transcription factors (Paolicchi et al. 2002). It has been hypothesized that GSH may also be involved as a physiological buffer for controlling cellular oxygen tension (Del Corso et al. 2002).

In a community-based study, cigarette smokers were found to have about 20% more glutathiolated proteins in their plasma, compared with nonsmokers (Muscat et al. 2004). Therefore, S-thiolation measurement has been hypothesized to be a prognostic marker for cigarette smoke-dependent oxidative stress. Similarly, cigarette smoking was associated with oxidation of GSH and cysteine in human plasma in smokers of ages 40–85 years, compared with nonsmokers (Moriarty et al. 2003). Cigarette smoke extract causes increased formation of S-adenosylmethionine and cystathionine by the transulfuration pathway in A549 lung epithelial cells (Panayiotidis et al. 2004). Analogous to ROS-dependent oxidative stress, Hausladen and Stamler (1999) have coined the term nitrosative stress for RNS-mediated oxidative stress. The excessive production of ROS or RNS or the failure of a cell's defense and repair mechanisms lead to a condition known as oxidative or nitrosative stress. Such a situation may lead to an irreversible loss or a reversible modulation of a protein function.

5.4.3.2 Cysteine Sulfoxidation as Protein Function Modulator

Cysteine thiolates (Cys-S$^-$) but not cysteine thiol (Cys-SH) can be readily oxidized to a sulfenic acid (-SOH), which is a relatively reactive form that can quickly form a disulfide with a nearby thiol. Strong oxidants will oxidize either Cys-S$^-$ or Cys-SH to sulfinic (Cys-SO$_2$H) and/or sulfonic (Cys-SO$_3$H) acid derivatives (Claiborne et al. 1999). This difference in the generation of a particular cysteine thiol species provides a basis for distinguishing redox signaling from oxidative stress. Whereas oxidative stress generally involves nonspecific oxidation of wide variety molecules, redox signaling is gradually being recognized to involve oxidation of those cysteines that are located in an environment promoting dissociation of thiols. The higher oxidation states in the form of sulfinic and sulfonic derivatives have essentially been considered as irreversible modifications under biologically relevant conditions and associated with oxidative injury. On the other hand, protein-cysteine-sulfenic acids are unstable and may be further oxidized to sulfinic or sulfinic species or scavenged by GSH or vicinal thiols to form intramolecular disulfides or mixed disulfides (Claiborne et al. 1993). Therefore, it is evident that cysteine may be recycled between a reduced (Cys-SH) and its oxidized forms (sulfonate, sulfinic, or sulfinic derivatives). This transition between the reduced and oxidized forms by itself may represent a regulatory mechanism of protein function. Most noteworthy examples of such a regulation are the ROS-dependent sulfinic acid formation-dependent inhibition of tyrosine phosphatase-IB (PTP-IB) and modulation of insulin receptor kinase activity (Denu et al. 1998; Lee et al. 1998). Recently GSSG reductase, cathepsin S-nitrosoglutathione (GSNO) and other NO· donors, and glyceraldehydes-3-P-dehydrogenase (GAPDH) have been identified as potential inducers of sulfinate species formation. Poole et al. (2004) have considered the idea that Cys-sulfenic acid might have an important role in the catalytic centers of the respective enzymes. These workers further suggest that Cys-sulfenates might be useful as sensors of both oxidative and nitrosative stress that affect enzymes and transcriptional regulators. Because the formation of sulfenic, sulfinic, or sulfonic species depends on the degree of oxidative stress, the presence and stoichiometry of these species may yield useful information regarding the exact status of the prevailing oxidative stress. However, much work is needed to establish emphatically protein function modulation via cysteine–sulfoxidation pathways.

5.4.3.3 Protein Function Modulation by Disulfide/Mixed Disulfide Formation: Role of Peroxiredoxin, Sulfiredoxin, and Thioredoxin

The concept that sulfinic and sulfonic acid derivatives of protein cysteines are irreversibly damaged has been contradicted by the work of Biteau et al. (2003), who have reported the presence of an enzyme capable of reducing sulfinic acid derivatives. These workers detected a protein in yeast that can reduce the sulfinic derivative of yeast peroxiredoxin Tsa1. This enzyme was termed sulfiredoxin, and is found to be highly conserved in eukaryotes. The evolutionary conservation of the enzyme might be an important indicator of its importance in the recovery of oxidatively modified proteins, which might be vital to cell signaling and/or functioning. Biteau et al. (2003) further proposed that sulfiredoxin might catalyze a multistep reduction process in view of its intrinsic phosphotransferase and thioltransferase activities. Sulfiredoxin may apparently overcome the energy barrier that normally prevents the reduction of protein-Cys-SO_2H by a transient introduction of a phosphate group in the peroxiredoxin–sulfinate moiety to make sulfinic phosphorylester in the presence of ATP and Mg^{2+}. Similarly, Woo et al. (2005) have shown that reduction of Cys-sulfinic acid by sulfiredoxin is specific to 2-Cys-peroxiredoxins, suggesting that the process is specifically reversible (Fig. 5.4). A thiolsulfinate disulfide is formed with another sulfiredoxin molecule, followed by replacement of the phosphate group to form reduced and stabler forms of the enzyme. The thiolsulfinate can also be reduced to peroxiredoxin-sulfenate and a sulfiredoxin-disulfide by reducing agents such as DTT or thioredoxin (Trx). Thus, peroxiredoxin inactivation may facilitate H_2O_2 signaling, whereas its reverse activation by sulfiredoxin may add a new dimension in the regulation of such a signaling. In contrast, disulfide bonds and protein sulfenic acid moieties can be easily reduced and are often considered as the mediators of redox signaling (Claiborne et al. 1999; Stamler and Hausladen 1998; Suzuki et al. 1997). Nonetheless, it is essential to the understanding of redox signaling to remember that not all cysteine residues are equal. GSH and most protein cysteines cannot react at a biologically significant rate with H_2O_2 unless they are in close association with a metal or exist in the form of a thiolate anion, $-S^-$ (Winterbourn and Metodiewa 1999). Indeed, the GSH peroxidase and peroxiredoxins that involve reaction of H_2O_2 with GSH never involve such a direct interaction. Instead, the GSH peroxidase reaction involves the interaction of H_2O_2 with the selenocysteine of that enzyme, whereas the peroxiredoxin reactions involve interaction of H_2O_2 with a Cys-thiolate residue of the peroxiredoxin. When ionized to the thiolate form, cysteine reacts quite rapidly with H_2O_2. The pK_a of cysteine being normally around 8.3, its ionization will only occur in unusual environments as a function of the surrounding residues. For example, when a cysteine is near a positively charged amino acid, its pK_a is lowered to below 5.0. Such a cysteine is deprotonated and becomes a prime target for H_2O_2 oxidation. Thus, only cysteine-containing proteins located in such an environment will be affected by H_2O_2 directly.

Cysteine in its thiolate form could also participate in thiol-disulfide exchange if there is no interference by steric hindrance:

$$R_1S^- + R_2SSR_3 \longleftrightarrow R_1SSR_3 + R_2S^- \quad (1)$$

In contrast, exchanges between thiols and disulfides are very slow and must be catalyzed by glutaredoxin or other protein disulfide isomerases that have a thioredoxin-like

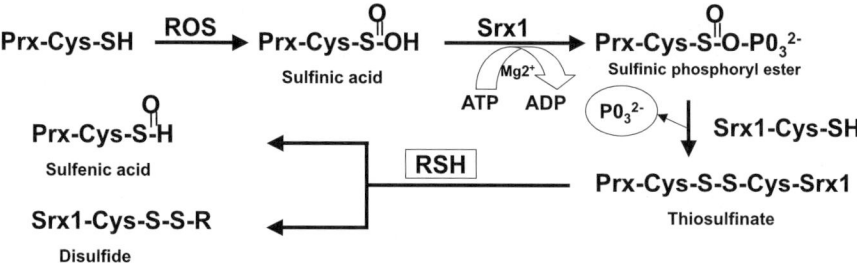

Fig. 5.4 The mechanism of peroxiredoxin sulfinic acid reversal by sulfiredoxin. The thermodynamic energy barrier for reduction of sulfinic acid species can be overcome by the help of a novel class of dual enzyme sulfiredoxin (*Srx*). This enzyme first catalyzes a phosphate group transfer from ATP to peroxiredoxin (*Prx*)-sulfinate (*Prx-Cys-SOH*) as a part of its phosphotransferase activity to form an intermediate disulfide (*Prx-Cys-S-S-Cys-Srx*). The latter is then reduced to a sulfenate and a corresponding disulfide, depending on the reducing group involved

structure in their active sites. Such disulfide exchange is a potential signaling mechanism because of its capacity for modifying cysteine residues in enzymes.

The redox status of proteins outside and within the cells is maintained by several different mechanisms. Whereas the proteins present on the extracellular face of a cell are stabilized by disulfide bonds (S-S) between two protein molecules, the proteins within the cells are redox stabilized by free sulfhydryl (-SH) moieties. Regulation of such redox states of proteins is carried out by a special class of proteins known as thioredoxins (Trx, mol. wt. 10–12) (Miranda-Vizuette et al. 1998). Trx are dithiol $[(SH)_2]$-disulfide oxidoreductases and catalyzes reduction of disulfides to their corresponding sulfhydryls. Trx systems comprises Trx and thioredoxin reductase (TrxR) components and need NADPH for their function. Mammalian TrxR are selenoenzymes that reduce oxidized thioredoxin and other protein disulfides. Trx of lower and higher animals are quite different, mammalian thioredoxins being closely related to the enzyme glutathione reductase. Along with GSH and glutaredoxin, Trx modulate the thiol:disulfide status of many signaling proteins (Holmgren 2003). Normally, Trx functions by reducing the disulfide bonds to dithiols [S-S to 2(-SH)]. However, Trx has been reported to introduce disulfides into proteins during oxidative stress (Watson et al. 2003). At the present juncture, this latter mechanism does not seem to be physiologically significant because such a reaction would possibly be inhibited by the presence of another dithiol motif at Cys-62 and Cys-69 of the Trx-1.

Trx are involved in a wide variety of cellular phenomena such as cell proliferation, reduction of ribonucleotide reductase, thioredoxin peroxidase, thiol–dithiol exchange between cysteine residues of key transcription factors, and protection against exogenous oxidants (Watson et al. 2004). In healthy lungs, Trx and TrxR are expressed in bronchial and alveolar macrophages. Their distribution may be altered in diseases such as usual interstitial pneumonia (UIP); desquamative interstitial pneumonia (DIP); UIP associated with collagen diseases, sarcoidosis, allergic alveolitis, granulomatous disease; and other lung disorders. Thioredoxin reduces the viscosity of sputum in cystic fibrosis patients. Exogenous thioredoxin has been shown to reduce ischemia reperfusion in the lungs. Trx also plays protective role against oxidative stress, bleomycin–induced lung damage, and doxorubicin-induced cardiotoxicity (Andoh et al. 2002). The major role of Trx appears to be through transcriptional modulation (Nishiyama et al. 2001). In one of the identified mechanisms, Trx in its reduced form reduces Ref-1, which in turn reduces Jun/Fos. Reduction of the dimer Jun/Fos facilitates NF-κB binding to the DNA. Because Trx is present in very low concentrations as compared with other cellular antioxidants, it probably exerts its influence via signaling pathways rather than scavenging mechanisms observed for other gross antioxidants (Watson et al. 2004). Interestingly, TRx enzyme activity can be ablated itself by introduction of a GSH-dependent disulfide bond at its Cys-72 position (Casagrande et al. 2002). Glutathiolated TRx then regains activity by an autodeglutathiolation mechanism. Thus, a reversible disulfidation mechanism is evident that might be an important adaptive and signaling cellular response during oxidative stress. A recent report has suggested that disulfide bond formation within particular families of cytoplasmic proteins may depend on the nature and extent of the oxidative stress and may serve as a focal point of control mechanisms involved in multiple physiological processes (Cummings et al. 2004).

5.4.3.4 Protein-S-Glutathiolation and Oxidative Stress

The term S-thiolation often refers to the phenomena wherein a mixed disulfide is formed between a protein and a cysteine or other thiols.

A cell may experience a redox imbalance either because of oxidative and or nitrosative stress, which can render a host of proteins nonfunctional. The adaptive response of a cell to such an environment is reflected by the modulation of structure and functions of its proteins. In addition to the mechanisms described in the preceding sections, to counter a general stress situation, a cell may employ a variety of other adaptive mechanisms such as acetylation, acylation, proteolytic processing, allosteric modulation, phosphorylation, alkylation, and a host of other mechanisms (Klatt and Lamas 2000). However, the mechanisms as to how proteins are protected and modulated during an oxidative or a nitrosative stress require deeper understanding. A large body of work in the past two decades has amply demonstrated the formation and accumulation of protein-mixed disulfides, both in intact tissues and cell cultures challenged with oxidative stress (Cotgreave and Gerdes 1998; Gilbert 1984; Thomas et al. 1995; Ziegler 1985). In addition, observation of accumulation of protein-mixed disulfides in rat lungs exposed to cigarette smoke further emphasizes the importance of these species in not only adaptive protection against oxidative stress, but also in cellular signaling (Park et al. 1998).

5.4.3.5 S-Glutathiolation-Dependent Redox—Adaptive and Signaling Mechanisms

5.4.3.5.1 Role of S-Glutathiolation in Cellular Resistance to Oxidative Stress

Physiological redox signaling disulfides are more likely formed by reaction of the thiolate with H_2O_2, forming a relatively unstable sulfenic acid intermediate followed by conjugation with GSH to form a mixed disulfide (Fig. 5.5). Apart from providing the proper cellular reducing environment, there is growing evidence that the GSH redox couple

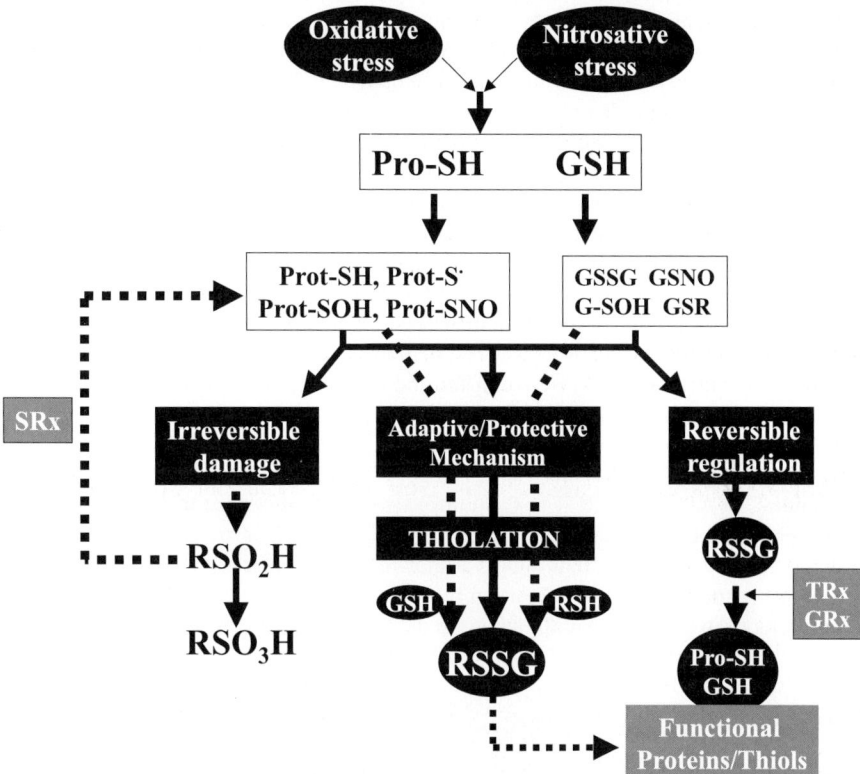

Fig. 5.5 Scheme summarizing protein thiolation. Oxidative or nitrosative stress oxidize thiols (*-SH*) of various proteins (*Pro-SH*) and glutathione (*GSH*). Two series of oxidized species arise, depending on the starting target. Oxidation/nitrosation of Pro-SH leads to the formation of Prot-S, Prot-SOH, Prot-SNO, and that of GSH yields GSNO, G-SOH, and GSR. All these oxidized species may (1) further be oxidized irreversibly to sulfinic (RSO_2H) and then sulfonic (RSO_3H) derivatives; (2) undergo *trans*-thiolation/reduction (*broken lines*) either by GSH or other thiol species (*RSH*) to form a mixed disulfide, RSSG; and (3) the RSSG formed may be reduced by various agents such as peroxiredoxin, thioredoxins, sulfiredoxins, or glutaredoxins to form active thiols (*Pro-SH/GSH*). The RSO_2H species, earlier thought to be irreversibly damaged, are now known to be reversibly modified by sulfiredoxins to form the unstable sulfenic species which may then be reduced back to their respective active forms. Formation of RSSG appears to be a protective mechanism during an oxidative/nitrosative stress and may be an important mechanism for preventing loss of important proteins because of oxidative damage

dynamically regulates protein function by a reversible formation of mixed disulfides between protein cysteines and GSH (Cotgreave and Gerdes 1998; Gilbert 1984; Thomas et al. 1995.). A specific mixed disulfide formation in conjunction with GSH is termed S-glutathiolation. Protein S-glutathiolation has been implicated in redox buffering of oxidative stress, extracellular protein stabilization, protection of proteins against irreversible oxidation of their critical cysteine residues, and regulation of enzyme activity (Cotgreave and Gerdes 1998; Thomas et al. 1995). ROS and RNS and alterations in intracellular redox potential have been reported to induce protein S-glutathiolation. These reversible chemical modifications of the thiols can result in a conformational change that may affect DNA binding of transcription factors or enzymatic activities or the formation or release of protein complexes. In addition, these changes are transient, with the duration of the intermediate determined by the ratio of GSH/GSSG and reduced/oxidized thioredoxin.

Classically, phosphorylation of proteins has been considered the major mechanism of cellular homeostasis. S-glutathiolation has now been recognized as a potential modulator of redox-sensitive thiol proteins, especially those involved in signal transduction and protein translocation pathways (Shelton et al. 2005). The role of cellular redox alterations is increasingly being recognized in the control of transcriptional factor binding to DNA (Klatt et al. 1999). Actin, PTP-1B, Ras, and several other proteins are now known to be regulated by S-glutathiolation. Decomposition of GSNO formed as a consequence of nitrosative stress, has been found to induce S-glutathiolation of various proteins such as human Cu,Zn superoxide dismutase (SOD), brain calbindin D, rabbit muscle GAPDH and bovine serum albumin (reviewed in Tao and English 2004), creatine kinase, carbonic anhydrase, actin, and glycogen phosphorylase b (reviewed in Klatt and Lamas 2000). ONOO⁻, a toxic product of NO·, has recently been implicated in inducing S-glutathiolation of proteins (Adachi et al. 2004). It was observed that sarcoplasmic/endoplasmic reticulum Ca^{2+} ATPase (SERCA or Ca-pump) activity was increased by S-glutathiolation of the enzyme because of ONOO⁻ derived from NO·. This is an interesting observation, especially in the light that NO· is a known smooth muscle relaxant. Involvement of ONOO⁻-dependent S-glutathiolation in muscle relaxation is therefore an important indication of the role of S-glutathiolation in oxidative stress response and cell signaling.

5.4.3.5.2 S-Glutathiolation and Phosphorylation/Dephosphorylation: a Possible Crosstalk

Protein tyrosine phosphatases play an important role in the dynamics of cell regulation because of phosphorylation–dephosphorylation mechanisms during extracellular signaling (Tonks and Neel 1996). Phosphorylation of tyrosine residues of various target proteins has been recorded in response to cytokines and growth factors and has been found to be at least partly mediated by the generation of ROS (Bae et al. 1997). A recent report has suggested that protein-tyrosine phosphatase 1B (PTB-1B) is oxidized at Cys-215 in a redox-dependent manner (Lee et al. 1998). This suggestion was later confirmed in a study wherein purified PTP-1B when treated with H_2O_2 was irreversibly inactivated, and reversibly inhibited when treated with O_2^-· (Barret et al. 1999a). It was observed during these experiments that PTP-1B was oxidized at its Cys-215 to sulfenic acid, which reacted with GSH to form a stable mixed disulfide (Barret et al. 1999b). Furthermore, the S-glutathiolated PTP-1B thus formed was found to undergo reduction to an active form when reacted with glutaredoxins (Barrett et al. 1999a). Importantly, S-glutathiolation of PTP-1B has also been demonstrated in intact cells (Barrett et al. 1999b). Interestingly, not only ROS, but also GSSG was found to induce PTP-S-glutathiolation (Degl'Innocenti et al. 1999). Overall, S-glutathiolation appears to be a protective/adaptive mechanism during oxidative stress and may also modulate signal transduction through the tyrosine phosphorylation pathway via modulation of the PTP-1B activity status. Several signal transduction pathways involving cell cycle progression, growth and differentiation, and cytoskeletal function have been found to be modulated by S-glutathiolation of proteins. A redox dependent β2-integrin (CD11b/CD18 or Mac-1)-mediated H_2O_2 and TNF-α promoted activation of neutrophil adhesion and recruitment was found to involve S-glutathiolation of a component of this signaling pathway (Blouin et al. 1999). Therefore, inactivation of PTP-1B by S-glutathiolation might be an important point of cellular signaling mechanisms where protein phosphorylation and oxidative stress may crosstalk.

5.4.3.5.3 S-Glutathiolation and the Proteasome Pathway

Ubiquitination of proteins is an important mechanism of posttranslational modification of proteins. Proteins, once ubiquitinated, are directed to the proteasomes for proteolytic cleavage in a cascade involving the action of three enzymes: E1, E2, and E3. It is now understood that ubiquitination of proteins protects the cell from accumulation of oxidatively damaged molecules via their degradation through this pathway (Kornitzer et al. 2000). Various components of cell cycle progression, differentiation, and death are also recognized to be regulated by ubiquitination. The ubiquitin–proteasome pathway is now known to be redox regulated and has been shown to be modulated by GSH (Figueiredo-Pereira et al. 1998). It has been demonstrated that the E1 and E2 components of the ubiquitin pathway are reversibly inhibited by S-glutathiolation (Jahngen-Hodge 1997; Obin et al. 1998). This protects and repairs the signaling functions of the ubiquitin pathway. Inhibition by S-glutathiolation of the ubiquitin–proteasome enzymes during oxidative stress is thus considered to prevent loss of reversibly oxidized and reparable proteins.

5.4.3.5.4 S-Glutathiolation Modulation of Transcription Factors

The evidence of S-glutathiolation involvement in transcription was first obtained from a study wherein it was shown that binding of the nuclear factor 1 (NF-1) to DNA required a particular ratio of GSH/GSSG, and that oxidative inactivation of NF-1 because of mixed disulfide formation was reversed by glutaredoxin (Bandyopadhyay et al. 1998). More information on the subject was provided by the work of Klatt et al. (1995) who showed that binding of AP-1–c-Jun subunit to the DNA depended on the cellular GSH/GSSG ratio. The GSH/GSSG ratio provided a redox potential that determined the oxidation of c-Jun via the formation of a mixed disulfide as well as its S-glutathiolation at the conserved cysteines of the dimerization domain of the DNA-binding site. Mixed disulfide formation led to the inhibition of DNA binding by c-Jun. Molecular characterizations have further revealed that the susceptibility of c-Jun to form mixed disulfide under mild oxidizing conditions depended on the structural environment of the target cysteine residue (Klatt et al. 1999). Interestingly, because various transcription factors such as NF-κB, members of Jun/Fos, activating factor (ATF)/cyclic AMP response element-binding proteins (CREB), and c-Myb exhibit a common putative GSH-binding domain, it appears that S-glutathiolation may represent a general mechanism of redox signal transduction leading to suppression of gene expression (Rokutan et al. 1998). The NF-κB subunit p50 has further been shown to be modulated by the GSH/GSSG ratio by a mixed disulfide formation at the cysteine residue of the DNA-binding domain. This observation was found to be in agreement with an in vitro finding of an inhibition of

AP-1 activation because of decrease in the GSH/GSSG ratio (Rokutan et al. 1998). The finding of a nuclear glutaredoxin has further emphasized the importance of a reversible and enzymatic modulation of mixed disulfide-dependent alterations of nuclear protein thiols. Thus, protein function modulation by S-glutathiolation spans a wide variety of cellular functions ranging from resistance to oxidative stress, phosphorylation-dependent signal transduction, and posttranslational protein modification to transcriptional activation and inhibition.

5.5 Involvement of Cigarette Smoke in Redox Signaling and Gene Transcription

5.5.1 Signal Transduction

ROS derived from both inflammatory cells and the environment can activate and phosphorylate a wide variety of signal transducing molecules via oxidation-prone cysteine-rich domains and the sphingomyelinase–ceramide pathway, leading to increased gene transcription (Adler et al. 1999; Guyton et al. 1996; Rahman and MacNee 1998; Sen 1998). These include the MAPK family, extracellular signal regulated kinase (ERK), c-Jun N-terminal kinase (JNK), p38 kinase, and PI-3K/Akt. Depending on the cell type and the cell's oxidative status, activation of members of the MAPK family leads to a complex array of transactivation of transcription factors, such as c-Jun, ATF-2, CREB-binding protein (CBP) and Elk-1 (Adler et al. 1999; Sen 1998; Thannickal and Fanburg 2000). This eventually results in chromatin remodeling, which in turn modulates the expression of a battery of distinct proinflammatory and antioxidant genes involved in several cellular events, including apoptosis, proliferation, transformation, and differentiation. Aldehydes, generated in part because of lipid peroxidation by cigarette smoke, have been shown to signal transcriptional activation and gene expression, leading to inflammatory responses (Parola et al. 1999; Uchida et al. 1999). Hoshino et al. (2005) showed that cigarette smoke extract specifically induces the JNK pathway, leading to endothelial cell injury. Stimulation of a metabolically important cellular signaling pathway mediated by protein kinase C (PKC) has been reported in response to cigarette smoke (Wyatt et al. 1999). Such activation may possibly be attributed to the formation of aldehyde/lipid peroxidation products in human bronchial epithelial cells.

5.5.2 NF-κB and AP-1 Activation

NF-κB regulates the expression of many inflammatory mediator genes, such as those for the cytokines, IL-8, TNFα, and NO· (Fig. 5.6). NF-κB, kept inactivated in the cytosol by its inhibitory subunit (IκB), may be stimulated by diverse stimuli including cytokines and oxidants. This results in ubiquitination, followed by dissociation of IκB from NF-κB and further destruction of IκB in the proteasome. These critical events during an inflammatory response are generally redox sensitive. Recently, Bai et al. (2005) have reported that ROS can directly activate receptor activator of NF-κB ligand (RANKL) and induce osteoclastic activity, leading to bone resorption in rats. It was found that ROS first promoted phosphorylation of CREB/ATF-2, which then binds to the CRE-binding

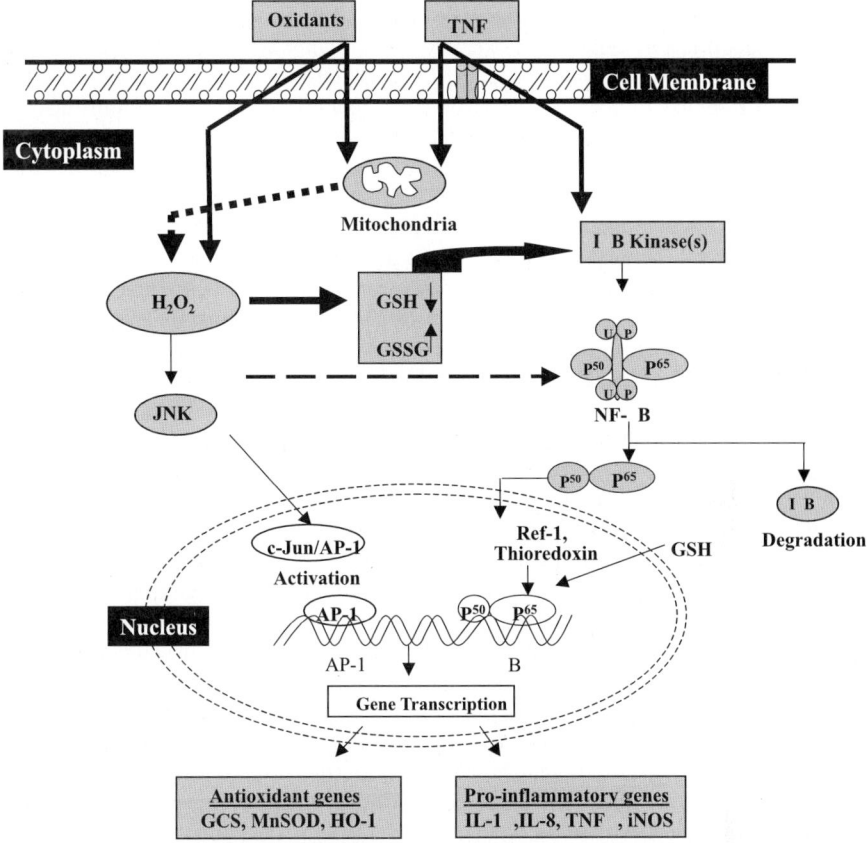

Fig. 5.6 Model for the mechanism of nuclear factor-κB (*NF-κB*) and activator protein-1 (*AP-1*) activation, leading to gene transcription. Tumor necrosis factor-α (TNF-α)/oxidants act on mitochondria to release hydrogen peroxide (and possibly peroxynitrite), which is involved in the activation of NF-κB and AP-1. Superoxide does not leave mitochondria unless generated by an outer mitochondrial membrane oxidoreductase. Hydrogen peroxide (H_2O_2) can leave mitochondria, as enough is generated to overcome the mitochondrial peroxidase activity. Activation of NF-κB involves the phosphorylation, ubiquitination, and subsequent proteolytic degradation of the inhibitory protein IκB. Free NF-κB then translocates into the nucleus and binds with its consensus sites. Intracellular redox ratio of glutathione (*GSH*)/oxidized GSH (*GSSG*) levels and intranuclear presence of Ref-1, and thioredoxin can modulate AP-1 and NF-κB activation. Similarly, AP-1 either c-Jun/c-Jun (homodimer) or c-Fos/c-Jun (heterodimer) is activated by the phosphorylation of c-Jun N-terminal kinase (*JNK*) pathway, leading to the activation AP-1, which binds with its TRE consensus region. Activation of NF-κB/AP-1 leads to the coordinate expression of protective antioxidant and proinflammatory genes

domain on the RANKL promoter. In the same study using human MG63 cells, it was revealed that ROS also triggered HSF2 binding to the heat shock element on the RANKL promoter domain. Thus, it appears that ROS can activate the NF-κB pathway via direct activation of RANKL via ERK/CREB-PKA and HSF2/ERK pathways in mouse and humans, respectively.

Activation of transcription factors and gene expression, leading to an inflammatory response, has been suggested to be because of the aldehydes, generated because of peroxidative alterations by cigarette smoke. A ten-fold higher activation of NF-κB was reported by Mochida-Nishimura et al. (2001) in bronchial alveolar lavage (BAL) cells from smokers in response to lipopolysaccharide (LPS), compared with that of nonsmokers. This was possibly because of enhanced release of inflammatory mediators that may activate NF-κB. However, a differential regulation of activation was recorded for MAPK-ERK, stress-activated protein kinase (SAPK), and p38. In contrast to ERK and SAPK, activation of p38 was found to be more rapid in BAL cells from smokers. The differences in activation of NF-κB and MAPKs in BAL cells from smokers and nonsmokers were attributed to the differences in their microenvironment, which is affected by chronic exposure to cigarette smoke. The activation of p38, therefore, may be responsible for the elevated levels of TNF-α and IL-8 seen in BAL fluid and sputum of patients with COPD (Keatings et al. 1996; Wesselius et al. 1997). In a study involving exposure of normal bronchial epithelial cells and A549 cells to Cigarette Smoke Condensate (CSC), Hellermann et al. (2002) showed an increased activation of NF-κB and phosphorylation of ERK1 and -2. The activation of NF-κB was confirmed by an increased reporter activity of NF-κB-luciferase promoter–reporter cassette transfected in A549 cells in response to CSC. The activation of NF-κB could further be associated with an increased expression of human soluble intercellular adhesion molecule-1 (sICAM-1), IL-1β, IL-8, and granulocyte-macrophage colony-stimulating factor (GM-CSF), suggesting that activation of NF-κB and MAPK pathways may play a role in the proinflammatory effects of CSC in epithelial cells. Involvement of IL-1β in cigarette smoke-mediated lung inflammation has recently been provided more impetus by the study of Castro et al. (2004). Similar effects of CSC via NF-κB activation were also observed in other cell lines, such as human histiocytic lymphoma U-937 Mono Mac 6 cells, Jurkat T cells, and H1299 lung cells (Anto et al. 2002; Yang et al. 2006). Furthermore, the activation of NF-κB by CSC corroborated well with time-dependent phosphorylation and degradation of IκBα and activation of IκBα kinase. In vitro experiments with CSC and cultured epithelial cells have revealed a distinct pattern of stress response in cultured epithelial cells, which may be related to the reported proinflammatory activities of CSC (via the formation of ROS/lipid peroxidation products) both in vitro and in vivo (Gebel and Muller 2001). Cigarette smoke exposure led to a decreased DNA binding of NF-κB during the first 2 h of exposure, followed by a further increase (>2-fold) over control after 4–6 h in Swiss 3T3 cells (Gebel and Muller 2001). This was independent of IκB-α, as evidenced by the lack of phosphorylation and degradation of IκB (Muller and Gebel 1998) In another elegant study, the DNA binding of NF-κB was effectively blocked by an anti-inflammatory celecoxib (Shishodia and Aggarwal 2004). In this study, it was observed that the celecoxib interfered with NF-κB binding to the COX-2 promoter region, inhibited p65 phosphorylation, nuclear translocation of NF-κB to the nucleus, and suppressed activation of IκBα and thus prevented activation of COX-2 by NF-κB and therefore, further inflammatory responses.

It has been shown that thioredoxin, a thiol-dependent protein, could regulate NF-κB DNA binding in a redox-dependent manner (Gebel and Muller 2001). Therefore, the initial loss of DNA-binding activity may also be because of the decreased level of reduced thioredoxin. However, within hours, the cells overcame the oxidative stress by induction of thioredoxin reductase mRNA, elevation of GSH levels, and restoration of NF-κB/thioredoxin complexes in nuclear extracts. An implication of this study is that the binding of NF-κB in response to cigarette smoke may be a redox-controlled mechanism depending on the availability of reduced thioredoxin in the nucleus and furthermore, that the redox status of thioredoxin or glutathione may be involved in the transcriptional regulation of gene expression by cigarette smoke. It is interesting to note that in vitro treatment with various constituents of cigarette smoke, such as nicotine, acrolein, hydroquinone, catechol, and 4-HNE, inhibits either basal or LPS-induced NF-κB activation and the expression of NF-κB-dependent genes such as *IL-1*, *IL-2*, *IF-γ*, *TNF-α*, and *IL-8* in the U937 cell line or peripheral blood-derived monocytes (Ouyang et al. 2000; Sugano et al. 1998). It is postulated that the inhibitory effects of nicotine may contribute to cigarette smoke-induced immunosuppression. Similarly, Vayssier et al. (1998) have shown that cigarette smoke itself inhibits both spontaneous and LPS-induced NF-κB activation and cytokine release in human peripheral blood monocytes, which may be related to the altered cytokine profile observed in alveolar macrophages of smokers. In line with this observation, Laan et al. (2004) have recently uncovered a novel mechanism wherein CSC was found to inhibit bacterial LPS-dependent neutrophil–chemotactic cytokine production via downregulation of AP-1 activation in airway epithelial cells. Thus, it appears that cigarette smoke-mediated regulation of NF-κB may be cell type specific.

The c-*fos* gene belongs to a family of growth and differentiation-related immediate early genes, the expression of which generally represents the first measurable response to a variety of chemical and physical stimuli (Luo 1994). Studies in various cell lines have shown enhanced expression of the c-*fos* gene in response to cigarette smoke (Luo 1994; Muller 1995). These effects of cigarette smoke can be mimicked by peroxynitrite and smoke-related aldehydes (4-HNE, acrolein, acetaldehyde) in concentrations that are present in aqueous cigarette preparations (Muller et al. 1997). AP-1 (c-Fos/c-Jun) DNA binding is increased in epithelial and endothelial cells in response to CSC (Rahman et al. 1996c; Wodrich and Volhm 1993) and NF-κB, AP-1, and various AP-1 components are increased in lungs of smokers and patients with COPD (Crowther et al. 1999). In a study employing rat lungs, cigarette smoke was found to trigger costimulation of both c-Fos and iNOS along with enhancement in protein-tyrosine phosphorylation and induction of MAPK-ERK kinase 1 (MEK1)/ERK2 pathways. The latter may then trigger processes leading to lung pathogenesis (Chang et al. 2001).

5.5.3 Gene Transcription

There is now a spate of evidence that oxidative stress may modulate the expression of both proinflammatory and protective antioxidant genes. A particular balance or a ratio of oxidants to antioxidants may therefore regulate the expression of pro- and anti-inflammatory genes in response to ROS and during inflammation (Rahman and MacNee 2000a). This oxidant/antioxidant ratio may therefore be critical to cell injury/protection against the aftermath of inflammation. It is likely that antioxidant genes expression during chronic inflammation might precede the expression of proinflammatory genes. The expression of the latter may overtake the adaptive/protective antioxidant responses with persistence of inflammation with a resultant irreversible lung damage seen in various chronic lung diseases including COPD.

5.5.3.1 Antioxidant Protective and Stress Response Genes

Among the antioxidant enzymes, GSH synthesizing and associated redox enzymes appear to play a crucial protective role in the airspaces and epithelial cells (Fig. 5.3). To this extent, the cytoprotective role of GSH has been amply demonstrated both in vivo in the rat and in vitro, using monolayer cultures of alveolar epithelial cells exposed to cigarette smoke/oxidants (Lannan et al. 1994; Li et al. 1994, 1996). This was evidenced by a profound increment in the GSH levels in response to acute intratracheal instillation of CSC in the rat, and exposure of epithelial cell monolayers to cigarette smoke in vitro (Li et al. 1996). This increment in GSH levels was further emphasized by a rebound adaptive increase of GSH levels and GCL heavy subunit (GCL-HS) mRNA expression in both rat lungs and epithelial cell lines (Lannan et al. 1994; Rahman et al. 1995). This finding was mirrored in humans, where GSH was found to be elevated in ELF associated with an increased expression of GCL mRNA in lungs of chronic cigarette smokers (Cantin et al. 1987; Morrison et al. 1999; Rahman and MacNee 2000b). Such a situation was not the case in acute smokers as compared with nonsmokers. Thus, cells respond to an oxidative stress, including that generated by cigarette smoking, by upregulation of an important antioxidant gene involved in the synthesis of GSH as an adaptive mechanism against subsequent oxidative stress. However, such an adaptive response may not entirely counteract the potential burden of proinflammatory mediators and oxidants released therein during inflammation.

A recent study has shown that the expression of GCL mRNA is elevated in smokers' lungs and is even more pronounced in smokers with COPD (Rahman et al. 2000c). This implies that GCL expression might be upregulated (GSH levels were not studied) in response to an ongoing inflammatory response and oxidative stress in lungs of smokers with and without COPD. However, Harju et al. (2002) have found that the GCL immunoreactivity was decreased (again, GSH levels were not measured) in the airways of smokers, compared with nonsmokers. This suggested that cigarette smoke predisposes lung cells to ongoing oxidant stress. Neurohr et al. (2003) showed that decreased GSH levels in BAL cells of chronic smokers were associated with a decreased expression of γ-GCS light subunit (γ-GCS-LS) without a change in γ-GCS-HS expression. This highlighted the fact that increased GSH levels in the ELF of chronic smokers were not associated with increased GSH levels in alveolar macrophages. Furthermore, rats exposed to cigarette smoke have shown increased expression of manganese superoxide dismutase (*MnSOD*), *NAO1*, *CINC-1*, metallothionein (*MT*), and *GPx* genes in the bronchial epithelial cells, suggesting the importance of the antioxidant gene adaptive response against the injurious effects of cigarette smoke (Gilks et al. 1998; Stringer et al. 2004). Therefore, from the above discussion, cell response to a given oxidant stress appears to be quite intricate and delicately balanced and therefore merits further investigation in lungs of smokers with and without COPD.

Comhair et al. (2000) showed over a 2-fold increase in extracellullar glutathione peroxidase (eGPx) mRNA in human airway epithelial cells and alveolar macrophages in response to cigarette smoke, but without any iNOS expression. On the other hand, hyperoxic exposure increased iNOS mRNA in airway epithelial cells by 2.5-fold, without an increase in eGPx mRNA. They suggested that molecular responses by the lung cells to an oxidant may vary with the type of inhaled ROS, which are likely to influence the susceptibility of the airway to oxidative injury in vivo. In view of the possible differential regulation of eGPx in acute and chronic smokers, it would be an interesting proposition to investigate the expression of eGPx in airway epithelial cells of smokers with and without COPD. In a recent study by the same group, eGPx was found to be increased in asthmatic airways (bronchial epithelial cells) in comparison to healthy controls, which might be an important defensive strategy of a cell against hydroperoxide-mediated injury to the airway surface in asthmatic individuals (Comhair et al. 2001). Comhair (2005) has further emphasized that induction of eGPx in the airways may be an important defense arsenal against oxidative injury to airway surface cells. Another antioxidant enzyme, GSH S-transferase P1 (GSTP1), was shown by Ishii et al. (2001) and coworkers to act in against cigarette smoke in the airway cells. Similarly, Maestrelli et al. (2001) have suggested that induction of heme oxygenase-1 (HO-1) in alveolar spaces of smokers may lead to increased levels of exhaled CO. Cigarette smoke also induces heat shock protein 70 (HS 70) in human monocytes and HO-1, which have been implicated in the regulation of cell injury and cell death and, in particular, modulation of apoptosis in human endothelial cells and monocytes (Favatier and Polla, 2001; Vayssier et al. 1998). The induction of HSP70 may stabilize IκBα, possibly through the inhibition of IκB kinase activation.

5.5.3.2 Pro- and Anti-Inflammatory Genes

TNF-α and LPS are important stimuli for inflammatory responses in COPD. Airway epithelial cells can respond to these stimuli by a concurrent increased generation of both intracellular ROS and RNS (MacNee and Rahman 1999; Rahman and MacNee 2000c; Rochelle et al. 1998). This intracellular production of oxidants and the subsequent changes in intracellular redox status are important in the molecular events (MAPK signaling and chromatin remodeling) controlling the expression of genes for inflammatory mediators (Richer et al. 1995). Animal studies have clearly demonstrated that cigarette smoking induces neutrophil influx to the airspace, increased IL-8 release, and NF-κB activation in the lungs. (Manwick et al. 2004) These observations were further supported by several other investigators who demonstrated that IL-8 release from human bronchial, alveolar epithelial, and endothelial cells increased in response to cigarette smoke, which led to airway inflammation (Masubuchi et al. 1998; Mio et al. 1997; Wang et al. 2000). The increased IL-8 paralleled the increased neutrophil counts in bronchial samples of BAL fluid. Abolition of these effects by recombinant SOD treatment suggested that cigarette smoke-mediated peroxidation/oxidative stress regulates the molecular events in lung inflammation (Nishikawa et al. 1999). Cigarette smoke-induced IL-8 release in turn may be mediated via oxidative stress because of a Fenton reaction–catalyzed peroxidation reaction, because aldehydes such as acrolein and acetaldehyde augmented IL-8 release (Masubuchi et al. 1998; Mio et al. 1997; Wang et al. 2000). A report by Saetta et al. (2002) lends credence to this observation by their demonstration of an increased expression of the chemokine receptor CXCR3 and its ligand CXCL10 in peripheral airways of smokers with COPD. Because the CXCR3/CXCL10 axis is associated with T-cell response, their increased expression might be involved in T-lymphocyte recruitment during airway inflammation because of increased levels of chemokines.

Another consequence of cigarette smoking is an increased adherence of leukocytes to vascular endothelial cells (Noguera et al. 1998). According to Shen et al. (1996), CSC induces leukocyte adherence by increasing the expression of a wide variety of cell adhesion molecules. Adhesion molecules such as ICAM-1, endothelial leukocyte adhesion molecule 1 (ELAM-1), and vascular cell adhesion molecule-1 (VCAM-1) in human umbilical vascular endothelial cells have been associated with an increase in the binding activity of NF-κB. Such an expression of adhesion molecules has been implicated in an increased transendothelial migration of monocytes by cigarette smoking. Exposure of bronchial epithelial cells cultured from biopsy from patients with COPD to cigarette smoke, exhibited increased release of proinflammatory mediators, such as IL-1β and sICAM-1, as compared with smokers (Rusznak et al. 2000). This implies that patients with COPD have a greater susceptibility to the effects of cigarette smoke.

Transforming growth factor-β_1 (TGF-β_1) is a multifunctional growth factor that modulates cellular proliferation, differentiation, and tissue repair (Border and Ruoslahti 1992; Clark and Cocker 1998). In addition, TGF-β_1 acts as a chemoattractant and mitogen for fibroblasts and fibroblast-like cells and stimulates the synthesis and deposition of extracellular matrix. Recently, increased TGF-β_1 expression was demonstrated in bronchiolar and alveolar epithelium in subjects with COPD (de Boer et al. 1998; Takizawa et al. 2001). Increased TGF-β_1 expression associated with fibrosis in the basement membrane in the lungs could be suggestive of an abnormal repair process after exposure to cigarette smoke (Chan-Yeung 1988). TGF-β_1, which decreases GSH synthesis, has been associated with increased ROS production in human alveolar epithelial cells and pulmonary artery endothelial cells in vitro (Das and Fanburg 1991; Jardine et al. 2002; White et al. 1992) and thus may a play a role in membrane lipid peroxidation (Fig. 5.7). Conversely, lipid peroxidation products may in turn affect the expression of TGF-β_1, as has been recorded in experiments with 4-HNE (Leonarduzzi et al. 1997; Parolla et al. 1999). 4-HNE has been shown to induce cellular stress responses via the MAPK pathways, leading to the induction of AP-1-mediated genes (Leonarduzzi et al. 2000) such as GCL mRNA in alveolar epithelial cells (Liu et al. 2001). Smokers and subjects with COPD have been found to express increased GCL in lung alveolar epithelial cells (Rahman et al. 1996c). Hence, 4-HNE may play a role in the regulation of AP-1-dependent TGF-β1 and *GCL* gene expression in patients with COPD. It may therefore be surmised that increased 4-HNE because of membrane lipid peroxidation may be one factor signaling the expression of TGF-β_1 and GCL in lungs of COPD patients. Such a possibility is based on the observation of increased levels of 4-HNE adducts being associated with increased levels of TGF-β_1 in bronchiolar and alveolar epithelium and macrophages in subjects with COPD as compared with those without COPD (MacNee and Rahman 1999; Rahman et al. 2002a). The observed induction of GCL may be an important adaptive response of the alveolar epithelium to oxidative stress. A recent study by Sano et al. (2002) has shown that another antioxidant gene, thioredoxin, is induced by 4-HNE in response to LPS challenge in mice and may impart endotoxin tolerance. This suggests that 4-HNE triggers a second messenger response that upregulates expression of the protective GCL and thioredoxin genes as well as a variety of other genes like TGF-β_1, matrix metalloproteinase-1, cyclooxygenase 2 (*COX-2*), monocyte chemoattractant protein-1 (*MCP-1*) and *VEGF*, all of which have been implicated in the pathogenesis of COPD (Belloeq et al. 1999; Kasahara et al. 2000; Kumgai et al. 2000; Sano et al. 2002) (Fig. 5.8). Similarly, 4-HNE has been also shown to induce VEGF expression in retinal pigment epithelial cells (Ayalasomayajula and Kompella 2002), and such an induction has been linked to the pathogenesis of inflammatory lung diseases such as emphysema and COPD (Kasahara et al. 2000). Cigarette smoke exposure resulted in increased expression of VEGF and its flk-1 receptor in main pulmonary arteries and in intraparenchymal arteries (Wright et al. 2002). Such an imbalance of an array of redox-regulated antioxidant versus pro-inflammatory genes therefore might be associated with the susceptibility or tolerance to disease (MacNee and Rahman 1999). Ward et al. (2000) have shown an upregulation of the protective antiapoptotic protein bcl-2 in response to transgenic IL-6 expression against hyperoxic acute lung injury and lipid peroxidation in animal models. Other investigators have reported that the activated Akt signaling pathway protects the lung from oxidant-induced injury in mice (Lu et al. 2001). However, the implications of these relatively novel antioxidant protective signaling mechanisms in various chronic lung inflammatory diseases are yet to be fully explored.

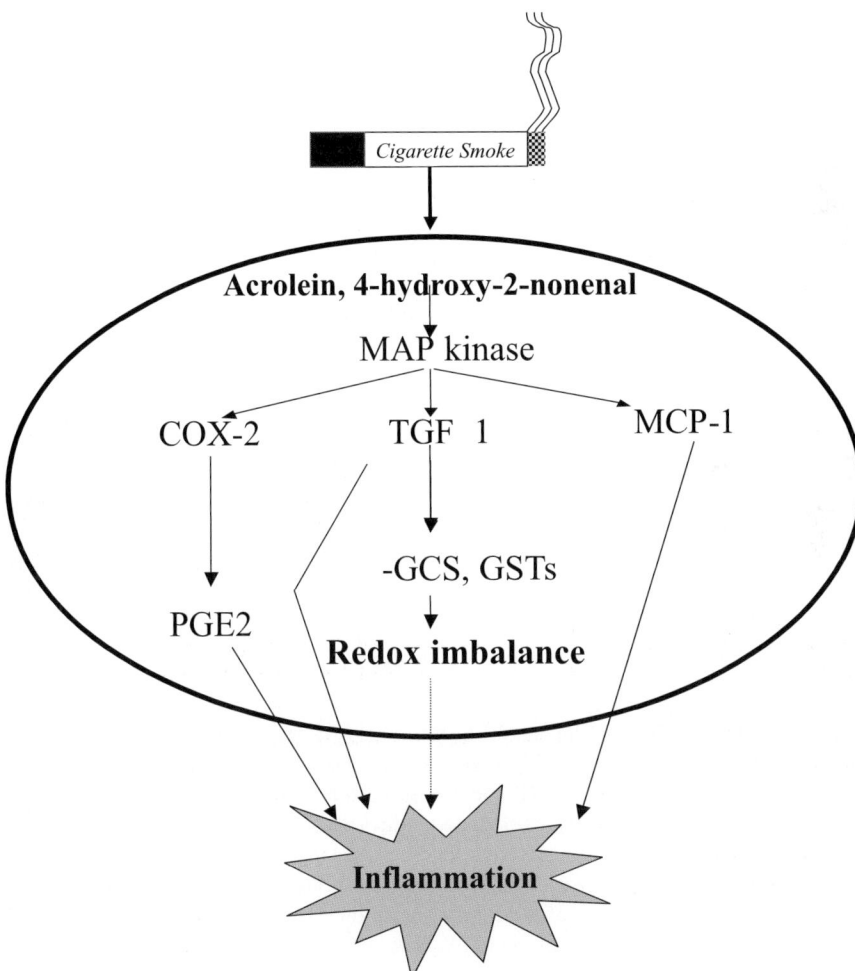

Fig. 5.7 Proposed model of the mechanism of cigarette smoke-mediated oxidative stress (formation of 4-hydroxy-2-nonenal) in redox-mediated lung inflammation

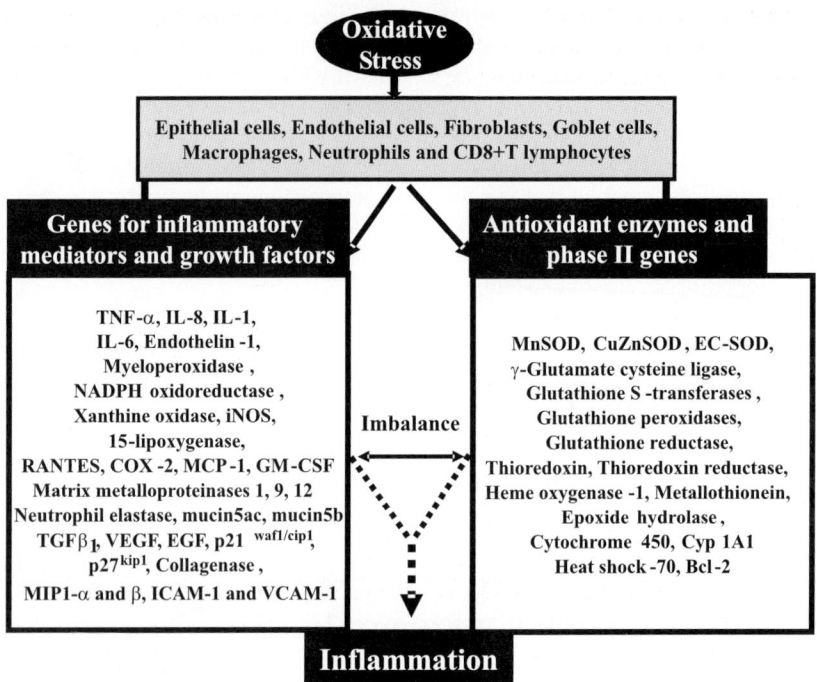

Fig. 5.8 Various inflammatory and structural cells are activated by oxidative stress, leading to transcription of various proinflammatory and antioxidant genes. It may be possible that induction of antioxidant enzymes might provide initial adaptive or protective responses against oxidative stress and inflammatory mediators. However, during sustained/chronic inflammation, the balance between genes for inflammatory mediators and antioxidant/phase II enzymes may be tipped in favor of proinflammatory mediators

5.5.3.3 Aldehyde/Lipid Peroxidation Product-Mediated Gene Expression

Acrolein, being an electrophilic agent, may induce a variety of genes regulated via the electrophilic response element or antioxidant response element (ARE). GCL and GST, which are under regulation by ARE, may be induced by acrolein (Biswal et al. 2002). Li et al. (1999) reported that acrolein-mediated induction of IκB occurred within 15 min of exposure to 5 μM acrolein in rat alveolar macrophages that subsequently led to the inhibition of NF-κB activity. However, acrolein did not induce IκB in A549 epithelial cells, suggesting that the inhibition of NF-κB activation by acrolein may be IκB independent and cell-type specific (Horton et al. 1999). Similarly, 4-HNE induction of JNK-mediated AP-1 activation may be involved in transcriptional activation of ARE-dependent xenobiotic-metabolizing genes. 4-HNE also inhibits NF-κB activation and LPS-induced TNF-α expression by inhibiting I-κB phosphorylation and subsequent proteolysis in THP-1 monocytic cells (Page et al. 1999) This role of 4-HNE has been refuted by Okada et al. (1999), who have shown that 4-HNE impairs ubiquitin/proteasome-dependent intracellular proteolysis, a mechanism involved in NF-κB activation. Later studies have shown that 4-HNE-mediated NF-κB inhibition was because of inhibition of IκB kinase in a human lung carcinoma cell line (H1299) (Ji et al. 2001) that may be accompanied by the inhibition of IκBα degradation. The differential activation of *NF-κB* and *AP-1* genes by aldehydes in cigarette smoke may reflect an imbalance of the genes induced by cigarette smoking.

5.5.3.4 Mucin Genes

Mucins are complex glycoproteins secreted by the goblet cells, which impart viscoelastic properties to the mucus and play a crucial role in airway defense. Although the regulation of mucins in lungs of COPD patients is not well understood, many chronic inflammatory diseases of the airway are associated with mucus hypersecretion. Smokers express more goblet cells than do nonsmokers, and activation of these cells results in mucus hypersecretion leading to airway plugging (Nadel 2001). Cigarette smoke can activate epidermal growth factor (EGF) receptors via tyrosine phosphorylation, resulting in the induction of *MUC5AC* gene expression leading to mucin hypersynthesis in epithelial cells and in lungs (Chang et al. 2005; Takeyama et al. 2001). Acrolein has been shown to induce the *MUC5AC* gene in the airway epithelial cell line NCI-H292 (Leikauf et al. 2002; Takeyama et al. 2001). This induction was accompanied by EGF ligand formation and the activation of EGF-dependent pathways by TNF-α-converting enzyme and amphiregulin (Lemjabbar et al. 2003; Shao et al. 2004). Neutrophil elastase also increases the expression of *MUC5AC* by enhancing mRNA stability (Fischer and Voynow 2002). Neutrophil release of elastase also impairs mucociliary clearance and stimulates goblet cell metaplasia and therefore, mucin production. Furthermore, inhibition of elastase-induced *MUC5AC* gene expression by antioxidants in human bronchial and alveolar epithelial cells suggests that neutrophil elastase-mediated *MUC5AC* gene expression is oxidant dependent (Kasahara 2000). Therefore, enhanced levels of lipid peroxidation products may be of etiological importance for mucus cell hyperplasia, as observed in smokers with airflow obstruction (Leikauf et al. 2002). This hypothesis is strengthened by the observation that cigarette smoke-mediated *MUC5AC* gene expression could be inhibited by selective EGFR tyrosine kinase inhibitors and antioxidants (Takeyama et al. 2001). In a recent study, it was reported that cigarette smoke-generated ROS upregulates *MUC5AC* gene expression via AP-1-JunD and Fra-2 or Fra-1 pathway (Gensch et al. 2004; Zhang et al. 2005). These transcription factors are known to require phosphorylation by upstream kinases such as JNK and ERK, respectively. Activation of JNK was found to be Src dependent and did not require EGFR. Understanding the EGF receptor signaling pathway in cigarette smoke-mediated upregulation of mucin gene expression could therefore lead to targeted inhibition of mucus hyper-production in epithelial cells.

5.5.3.5 DNA Microarray Profile: Cigarette Smoke-Mediated Gene Expression

A comprehensive gene expression profile of COPD has been carried out by Ning et al. (2004). Serial analysis of gene expression (SAGE) and microarray analysis were used to compare the gene expression patterns of lung tissues from smokers with and without COPD. A total of 261 transcripts were differentially expressed in a total of 26,502 transcripts that were sequenced. The genes encoding for transcription factors (*EGR1* and *FOS*), growth factors, or related proteins (*CTGF, CYR61, CX3CL1, TGFB1,* and *PDGFRA*) and extracellular matrix proteins (*COL1A1*) were induced. Most recently, Shah et al. (2005) have compiled and analyzed over 22,500 transcripts of human thoracic airway cells in a study termed SIEGE (Smoking-Induced Epithelial Gene Expression database), using Affymetrix HG-U133A gene chips. (This microarray data along with relevant patient information is available on http://pulm.bumc.bu.edu/siegeDB.) Similarly, Golpon et al. (2004) have demonstrated a global decrease in gene expression associated with increased abundance of genes encoding proteins involved in inflammation, immune responses, and proteolysis in emphysematous lung tissues. Zhang et al. (2001) have also identified a number of genes that are modulated by nicotine in human coronary artery endothelial cells, using a cDNA microarray approach to evaluate over 4,000 genes. This observation is particularly interesting because nicotine can induce CBP coactivator and MAPK cascade genes that are also involved in cigarette smoke-related pathologies. Izzotti et al. (2004) have shown alterations of gene expression in skin and lungs of mice exposed to light and cigarette smoke. It has been shown that sunlight-mimicking light induces genotoxic damage not only in skin, but also in lung, bone marrow, and peripheral blood of mice. By using cDNA-arrays of 746 toxicologically relevant genes, they have identified glutathione-*S*-transferase-Pi, catalase, and COX-2 expression in both skin and lung. In another elegant study, Basio et al. (2002) described the kinetics of gene expression profiling up to 24 h, using glass chips containing 513 different cDNA probes in Swiss 3T3 cells exposed to aqueous extracts of cigarette smoke. The cigarette smoke-induced stress response genes related to antioxidant response elements studied were heme oxygenase-1, metallothionein 1 and 2, and heat shock proteins (*hsp90* and *hsp105*), genes coding for transcription factors, e.g., JunB, c-*maf*, sarp1 (antiapoptotic protein, secreted apoptosis-related protein) and CAAT/enhancer protein (*C/EBP*), cell cycle-related genes, e.g., *gadd34* and *gadd45*, and genes for inflammatory/immune-regulatory response, e.g, *st2* (IL-1-like receptor), *kc* (chemoattractant cytokine involved in neutrophil activation), and *id3* (induction of growth arrest/apoptosis in B-lymphocyte progenitor cells). Gebel and colleagues (2004), by using DNA microarray chips covering 2,031 cDNA probes, demonstrated a differential gene expression in tissues of rat respiratory tract after acute and subchronic cigarette smoke exposures. They show the induction of oxidative stress-responsive and phase II drug-metabolizing enzymes, such as heme oxygenase-1, NAD(P)H-quinine oxidoreductase, and Nrf2, without any change in phase I genes cytochrome P450 1A1 and aldehyde dehydrogenase 3 after acute cigarette smoke exposure. Taken together, these studies lay further emphasis on the potential imbalance of pro- and anti-inflammatory/antioxidant genes induced by cigarette smoking. It may now be possible in the near future to study the gene expression profile in a specific region of inflamed lungs by laser capture microdissection combined with real-time reverse transcriptase-polymerase chain reaction (Betsuyaku et al. 1996).

5.6 Role of ROS and Cigarette Smoke-Induced Oxidative Stress in Chromatin Modeling: Role for Histone Acetylation/Deacetylation and DNA Methylation

5.6.1 Role of ROS in Chromatin Remodeling and Gene Transcription: Epigenetics

Epigenetics is defined as the inheritance of information based on gene expression, in contrast to *genetics*, which is described as the inheritance of information based on DNA sequence. Histone acetylation/deacetylation and DNA methylation are two important epigenetic events that play an important role in inflammatory lung responses.

5.6.1.1 Chromatin Remodeling (Histone Acetylation and Deacetylation)

Many factors, including specific DNA sequences, histones, nonhistone chromosomal proteins, transcriptional activators/repressors, and the transcription machinery are all necessary for the assembly of an active transcriptional complex (Sternglanz 1996). Condensation of eukaryotic DNA as a tightly coiled structure in chromatin suppresses gene activity through the coiling of DNA on the surface of the nucleosome core and folding of nucleosome assemblies, thus denying accessibility to the transcriptional apparatus (Wu 1997). Tightly bound DNA around a nucleosome core (by histone residues H2A, H2B, H3, and H4) suppresses gene transcription by decreasing the accessibility of transcription factors, such as NF-κB and AP-1, to the transcriptional complex. Uncoiling of the DNA via acetylation of lysine (K) residues in the N-terminal tails of the core histone proteins allows increased accessibility for transcription factor binding (Imhof and Wolffe 1998). Acetylation of K residues on histone 4 (K5, K8, K12, K16) is thought to be directly related to the regulation of gene transcription (Bannister and Miska 2000; Imhof and Wolffe 1998). Histone acetylation is reversible and is regulated by a group of histone acetyltransferases (HATs), which promote acetylation, and histone deacetylases (HDACs), which promote deacetylation.

The nuclear receptor coactivators, steroid receptor coactivator 1 (SRC-1), CBP/adenoviral protein E1A (p300) protein, CBP/p300-associated factor (P/CAF), and ATF-2, all possess intrinsic HAT activity (Fig. 5.9) (Kawasaki et al. 2000; Ogryzko et al. 1996; Pham and Sauer 2000). Of these, CBP/p300 and ATF-2 are vital for the coactivation of several transcription factors, including NF-κB and AP-1, and are regulated by the p38-MAPK pathway (Kawasaki et al. 2000; Ogryzko et al. 1996; Pham and Sauer 2000; Thomson et al. 1999). These activation complexes act in consonance with RNA polymerase II to initiate transcription (Carrero et al. 2000; Kamei et al. 1996; Ng et al. 1997). Thus, it is likely that histone acetylation of H4 via CBP/p300 and/or ATF-2 has a significant role in the activation of NF-κB/AP-1-mediated gene expression of proinflammatory mediators (Carrero et al. 2000; Kamei et al. 1996; Kawasaki et al. 2000). However, the precise molecular mechanisms involved in such transcriptional regulation warrant more investigations.

The family of HDAC enzymes consists of at least ten distinct deacetylases (Tong et al. 2002). Several distinct HDACs are now recognized, and these are differentially expressed and regulated in different cell types. HDACs catalyze the removal of the acetyl moieties from the ε-acetamido groups of lysine residues of histones, causing DNA rewinding and silencing of gene transcription. Recently, it has been shown that HDACs (1 and 2) play a crucial role in the regulation of cell proliferation and corticosteroid-mediated inhibition of proinflammatory mediators (Ito et al. 2000; Sambucetti et al. 1999). Disruption of the nucleosome or DNA unwinding caused by deacetylation inhibitors has been shown to facilitate AP-1 binding. HDACs not only cause the inhibition of gene transcription by deacetylation and, therefore, limiting coactivator access to target sites of DNA, but also directly affect the nuclear activity of transcription factors such as NF-κB. The duration of the NF-κB nuclear activation has been shown to be dependent on the activity of HDAC3, which provides an acetylation balance-dependent mechanism for the regulation of NF-κB mediated transcription (Chen et al. 2001).

It has been suggested that oxidant-generating systems and proinflammatory mediators influence histone acetylation/phosphorylation via a mechanism dependent on the

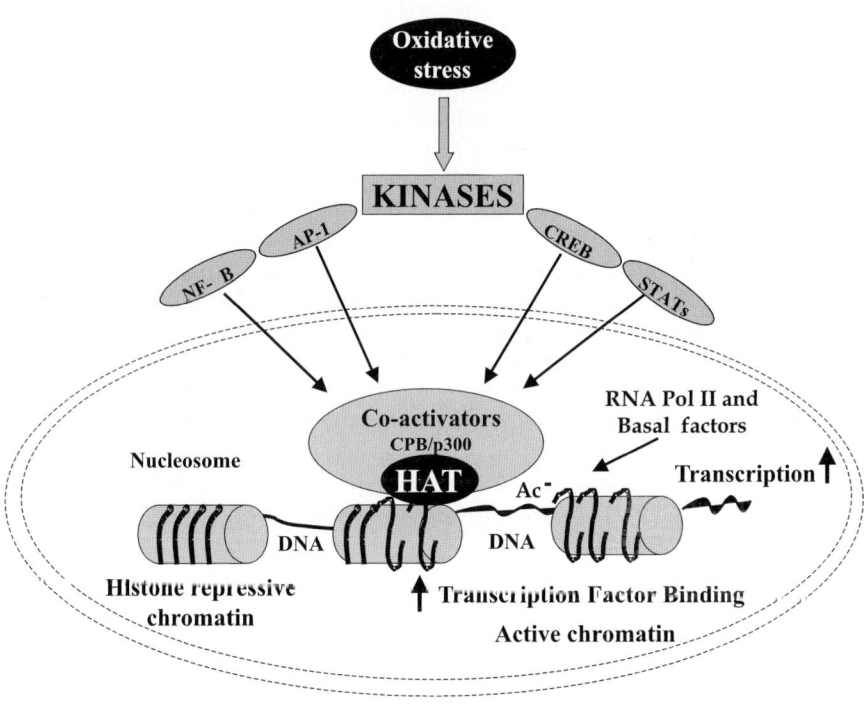

Fig. 5.9 Histone acetylation and deacetylation: oxidative stress and other stimuli, such as cytokines, activate various signal transduction pathways (Janus kinase [JAK], c-Jun N-terminal kinase [JNK], and IκB kinase [IKK]), leading to activation of transcription factors, such as nuclear factor-κB (*NF-κB*), activator protein-1 (*AP-1*), cyclic AMP response element-binding proteins (*CREB*), and signal transducers and activators of transcription (*STAT*) proteins. Binding of these transcription factors leads to recruitment of CREB-binding protein (*CBP*) and/or other coactivators to the transcriptional initiation complex on promoter region of various genes. Activation of CBP leads to acetylation (*Ac*) of specific core histone lysine residues by an intrinsic acetyltransferase activity (histone transacetylase [*HAT*]). Histone acetylation (active chromatin) leads to loosening of nucleosome, which enables access to basal factors and RNA polymerase II for gene transcription to occur

activation of the MAPK pathway (Bohm et al. 1997; Miyata et al. 2001; Tikoo et al. 2001). Recent evidence has shown that oxidative stress induced by H_2O_2 and TNF-α increases the activation of AP-1 and NF-κB and may regulate chromatin remodeling, leading to IL-8 expression (Rahman et al. 2002b). This may be pivotal in cell proliferation, apoptosis, and imbalance in gene transcription for proinflammatory mediators and antioxidant protective genes.

5.6.1.1.1 Gene Transcription

Inflammatory mediators play a crucial role in chronic inflammatory processes and appear to determine and direct the nature of the inflammatory responses via selective recruitment and activation of inflammatory cells and their perpetuation within the lungs. In several in vitro studies employing macrophages, alveolar, and bronchial epithelial cells, ROS have been shown to cause increased gene expression of inflammatory mediators, such as IL-1 and TNF-α. Direct or indirect oxidant challenge to the airway epithelium and alveolar macrophages is also known to generate cytokines, such as TNF-α (which in turn can affect airway epithelial cells to induce proinflammatory genes), TNF-α, IL-8, IL-1, inducible nitric oxide synthase (iNOS), COX-2, ICAM-1, IL-6, macrophage inflammatory protein 1 (MIP-1), GM-CSF, stress response genes (*HSP-27, -70, -90, HO-1*), and antioxidant enzymes (γ-glutamylcysteine synthetase γ-GCS, MnSOD, and thioredoxin) (Gutteridge and Halliwell 2000) (Fig. 5.8). The genes for these inflammatory mediators are regulated by redox-sensitive transcription factors, such as NF-κB and AP-1 (Anto et al. 2002; Hellerman et al. 2002). However, the expression/induction of these genes is now known to be regulated by their acetylation/deacetylation status. Acetylation of histones has been associated with the transcription of a range of inflammatory mediators including IL-8 (Hoshimoto et al. 2002), eotaxin, IL-1β, and GM-CSF (Adcock and Caramori 2001), MIP-2 (Ohno et al. 1997), and IL-6 (Berghe et al. 1999). Acetylation can occur specifically at the promoter sites of these genes as shown by chromatin immunoprecipitation (CHiP) assays for IL-8 (Ashburner et al. 2001), CYP1A1 (Ke et al. 2001), myeloperoxidase (Miyata et al. 2001), and 15-lox-1 (Shankaranarayanan et al. 2001) gene promoters, indicating acetylation specificity.

5.6.1.2 Mechanisms of Transcriptional Regulation

5.6.1.2.1 MAPK- and NF-κB-Mediated Histone Acetylation and Deacetylation

Oxidative stress and proinflammatory mediators have been suggested to influence histone acetylation and phosphorylation by ADP ribosylation, via a mechanism dependent on the activation of a MAPK pathway (Bohm et al. 1997; Miyata et al. 2001; Tikoo et al. 2001). Recently, work in our laboratory and by other investigators has shown that both H_2O_2 and TNF-α caused an increase in HAT activity in alveolar epithelial cells (Ito et al. 2001a; Moodie et al. 2004; Rahman et al. 2002b). The exact mechanism of increased histone acetylation in response to these agents is, however, yet to be fully decrypted. Reports are nonetheless available wherein oxidants and TNF-α have been shown to activate MAPK pathways, specifically ERK and JNK. Activation of these redox-dependent pathways may then modulate ATF-2 and CBP coactivators that possess intrinsic HAT activity (Carrero et al. 2000; Kawasaki et al. 2000; Tong et al. 2002). ROS and TNF-α increase the activation of AP-1 and NF-κB and regulate chromatin remodeling, leading to IL-8 expression in lung cells (Berghe et al. 1999; Lakshminarayan et al. 1998; Rahman et al. 2002b). Recently, Ito and coworkers (2001b) have shown a role for histone acetylation and deacetylation in IL-1β-induced TNF-α release in alveolar macrophages derived from cigarette smokers. They have also suggested that oxidants may play an important role in the modulation of HDAC and inflammatory cytokine gene transcription. They further demonstrated increased expression of p65 protein of NF-κB in bronchial epithelium of smokers and patients with COPD (Di Stefano et al. 2002). The increased expression of p65 in epithelial cells was correlated with the degree of airflow limitation in patients with COPD. NF-κB is known to be associated with coactivators such as CBP and p300 that have HAT activity (Berghe et al. 1999). Their recruitment by transcription factors is thus an important link between promoter activation and transcriptional machinery. Shenkar et al. (2001) have shown that the p65 subunit of NF-κB interacts with CBP after hemorrhage and endotoxemia-induced acute lung injury. However, it is still unclear as to the status of the NF-κB signaling pathway and chromatin remodeling in small airways and parenchyma of COPD patients. We have also shown that CSC increased the acetylation of histone 4 associated with decreased levels of HDAC-2 levels in alveolar epithelial cells, monocytes and in vivo in rat lungs in response to cigarette smoke exposure (Marwick et al. 2004; Moodie et al. 2004; Yang et al. 2006). We also showed that inhibiting HDACs alone resulted in enhanced activation of AP-1 and NF-κB and increased histone acetylation, culminating in increased IL-8 release (Rahman et al. 2002, 2004) (Fig. 5.10). This observation is corroborated by previous studies showing that acetylation of histone proteins is associated with increased binding of the transcription factors AP-1 and NF-κB (Fusunyan et al. 1999; Ng et al. 1997). IL-8 release was also augmented on histone deacetylase inhibition by trichostatin A, when combined with TNF-α or H_2O_2. This increase in IL-8 release was associated with NF-κB binding, suggesting that inhibition of HDAC may promote NF-κB retention in the nucleus, triggering augmented TNF-α or H_2O_2-mediated gene transcription. In addition, NF-κB itself can be acetylated while in the nucleus by virtue of its interaction with CBP, which may lead to further transcriptional activation (Saccani et al. 2001). Once the acetylated active NF-κB dimers are localized in the nucleus, they scan the chromatin for any exposed transcriptional sites. This mechanism was supported by Saccani et al. (2002), who have shown bimodal (two temporally distinct phases) recruitment of NF-κB to target promoters by LPS stimulation in the Raw 264.7 murine macrophage cell line. They suggested that a subset of target genes, whose promoters are already heavily acetylated (H4 acetylation) before stimulation, are constitutively and immediately accessible to NF-κB. Such genes (*MnSOD, MIP2, IκB-α, IL-2*) are subject to immediate transcription post-NF-κB recruitment, whereas other target genes (*MCP-1, RANTES, IL-6*) are not immediately accessible. Recruitment of NF-κB (p38 dependent) to late accessible gene promoters occurs after nuclear entry and is preceded by the formation of an initial transcription factor complex that directs the hyperacetylation of the promoter and makes it accessible to NF-κB. This shows the selectivity of stimulus-specific p38-dependent and NF-κB-mediated histone acetylation, leading to a subset of gene transcription.

It is known that p65, a component of the NF-κB transcription factor, has intrinsic HAT activity, and transactivation of p65 is independent of nuclear translocation (Ashburner et al. 2001; Chen et al. 2001; Pham and Sauer 2000). It has been shown that

HDAC1 can interact directly with the p65 subunit of NF-κB to exert its corepressor function in the nucleus (Ito et al. 2001; Yang et al. 2006). Therefore, NF-κB interaction with HDAC (Rahman and MacNee 2000b; Rahman et al. 2004) proteins may be an additional mechanism whereby NF-κB can regulate transcription (Zhong 2002). HDACs may be prevented from binding to nuclear p65 by cigarette smoke/oxidants, leading to enhanced p65 acetylation/phosphorylation, resulting in *IL-8* gene expression (Fig. 5.10). Zhong et al. (2002) have demonstrated yet another mechanism whereby the phosphorylation status of NF-κB determines its association with HAT (CBP/p300) or HDAC-1, a leading to gene transcription of various proinflammatory mediators in transformed human embryonic kidney HEK293 cells. These workers have proposed that transcriptionally inactive nuclear NF-κB in resting cells consists of homodimers of either p65 or p50 complexed with HDAC-1. Only the p50–HDAC-1 complex binds to the DNA and suppresses NF-κB-dependent gene expression in unstimulated cells. Activation of cells with NF-κB-inducing agents leads to nuclear localization of active phosphorylated p65 that associates with CBP and displaces the p50–HDAC-1 complexes, leading to gene transcription. It remains to be determined, however, whether the above-proposed mechanisms for NF-κB activation (phosphorylation of p65/depletion of HDAC-1 or displacement of p50–HDAC-1 complex) are also operative under oxidative stress. Furthermore, the transactivation of NF-κB may not necessarily require the classical NF-κB/IκB kinase

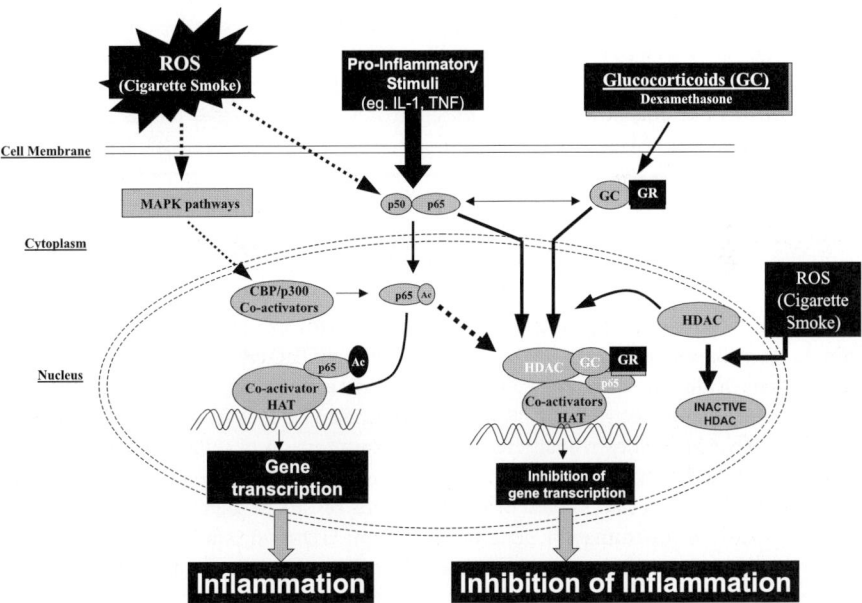

Fig. 5.10 Model showing the possible mechanism of histone acetylation by oxidative stress and its repression by corticosteroids (glucocorticoids [*GC*]), leading to inhibition of gene transcription. Mitogen-activated protein kinase (*MAPK*) signaling pathways may be activated by oxidative stress, leading to histone acetylation. Direct interaction between coactivators (histone transacetylase [*HAT*]), histone deacetylase, and the glucocorticoid receptor (*GR*) may result in repression of the expression of proinflammatory genes. Histone deacetylase (*HDAC*) forms a bridge with HAT to inhibit gene transcription. However, when the HDAC is inhibited by oxidants or the NF-κB subunit p65 is acetylated, steroids may not be able to recruit HDACs into the transcriptional complex to inhibit proinflammatory gene expression

pathway (Ashburner et al. 2001; Ito et al. 2001; Madrid et al. 2001; Pham and Sauer 2000; Saccani et al. 2002; Zhong et al. 2002). IL-8 and IL-6 release have been reported to be enhanced by HDAC inhibitors in intestinal epithelial cells and in murine fibrosarcoma L929sA cells (Gerritsen et al. 1997; Pender et al. 2000). The HDAC inhibitors were also found to prime the effect of IL-1 or TNF-α treatments and enhanced pulmonary cells responsiveness to H_2O_2 and TNF-α, leading to increased transcription factor DNA-binding and enhanced gene expression (Kuscher et al. 1996). On similar lines, Pender and coworkers (2002) have demonstrated that HDAC inhibitors enhance the levels of stromelysin-1 (matrix metalloproteinase 3) by augmenting histone acetylation by TNF-α or IL-1-stimulated mesenchymal cells. Similarly, IL-4 production from activated peripheral blood T cells was enhanced by the histone deacetylase inhibitor trichostatin A, and overexpression of HDACs 1, 2, and 3 inhibited transcription driven by the *IL-4* promoter in Jurkat T cells (Valapour et al. 2002). Potentiation of *IL-4* promoter activity because of cotransfection of HAT-CBP suggested that IL-4 expression is controlled at the transcriptional level by chromatin remodeling. It has been shown that *IL-4* gene expression was increased in lung cells obtained from smokers with COPD (Zhu et al. 2001). Thus, the gene expression of these proinflammatory mediators has important implications for inflammatory lung disease states where the HDAC enzyme is inactivated (Cosio et al. 2004; Ito et al. 2001). In these cases, ROS and TNF-α would lead to an augmented inflammatory response from the tissue. However, it is important to bear in mind that another HDAC inhibitor, suberoylanilide hydroxamic acid (SAHA), inhibited release of key proinflammatory cytokines, such as TNF-α, IL-1β, IL-6, and IFN-γ, in monocytes/macrophages both in vitro and in vivo (Leoni et al. 2002). Thus, HDAC inhibitors may also exhibit anti-inflammatory properties through suppression of cytokine expression. At present, however, the molecular mechanism for the inhibition of these cytokines by SAHA is not yet known.

5.6.1.2.2 Glucocorticoids and Chromatin Remodeling

Corticosteroids are potent anti-inflammatory agents. However, they do not significantly inhibit the inflammatory responses in patients with COPD. Recently, it has been suggested that oxidative stress may induce inflammation and influence glucocorticoid sensitivity via remodeling of the chromatin structure (Adcock et al. 2005; Rahman et al. 2004). It has been shown that glucocorticoid suppression of inflammatory genes requires recruitment of HDAC-2 to the transcription activation complex by the glucocorticoid receptor (Fig. 5.10) (Berghe et al. 1999). This results in deacetylation of histones and a decrease in inflammatory gene transcription. HDAC-2 is inhibited by ROS and CSC, which is reflected by an increase in the expression of various proinflammatory mediators, such ICAM-1, IL-8, IL-6, TNF-α, IL-1β, monocyte chemoattractant protein-1, matrix metalloproteinases, and heat shock proteins, in BAL fluid of smokers (McCrea et al. 1994; Ragione et al. 2001) and in various other cells (Berghe et al. 1999; Pender et al. 2000; Rahman et al. 2001). A reduced level of HDAC-2 was associated with increased proinflammatory response and reduced responsiveness to glucocorticoids in alveolar macrophages obtained from smokers and in rat lungs in response to cigarette smoke exposure (Ito et al. 2001a: Marwick et al. 2004). Similarly, reduced levels of HDAC activity and HDAC1 and HDAC2 proteins were found in bronchial biopsies obtained from asthmatics (Ito et al. 2002). This was partially restored in patients who received inhaled steroids, suggesting that steroids either induce HDAC or decrease HAT activity in asthmatics. However, this mechanism may not be fully operational in case of COPD. In a recent study, Culpitt and coworkers (2002) have shown that release of IL-8 and GM-CSF was not inhibited in cigarette smoke solution-stimulated alveolar macrophages obtained from COPD subjects, compared with that of smokers. They suggested that the lack of efficacy of corticosteroids in COPD might be because of steroid insensitivity of macrophages in the respiratory tract. Thus, the cigarette smoke/oxidant-mediated reduction in HDAC-2 levels in alveolar epithelial cells and macrophages will not only increase inflammatory gene expression, but will also cause a decrease in glucocorticoid function in patients with COPD (Cosio et al. 2004; Rahman et al. 2004). This may be one of the potential reasons for the failure of glucocorticoids to function effectively in reducing inflammation in COPD (Fig 5.10). Other plausible mechanisms that would explain glucocorticoid inefficacy in COPD may be p65 acetylation by cigarette smoke-derived oxidants, elevated levels of hepatocyte nuclear factor-6, or enhancement of macrophage migration inhibitory factor (MIF), which can antagonize/override glucocorticoid-stimulated gene transcription (Chen et al. 2001; Ito et al. 2001b; Lolis 2001; Pierreux et al. 1999). It is also interesting to note that certain other translocatory HDACs, such as HDAC3 and HDAC5, which shuttle between cytoplasm and the nucleus, may also be important in regulating the transcriptional initiation complex by the glucocorticoid receptor. The exact signaling mechanisms that may be involved in the cigarette smoke-mediated chromatin remodeling and glucocorticoid insensitivity are currently unknown. It may be possible that cigarette smoke-mediated formation of aldehydes could be responsible for oxidation/nitrosylation/phosphorylation of HDACs 1, 2, and 5 during inflammation (Manwick et al. 2004; Yang et al. 2006). This line of thought is supported by a report of the ability of theophylline, a polyphenol antioxidant, to restore HDAC activity in alveolar macrophages from patients with COPD (Cosio et al. 2004). Furthermore, theophylline improved the response to dexamethasone in these subjects. Nevertheless, in general, oxidative stress that results in an imbalance between histone acetylation and deacetylation may account for the enhanced expression of inflammatory mediators, leading to amplified lung inflammation. This may serve as a potential mechanism for therapeutic intervention to ameliorate chronic inflammatory response that occurs in the development of smoking-induced chronic inflammatory lung diseases, such as COPD.

5.6.1.2.3 Coactivator Adenoviral E1A and Chromatin Remodeling

Adenoviral DNA can integrate itself into the human genome, and this can lead to the amplification of viral oncoproteins, such as adenoviral protein (E1A). The major role of E1A is to induce entry into the S phase of the cell cycle so that the conditions are optimal for viral replication. CBP and adenovirus E1A-associated protein p300 play essential coactivator roles for a number of transcription factors, including CREB, NF-κB, and signal transducers and activators of transcription (STAT). Therefore, the presence of E1A has been suggested to be a possible factor in susceptibility to inflammation caused by cigarette smoke. It is understood that E1A subverts cellular processes by displacing cellular transcription factors from CBP (Yang et al. 1996). The *E1A* gene has been found to be expressed at a higher frequency in the lungs of COPD patients than in smokers without COPD (Hogg 1999). Retamales and colleagues (2001) suggests that cigarette smoke-induced inflammatory processes that underlie emphysematous destruction of the lung in COPD are amplified in smokers with advanced disease, compared with those with similar smoking histories and preserved lung structure and function. This enhanced response to a similar degree of stimulation was attributed to a latent adenoviral infection of the alveolar surface epithelium. The presence of E1A also enhances the inflammatory response of cells to endotoxins and oxidative stress (Keicho et al. 1999). NF-κB activation, expression of IL-8, TGF-β and ICAM-1 were all enhanced in E1A+ve lung epithelial cells in response to oxidative stress, compared with E1A–ve cells (Gilmour et al. 2001; Higashimoto et al. 2002). Stimulation of E1A-transfected cell lines (THP-1 and Jurkat) led to an increased synthesis of TNF-α, compared with cells transfected with a control plasmid, suggesting that the presence of E1A may induce histone acetylation by increasing the intrinsic HAT activity of CBP. Thus, the presence of transactivating E1A primes the transcriptional machinery for oxidative stress signaling and in turn facilitates persistent amplification of proinflammatory responses. This may also interfere in the action of glucocorticoids in reducing the inflammatory responses in COPD.

5.7 Conclusions

Cigarette smoke-derived ROS are important in the pathogenesis of COPD and may be critical not only to the inflammatory response to cigarette smoke/environmental oxidants, through the activation of redox-sensitive transcription factors, DNA nicking, alteration in histone acetylation/deacetylation and hence, proinflammatory gene expression, but may also be involved in the protective mechanisms against the effects of cigarette smoke by the induction of antioxidant genes. Further understanding of the effects and roles of cigarette smoke-mediated ROS in basic cellular redox functions, such as amplification of proinflammatory and immunological responses, signaling pathways, activation of transcription factors, chromatin modeling (histone acetylation and deacetylation) and gene expression, will provide important information regarding basic pathological processes contributing to smoking-induced lung diseases.

GSH is an important protective antioxidant in the lungs, which is altered in lining fluid in several inflammatory diseases. The glutathione redox status plays an important role in protein modifications and signaling pathways, including a dual effect on redox-sensitive transcription factors. Protein S-glutathiolation and mixed disulfide formation as candidate mechanisms for protein regulation during intracellular oxidative stress have gained a renewed impetus in view of the involvement of oxidants/antioxidants in various disease processes. The upstream regulation of the MAPKs, involvement of the oxidative species in cell proliferative mechanisms, and transient silencing of various protein function by sulfenic-species formation are all important indicators as to how thiol-dependent reactions involving GSH, cysteine, methionine, and other small-molecular-weight thiols may determine the overall outcome of an oxidative stress imposed by cigarette smoke-derived. ROS can influence the inflammatory response through its impact on signal transduction mechanisms, activation of NF-κB, and chromatin modifications resulting in pro-inflammatory gene expression. Understanding of the molecular mechanisms of ROS-mediated cell signaling pathways could provide information for development of novel antioxidant therapeutic targets to prevent smoking-induced diseases. As our understanding of gene expression/epigenetics/genomics increases, further clinical targets and therapeutic strategies are likely to emerge.

Acknowledgements

This study was supported by the Environmental Health Sciences Center Support ES01247. The author would like to thank Dr. Saibal Biswas for his helpful suggestions and comments.

References

Adachi T, Weisbrod RM, Pimentel DR, Ying J, Sharov VS, Schoneich C and Cohen RA (2004) S-glutathiolation by peroxynitrite activates SERCA during arterial relaxation by nitric oxide. Nat Med 10:1200–1207

Adcock IM, Caramori G (2001) Cross-talk between pro-inflammatory transcription factors and glucocorticoids. Immunol Cell Biol 79:376–384

Adcock IM, Cosio B, Tsaprouni L, Barnes PJ, Ito K (2005) Redox regulation of histone deacetylases and glucocorticoid-mediated inhibition of the inflammatory response. Antioxid Redox Signal 7:144–152

Adler V, Yin Z, Tew KD, Ronai Z (1999) Role of redox potential and reactive oxygen species in stress signaling. Oncogene 18:6104–6111

Andoh T, Chock PB, Chiueh CC (2002) The role of thioredoxins in protection against oxidative stress-induced apoptosis in SH-SY5Y cells. J Biol Chem 277:9655-9660

Anto RJ, Mukhopadhyay A, Shishodia S, Gairola CG, Aggarwal BB (2002) Cigarette smoke condensate activates nuclear transcription factor κB through phosphorylation and degradation of IκBα: correlation with induction of cyclooxygenase-2. Carcinogenesis 23:1511–1518

Arumugam N, Sivakumar V, Thanislass J, Pillai KS, Devaraj SN, Devaraj H (1999) Acute pulmonary toxicity of acrolein in rats—underlying mechanism. Toxicol Lett 104:189194

Ashburner BP, Westerheide SD, Baldwin AS Jr (2001) The p65 (RelA) subunit of NF-kappaB interacts with the histone deacetylase (HDAC) corepressors HDAC1 and HDAC2 to negatively regulate gene expression. Mol Cell Biol 21:7065–7077

Ayalasomayajula SP, Kompella UB (2002) Induction of vascular endothelial growth factor by 4-hydroxynonenal and its prevention by glutathione precursors in retinal pigment epithelial cells. Eur J Pharmacol 449:213–220

Bae YS, Kang SW, Seo MS, Baines IC, Tekle E, Chock PB, Rhee SG (1997) Epidermal growth factor (EGF)-induced generation of hydrogen peroxide. Role in EGF receptor-mediated tyrosine phosphorylation. J Biol Chem 272:217–221

Bai XC, Lu D, Liu A, Zhang Z, Li X, Zou Z, Zeng W, Cheng B, Luo S (2005) Reactive oxygen species stimulates receptor activator of NF-κB Ligand expression in osteoblast. J Biol Chem 280:17497–17506

Bandyopadhyay S, Starke DW, Mieyal JJ, Gronostajski RM (1998) Thioltransferase (glutaredoxin) reactivates the DNA-binding activity of oxidation-inactivated nuclear factor 1. J Biol Chem 273:392–397

Bannister AJ, Miska EA (2000) Regulation of gene expression by transcription factor acetylation. Cell Mol Life Sci 57:1184–1192

Barrett WC, DeGnore JP, Konig S, Fales HM, Keng YF, Zhang ZY, Yim MB, Chock PB (1999a) Regulation of PTP1B via glutathionylation of the active site cysteine 215. Biochemistry 38:6699–6705

Barrett WC, DeGnore JP, Keng YF, Zhang ZY, Yim MB, Chock PB (1999b) Roles of superoxide radical anion in signal transduction mediated by reversible regulation of protein-tyrosine phosphatase 1B. J Biol Chem 274:34543–34546

Basio A, Knorr C, Janssen U, Gebel S, Haussmann HJ, Muller T (2002) Kinetics of gene expression profiling in Swiss 3T3 cells exposed to aqueous extracts of cigarette smoke. Carcinogenesis 23:741–748

Basu-Modak S, Luscher P, Tyrrell RM (1996) Lipid metabolite involvement in the activation of human heme oxygenase-1 gene. Free Radic Biol Med 20:887–897

Beeh KM, Beier J, Koppenhoefer N, Buhl R (2004) Increased glutathione disulfide and nitrosothiols in sputum of patients with stable COPD. Chest 126:1116–1122

Bellocq A, Azoulay E, Marullo S, Flahault A, Fouqueray, Philippe C, Cadranel J, Baud L (1999) Reactive oxygen and nitrogen intermediates increase transforming growth factor-β1 release from human epithelial alveolar cells through two different mechanisms. Am J Respir Cell Mol Biol 21:128–136

Berghe WV, Bosscher KD, Boone E, Plaisance S, Haegeman G (1999) The nuclear factor-κB engages CBP/p300 and histone acetyltransferase activity for transcriptional activation of the interleukin-6 gene promoter. J Biol Chem 274:32091–32098

Betsuyaku T, Griffin GL, Watson MA, Senior RM (2001) Laser capture microdissection and real-time reverse transcriptase/polymerase chain reaction of bronchiolar epithelium after bleomycin. Am J Respir Cell Mol Biol 25:278–284

Biswal S, Acquaah-Mensah G, Datta K, Wu X, Kehrer JP (2002) Inhibition of cell proliferation and AP-1 activity by acrolein in human A549 lung adenocarcinoma cells due to thiol imbalance and covalent modifications. Chem Res Toxicol 15:180–186

Biteau B, Labarre J, Toledano MB (2003) ATP-dependent reduction of cysteine-sulfinic acid by S. cerevisiae sulfiredoxin. Nature 425:980–984

Blouin E, Halbwachs-Mecarelli L, Rieu P (1999) Redox regulation of beta2-integrin CD11b/CD18 activation. Eur J Immunol 29:3419–3431

Bohm L, Schneeweiss FA, Sharan RN, Feinendegen LE (1997) Influence of histone acetylation on the modification of cytoplasmic and nuclear proteins by ADP-ribosylation in response to free radicals. Biochim Biophys Acta 1334:149–154

Border WA, Ruoslahti E (1992) Transforming growth factor-b1 in disease: the dark side of tissue repair. J Clin Invest 90:1–7

Bosken CH, Hards J, Gatter K, Hogg JC (1992) Characterization of the inflammatory reaction in the peripheral airways of cigarette smokers using immunocytochemistry. Am Rev Respir Dis 145:911–917

Cantin AM, North SL, Hubbard RC, Crystal RG (1987) Normal alveolar epithelial lining fluid contains high levels of glutathione. Am J Physiol 63:152–157

Carp H, Janoff A (1978) Possible mechanisms of emphysema in smokers: in vitro suppression of serum elastase-inhibitory capacity by fresh cigarette smoke and its prevention by anti-oxidants. Am Rev Respir Dis 118:617–621

Carrero P, Okamoto K, Coumailleau O'Brien S, Tanaka H, Poellinger L (2000) Redox regulated recruitment of the transcriptional coactivators CREB-binding protein and SRC-1 to hypoxia-inducible factor 1-alpha. Mol Cell Biol 20:402–415

Casagrande S, Bonetto V, Fratelli M, Gianazza E, Eberini I, Massigna T, Salmona M, Chang G, Holmgren A, Ghezzi P (2002) Glutathiolation of human thioredoxin: a possible crosstalk between the glutathione and thioredoxin systems. Proc Natl Acad Sci U S A 99:9745–9749

Cassee FR, Groten JP, Feron VJ (1996) Changes in the nasal epithelium of rats exposed by inhalation to mixtures of formaldehyde, acetaldehyde, and acrolein. Fundam Appl Toxicol 29:208–218

Castro P, Legora MA, Cardilo RL, Valenca S, Porto LC, Walker C, Zuany AC, Koatz VL (2004) Inhibition of interleukin-1-beta reduces mouse lung inflammation induced by exposure to cigarette smoke. Eur J Pharmacol 498:279–286

Chang WC, Lee YC, Liu CL, Hsu JD, Wang HC, Chen CC, Wang CJ (2001) Increased expression of iNOS and c-fos via regulation of protein tyrosine phosphorylation and MEK1/ERK2 proteins in terminal bronchiole lesions in the lungs of rats exposed to cigarette smoke. Arch Toxicol 75:28–35

Chan-Yeung M, Dybuncio A (1984) Leucocyte count, smoking and lung function. Am J Med 76:31–37

Chan-Yeung M, Abboud R, Dybuncio A, Vedal S (1988) Peripheral leukocyte count and longitudinal decline in lung function. Thorax 43:426–468

Chen LF, Fischle W, Verdin E, Greene WC (2001) Duration of nuclear NF-κB action regulated by reversible acetylation. Science 293:1653–1657

Church T, Pryor WA (1985) Free radical chemistry of cigarette smoke and its toxicological implications. Environ Health Perspect 64:111–126

Claiborne A, Miller H, Parsonage D, Ross PR (1993) Protein sulfenic acid stabilization and function in enzyme catalysis and gene regulation. FASEB J 7:1483–1490

Claiborne A, Yeh JI, Mallett TC, Luba J, Crane EJ, Charrier V, Parsonage D (1999) Protein-sulfenic acids: diverse roles for an unlikely player in enzyme catalysis and redox regulation. Biochemistry 38:15407–15416

Clark DA, Coker R (1998) Transforming growth factor-beta (TGF-beta). Int J Biochem Cell Biol 30:293–298

Comhair SA, Thomassen MJ, Erzurum SC (2000) Differential induction of extracellular glutathione peroxidase and nitric oxide synthase 2 in airways of healthy individuals exposed to 100% O_2 or cigarette smoke. Am J Respir Cell Mol Biol 23:350–354

Comhair SA, Bhathena PR, Farver C, Thunnissen FBJM, Erzurum SC (2001) Extracellular glutathione peroxidase induction in asthmatic lungs: evidence for redox regulation of expression in human airway epithelial cells. FASEB J 15:70–78

Comhair SAA (2005) The regulation and role of extracellular glutathione peroxidase. Antioxid Redox Signal 7:72–79

Cosio BG, Tsaprouni L, Ito K, Jazrawi E, Adcock IM, Barnes PJ (2004). Theophylline restores histone deacetylases activity and steroid responses in COPD macrophages. J Exp Med 200:689–695

Cotgreave IA Gerdes RG (1998) Recent trends in glutathione biochemistry: glutathione–protein interactions: a molecular link between oxidative stress and cell proliferation. Biochem Biophys Res Commun 242:1–9

Crabb JW, O'Neil J, Miyagi M, West K, Hoff HF (2002). Hydroxynonenal inactivates cathepsin B by forming Michael adducts with active site residues. Protein Sci 11:831–840

Crowther A, Rahman I, Antonicelli F, Jimenez LA, Salter D, MacNee W (1999) Oxidative stress and transcription factors AP-1 and NF-κB in human lung tissue. Am Rev Respir Crit Care Med 169:A816

Culpitt SV, Rogers DF, Shah P, De Matos C, Russel RE, Donnelly LE, Barnes PJ (2002) Impaired inhibition by dexamethasone of cytokine release by alveolar macrophages from COPD patients. Am J Respir Crit Care Med 167:24–31

Cummings RC, Andon NL, Haynes PA, Park M, Fischer WH Schubert D (2004). Protein disulfide bond formation in the cytoplasm during oxidative stress. J. Biol Chem 279:21749–21758

Das KC, Lewis-Molock Y, White CW (1995) Activation of NF-κB and elevation of *MnSOD* gene expression by thiol-reducing agents in lung adenocarcinoma (A549) cells. Am J Physiol 269: L588–L602

Das KC (2001) c-Jun NH_2-terminal kinase-mediated redox dependent degradation of IkB: role of thioredoxin in NF-KB activation. J Biol Chem 276:4662–4670

Das SK, Fanburg BL (1991) TGF-β1 produces a "prooxidant" effect on bovine pulmonary artery endothelial cells in culture. Am J Physiol 262:L249–L254

de Boer WI, van Schadewijk A, Sont JK, Sharma HS, Stolk J, Hiemstra PS, van Krieken JHJM (1998) Transforming growth factor-β1 and recruitment of macrophages and mast cells in airways in chronic obstructive pulmonary disease. Am J Respir Crit Care Med 158:1951–1957

Degl'Innocenti D, Caselli A, Rosati F, Marzocchini R, Manao G, Camici G, Ramponi G (1999) Thiolation of low-M_r phosphotyrosine protein phosphatase by thiol-disulfides. IUBMB Life 48:505–511

Del Corso A, Vilardo PG, Cappiello M, Cecconi I, Dal Monte M, Barsacchi D, Mura U (2002) Physiological thiols as promoters of glutathione oxidation and modifying agents in protein S-thiolation. Arch Biochem Biophys 397:392–398

Denu JM, Tanner KG (1998) Specific and reversible inactivation of protein tyrosine phosphatases by hydrogen peroxide: evidence for a sulfenic acid intermediate and implications for redox regulation. Biochemistry 37:5633–5642

Di Simplicio P, Franconi F, Frosali S, Giuseppe D (2003) Thiolation and nitrosation of cysteines in biological fluids and cells. Amino Acids 25:323–339

Di Stefano A, Caramore G, Oates T, Capelli A, Lusuardi M, Gnemmi I, Ioli F, Chung KF, Donner CF, Barnes PJ, Adcock IM (2002) Increased expression of nuclear factor-kB in bronchial biopsies from smokers and patients with COPD. Eur Respir J 20:556–563

Dominici S, Valentini M, Maellaro E, Del Bello B, Paolicchi A, Lorenzini E, Tongiani R, Comporti M, Pompella A (1999) Redox modulation of cell surface protein thiols in U937 lymphoma cells: the role of gamma-glutamyl transpeptidase-dependent H_2O_2 production and S-thiolation Free Radic Biol Med 27:623–635

Euler DE, Dave SJ, Guo H (1996) Effect of cigarette smoking on pentane excretion in alveolar breath. Clin Chem 42:303–308

Favatier F, Polla BS (2001) Tobacco-smoke-inducible human haem oxygenase-1 gene expression: role of distinct transcription factors and reactive oxygen intermediates. Biochem J 353:475–482

Figueiredo Pereira, ME, Yakushin S, Cohen, G (1998) Disruption of the intracellular sulfhydryl homeostasis by cadmium-induced oxidative stress leads to protein thiolation and ubiquitination in neuronal cells. J Biol Chem 273:12703–12709

Fischer BM, Voynow JA (2002) Neutrophil elastase induces *MUC5AC* gene expression in airway epithelium via a pathway involving reactive oxygen species. Am J Respir Cell Mol Biol 26:447–452

Forman HJ, Dickinson DA (2003) Oxidative signaling and glutathione synthesis. Biofactors 17:1–12

Fusunyan RD, Quinn JJ, Fujimoto M, MacDermott RP, Sanderson IR (1999) Butyrate switches the pattern of chemokine secretion by intestinal epithelial cells through histone acetylation. Mol Med 5:631–640

Gebel S, Muller T (2001) The activity of NF-kappa B in Swiss 3T3 cells exposed to aqueous extracts of cigarette smoke is dependent on thioredoxin. Toxicol Sci 59:75–81

Gebel S, Gerstmayer B, Bosio A, Haussmann HJ, Van Miert E, Muller T (2004). Gene expression profiling in respiratory tissues from rats exposed to mainstream cigarette smoke. Carcinogenesis 25:169–178

Gensch E, Gallup M, Sucher A, Li D, Gebremichael A, Lemjabbar H, Mengistab A, Dasari V, Hotchkiss J, Harkema J Basbaum C (2004) Tobacco smoke control of mucin production in lung cells requires oxygen radicals AP-1 and JNK. J Biol Chem 279:39085–39093

Gerritsen ME, Williams AJ, Neish AS, Moore S, Shi Y, Collins T (1997) CREB-binding protein/p300 are transcriptional coactivators of p65. Proc Natl Acad Sci U S A 94:2927–2932

Gilbert HF (1984) Redox control of enzyme activities by thiol/disulfide exchange. Methods Enzymol 107:330–351

Gilks CB, Price K, Wright JL, Churg A (1998) Antioxidant gene expression in rat lung after exposure to cigarette smoke. Am J Path 152:269–278

Gilmour PS, Rahman I, Hayashi S, Hogg JC, Donaldson K, MacNee W (2001). Adenoviral E1A renders alveolar epithelial cells susceptible to environmental particle-induced transcription of interleukin-8. Am J Physiol 281:L598–L606

Golpon HA, Coldren CD, Zamora MR, Cosgrove GP, Moore MD, Tuder RM, Geraci MW, Voelkel NF (2004). Emphysema lung tissue gene expression profiling. Am J Respir Cell Mol Biol 31:595–600

Gutteridge JM, Halliwell B (2000) Free radicals and antioxidants in the year 2000. A historical look to the future. Ann N Y Acad Sci 899:136–147

Gutteridge JMC, Halliwell B (1990) The measurement and mechanism of lipid peroxidation in biological systems. Trends Biochem Sci 15:129–135

Gutteridge JMC (1995) Lipid peroxidation and antioxidants as biomarkers of tissue damage. Clin Chem 41:1819–1828

Guyton KZ, Liu Y, Gorospe M, Xu Q, Holbrook NJ (1996) Activation of mitogen-activated protein kinase by H_2O_2. J Biol Chem 271:4138–4142

Harats D, Ben-Naim M, Dabach Y, Hollander G, Stein O, Stein Y (1989) Cigarette smoking renders LDL susceptible to peroxidative modification and enhanced metabolism by macrophages. Atherosclerosis 79:245–252

Harju T, Kaarteenaho-Wiik R, Soini Y, Sormunen R, Kunnula VL (2002) Diminished immunoreactivity of γ-glutamylcysteine synthetase in the airways of smokers' lung. Am J Respir Crit Care Med 166:754–759

Hausladen A, Stamler JS (1999) Nitrosative stress. Methods Enzymol 300:389–395

Hellermann GR, Nagy SB, Kong X, Lockey RF, Mohapatra SS (2002) Mechanism of cigarette smoke condensate-induced acute inflammatory response in human bronchial epithelial cells. Respir Res 3:22–30

Higashimoto Y, Elliott WM, Behzad AR, Sedgwick EG, Takei T, Hogg JC, Hayashi S (2002) Inflammatory mediator mRNA expression by adenovirus E1A-transfected bronchial epithelial cells. Am J Respir Crit Care Med 166:200–207

Hogg JC (1999) Childhood viral infection and the pathogenesis of asthma and chronic obstructive lung disease. Am J Respir Crit Care Med 160:S26–S28

Holmgren A (2003) Thiols of thioredoxin and glutaredoxin in redox signaling. In: Forman HJ, Fukuto J, Torres M (eds) Signal transduction by reactive oxygen and nitrogen species: pathways and chemical principles. Kluwer, Dordrecht, pp 33–52

Horton ND, Biswal SS, Corrigan LL, Bratta J, Kehrer JP (1999) Acrolein causes inhibitor kappaB-independent decreases in nuclear factor kappaB activation in human lung adenocarcinoma (A549) cells. J Biol Chem 274:9200–9206

Hoshimoto A, Suzuki Y, Katsuno T, Nakajima H, Saito Y (2002) Caprylic acid and medium-chain triglycerides inhibit *IL-8* gene transcription in Caco-2 cells: comparison with the potent histone deacetylase inhibitor trichostatin A. Br J Pharmacol 136:280–286

Hoshino S, Yoshida M, Inoue K, Yano Y, Yanagita M, Mawatari H, Yamane H, Kijima T, Kumagai T, Osaki T, Tachiba I, Kawase I (2005). Cigarette smoke extract induces endothelial cell injury via JNK pathway. Biochem Biophys Res Commun 329:58–63

Huang CS, Chang LS, Anderson ME, Meister A (1993) Catalytic and regulatory properties of the heavy subunit of rat kidney γ-glutamylcysteine synthetase. J Biol Chem 268:19675–19680

Humphries KM, Szweda LI (1998) Selective inactivation of alpha-ketoglutarate dehydrogenase and pyruvate dehydrogenase: reaction of lipoic acid with 4-hydroxy-2-nonenal. Biochemistry 37:15835–15841

Imhof A, Wolffe AP (1998) Transcription: gene control by targeted histone acetylation. Curr Biol 8:R422–R424

Ishii T, Matsuse T, Igarashi H, Masuda M, Teramoto S, Ouchi Y (2001) Tobacco smoke reduces viability in human lung fibroblasts: protective effect of glutathione *S*-transferase P1. Am J Physiol 280:L1189–L1195

Ito K, Barnes PJ, Adcock IM (2000) Glucocorticoid receptor recruitment of histone deacetylase 2 inhibits interleukin-1beta-induced histone H4 acetylation on lysines 8 and 12. Mol Cell Biol 20:6891–6903

Ito K, Lim G, Caramori G, Chung KF, Barnes PJ, Adcock IM (2001a) Cigarette smoking reduces histone deacetylase 2 expression, enhances cytokine expression, and inhibits glucocorticoid actions in alveolar macrophages. FASEB J 15:1110–1112

Ito K, Jazrawi E, Cosio B, Barnes PJ, Adcock IM (2001b) p65-activated histone acetyltransferase activity is repressed by glucocorticoids: mifepristone fails to recruit HDAC2 to the p65–HAT complex. J Biol Chem 276:30208–30215

Ito K, Caramori G, Lim S, Oates T, Chung KF, Barnes PJ, Adcock IM (2002) Expression and activity of histone deacetylases in human asthmatic airways. Am J Respir Crit Care Med 166:392–396

Izzotti A, Cartiglia C, Longobardi M, Balansky RM, D'Agostini F, Lubet RA, De Flora S (2004). Alterations of gene expression in skin and lung of mice exposed to light and cigarette smoke. FASEB J 18:1559–1561

Jahngen-Hodge J, Obin MS, Gong X, Shang F, Nowell TR, Gong J, Abasi H, Blumberg J, Taylor A (1997) Regulation of ubiquitin-conjugating enzymes by glutathione following oxidative stress. J Biol Chem 272:28218–28226

Jardine H, MacNee W, Donaldson K, Rahman I (2002) Molecular mechanism of transforming growth factor (TGF)-beta1-induced glutathione depletion in alveolar epithelial cells. Involvement of AP-1/ARE and Fra-1. J Biol Chem 277:21158–21166

Ji C, Kozak KR, Marnett LJ (2001) IkB kinase, a molecular target for inhibition of 4-hydroxy-2-nonenal. J Biol Chem 276:18223–18228

Kamei Y, Xu L, Heinzel T, Torchia J, Kurokawa R, Gloss B, Lin SC, Heyman RA, Rose DW, Glass CK, Rosenfeld MG (1996) A CBP integrator complex mediates transcriptional activation and AP-1 inhibition by nuclear receptors. Cell 85:403–414

Kasahara Y, Tuder RM, Taraseviciene-Stewart L, Le Cras TD, Abman S, Hirth PK, Waltenberger J, Voelkel NF (2000) Inhibition of VEGF receptors causes lung cell apoptosis and emphysema. J Clin Invest 106:1311–1319

Kawasaki H, Schiltz L, Chiu R, Itakura K, Taira K, Nakatani Y, Yokoyama KK (2000) ATF-2 has intrinsic histone acetyltransferase activity which is modulated by phosphorylation. Nature 405:195–200

Ke S, Rabson AB, Germino JF, Gallo MA, Tian Y (2001) Mechanism of suppression of cytochrome P-450 1A1 expression by tumor necrosis factor-alpha and lipopolysaccharide. J Biol Chem 276:39638–39644

Keatings VM, Collins PD, Scott DM, Barnes PJ (1996) Differences in interleukin-8 and tumor necrosis factor-alpha in induced sputum from patients with chronic obstructive pulmonary disease or asthma. Am J Respir Crit Care Med 153:530–534

Kehrer JP, Biswal SS (2000) The molecular effects of acrolein. Toxicol Sci 57:6–15

Keicho N, Higashimoto Y, Bondy GP, Elliott WM, Hogg JC, Hayashi S (1999) Endotoxin-specific NF-kappaB activation in pulmonary epithelial cells harboring adenovirus E1A. Am J Physiol 277:L523–L532

Klatt P, Molina EP, de Lacoba MG, Padilla CA, Martinez-Galisteo E, Barcena JA, Lamas S (1999) Redox regulation of c-Jun DNA binding by reversible I-glutathiolation. FASEB J 13:1481–1490

Klatt P and Lamas S (2000) Regulation of protein function by S-glutathiolation in response to oxidative and nitrosative stress. Eur J Biochem 267:4928–4944

Kornitzer D, Ciechanover A (2000) Modes of regulation of ubiquitin-mediated protein degradation. J Cell Physiol 182:1–11

Krzywanski DM, Dickinson DA, Iles KE, Wigley AF, Franklin CC, Liu RM, Kavanagh TJ, Forman HJ (2004) Variable regulation of glutamate cysteine ligase subunit proteins affects glutathione biosynthesis in response to oxidative stress. Arch Biochem Biophys 423:116–125

Kumagai T, Kawamoto Y, Nakamura Y, Hatayama I, Satoh K, Osawa T, Uchida K (2000) 4-hydroxy-2-nonenal, the end product of lipid peroxidation, is a specific inducer of cyclooxygenase-2 gene expression. Biochem Biophys Res Commun 273:437–441

Kumagai T, Matsukawa N, Kaneko Y, Kusumi Y, Mitsumata M, Uchida K (2004) A lipid peroxidation-derived inflammatory mediator: identification of 4-hydroxy-2-nonenal as a potential inducer of cyclooxygenase-2 in macrophages. J Biol Chem 279:48389–48396

Kuscher WG, D'Alexandro A, Wong H, Blanc PD (1996) Dose-dependent cigarette smoking-related inflammatory responses in healthy adults. Eur Respir J 10:1989–1994

Laan M, Bozinovski S, Anderson GP (2004) Cigarette smoke inhibits lipopolysaccharide-induced production of inflammatory cytokines by suppressing the activation of activator protein-1 in bronchial epithelial cells. J Immunol 173:4164–4170

Lagrue G, Branellec A, Lebargy F (1993) Toxicology of tobacco. Rev Prat 43:1203–1207

Lakshminarayanan V, Drab-Weiss EA, Roebuck KA (1998) H_2O_2 and TNF induce differential binding of the redox-responsive transcription factor AP-1 and NF-kB to the interleukin-8 promoter in endothelial and epithelial cells. J Biol Chem 273:32670–32678

Lam CW, Casanova M, Heck HA (1985) Depletion of nasal mucosal glutathione by acrolein and enhancement of formaldehyde-induced DNA-protein cross-linking by simultaneous exposure to acrolein. Arch Toxicol 58:67–71

Lannan, S, Donaldson K, Brown D, MacNee W (1994) Effects of cigarette smoke and its condensates on alveolar cell injury in vitro. Am J Physiol 266:L92–L100

Lawson JA, Rokach J, FitzGerald GA (1999) Isoprostanes: formation, analysis and use as indices of lipid peroxidation in vivo. J Biol Chem 274:24441–24444

Lee SR, Kwon KS, Kim SR, Rhee SG (1998) Reversible inactivation of protein-tyrosine phosphatase 1B in A431 cells stimulated with epidermal growth factor. J Biol Chem 273:15366–15372

Leikauf GD, Borchers MT, Prows DR, Simpson LG (2002) Mucin apoprotein expression in COPD. Chest 121:S166–S182

Lemjabbar H, Li D, Gallup M, Sidhu S, Drori E, Basbaum C (2003). Tobacco smoke-induced lung cell proliferation mediated by tumor necrosis factor alpha-converting enzyme and amphiregulin. J Biol Chem 278:26202–26207

Leonarduzzi G, Arkan MC, Basaga H, Chiarpotto E, Sevanian A, Poli G (2000) Lipid oxidation products in cell signaling. Free Radic Biol Med 28:1760–1768

Leonarduzzi G, Scavazza A, Biasi F, Chiarpotto E, Camandola S, Vogl S, Dargel R, Poli G (1997) The lipid peroxidation end product 4-hydroxy-2,3-nonenal up-regulates transforming growth factor-β1 expression in the macrophage lineage: a link between oxidative injury and fibrosclerosis. FASEB J 11:851–857

Leoni F, Zaliani A, Bertolini G, Porro G, Pagani P, Pozzi P, Dona G, Fossati G, Sozzani S, Azam T, Bufler P, Fantuzzi G, Goncharov I, Kim SH, Pomerantz BJ, Reznikov LL, Siegmund B, Dinarello CA, Mascagni P (2002) The antitumor histone deacetylase inhibitor suberoylanilide hydroxamic acid exhibits antiinflammatory properties via suppression of cytokines. Proc Natl Acad Sci U S A 99:2995–3000

Li L, Hamilton RF Jr, Holian A (1999) Effect of acrolein on human alveolar macrophage NF-kappaB activity. Am J Physiol 277:L550–L557

Li XY, Donaldson K, Rahman I, MacNee W (1994) An investigation of the role of glutathione in the increased permeability induced by cigarette smoke in vivo and in vitro. Am Rev Respir Crit Care Med 149:1518–1525

Li XY, Rahman I, Donaldson K, MacNee W (1996) Mechanisms of cigarette smoke induced increased airspace permeability. Thorax 51:465–471

Liu RM, Borok Z, Forman HJ (2001) 4-Hydroxy-2-nonenal increases γ-glutamylcysteine synthetase gene expression in alveolar epithelial cells. Am J Respir Cell Mol Biol 24499–505

Liu W, Akhand AA, Kato M, Yokoyama I, Miyata T, Kurokawaka K. Uchida K, Nakashima I (1999) 4-Hydroxynonenal triggers an epidermal growth factor receptor-linked signal pathway for growth inhibition. J Cell Sci 112:2409–2417

Liu W, Kato M, Akhand AA, Hayakawa A, Suzuki H, Miyata T, Kurokawa K, Hotta Y, Ishikawa N, Nakashima I (2000) 4-Hydroxynonenal induces a cellular redox status-related activation of the caspase cascade for apoptotic cell death. J Cell Sci 113:635–641

Rui-Ming L, Gao L, Choi J, Forman HJ (1998) γ-Glutamylcysteine synthetase: mRNA stabilization and independent subunit transcription by 4-hydroxy-2-nonenal. Am J Physiol 19:L861–L869

Lolis E (2001) Glucocorticoid counter-regulation: macrophage migration inhibitory factor as a target for drug discovery. Curr Opin Pharmacol 1:662–668

Lu Y, Parkyn L, Otterbein LE, Kureishi Y, Walsh K, Ray A, Ray PJ (2001) Activated Akt protects the lung from oxidant-induced injury and delays death of mice. J Exp Med 193:545–549

Luo GAG, Lao P, Shea J, Chuu YJ, Wu R (1994) Transcriptional activation of squamous cell differentiation marker, *spr1* gene, by cigarette smoke in conducting airway epithelium. Am J Respir Crit Care Med 149:A446

MacNee W, Rahman I (1999) Oxidants and antioxidant in COPD: therapeutic targets. Am J Respir Crit Care Med 160:S1–S8

Madrid LV, Mayo MW, Reuther JY, Baldwin AS Jr (2001) Akt stimulates the transactivation potential of the RelA/p65 subunit of NF-kappa B through utilization of the Ikappa B kinase and activation of the mitogen-activated protein kinase p38. J Biol Chem 276:18934–18940

Maestrelli P, Messlemani AHE, Fina OD, Nowicki Y, Saetta M, Mapp C, Fabbri LM (2001) Increased expression of heme oxygenase (HO)-1 in alveolar spaces and HO-2 in alveolar walls of smokers. Am J Respir Crit Care Med 164:1508–1513

Martey CA, Pollock SJ, Turner CK, O'Reilly KM, Baglole CJ, Phipps RP, Sime PJ (2004) Cigarette smoke induces cyclooxygenase-2 and microsomal prostaglandin E2 synthase in human lung fibroblasts: implications for lung inflammation and cancer. Am J Physiol 287:L981–L991

Marwick JA, Giddings J, Butler K, Kirkham P, Donaldson K, MacNee W, Rahman I (2004) Cigarette smoke induces inflammatory response and alters chromatin remodeling in rat lungs. Am J Respir Cell Mol Biol 31:633–642

Masubuchi T, Koyama S, Sato E, Takamizawa A, Kubo K, Sekiguchi M, Nagai S, Izumi T (1998) Smoke extract stimulates lung epithelial cells to release neutrophil and monocyte chemotactic activity. Am J Pathol 153:1903–1912

McCrea KA, Ensor JE, Nall K, Bleecker ER, Hasday JD (1994) Altered cytokine regulation in the lungs of cigarette smokers. Am J Respir Crit Care Med 150:696–703

Mio T, Romberger DJ, Thompson AB, Robbins RA, Heires A, Rennard SI (1997) Cigarette smoke induces interleukin-8 release from human bronchial epithelial cells. Am J Respir Crit Care Med 155:1770–1776

Miranda-Vizuette A, Gustafsson J, Spyrou G (1998) Molecular cloning and expression of a cDNA encoding a human thioredoxin-like protein. Biochem Biophys Res Commun 243:284–288

Miyata Y, Towatari M, Maeda T, Ozawa Y, Saito H (2001) Histone acetylation induces by granulocyte colony-stimulating factor in a MAP kinase-dependent manner. Biochem Biophys Res Commun 283:655–660

Mochida-Nishimura K, Sureweicz K, Cross JV, Hejal R, Templeton D, Rich EA, Toossi Z (2001) Differential activation of MAP kinase signaling pathways and nuclear factor-kappaB in bronchoalveolar cells of smokers and nonsmokers. Mol Med 7177–185

Montuschi P, Collins JV, Ciabattoni G, Lazzeri N, Corradi M, Kharitonov SA, Barnes PJ (2000) Exhaled 8-isoprostane as an in vivo biomarker of lung oxidative stress in patients with COPD and healthy smokers. Am J Respir Crit Care Med 1621175–1177

Morrison D, Rahman I, Lannan S, MacNee W (1999) Epithelial permeability, inflammation and oxidant stress in the airspaces of smokers. Am J Respir Crit Care Med 159:473–479

Morrow JD, Hill KE, Burk RF, Nammour TM, Badr KF, Roberts LJ (1990) A series of prostaglandin F2-like compounds are produced in vivo in humans by a noncyclooxygenase, free radical-catalyzed mechanism. Proc Natl Acad Sci U S A 87:9383–9387

Morrow JD, Awad JA, Boss HJ, Blair IA, Roberts LJ (1992) Non-cyclooxygenase derived prostanoids (F2-isoprostanes) are formed in situ on phospholipids. Proc Natl Acad Sci U S A 89:10721–10725

Morrow JD, Roberts LJ (1997) The isoprostanes: unique bioactive products of lipid peroxidation. Prog Lipid Res 36:1–21

Moriarty SE, Shah JH, Lynn M, Jiang S, Openo K, Jones DP, Sternberg P (2003). Oxidation of glutathione and cysteine in human plasma associated with smoking. Free Radic Biol Med 35:1582–1588

Moodie F, Marwick JA, Anderson C, Szulakowski P, Biswas S, Kilty I, Rahman I (2004) Oxidative stress and cigarette smoke alter chromatin remodeling but differentially regulate NF-κB activation and pro-inflammatory cytokine release in alveolar epithelial cells. FASEB J 18:1897–1899

Muller K, Hardwick SJ, Marchant CE, Law NS, Waeg G, Esterbauer H, Carpentar KL, Mitchinson MJ (1996) Cytotoxic and chemotactic potencies of several aldehydic components of oxidised low density lipoprotein for human monocyte-macrophages. FEBS Lett 388:165–168

Muller T (1995) Expression of c-fos in quiescent Swiss 3T3 cells exposed to aqueous cigarette smoke fractions. Cancer Res 55:1927–1932

Muller T, Haussmann HJ, Schepers G (1997) Evidence for peroxynitrite as an oxidative stress-inducing compound of aqueous cigarette smoke fractions. Carcinogenesis 18:295–301

Muller T, Gebel S (1998) The cellular stress response induced by aqueous extracts of cigarette smoke is critically dependent on the intracellular glutathione concentration. Carcinogenesis 19:797–801

Muns G, Rubinstein I, Bergmann KC (1995) Phagocytosis and oxidative bursts of blood phagocytes in chronic obstructive airway disease. Scand J Infect Dis 27:369–373

Muscat JE, Kleinman W, Colosimo S, Muir A, Lazarus P, Park J, Richie JP Jr (2004) Enhanced protein glutathiolation and oxidative stress in cigarette smokers. Free Radic Biol Med 36:464–470

Nadel JA (2001) Role of epidermal growth factor receptor activation in regulating mucin synthesis. Respir Res 2:85–89

Nakayama T, Church DF, Pryor WA (1989) Quantitative analysis of the hydrogen peroxide formed in aqueous cigarette tar extracts. Free Radic Biol Med 7:9–15

Neurohr C, Lenz AG, Ding I, Leuchte H, Kolbe T, Behr J (2003). Glutamate-cysteine ligase modulatory subunit in BAL alveolar macrophages of healthy smokers. Eur Respir J 22:82–87

Ng KW, Ridgway P, Cohen DR, Tremethick DJ (1997) The binding of a Fos/Jun heterodimer can completely disrupt the structure of a nucleosome. EMBO J 16:2072–2085

Ning W, Li CJ, Kaminski N, Feghali-Bostwick CA, Alber SM, Di YP, Otterbein SL, Song R, Hayashi S, Zhou Z, Pinsky DJ, Watkins SC, Pilewski JM, Sciurba FC, Peters DG, Hogg JC, Choi AM (2004) Comprehensive gene expression profiles reveal pathways related to the pathogenesis of chronic obstructive pulmonary disease. Proc Natl Acad Sci U S A 101:14895–14900

Nishikawa M, Nobumasa K, Ito T, Kudi M, Kaneeko T, Suzuki M, Udaka N, Ikeda H, Okubo T (1999) Superoxide mediates cigarette smoke-induced infiltration of neutrophils into the airways through nuclear factor-kB activation and IL-8 mRNA expression in guinea pigs in vivo. Am J Respir Cell Mol Biol 20:189–198

Nishiyama A, Masutani H, Nakamura H, Nishinaka Y, Yodoi J (2001) Redox regulation by thioredoxin and thioredoxin-binding proteins. IUBMB Life 52:29–33

Noguera A, Busquets X, Sauleda J, Villaverde JM, MacNee W, Agusti AG (1998) Expression of adhesion molecules and G-proteins in circulating neutrophils in COPD. Am J Respir Crit Care Med 158:1664–1668

Obin M, Shang F, Gong X, Handelman G, Blumberg J, Taylor A (1998) Redox regulation of ubiquitin-conjugating enzymes: mechanistic insights using the thiol-specific oxidant diamide. FASEB J 12:561–569

Ogryzko VV, Schiltz RL, Russanova V, Howard BH, Nakatani Y (1996) The transcriptional coactivators p300 and CBP are histone acetyltransferases. Cell 87:953–959

Ohno Y, Lee J, Fusunyan RD, MacDermott RP, Sanderson RI (1997) Macrophage inflammatory protein-2: chromosomal regulation in rat small intestinal epithelial cells. Proc Natl Acad Sci U S A 94:10279–10284

Okada K, Wangpoengtrakul C, Osawa T, Toyokuni S, Tanaka K, Uchida K (1999) 4-Hydroxy-2-nonenal-mediated impairment of intracellular protolysis during oxidative stress: identification of proteosomes as target molecules. J Biol Chem 274:23787–23793

Ouyang Y, Virasch N, Hao P, Aubrey MT, Mukerjee N, Bierer BE, Freed BM (2000) Suppression of human IL-1beta, IL-2, IFN-gamma, and TNF-alpha production by cigarette smoke extracts. J Allergy Clin Immunol 16:280–287

Page S, Fischer C, Baumgartner B, Haas M, Kreusel U, Loidl G, Hayn M, Ziegler-Heitbrock HWL, Neumeier D, Brand K (1999) 4-Hydroxynonenal prevents NF-κB activation and tumor necrosis factor expression by inhibiting IkB phosphorylation and subsequent proteolysis. J Biol Chem 274:11611–11618

Panayiotidis MI, Stabler SP, Allen RH, Ahmad A, White CW (2004). Cigarette smoke extract increases S-adenosylmethionine and cystathionine in human lung epithelial-like (A549) cells. Chem Biol Interact 147:87–97

Paolicchi A, Dominici S, Pieri L, Maellaro E, Pompella A (2002) Glutathione catabolism as signaling mechanism. Biochem Pharmacol 64:1027–1035

Paredi P, Kharitonov SA, Leak D, Ward S, Cramer D, Barnes PJ (2000) Exhaled ethane, a marker of lipid peroxidation, is elevated in chronic obstructive pulmonary disease. Am J Respir Crit Care Med 161:369–373

Park EM, Park YM, Gwak YS (1998) Oxidative damage in tissues of rats exposed to cigarette smoke. Free Radic Biol Med 25:79–-86

Parola M, Bellomo G, Robino G, Barrera G, Dianzani MU (1999) 4-Hydroxynonenal as a biological signal: molecular basis and pathophysiological implications. Antioxid Redox Signal 1:255–284

Parola M, Pinzani M, Casini A, Albano E, Poli G, Gentilini A, Gentilini P, Dianzani MU (1993) Stimulation of lipid peroxidation or 4-hydroxynonenal treatment increases procollagen a1 (1) gene expression in human liver fat-storing cells. Biochem Biophys Res Commun 194:1044–1050

Pender SLF, Quinn JJ, Sanderson IR, MacDonald TT (2000) Butyrate upregulates stromelysin-1 production by intestinal mesenchymal cells. Am J Physiol 279:G918–G924

Pham A, Sauer F (2000) Ubiquitin-activating/conjugating activity of TAFII250, a mediator of activation of gene expression in *Drosophila*. Science 289:2357–2360

Pierreux CE, Stafford J, Demonte D, Scot DK, Vandenhaute J, O'Brien RM, Granner DK, Rousseau GG, Lemaigre FP (1999) Antiglucocorticoid activity of hepatocyte nuclear factor-6. Proc Natl Acad Sci U S A 96: 8961–8966

Poole LB, Karplus PA, Claiborne A (2004) Protein sulfenic acids in redox signaling. Annu Rev Pharmacol Toxicol 44:325–347

Pryor WA, Stone K (1993) Oxidants in cigarette smoke: radicals, hydrogen peroxides, peroxynitrate, and peroxynitrite. Ann N Y Acad Sci 686:12–28

Ragione FD, Criniti V, Pietra VD, Borriello A, Oliva A, Indaco S, Yamamoto T, Zappia V (2001) Genes modulated by histone acetylation as new effectors of butyrate activity. FEBS Letts 99:199–204

Rahman I, Li XY, Donaldson K, Harrison DJ, MacNee W (1995) Glutathione homeostasis in alveolar epithelial cells in vitro and lung in vivo under oxidative stress. Am J Physiol 269:L285–L292

Rahman I, MacNee W (1996a) Role of oxidants/antioxidants in smoking-induced airways diseases. Free Radic Biol Med 21:669–681

Rahman I, Morrison D, Donaldson K, MacNee W (1996b) Systemic oxidative stress in asthma, COPD, and smokers. Am J Respir Crit Care Med 154:1055–1060

Rahman I, Lawson MF, Smith CAD, Harrison DJ, MacNee W (1996c) Induction of γ-glutamylcysteine synthetase by cigarette smoke is associated with AP-1 in human alveolar epithelial cells. FEBS Lett 396:21–25

Rahman I, Skwarska E, MacNee W (1997) Attenuation of oxidant/antioxidant imbalance during treatment of exacerbations of chronic obstructive pulmonary disease. Thorax 52:565–568

Rahman I, MacNee W (1998) Role of transcription factors in inflammatory lung diseases. Thorax 53:601–612

Rahman I, MacNee W (1999) Lung glutathione and oxidative stress: implications in cigarette smoke-induced airways disease. Am J Physiol 277:L1067–L1088

Rahman I, MacNee W (2000a) Regulation of redox glutathione levels and gene transcription in lung inflammation: therapeutic approaches. Free Radic Biol Med 28:1405–1420

Rahman I, Van Schadewijk AAM, Hiemstra PS, Stolk J, Van Krieken JHJM, MacNee W, De Boer WI (2000b) Localization of γ-glutamylcysteine synthetase messenger RNA expression in lungs of smokers and patients with chronic obstructive pulmonary disease. Free Radic Biol Med 28:920–925

Rahman I, MacNee W (2000c) Oxidative stress and regulation of glutathione synthesis in lung inflammation. Eur Respir J 16:534–554

Rahman I, Mulier B, Gilmour PS, Watchorn T, Donaldson K, Jeffery PK, MacNee W (2001) Oxidant-mediated lung epithelial cell tolerance: the role of intracellular glutathione and nuclear factor-κB. Biochem Pharmacol 62:787–794

Rahman I, Van Schadewijk AA, Crowther A, Hiemstra PS, Stolk J, MacNee W. De Boer WI (2002a) 4-Hydroxy-2-nonenal, a specific lipid peroxidation product is elevated in lungs of patients with chronic obstructive pulmonary disease (COPD). Am J Respir Crit Care Med 166:490–495

Rahman I, Gilmour P, Jimenez LA, MacNee W (2002b) Oxidative stress and TNF-α induce histone acetylation and AP-1/NF-κB in alveolar epithelial cells: potential mechanism in inflammatory gene transcription. Mol Cell Biochem 234/235:239–248

Rahman I, Marwick JA, Kirkham PA (2004) Redox modulation of histone acetylation and deacetylation in vitro and in vivo: modulation of NF-κB and pro-inflammatory genes. Biochem Pharmacol 68:1255–1267

Rahman I, Biswas SK, Jimenez LA, Torres M, Forman J (2005) Glutathione, stress responses, and redox signaling in lung inflammation. Antioxid Redox Signal 7:42–59

Retamales I, Elliott WM, Meshi B, Coxson HO, Pare PD, Sciurba FC, Rogers RM, Hayashi S, Hogg JC (2001) Amplication of inflammation emphysema its association with latent adenoviral infection. Am J Respir Crit Care Med 164:469-473

Reynaert NL, Ckless K, Wouters EF, van der Vliet A, Janssen-Heininger YM (2005) Nitric oxide and redox signaling in airway inflammation. Antioxid Redox Signal 7:129–143

Richards GA, Theron AJ, van der Merwe CA, Anderson R (1989) Spirometric abnormalities in young smokers correlate with increased chemiluminescence responses of activated blood phagocytes. Am Rev Respir Dis 139:181–187

Richer C, Cogvadze V, Laffranchi R, Schlapbach R, Schweizer M, Suter M (1995) Oxidants in mitochondria: from physiology to diseases. Biochim Biophys Acta 127:67–74

Rochelle LG, Fischer BM, Adler KB (1998) Concurrent production of reactive oxygen and nitrogen species by airway epithelial cells in vitro. Free Radic Biol Med 24:863–868

Rokutan K, Teshima S, Miyoshi M, Kawai T, Nikawa T, Kishi K (1998) Glutathione depletion inhibits oxidant-induced activation of nuclear factor-kappa B, AP-1, and c-Jun/ATF-2 in cultured guinea-pig gastric epithelial cells. J Gastroenterol 33:646–655

Rusznak C, Mills PR, Devalia JL, Sapsford RJ, Davies RJ, Lozewicz S (2000) Effect of cigarette smoke on the permeability and IL-1beta and sICAM-1 release from cultured human bronchial epithelial cells of never-smokers, smokers, and patients with chronic obstructive pulmonary disease. Am J Respir Cell Mol Biol 23:530–536

Saccani S, Pantano S, Natoli G (2002) p38-dependent marking of inflammatory genes for increased NF-κB activation. Nature Immunol 3:69–75

Saccani S, Pantano S, Natoli G (2001) Two waves of nuclear factor κB recruitment to target promoters. J Exp Med 193:1351–1359

Saetta M, Mariani M, Panina-Bordignon P, Turato G, Buonsanti C, Baraldo S, Bellettato CM, Papi A, Corbetta L, Zuin R, Sinigaglia F, Fabbri LM (2002) Increased expression of the chemokine receptor CXCR3 and its ligand CXCL10 in peripheral airways of smokers with chronic obstructive pulmonary disease. Am J Respir Crit Care Med 165:1404–1409

Sambucetti LC, Fischer DD, Zabludoff S, Kwon PO, Chamberlin H, Trogani N, Xu H, Cohen D (1999) Histone deacetylase inhibition selectively alters the activity and expression of cell cycle proteins leading to specific chromatin acetylation and antiproliferative effects. J Biol Chem 274:34940–34947

Sano H, Sata T, Nanri, H, Ikeda M, Shigematsu A (2002) Thioredoxin is associated with endotoxin tolerance in mice. Crit Care Med 30:190–194

Schaur RJ, Dussing G, Kink E, Schauenstein E, Posch W, Kukovetz E, Egger, G (1994) The lipid peroxidation product 4-hydroxynonenal is formed by—and is able to attract—rat neutrophils in vivo. Free Radic Res 20:365–373

Sen CK (1998) Redox signaling and the emerging therapeutic potential of thiol antioxidants. Biochem Pharmacol 55:1747–1758

Shah V, Sridhar S, Beane J, Brody JS, Spira A (2005) SIEGE: Smoking-Induced Epithelial Gene Expression database. Nucleic Acids Res 33:D573–D579

Shankaranarayanan P, Chaitidis P, Kuhn H, Nigam S (2001) Acetylation by histone acetyltransferase CREB-binding protein/p300 of STAT6 is required for transcriptional activation of the 15-lipoxygenase-1 gene. J Biol Chem 276: 42753–42760

Shao MX, Nakanaga T, Nadel JA (2004) Cigarette smoke induces MUC5AC mucin overproduction via tumor necrosis factor-alpha-converting enzyme in human airway epithelial (NCI-H292) cells. Am J Physiol 287:L420–L427

Shelton MD, Chock PB, Mieyal JJ (2005) Glutaredoxin: role in reversible protein S-glutathiolation and regulation of redox signal transduction and protein translocation. Antioxid Redox Signal 7:348–366

Shen Y, Rattan V, Sultana C, Kalra VK (1996) Cigarette smoke condensate-induced adhesion molecule expression and transendothelial migration of monocytes. Am J Physiol 39:H1624–H1633

Shenkar R, Yum H, Arcaroli J, Kupfner J, Abraham E (2001) Interactions between CBP, NF-κB and CREB in the lungs after hemorrhage and endotoxemia. Am J Physiol 281:L418–LL426

Shishodia S, Aggarwal BB (2004) Cyclooxygenase (COX-2) inhibitor celecoxib abrogates activation of cigarette smoke-induced nuclear factor (NF)-kappaB by suppressing activation of IkappaBalpha kinase in human non-small cell lung carcinoma: correlation with suppression of cyclinD1, COX-2 and matrix metalloproteinase-9. Cancer Res 64:5004–5012

Spycher SE, Tabataba-Vakili S, O'Donnell VB, Palomba L, Azzi A (1997) Aldose reductase induction: a novel response to oxidative stress of smooth muscle cells. FASEB J 11:181–188

Stamler JS, Hausladen A (1998) Oxidative modifications in nitrosative stress. Nat Struct Biol 5:247–249

Steinerova A, Racek J, Stozicky F, Zima T, Fialova L (2001) Antibodies against oxidised LDL—theory and clinical use. Physiol Res 50:131–141

Sternglanz R (1996) Histone acetylation: a gateway to transcriptional activation. Trends Biol Sci 21:357–358

Stringer KA, Freed BM, Dunn JS, Sayers S, Gustafson DL, Flores SC (2004). Particulate phase cigarette smoke increases MnSOD, NQO1, and CINC-1 in rat lungs. Free Radic Biol Med 37:1527–1533

Sugano N, Shimada K, Ito K, Murai S (1998) Nicotine inhibits the production of inflammatory mediators in U937 cells through modulation of nuclear factor-kappaB activation. Biochem Biophys Res Commun 252:25–28

Takeyama K, Jung B, Shim JJ, Burgel PR, Dao-Pick T, Ueki IF, Protin U, Kroschel P, Nadel JA (2001) Activation of epidermal growth factor receptors is responsible for mucin synthesis induced by cigarette smoke. Am J Physiol 280:L165–L172

Takizawa H, Tanaka M, Takami K, Ohtoshi T, Ito K, Satoh M, Okada Y, Yamasawa F, Nakahara K, Umeda A (2001) Increased expression of transforming growth factor-β1 in small airway epithelium from tobacco smokers and patients with chronic obstructive pulmonary disease (COPD). Am J Respir Crit Care Med 163:1476–1483

Tao L, English AM (2004) Protein S-glutathiolation triggered by decomposed S-nitrosoglutathione. Biochemistry 43:4028–4038

Thannickal VJ, Fanburg BL (2000) Reactive oxygen species in cell signaling. Am J Physiol 279: L1005–L1028

Thomas JA, Poland B, Honzatko R (1995) Protein sulfhydryls and their role in the antioxidant function of protein S-thiolation. Arch Biochem Biophys 319:1–9

Thomson S, Mahadevan LC, Clayton AL (1999) MAP kinase-mediated signaling to nucleosomes and immediate-early gene induction. Cell Dev Biol 10:205–214

Tikoo K, Lau SS, Monks TJ (2001) Histone H3 phosphorylation is coupled to poly-(ADP-ribosylation) during reactive oxygen species-induces cell death in renal proximal tubular epithelial cells. Mol Pharmacol 60:394–402

Tjalkens RB, Cook LW, Peterson DR (1999) Formation and export of glutathione conjugate of 4-hydroxy-2,3-E-nonenal (4-HNE) in hepatoma cells. Arch Biochem Biophys 361:113–119

Tong JJ, Liu J, Bertos NR, Yang XJ (2002) Identification of HDAC10, a novel class II human histone deacetylase containing a leucine-rich domain. Nucleic Acid Res 30:1114–1123

Tonks NK, Neel BG (1996) From form to function: signaling by protein tyrosine phosphatases. Cell 87:365–368

Uchida K, Shiraishi M, Naito Y, Torii N, Nakamura Y, Osawa T (1999) Activation of stress signaling pathways by the end product of lipid peroxidation. J Biol Chem 274:2234–2242

Valapour M, Gui J, Schroeder JT, Keen J, Cianferoni A, Casolaro V, Georas SN (2002) Histone deacetylation inhibits *IL4* gene expression in T cells. J Allergy Clin Immunol 109:238–245

Van Antwerpen VL, Theron AJ, Richards GA, Steenkamp KJ, Van der Merwe CA, Van der Walt R, Anderson R (1995) Vitamin E, pulmonary functions, and phagocyte-mediated oxidative stress in smokers and nonsmokers. Free Radic Biol Med 18:935–943

Vayssier M, Banzet N, Francois D, Bellmann K, Polla BS (1998) Tobacco smoke induces both apoptosis and necrosis in mammalian cells: differential effects of HSP70. Am J Physiol 275: L771–L779

Vayssier M, Favatier F, Pinot F, Bachelet M, Poll BS (1998) Tobacco smoke induces coordinate activation of HSF and inhibition of NF-κB in human monocytes: effects on TNF-alpha release. Biochem Biophys Res Commun 252:249–256

Wang H, Ye Y, Zh M, Cho C (2000) Increased interleukin-8 expression by cigarette smoke extract in endothelial cells. Environ Toxicol Pharmacol 9:19–23

Ward NS, Waxman AB, Homer RJ, Mantell LL, Einarsson O, Du Y, Elias JA (2000) Interleukin-6-induced protection in hyperoxic acute lung injury. Am J Respir Cell Mol Biol 22:535–542

Watson WH, Pohl J, Montfort WR, Stuchlik O, Powis G, Jones DP (2003) Redox potential of human thioredoxin-1 and identification of a second dithiol/disulfide motif. J Biol Chem 278:33408–33415

Watson WH, Yang X, Choi YE, Jones DP, Kehree JP (2004) Thioredoxin and its role in toxicology. Toxicol Sci 78:3–14

Wesselius LJ, Nelson ME, Bailey K, O'Brien-Ladner AR (1997) Rapid lung cytokine accumulation and neutrophil recruitment after lipopolysaccharide inhalation by cigarette smokers and non-smokers. J Lab Clin Med 129:106–114

White AC, Das SK, Fanburg BL (1992) Reduction of glutathione is associated with growth restriction and enlargement of bovine pulmonary artery endothelial cells produced by transforming growth factor-β1. Am J Respir Cell Mol Biol 6:364–368

Winterbourn CC, Metodiewa D (1999) Reactivity of biologically important thiol compounds with superoxide and hydrogen peroxide. Free Radic Biol Med 27:322–328

Wodrich W, Volhm M (1993) Overexpression of oncoproteins in non-small cell lung carcinomas of smokers. Carcinogenesis 14:1121–1124

Woo HA, Jeong W, Chang TS, Park KJ, Park SJ, Yang JS, Rhee SG (2005). Reduction of cysteine sulfinic acid by sulfiredoxin is specific to 2-Cys peroxiredoxins. J Biol Chem 280:3125–3128

Wright JL, Tai H, Dai J, Churg A (2002) Cigarette smoke induces rapid changes in gene expression in pulmonary arteries. Lab Invest 82:1391–1398

Wu C (1997) Chromatin remodeling and the control of gene expression. J Biol Chem 272:28171–28174

Wyatt TA, Heires AJ, Sanderson SD, Floreani AA (1999) Protein kinase C activation is required for cigarette smoke-enhanced C5a-mediated release of interleukin-8 in human bronchial epithelial cells. Am J Respir Cell Mol Biol 21:283–288

Yang XJ, Ogryzko VV, Nishikawa J, Howard BH, Nakatani Y (1996) A p300/CBP-associated factor that competes with the adenoviral oncoprotein E1A. Nature 25:319–324

Yang SR, Chida AS, Bauter M, Shafiq N, Seweryniak K, Maggirwan SB, Kilty I, Rahman I. (2006) Cigarette smoke induces pro-inflammatory cytokine release by activation of NF-κB and post-translational modifications of histone deacetylase in monocytes. Am. J. Physiol Lung Cell Mol Physiol (Epub ahead of print).

Yoo CG, Lee S, Lee CT, Kim YW, Han SK, Shim YS (2000) Anti-inflammatory effect of heat shock protein induction is related to stabilization of I kappa B alpha through preventing I kappaB kinase activation in respiratory epithelial cells. J Immunol 164:5416–5423

Zang LY, Stone K, Pryor WA (1995) Detection of free radicals in aqueous extracts of cigarette tar by electron spin resonance. Free Radic Biol Med 19:161–167

Zhang S, Day IN, Ye S (2001) Microarray analysis of nicotine-induced changes in gene expression in endothelial cells. Physiol Genomics 5:187–192

Zhong H, May HJ, Jimi E, Ghosh S (2002) The phosphorylation status of nuclear NF-kappaB determines its association with CBP/p300 or HDAC-1. Mol Cell 9:625–636

Zhang Q, Adiseshaiah P, Reddy SP (2005). Matrix metalloproteinase/epidermal growth factor receptor/mitogen-activated protein kinase signaling regulate fra-1 induction by cigarette smoke in lung epithelial cells. Am J Respir Cell Mol Biol 32:72–81

Zhu J, Majumdar S, Qiu Y, Ansari T, Oliva A, Kips JC, Pauwels RA, De Rose V, Jeffery PK (2001) Interleukin-4 and interleukin-5 gene expression and inflammation in the mucus-secreting glands and subepithelial tissue of smokers with chronic bronchitis. Lack of relationship with CD8[+] cells. Am J Respir Crit Care Med 164:2220–2228

Ziegler DM (1985) Role of reversible oxidation-reduction of enzyme thiols-disulfides in metabolic regulation. Annu Rev Biochem 54:305–329

Chapter 6

Oxidative Stress in the Pathogenesis of Chronic Obstructive Pulmonary Disease

Irfan Rahman

Contents

6.1	Introduction	166
6.2	Sources of Oxidants in the Lungs	167
6.2.1	Cell-Derived ROS/Oxidants	167
6.2.2	Inhaled Oxidants and Cigarette Smoke	168
6.3	COPD	168
6.3.1	Clinical Features	168
6.4	Morphological/Cellular Alterations in COPD	170
6.4.1	Airspace Epithelial Injury/Permeability	170
6.4.2	Neutrophil Sequestration and Migration in the Lungs	170
6.5	Biochemical Features of COPD	171
6.5.1	Antioxidant Status in COPD	171
6.5.1.1	Systemic and Local Depletion of Antioxidants	171
6.5.1.2	Depletion of Lung GSH	171
6.6	Oxidants and Oxidative Stress in COPD	172
6.6.1	Oxidative Stress in the Alveolar Space	172
6.6.2	Alterations in Lung Tissue	173
6.6.3	Systemic Oxidative Stress	174
6.7	Noninvasive Biomarkers of Oxidative Stress	174
6.7.1	ROS and RNS as Surrogate Markers in Plasma and Exhaled Breath Condensate	174
6.7.2	H_2O_2	176
6.7.3	Lipid Peroxidation Products	176
6.8	Consequences of Oxidative Stress in COPD	177
6.8.1	Protease/Antiprotease Imbalance	177

Contents

6.8.2	Mucus Hypersecretion	178
6.8.3	Remodeling of Extracellular Matrix	179
6.8.4	Apoptosis	179
6.8.5	Muscle Dysfunction	181
6.9	Oxidative Stress and the Development of Airways Obstruction	181
6.10	Molecular Mechanisms of Oxidative Stress effects in COPD	182
6.10.1	NF-κB Activation	182
6.10.2	Proinflammatory Genes	183
6.10.3	Antioxidant and Stress Response Genes	183
6.11	Chromatin Remodeling (Histone Acetylation and Deacetylation) and Glucocorticoid Inefficacy in Response to Smoking and in Patients with COPD	184
6.12	Genetic Polymorphisms as Markers of COPD	187
6.13	Models for Studying COPD	188
6.14	Conclusions	189
	References	190

6.1 Introduction

The lung is the only organ that has the highest exposure to atmospheric oxygen and together with its large surface area and blood supply is susceptible to injury mediated by reactive forms of oxygen species.

In situ lung injury because of reactive oxygen species (ROS) is linked to oxidation of proteins, DNA, and lipids. These oxidized biomolecules may also induce a variety of cellular responses through the generation of secondary metabolic reactive species. Physiologically, ROS inflict their effects by altering remodeling of extracellular matrix and blood vessels and stimulate mucus secretion and alveolar repair responses. On the biochemical level, ROS inactivate antiproteases, cause apoptosis, and regulate cell proliferation (Rahman and MacNee 1996, 1999) (Fig. 6.1) and modulate the immune system in the lungs. At the molecular level, increased ROS levels have been implicated in initiating inflammatory responses in the lungs through the activation of transcription factors such as nuclear factor-kappaB (NF-κB) and activator protein 1 (AP-1), signal transduction, chromatin remodeling, and gene expression of proinflammatory mediators (Rahman and MacNee 1998).

This chapter brings forth the evidence for the role of ROS pertaining to chronic obstructive pulmonary disease (COPD) and attempts to unravel the cellular and molecular mechanisms and pathophysiological consequences of increased ROS release in COPD.

The relevance of noninvasive oxidative stress biomarkers in the pathophysiology of COPD is also discussed.

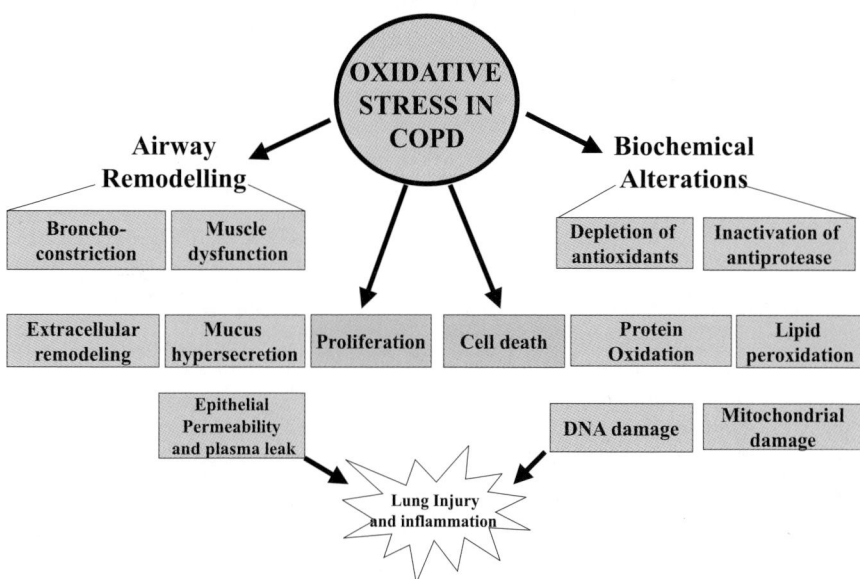

Fig. 6.1 Reactive oxygen species (ROS)-mediated cellular responses in chronic obstructive pulmonary disease (*COPD*)

6.2 Sources of Oxidants in the Lungs

6.2.1 Cell-Derived ROS/Oxidants

COPD is pathologically characterized by an inflammatory response, involving activation of epithelial cells, resident macrophages, and the recruitment and activation of pulmonary phagocytic cells and lymphocytes. Once recruited in the airspace, these cells become activated and generate ROS in response to inflammatory mediators. The primary ROS-generating enzyme is NADPH oxidase, a complex enzyme system that is present in phagocytes and epithelial cells. Following activation, macrophages, neutrophils, and eosinophils generate $O_2^-\cdot$, which is rapidly converted to hydrogen peroxide (H_2O_2) under the influence of superoxide dismutase (SOD). $\cdot OH$ may be formed nonenzymatically in the presence of free catalytic iron (Fe^{2+}) as a secondary reaction. ROS and reactive nitrogen species (RNS) can also be generated intracellularly from several sources such as mitochondrial respiration, the NADPH oxidase system, and xanthine/xanthine oxidase. In addition to NADPH oxidase, phagocytes employ other enzymes to produce ROS and other potent oxidants such as hypochlorous acid (HOCl) and hypobromous acid (HOBr). The later two species are generated by the action of heme peroxidases (myeloperoxidase [MPO] or eosinophil peroxidase [EPO]).

6.2.2 Inhaled Oxidants and Cigarette Smoke

A direct consequence of cigarette smoking, inhalation of airborne pollutants, such as oxidant gases (ozone, nitrogen dioxide [NO_2], sulphur dioxide [SO_2]) or particulate in air, is lung damage and elevated inflammatory responses in the lungs. These environmental noxious agents are implicated in the pathogenesis and exacerbations of COPD. In the gas phase, the smoke contains high concentrations of oxidants/free radicals (>10^{15} molecules per puff) (Church and Pryor 1985), short-lived oxidants such as $O_2^{-}\cdot$, and nitric oxide (NO). NO and $O_2^{-}\cdot$ immediately react to form the highly reactive peroxynitrite ($ONOO^{-}$) molecule. The tar phase of cigarette smoke contains organic radicals, such as long-lived semiquinone radicals, which can react with molecular oxygen in a redox-dependent manner to form $O_2^{-}\cdot$ to form $\cdot OH$ and H_2O_2 (Nakayama et al. 1989). The cycle can be sustained by biological reducing equivalents (ascorbate, NAD[P]H, glutathione [GSH], etc.), which reduce the oxidized quinoid substances back to their reduced states, enabling them to reproduce the superoxide radical. The aqueous phase of cigarette smoke condensate may undergo redox recycling for a considerable period of time in the epithelial lining fluid (ELF) of smokers (Nakayama et al. 1989). The tar phase is also an effective metal chelator wherein iron is chelated to produce tar semiquinone plus tar Fe^{2+}, which can generate H_2O_2 continuously (Nakayama et al. 1989). Sidestream cigarette smoke contains more than 10^{17} reactive organic compounds per puff, such as carbon monoxide, nicotine, ammonia, formaldehyde, acetaldehyde, crotonaldehyde, acrolein, *N*-nitrosamines, benzo[*a*]pyrene, benzene, isoprene, ethane, pentane, and other genotoxic and carcinogenic organic compounds. The concentrations of these reactive compounds present in the ELF following inhalation of cigarette smoke have been calculated by other workers (Eiserich et al. 1995).

6.3 COPD

6.3.1 Clinical Features

COPD is a gradually progressing condition characterized by airflow limitation, which is largely irreversible (Pauwels et al. 2001), and its diagnosis usually is based on the history of exposure to toxic stimuli (mainly tobacco smoke) and abnormal lung function tests. Because of variable pathology and only partial understanding of the molecular mechanisms involved in the disease process, a straightforward definition of COPD is yet to be understood. However, the diagnosis of COPD still based on the persistent presence of airflow obstruction in a cigarette smoker (Celli et al. 2004).

Cigarette smoking has been implicated as the major etiological factor underlying the disease. Although more than 90% of patients with COPD are smokers, not all smokers develop COPD (Pauwels et al 2001). However, 15–20% of smokers appear to be susceptible to the ill effects of smoking and show a rapid decline in lung function measured as forced expiratory volume in one second (FEV_1). This category of smokers is at an increased risk of developing the disease. Other factors that may exacerbate COPD are air pollutants, infections, and occupational dusts, which also have the potential to produce oxidative stress (Fig. 6.2). Based primarily on FEV_1, the Global Initiative for Chronic

Obstructive Lung Disease (GOLD) guidelines have classified the severity of COPD into four stages (Pauwels et al 2001). However, mere emphasis on FEV_1 alone as an index of severity for COPD has been criticized. A composite measure essentially based on clinical parameters (Body-Mass Index, Airflow Obstruction, Dyspnea, and Exercise Capacity [BODE] Index) has been shown to be better at predicting mortality than does FEV_1 (Celli et al. 2004).

Although the development of COPD in terms of deterioration of FEV_1 is yet to be confirmed, there is, however, a tendency to classify the stages as evolving from stage 0 to stage 4. In the context that not all smokers develop COPD, it is similarly possible that the disease may not progress from one stage to the next in an established sequence. In relatively young patients with severe COPD, it is yet to be established if early stages of their disease are similar to those found in patients with mild COPD. With COPD being a heterogeneous disease, several outcomes may be seen at each of the stages. For example, recently, Hogg and coworkers (2004) have shown that the progression of COPD was strongly associated with an increase in the volume of tissue in the wall and the accumulation of inflammatory mucous exudates in the lumen of the small airways. The percentage of the airways that contained polymorphonuclear neutrophils, macrophages,

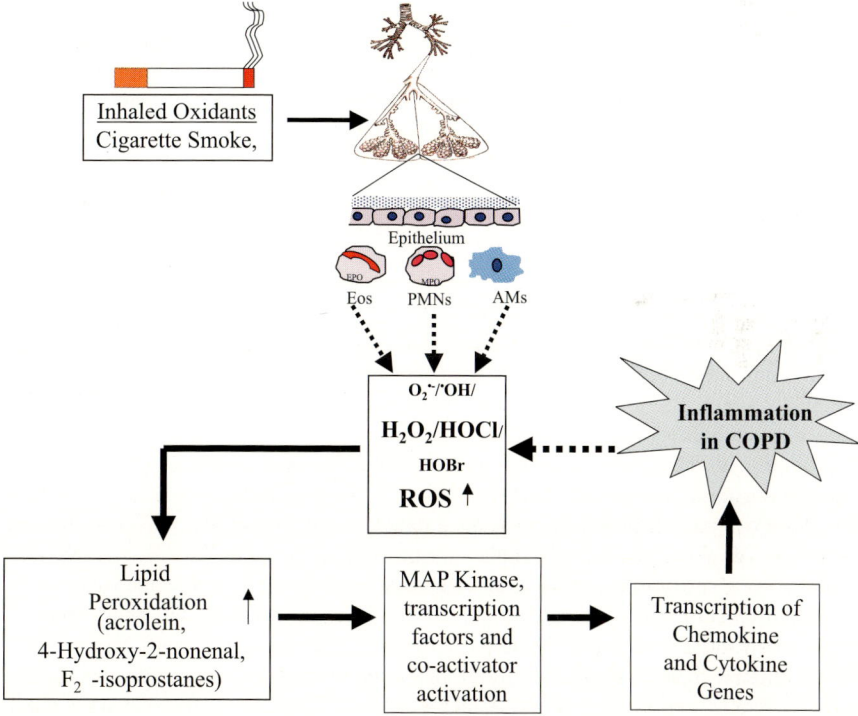

Fig. 6.2 Mechanisms of reactive oxygen species (ROS)-mediated lung inflammation in chronic obstructive pulmonary disease (*COPD*). Inflammatory response is mediated by oxidants either inhaled and/or released by the activated neutrophils, alveolar macrophages, eosinophils, and epithelial cells, leading to production of ROS and membrane lipid peroxidation. Activation of transcription of the proinflammatory cytokine and chemokine genes, upregulation of adhesion molecules, and increased release of proinflammatory mediators are involved in the inflammatory responses in patients with COPD

CD4, CD8, and B cells increases as COPD progresses. Systematic experimental modeling of each stage of severity might provide a better insight into this issue (Groneberg and Chung 2004).

6.4 Morphological/Cellular Alterations in COPD

6.4.1 Airspace Epithelial Injury/Permeability

An important early consequence of inflammation because of cigarette smoke is airspace epithelial injury that leads to an increase in airspace epithelial permeability. ^{99m}Technetium-diethylenetriaminepentacetate (^{99m}Tc-DTPA) lung clearance studies in humans have revealed increased epithelial permeability in chronic smokers, compared with nonsmokers. ^{99m}Tc-DTPA clearance was further increased following acute smoking (Morrison et al. 1999). Extra- and intracellular levels of GSH appear to be critical for the maintenance of epithelial integrity following exposure to cigarette smoke. Studies involving epithelial cell monolayers in vitro and in rat lungs in vivo following exposure to cigarette smoke condensate have demonstrated increased epithelial permeability. This increase in epithelial permeability was related to profound changes in the antioxidant GSH (Rahman and MacNee 1999, 2000). Treatment of cells with GSH markedly diminished cigarette smoke-induced epithelial injury/permeability, suggesting that the injurious effects were in part oxidant-mediated (Rahman and MacNee 1999).

6.4.2 Neutrophil Sequestration and Migration in the Lungs

The pathophysiology of COPD includes an important role of neutrophils. These cells can release a multitude of mediators and tissue-degrading enzymes such as elastases, which can orchestrate tissue destruction and chronic inflammation (Chung 2001; Stockley 2002). A large number of mediators including cytokines released from resident lung cells, alveolar macrophages, epithelial, and endothelial cells can activate neutrophils while in transit in the pulmonary microcirculation. Inhaled oxidants such as those contained in cigarette smoke and other air pollutants could influence the transit of cells in the pulmonary capillary bed by decreasing neutrophil deformability (shape alterations in neutrophils to pass the smaller capillary segments).

Increased neutrophils and macrophages have been reported in bronchoalveolar lavage fluid (BALF) from cigarette smokers (Hunninghake and Crystal 1983). Induced sputum neutrophilia has been found to be higher in patients with a high degree of airflow limitation than in subjects without airflow limitation. Increased sputum neutrophilia is also related to an accelerated decrease in FEV_1. Subjects with chronic cough and sputum production have a greater incidence of sputum neutrophilia (Stanescu et al. 1996). Studies in humans, using radiolabeled neutrophils and red cells, show a transient increase in neutrophil sequestration and decreased neutrophil deformability in the lungs during smoking/oxidative stress (Rahman and MacNee 1996) and returns to normal on cessation of smoking. A similar decrease in deformability is demonstrated in vivo for neutrophils from the blood of subjects who are actively smoking (Rahman and MacNee 1996). Activation of neutrophils sequestered in the pulmonary microvasculature could induce the release of ROS and proteases within the microenvironment, leading to destruction of the alveolar wall that occurs in emphysema.

6.5 Biochemical Features of COPD

6.5.1 Antioxidant Status in COPD

6.5.1.1 Systemic and Local Depletion of Antioxidants

The antioxidants armamentarium of ELF is composed of low-molecular-weight antioxidants, metal-binding proteins, antioxidant enzymes, sacrificial reactive proteins, and unsaturated lipids. The major antioxidants in ELF include mucin, reduced GSH, uric acid, protein (largely albumin), ceruloplasmin, and ascorbic acid (Cross et al. 1994). Depending on the redox environment, the concentrations of nonenzymatic antioxidants may vary in ELF. Some of these antioxidants, such as GSH and ascorbate, are concentrated in ELF, compared with plasma. This indicates their relative importance in the antioxidant defenses of ELF. Smoking and exacerbations of COPD are reflected in the plasma by decreased antioxidant capacity, associated with depleted protein sulfhydryls in the plasma (Rahman et al. 1996, 1997). The decrease in antioxidant capacity in smokers occurred transiently during smoking and resolved rapidly after smoking cessation (Rahman et al. 1996). In exacerbations of COPD, however, diminished antioxidant capacity continued for several days after the onset of the exacerbation. The levels tended towards controls only at the time of recovery from the exacerbation (Rahman et al. 1997). The depletion of antioxidant capacity could be partially explained by increased release of ROS from peripheral blood neutrophils. ROS thus released are neutralized by the antioxidants, which leads to the reduction of antioxidant levels. This observation is further emphasized by a significant negative correlation between neutrophil superoxide anion release and plasma antioxidant capacity (Rahman et al. 1996).

Depletion of total antioxidant capacity in smokers is associated with depletion of major plasma antioxidants, i.e., ascorbic acid, vitamin E, β-carotene, and selenium in the serum of chronic smokers (Mezzetti et al. 1995). No such consensus has been established for changes in other antioxidants and antioxidant enzymes in response to cigarette smoke. Reduced levels of vitamin E in the BALF of smokers and a marginal increase in vitamin C in BALF of smokers, compared with nonsmokers have been shown (Rahman and MacNee 1996). Thus, there is clear evidence that oxidants in cigarette smoke markedly decrease plasma and BALF antioxidants.

6.5.1.2 Depletion of Lung GSH

GSH homeostasis may play a pivotal role in maintaining the integrity of lung airspace epithelial barrier. This is supported by the observation that a decrease in the levels of GSH in epithelial cells alters barrier function and increases epithelial permeability (Morrison et al. 1999; Rahman and MacNee 2000; Rahman et al. 1995). There is, however, limited information as to the status of respiratory epithelial antioxidant defenses in smokers, and even less for patients with COPD. Several studies have shown that GSH is elevated in BALF in chronic smokers (Cantin et al. 1987; Morrison et al. 1999). However, this increase is not observed immediately after acute cigarette smoking (Morrison et al. 1999). Interestingly, Harju and colleagues (2002) have found that γ-glutamylcysteine synthetase, ([γ-GCS] now called γ-glutamale cysteine ligase [GCL]) immunoreactivity was decreased (GSH levels were not measured) in the airways of smokers, compared with nonsmokers, suggesting that cigarette smoke predisposes lung cells to ongoing oxidant stress. GCL has light regulatory and heavy catalytic subunits. This indicates that a twofold increase of GSH in BALF in chronic smokers may not suffice for the excessive oxidant burden recorded during smoking. In such a condition, an acute depletion of GSH may be observed (Morrison et al. 1999; Rahman and MacNee 2000). Neurohr and colleagues (2003) recently attributed decreased GSH levels in BALF cells of chronic smokers to a decreased expression of the GCL light subunit. However, no change was observed in GCL heavy subunit expression. This highlight the fact that increased GSH level in ELF of chronic smokers may not be associated with increased GSH levels in alveolar macrophages. Thus, further in-depth studies are needed to understand the regulation of GSH levels in the lungs of smokers and COPD subjects in order to devise appropriate antioxidant GSH therapy.

6.6 Oxidants and Oxidative Stress in COPD

6.6.1 Oxidative Stress in the Alveolar Space

Increased oxidant burden in the lungs is characteristic of COPD. In smokers, the oxidant load is enhanced by the release of ROS from macrophages and neutrophils, which are known to migrate in increased numbers into the lungs of cigarette smokers. Once activated in the lungs, these cells can generate ROS via the NADPH oxidase system (also known as respiratory burst oxidase). The respiratory burst is an important step implicated in a sudden surge in the generation of $O_2^-\cdot$. Circulating neutrophils from cigarette smokers and patients with COPD release more $O_2^-\cdot$ (Rahman et al 1996). Increased content of MPO in neutrophils from smoker has been found to correlate with the degree of pulmonary dysfunction (Gompertz et al. 2001), suggesting that neutrophil MPO-mediated oxidative stress may be important in the pathogenesis of COPD. Macrophages obtained from BALF of smokers are activated, compared with those from nonsmokers. One manifestation of this is the release of increased amounts of ROS such as $O_2^-\cdot$ and H_2O_2 (Morrison et al. 1999; Rahman and MacNee 1996).

COPD subjects manifest higher intracellular iron content in alveolar macrophages, which is increased in cigarette smokers. The iron level is further increased in chronic bronchitis, compared with nonsmokers (Lapenna et al. 1995). High iron levels augment the generation of ROS in ELF in the airspaces of smokers and COPD subjects. This is further supported by the observation that lungs of smokers contain darkly pigmented areas. These pigmented areas yield high electron spin resonance (ESR) signals because of heme/nonheme iron and carbon-centered radicals (Church and Pryor 1985). This may relate to excessive iron accumulation in the alveolar macrophages of smokers and COPD subjects.

6.6.2 Alterations in Lung Tissue

An important link between oxidative stress and the pathogenesis of COPD has emerged from the demonstration of ROS-dependent oxidative modification of target molecules and their presence in increased amounts in the lungs of smokers, particularly those who develop COPD. ROS such as $O_2^-\cdot$ and $\cdot OH$, generated and released by activated immune and inflammatory cells, are highly reactive and when generated in close vicinity to cell membranes, initiate membrane phospholipids peroxidation (lipid peroxidation). Lipid peroxidation then may continue as a chain reaction, leading to membrane and cell damage. Many of the effects of ROS in airways may be mediated by the secondary release of inflammatory lipid mediators such as 4-hydroxy-2-nonenal (4-HNE), a footprint of oxidative stress/lipid peroxidation. 4-HNE, a highly reactive and diffusible end product of lipid peroxidation, is known to induce/regulate various cellular events, such as proliferation, apoptosis, and activation of mitogen-activated protein kinase (MAPK) signaling pathways (Uchida et al. 1999). 4-HNE has a high affinity towards cysteine, histidine, and lysine residues and also conjugates with GSH. Conjugation of 4-HNE with amino acid residues in proteins may render a protein nonfunctional. It is also chemotactic to neutrophils in vitro and in vivo. The levels of 4-HNE-modified protein were increased in airway and alveolar epithelial cells, endothelial cells, and neutrophils in subjects with airway obstruction, compared with otherwise normal subjects (Rahman et al. 2002) (Fig. 6.3). Furthermore, Aoshiba and colleagues (2003a) have demonstrated that cigarette smoking enhanced the levels of 4-HNE adducts in bronchiolar epithelial and alveolar type cells in mice. Thus, evidence is accumulating that cigarette smoke triggers oxidative

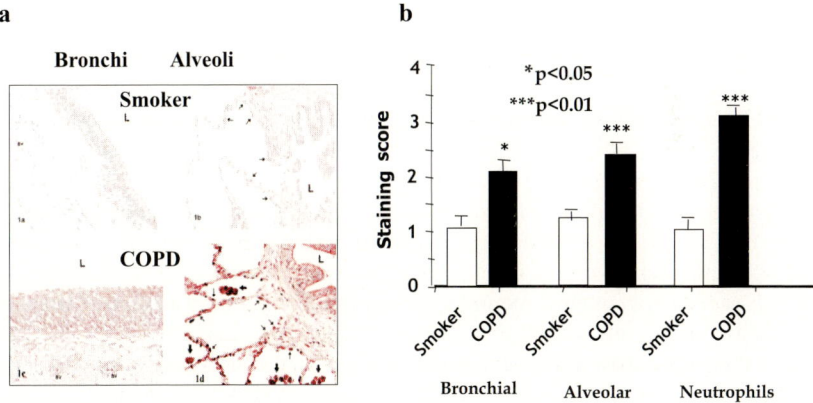

Photographs from immunostaining for 4-HNE in lung tissue from subjects with and without COPD. 1b: Non-COPD; 2b: COPD, L=Lumen. Original magnification: 200X

Fig. 6.3 a Photographs from immunostaining for 4-hydroxy-2-nonenal (*4-HNE*) in lung tissue from subjects with and without chronic obstructive pulmonary disease (*COPD*). *1a* Non-COPD, bronchial; *1b* Non-COPD, alveolar; *2a* COPD, bronchial; *2b* COPD, alveolar. *L* lumen. Original magnification, ×200. b Individual immunostaining scores for 4-HNE-adducts in bronchial and alveolar lung tissue in epithelial cells, endothelial cells, and neutrophils. The mean is indicated, as well significance levels (*p*) for differences between the indicated groups stress, leading to lipid peroxidation in lungs of smokers and patients with COPD. Lipid peroxidation may further herald extensive damage to the lung architecture.

6.6.3 Systemic Oxidative Stress

In addition to in the lungs, COPD is now considered to have systemic manifestations. One manifestation of a systemic effect is the presence of markers of oxidative stress in the blood in patients with COPD. Various studies have demonstrated increased production of $O_2^-\cdot$ from peripheral blood neutrophils obtained from patients during acute exacerbations of COPD, which returned to normal when the patients were clinically stable (Noguera et al. 1998; Rahman et al. 1996, 1997). Another biological source of $O_2^-\cdot$ and H_2O_2 is the cellular xanthine/xanthine oxidase (XO) system, which has been shown to be increased in cell free BALF and plasma from COPD patients. (Rahman et al.1996) This observation has been further associated with increased $O_2^-\cdot$ and lipid peroxide levels in COPD subjects (Pinamonti et al. 1998).

6.7 Noninvasive Biomarkers of Oxidative Stress

6.7.1 ROS and RNS as Surrogate Markers in Plasma and Exhaled Breath Condensate

Assessment of oxidative end products as biomarkers by both noninvasive and semi-invasive techniques has recently emerged to be of interest for understanding the status of COPD. Measurements of surrogate biomarkers oxidative stress have been made in blood, urine, breath, or exhaled breath condensate or in induced or spontaneously produced sputum of smokers and patients with COPD. Oxidative stress biomarker assessment in exhaled breath condensate (EBC) is emerging as a promising area of future research in COPD (Kharitonov and Barnes 2001; Rahman and Kelly 2003). The relative concentrations of various oxidant/antioxidant biomarkers detected in EBC are listed in Table 6.1 (Kharitonov and Barnes 2001; Rahman and Kelley 2003) There is, however, a limitation of oxidative stress biomarkers at present because of the lack of correlation with disease severity or outcome and the variations in the control subjects. Furthermore, the validity of EBC as a tool for the assessment of airway oxidative stress is still questionable, owing to limitations in the reproducibility of analyzed oxidative biomarkers, with respect to intra- and interindividual variability, sampling time, and variability in dilution of respiratory droplets by water vapor, sensitivity, and specificity of the assays used (Rahman 2004; Rahman and Biswas 2004). Other confounding factors contributing to variation include smoking, consumption of caffeine, alcohol, and intake of diet rich in antioxidants. Identification of specific and reproducible biomarkers of oxidative stress and inflammation in EBC would be of great value for noninvasive investigations of the natural history and epidemiology of COPD and for phenotyping in genetic perspectives. Exhaled NO has also been used as a marker of airway inflammation and as an alternate measure of oxidative stress. Sporadic reports of increased levels of NO in exhaled breath in patients with COPD are available, but not to the extent reported in asthmatics (Rahman et al. 1996). Although smoking increases NO levels in breath, the spontaneously rapid reaction of NO with $O_2^-\cdot$ (which forms $ONOO^-$), however, limits the usefulness of this marker in COPD. Generation of RNS because of cigarette smoke results in nitration and oxidation of various cellular and plasma proteins at their tyrosine residues. The levels of nitrated proteins (3-nitrotyrosine) were conspicuously higher in smokers, compared with nonsmokers (Petruzzelli et al. 1997). NO and $ONOO^-$-mediated formation of 3-nitrotyrosine in plasma and Fe^{2+} levels in ELF) are elevated in chronic smokers (Ichinose et al. 2000; Kanazawa et al. 2003). The levels of nitrotyrosine were negatively correlated with the $FEV_1\%$. Also, NO generated in the cells has been found to be involved in the depletion of GSH levels and may be important because their binding to the thiol to form S-nitrosoglutathione (GSNO). Of interest is the recent finding that sputum concentrations of nitrosothiols and oxidized GSH (GSSG) are increased in patients with COPD and associated to neutrophilic inflammation (Beeh et al. 2004).

These data further underline the role of oxidative stress in the pathogenesis of COPD and suggest that GSH is important to scavenge both reactive oxygen and nitrogen species. Because GSSG and nitrosothiols can be detected in sputum, this could be a simple, noninvasive source of a COPD marker. $ONOO^-$, on the other hand, can bring about thiol oxidation, lysosomal degranulation, and various oxidative changes that are potentially injurious to the cells. This indicates that the increased level of RNS plays a role in

Table 6.1 Oxidant/antioxidant biomarkers in exhaled breath condensate and their measurements

Biomarker	Analysis	Values in EBC		
		Nonsmoker	Smoker	COPD
Reactive oxygen species Hydrogen peroxide (μM)	Spectroscopy, Fluorometry, chemiluminesce	0.01–0.09	0.10–0.75	0.2–2.6
Reactive nitrogen species Nitrite (μM) Nitrite and nitrate (μM) Nitrotyrosine (ng/ml) Nitrosothiols (μM)	Electrometry, spectroscopy, ELISA, GC/MS, HPLC	0.64 20.2 0.66–6.3 –	0.44–2.4 20.2–29.2 7.2 0.1–0.46	2.6 – – 0.24
Lipid peroxidation products TBARS (μM) Malondialdehydes (nmol/l) F_2-Isoprostanes (pg/ml)	Colorimetry, ELISA EIA, GC/MS, HPLC LC/MS	– 17.2–19.4 nmol/l by LC/MS 3.9–15.8 by EIA, and 7±4 by GC/MS	– – –	0.48 57.2 by LC/MS 42.5
Antioxidant Glutathione, nM	Spectrophotometry, HPLC, LC/MS	14.1	–	–

Values are adapted in part from Rahman and Biswas 2004

EBC exhaled breath condensate, *COPD* chronic obstructive pulmonary disease, *ELISA* enzyme-linked immunosorbent assay, *GC/MS* gas chromatography/mass spectrometry, *HPLC* high-performance liquid chromatography, *TBARS* thiobarbituric acid reactive substances, *EIA* enzyme immunoassay, *LC/MS* liquid chromatography-tandem mass spectrometry the abnormal inflammatory response that occurs in COPD and may be involved in tissue damage.

6.7.2 H_2O_2

H_2O_2, measured in EBC, is a direct measurement of oxidant burden in the airspaces. The source of H_2O_2 in EBC is unknown, but may in part derive from the release of $O_2^{-\cdot}$ from alveolar macrophages. Smokers and patients with COPD have higher levels of exhaled H_2O_2 than do nonsmokers, and levels are even higher during exacerbations of COPD (Kharitonov and Barnes 2001; Rahman and Kelly 2003). However, H_2O_2 levels vary considerably in healthy, young nonsmokers and smokers from 0.01 to 0.09 μM and 0.10 to 0.75 μM, respectively (Rahman 2004). This variation (60–80%) in H_2O_2 concentrations may be attributed to different storage conditions and/or analytical techniques used for EBC H_2O_2 assay. Thus, the variability of the measurement of exhaled H_2O_2 because of its highly volatile nature, along with the presence of other confounding factors, e.g., increased generation of ROS by cigarette smoke-mediated redox cycling, has led to concerns about its reproducibility as a marker of oxidative stress in smokers and in patients with COPD (Rahman 2004; Rahman and Biswas 2004). Recently, Gerristen et al. (2005) have demonstrated increased levels of exhaled H_2O_2, interleukin 8 (IL-8) and the soluble cell adhesion molecule (sICAM), and sE-selectin in serum of freshly admitted COPD patients. On medication with prednisolone, the levels of H_2O_2 were found to be significantly reduced in the exhaled breath and a concomitant decrease in the serum levels of IL-8 and sICAM was found. However, no appreciable alterations were observed for sE-selectins and spirometry. This further emphasizes the importance of certain cell adhesion molecules as biomarkers of COPD for diagnosis and prognosis of the disease (Gerritsen et al. 2005). A study characterizing the relationship between oxidative stress and inflammatory components in induced sputum and blood of COPD patients has been conducted by Sadowska et al. (2005). In their study, the authors have established a correlation between inflammatory markers such as IL-8, eosinophil cationic protein (ECP), sICAM-1, and oxidative stress markers such as SOD, GSH peroxidase (GPx), Trolox-equivalent antioxidant capacity (TEAC), albumin, vitamins E, and A. Treatment with N-acetyl-L-cysteine and/or inhaled corticosteroids was found to significantly modulate the correlation of these markers of COPD.

6.7.3 Lipid Peroxidation Products

Evidence of aldehydes being generated endogenously during the process of lipid peroxidation has been amply demonstrated. These aldehydes are being implicated in many pathophysiological processes and are associated with oxidative stress in cells and tissues. In addition to their cytotoxic properties, lipid peroxides are now recognized as mediators of inflammatory response via the signal transduction pathways.

Isoprostanes are products of nonenzymatic lipid peroxidation. They have also been used as markers of oxidative stress. The levels of 8-iso-prostaglandin F_2 (8-isoprostane) in EBC are elevated in healthy smokers and more markedly in patients with COPD reflecting the degree of oxidative stress (Kharitonov and Barnes 2001; Montuschi et al.

2000). 8-Isoprostane levels were elevated in the plasma and BALF in chronic smokers and patients with stable COPD, as compared with healthy, age-matched nonsmoking subjects (Rahman and Biswas, 2004). Furthermore, F_2-isoprostanes were even higher in plasma of patients with acute exacerbations of COPD than in patients with stable COPD, indicating that increased oxidative stress occurs in exacerbations. Increased levels of these markers of lipid peroxidation products have been further correlated with airway obstruction. Because of its consistent association with the disease process, 8-isoprostane is currently considered to be a reliable oxidative stress biomarker that can be easily detected in plasma, EBC, and BALF of patients with COPD. In a more recent study, Santus et al. (2004) have reported an increased urinary excretion of the isoprostane 8-iso-prostaglandin $F_2\alpha$ as an index of in vivo oxidant stress. Overnight urinary excretion of the isoprostane was found to be significantly higher in COPD patients than in controls. Treatment with polyphenol extract resulted in a significant decrease in isoprostane excretion, which was found to be correlated with significant increase of partial pressure of arterial oxygen. Furthermore, changes in FEV_1 significantly correlated with the changes in isoprostane urinary excretion observed from enrollment to the end of treatment.

Indirect and nonspecific measurements of lipid peroxidation products, such as thiobarbituric acid reactive substances (TBARS) have also been shown to be elevated in breath condensate and in lungs of patients with stable COPD (Fahn et al. 1998; Nowak et al. 1999). The level of plasma lipid peroxides (TBARS) is elevated in COPD and has been negatively correlated with the FEV_1. Other specific products of lipid peroxidation such as malondialdehyde (MDA) and 4-HNE, derivatized immediately after sampling, can be measured successfully by a more reliable method employing high-performance liquid chromatography (HPLC). Using liquid chromatography-tandem mass spectrometry (LC/TMS), Corradi and coworkers (2003) have recently shown higher concentrations of MDA in the EBC of COPD. Further longitudinal and cross-sectional studies of well-characterized smokers with and without COPD are needed to evaluate the correlation of a broad array of putative oxidative markers of COPD to susceptibility, severity, exacerbations, progression, and status of the disease.

6.8 Consequences of Oxidative Stress in COPD

6.8.1 Protease/Antiprotease Imbalance

An imbalance between protease and antiprotease enzymes has been hypothesized with respect to the pathogenesis of emphysema (Shapiro 2003). This hypothesis was based on the observation that α1-antitrypsin (α_1-AT)-deficient subjects develop severe emphysema and that protease–antiprotease imbalance was later demonstrated in animal models of COPD (Hautamaki et al. 2004; Shapiro et al. 2003). Although α_1-AT deficiency is a very rare cause of emphysema (Parfrey et al. 2003), it implies the importance of proteases and proteolysis in COPD (Barnes et al. 2003). Studies have shown that mice deficient in neutrophil elastase were significantly protected from emphysema from chronic cigarette smoke exposure (Shapiro et al. 2003). Similarly, mice deficient in the macrophage elastase gene also were protected from emphysema induced by cigarette smoke (Hautamaki et al. 1997). Each of these elastases were found to cross-inactivate the endogenous inhibitor of the other, with macrophage elastase degrading α_1-AT and neutrophil elastase degrading tissue inhibitor of metalloproteinase-1 (Shapiro et al. 2003). Animals with elastase gene-deficiency when exposed to cigarette smoke showed impaired recruitment of neutrophils and monocytes. In addition, decreased macrophage elastase activity was observed, which was attributed to a decreased macrophage influx in these animals. Thus, it appears that neutrophil and macrophage elastase may play a major role in the mediation of alveolar destruction in response to cigarette smoke (Hautamaki et al. 1997; Shapiro et al. 2003).

In the case of smokers having normal levels of α_1-AT, the elastase burden may be increased as a result of increased recruitment of leukocytes into the lungs. A further functional deficiency of α_1-AT may be developed because of oxidative inactivation of α_1-AT in the lungs because of oxidative modification of methionine at the active site of the enzyme. Such oxidative inactivation may be carried out by the oxidants present in the cigarette smoke. Furthermore, oxidation of the methionine residue in α_1-AT was confirmed in the lungs of healthy smokers (Carp et al. 1982). These studies supported the concept of inactivation of α_1-AT by oxidation of the active site of the protein. Early studies showed that the function of α_1-AT in BALF was decreased by approximately 40% in smokers, compared with nonsmokers (Gadek et al. 1979). Secretory leukoprotease inhibitor (SLPI), another major inhibitor of neutrophil elastase (NE), can also be inactivated by oxidants. In vitro studies have also shown loss of α_1-AT inhibitory capacity from oxidants or cigarette smoke. All the above studies and many more reports have thus supported the hypothesis that α_1-AT pays an important role in the early pathogenesis of emphysema in COPD subjects.

6.8.2 Mucus Hypersecretion

Mucins are complex glycoproteins that provide viscoelastic properties to the mucus and form an essential protective mechanism in the upper airways. Mucins are secreted by goblet cells in the airway tracts and are responsible for removal of many types of substances from the lungs. The regulation of mucin production has been found to be altered in the lungs of COPD patients. Goblet cell hyperplasia has been documented in smokers. Goblet cell activation results in mucus hypersecretion, leading to airway plugging. Cigarette smoke has been found to activate epidermal growth factor (EGF) receptors by tyrosine phosphorylation. This results in the induction of mucin gene (*MUC5AC*) expression and synthesis in epithelial cells and in vivo in lungs (Takeyama et al. 2001). Tobacco smoke-induced mucin transcription was directly controlled by an AP-1-containing response element located at $-3700/-3337$ in the *MUC5AC* 5' flanking region. Site-specific mutagenesis revealed that the major functional components of this region were two AP-1 sites. The ability of smoke to stimulate *MUC5AC* through AP-1 strongly depends on both c-Jun N-terminal kinase (JNK) and extracellular signal-regulated kinase (ERK) for transcriptional activity. Although ERK activation was a consequence of epidermal growth factor receptor (EGFR) activation, JNK activation by smoke was mediated by Src in an EGFR-independent manner triggered by ROS (Gensch et al. 2004). Inhibition of tyrosine phosphorylation by selective EGFR tyrosine kinase inhibitors and antioxidants inhibits cigarette smoke-mediated *MUC5AC* gene expression. This suggests that ROS have a role in the mucin gene expression (Takeyama et al. 2001). 4-HNE, a lipid peroxidation product, has been shown to induce release of mucus from airway epithelial cells and fibroblasts via activation of extracellular signal-related kinases (ERK1/2) (Tsukagoshi et al. 2002). Furthermore, elastase released from neutrophils has been shown to impair mucociliary clearance and stimulates goblet cell metaplasia and mucin production. Neutrophil elastase increases the expression of *MUC5AC* by enhancing mRNA stability in the cytosol (Fischer and Voynow 2002). Detailed understanding of EGFR signaling pathway and regulation of *MUC5AC* expression by cigarette smoke could lead to targeted inhibition of mucus hyperproduction in epithelial cells.

6.8.3 Remodeling of Extracellular Matrix

Oxidative stress has been implicated in the remodeling of extracellular matrix in lung injury. Treatment of alveolar macrophages, obtained from COPD subjects with cigarette smoke, induced increased release of matrix metalloproteinase 9 (MMP-9), compared with that of nonsmokers. MMP-9 has extracellular matrix-degrading activity, thus suggesting the role of oxidative component of cigarette smoke in increased elastolytic enzyme activity (Russell et al. 2002). This increase in the elastolytic activity may have its genesis in the generation of hypochlorous acid or peroxynitrite by the alveolar macrophages, leading to extracellular matrix breakdown (Kirkham et al. 2003). MMP-9 synthesis and secretion has very recently been found to be triggered by IL-17 released by T lymphocytes (Prause et al. 2004). However, increased proteolytic load because of MMP-9 has been attributed to increased neutrophil recruitment in the lungs that triggers degradation of extracellular matrix and basement membrane in the airways and lungs. Factors other than oxidative stress, such as ozone and lipid peroxides, also induce matrix protein type I collagen and *MMP-1* gene expression (Choi et al. 1994). Other forms of oxidative stress derived from *tert*-butyl hydroperoxide and iron can also modify collagen synthesis by a mechanism presumably involving redox sensor/receptor. Wang and colleagues (2003) have recently documented that cigarette smoke produces airway wall remodeling in rat tracheal explants by induction of procollagen and NF-κB activation via a ROS-dependent mechanism. They suggested that transactivation of EGFR, rather than MAPK activation, was involved in airway remodeling. Furthermore, cigarette smoke-mediated activation of EGFR was found to be oxidant dependent.

Another important extracellular component is hyaluronan (HA) (Dentener et al. 2005). Extracellular matrix HA has proinflammatory role and has been found increased in sputum of COPD patients. Two categories of COPD subjects have been identified, one group having high HA levels and the other having moderate levels. COPD subjects exhibiting higher HA levels had low FEV_1 as compared with moderated and control categories. Furthermore, increased breakdown and therefore increased HA levels were further correlated with an increased expression of the *HYAL2* gene, and increased HA breakdown has been associated with local inflammation and severity of COPD.

6.8.4 Apoptosis

Alveolar epithelial lining cells have been found to undergo apoptosis in response to cigarette smoking, with consequent progressive cell loss and development of emphysema. Recent in vitro and in vivo studies in animals and humans have provided evidence of induction of apoptosis in cigarette smoke-treated macrophages, airway epithelial, dendritic cells, and lung fibroblasts (Carnevali et al. 2003; Hoshino et al. 2001). Therefore, it appears that oxidative stress may mediate apoptotic processes, particularly in airway epithelial cells. Cigarette smoke extract damages vascular endothelial cells through the JNK pathway, which is activated by oxidative stress (Hoshino et al. 2005). This may be because of oxidant dependent activation of caspases and/or apoptosis signal-regulating kinase-1 (ASK-1). The latter is held in an inactive form by thioredoxin, a redox-sensitive enzyme. Oxidant burden because of ROS triggers oxidation of thioredoxin, leading to an apoptotic cascade (Saitoh et al. 1998). Recently, both in vivo and in vitro investigations have revealed that cigarette smoke triggers endothelial cell apoptosis (Kasahara et al. 2000, 2001; Mullick et al. 2002; Wang et al. 2001), and that pulmonary vascular endothelial cell apoptosis is present in emphysematous lungs (Kasahara et al. 2003). Tuder and colleagues (2003) have shown that general inhibition of vascular endothelial growth factor receptor 2 (VEGF-KDR) leads to an increased oxidative stress that is mediated by reactive carbonyls and aldehydes (4-hydroxy-2-nonenal), leading to emphysema. They have further shown that both caspase inhibitor (Z-Asp-CH2) and a superoxide dismutase mimetic (M40419) blocked the development of emphysema and significantly reduced lung markers of oxidative stress and apoptosis (Mullick et al. 2002). However, Mansick et al. (2006) have shown that cigarette smoke decreased VEGFR2 but it was not assonated with emphysema in that lungs or in patients with COPD. In a more recent study, Karnenburg et al. (2005) have demonstrated that VEGF and its receptors Flt-1 and KDR/Flk-1 may induce peripheral vascular and airway remodeling processes via an autocrine or paracrine mechanism. The expression of VEGF and its receptors were greatly enhanced in the vascular and airway smooth muscles (VSM and ASM) bronchial, bronchiolar and alveolar epithelium, and alveolar macrophages COPD subjects as compared with control subjects. Whereas KDR/Flk-1 was markedly enhanced in endothelial cells and intimal and medial VSMs, Flt-1 was more intensively expressed in the endothelial cells. VEGF expression was found to be high in pulmonary microvasculature and intimal and medial VSMs. The enhanced expression of VEGF and its receptors correlated inversely with FEV_1.

Tsuji and his colleagues (2004) have reported that sublethal concentrations of CS induce senescence phenotypes in alveolar epithelial cells both in vitro and in vivo. Cellular senescence may be involved in the cigarette smoke-related pulmonary diseases associated with chronic epithelial damage. Cigarette smoking may induce the senescence of alveolar epithelial cells. In addition, the continuous proliferation of alveolar epithelial cells required to regenerate their loss as a result of apoptosis or necrosis accelerates telomere shortening, which in turn leads to the senescence of alveolar epithelial cells. When the alveolar epithelial cells reach the senescence stage, epithelial proliferation ceases, and the alveolar damage in cigarette smokers is no longer repaired. This model provides a plausible explanation for the chronic nature of cigarette smoke-related pulmonary diseases, such as pulmonary emphysema and fibrosis, which evolve slowly over many years.

Investigations in various cell models have led to the proposal that cigarette smoke may induce necrosis by inhibition of caspase activation and hence, may prevent apoptosis (Wickenden et al. 2003). Aoshiba and colleagues (2003a) have shown that single intratracheal injection of active caspase-3 resulted in epithelial cell apoptosis and enhanced elastolytic activity in mice. Further confirmation of the role of apoptosis in emphysematous changes in a murine model was obtained by an intratracheal injection of nodularin, a proapoptotic serine/threonine kinase inhibitor (Aoshiba et al. 2004b). Surprisingly, this approach did not cause inflammation or other forms of lung pathology, a hallmark of emphysema. Nevertheless, it is more or less now clear that cells involved in the lung architecture undergo apoptosis by cigarette smoke. However, the scenario may not be the same for inflammatory cells. It is likely that cigarette smoke and its constituents through their interaction with extracellular matrix may inhibit inflammatory cell (neutrophils) apoptosis, which renders them not to be recognized by macrophages. This phenomenon would then enhance or promote the inflammatory response in the lungs (Kirkham et al. 2004). Further studies are required to understand the mechanism of cigarette smoke-induced cell death, using both in vitro and in vivo models so as to define strategy for safe resolution of inflammation or inhibit alveolar wall destruction.

6.8.5 Muscle Dysfunction

Dysfunction of the respiratory and peripheral skeletal muscles along with weight loss and exercise limitations has been increasingly recognized as an important feature of systemic effects of COPD. Oxidative stress occurs in skeletal muscle during skeletal muscle fatigue, weakness, and sepsis, accompanied by an increased load imposed on the diaphragm in patients with severe COPD (Rabinovich et al. 2001). Hypoxia, impaired mitochondrial metabolism, and increased cytochrome C oxidase activity in skeletal muscle in patients with COPD have been implicated in the etiology of the aforementioned anomalies (Engelen et al 2000; Heunks and Dekhuijzen 2000). Ribera and colleagues (2003) have recently shown that mitochondrial electron transport chain (ETC) function is enhanced in inspiratory muscles of patients with COPD. Increased ETC activity was associated with an increase in functional demand on the muscles to endure training-like effects, leading to increased oxidative stress. Engelen and coworkers (2000) have correlated reduced muscle glutamate levels to increased muscle glycolytic metabolism in patients with severe COPD. Reduced glutamate levels (a precursor for GSH) were therefore associated with decreased GSH levels, suggesting that oxidant/antioxidant balance may be compromised in skeletal muscle dysfunction in patients with COPD (Agusti et al. 2002; Rabinovich et al. 2001). Apoptotic pathways have been implicated in skeletal muscle atrophy in patients with COPD (Agusti et al. 2002), linking oxidative stress-mediated muscle atrophy to apoptosis of skeletal myocytes/myofibers in patients with COPD. However, it still remains to be determined whether oxidative stress and/or poor nutrition (alterations in calorie intake or lowered basal metabolic rate) play a central role in mediating muscle mass wasting/apoptosis, particularly in susceptible subsets of patients with COPD. Whether susceptibility of subgroups of COPD patients to oxidative stress and injury in muscle wasting is because of their inability to boost endogenous protective and defect repair mechanisms warrants further examination.

6.9 Oxidative Stress and the Development of Airways Obstruction

Various epidemiological studies have shown a relationship between circulating neutrophil numbers and FEV_1 (Rahman and MacNee 1996; Rahman et al. 1996). Oxidative stress, measured as lipid peroxidation products in plasma, has also been shown to correlate inversely with the predicted FEV_1 in a population study (Celli et al. 2004). It is possible that differences in interindividual antioxidant capacity may contribute to the differences in the susceptibility against cigarette smoke-induced COPD. An association between dietary intake of antioxidant vitamins and lung function has been established in general population. However, some epidemiological studies have demonstrated negative associations of dietary antioxidant intake with pulmonary function and obstructive airway disease (Grievink et al. 1998). Another study (Britton et al. 1995) involving 2,633 subjects has shown an association between dietary intake of the antioxidant vitamin E and lung function, supporting the hypothesis that vitamin E may have a protective role in the development of COPD. Another study has suggested that antioxidant levels in the diet could be a possible explanation for differences in COPD mortality in different populations (Sargeant et al. 2000). Furthermore, dietary polyunsaturated fatty acids have also been found protective against the development of COPD in cigarette smokers (Shahar et al. 1999). These studies support the concept that dietary antioxidant supplementation including polyphenols may be a possible therapy to prevent of oxidative stress and inflammatory response in COPD.

6.10 Molecular Mechanisms of Oxidative Stress effects in COPD

6.10.1 NF-κB Activation

NF-κB is an important cytosolic transcription factor that can translocate to the nucleus on activation. In normally growing cells, NF-κB is maintained in an inactive state in the cytoplasm by the inhibitor IκBα, which prevents NF-κB from binding DNA. However, because both NF-κB and IκBα are shuttling proteins that rapidly move back and forth between the cytoplasm and the nucleus, the apparent cytoplasmic retention of NF-κB may simply represent an equilibrium state of a highly dynamic process. There are several pathways that can trigger NF-κB activation, the classical one that occurs in the cytoplasm and finally ends the nucleus. NF-κB activators such as tumor necrosis factor-α (TNF-α) and IL-1β engage cell surface receptors and transmit signals through the cytoplasm to the IκB kinase (IKK) complex. Activation of the IKK complex results in post-translational modification and proteasome-dependent degradation of IκBα; as a result, NF-κB is then free to activate transcription of responsive genes.

It is now generally accepted that NF-κB regulates the expression of various inflammatory genes, such as those for the cytokines, IL-8, TNF-α, and inducible nitric oxide (iNOS). Di Stefano and colleagues (2002) have demonstrated an increased expression of p65 protein of NF-κB in bronchial epithelium of smokers and patients with COPD, which was negatively correlated with the degree of airflow limitation in patients with COPD. Similarly, Caramori and coworkers (2003) have reported increased levels of p65 subunit of NF-κB in sputum macrophages but not in sputum neutrophils during exacerbations of COPD. This suggests that inflammatory responses may vary with the cell type. The activation of NF-κB in monocytes/macrophages may then, via release of proinflammatory mediators in lung epithelial fluid, trigger an amplified inflammatory cascade by activation of epithelial cells and recruitment of neutrophils in the airways.

Mochida-Nishimura and coworkers (2001) have shown that cells obtained from BALF of smokers exhibited tenfold higher activation of NF-κB in response to lipopolysaccharide (LPS), compared with that of nonsmokers. This may be because of the amplification of inflammatory mediators that may activate NF-κB. However, activation of the MAPK pathways, ERK, stress-activated protein kinase (SAPK), and p38 was differentially regulated. Activation of p38 was more rapid in BAL cells from smokers, compared with the activity of ERK and SAPK. They further suggested that the differences in activation of NF-κB and MAPKs in BAL cells from smokers and nonsmokers may be related to the differences in their microenvironment, which is affected by chronic exposure to cigarette smoke.

6.10.2 Proinflammatory Genes

A large number of studies have indicated that COPD is associated with airway/airspace inflammation and with the presence of markers of inflammation, including IL-8 and TNF-α, which are elevated in the sputum of patients with COPD (Keatings et al. 1996). In vitro treatment of macrophages, alveolar, and bronchial epithelial cells with oxidants has resulted in the release of inflammatory mediators such as IL-8, IL-1, and NO. The enhanced levels of these inflammatory markers paralleled increased transcription of their respective genes, and increased nuclear binding and activation of NF-κB (Antonicelli et al. 2002; Parmentier et al. 2000). Similarly, cigarette smoke-induced IL-8 release from human bronchial and endothelial cells, which may contribute to airway inflammation in smokers (Mio et al. 1997; Mochida-Nishimura et al. 2001). Increased IL-8 expression and release in COPD was found to parallel the increase in neutrophil counts in bronchial samples of BALF (Mochida-Nishimura et al. 2001).

Cigarette smoke has been implicated in vivo as a cause of increased leukocyte adhesion to vascular endothelium. Shen and coworkers (1996) have shown that cigarette smoke condensate induces the expression of a subset of cell adhesion molecules, such as ICAM-1, endothelial leukocyte adhesion molecule 1 (ELAM-1), and vascular cell adhesion molecule (VCAM-1) in human umbilical vascular endothelial cells associated with an increase in the binding activity of NF-κB. This suggests that increased transendothelial migration of monocytes occurs from cigarette smoking. The release of proinflammatory mediators, such as IL-1β and sICAM-1, was increased by cigarette smoke exposure to bronchial epithelial cells cultured from biopsy materials obtained from patients with COPD, compared with smokers (Rusznak et al. 2000; Witherden et al. 2004). Similarly, primary cultured human alveolar and bronchial epithelial cells obtained from patients COPD showed higher levels of TNF-α-induced release of IL-6 and IL-8, compared with nonstimulated COPD cells (Patel et al. 2003). These studies suggest that patients with COPD have a greater susceptibility to the effects of cigarette smoke.

6.10.3 Antioxidant and Stress Response Genes

An important effect of oxidative stress in the lungs is the upregulation of protective antioxidant and stress response genes. One of the important factors in this series is the upregulation of GSH levels in ELF in chronic smokers. Increased GSH has been correlated to the transcriptional activation of the gene for GSH synthesis (*GCL*) induced in the epithelial cells by cigarette smoke components (Cantin et al. 1987; Rahman and MacNee

2000; Rahman et al. 1995). Thus, upregulation of the gene(s) involved in GSH synthesis in response to oxidative stress, and cigarette smoke, may be protected by the cells. However, cigarette smoke may inflict injurious effects during intermittent smoking when the lung is already depleted of antioxidants because of earlier smoking. Importantly, GSH may also be one of the depleted antioxidants during such conditions.

TNF-α, which is an outcome of inflammation in COPD, has been shown to increase GCL mRNA expression in alveolar epithelial cells (Rahman et al. 1999). On the other hand, transforming growth factor-$β_1$ (TGF-$β_1$) has been shown to decrease antioxidant glutathione synthesis and is associated with increased ROS production in human alveolar epithelial cells and pulmonary artery endothelial cells in vitro (Jardine et al. 2002). Increased TGF-$β_1$ expression was associated with fibrosis in the basement membrane in the lungs and depletion of GSH, suggesting that cigarette smoking interferes in normal repair (Fig. 6.4).

Extracellular GPx (eGPx), another important antioxidant in the lungs, may be secreted by epithelial cells and macrophages, particularly in response to cigarette smoke or oxidative stress (Avissar et al. 1996). Ishii and coworkers (2001) have demonstrated the protective role of GSH S-transferase P1 (GSTP1) against cigarette smoke in the airway cells. Similarly, Maestrelli and coworkers have recently shown the induction of heme oxygenase-1 (HO-1) in alveolar spaces in response to smoking. This indicates that oxidative stress because of cigarette smoke may increase the gene expression of HO-1 (Maestrelli et al. 2001). Cigarette smoke also induces heat shock protein 70 (HS70) and HO-1 in human monocytes and has been implicated in the regulation of cell injury and cell death. In particular, HS70 and HO-1 has been implicated in the modulation of apoptosis in human endothelial cells and monocytes (Vayssier et al. 1998).

Thus, oxidative stress, including that produced by cigarette smoke, causes transcriptional activation of both proinflammatory genes and also of antioxidant and stress response genes. Therefore, a balance between proinflammatory and antioxidant gene expression may determine the susceptibility of a cell to injury in response to cigarette smoking. Such an imbalance of an array of redox-regulated antioxidant versus proinflammatory genes might therefore be associated with the susceptibility or tolerance to disease. It is possible that induction of antioxidant enzymes may provide initial adaptive or protective responses against oxidative stress and inflammatory mediators. However, during sustained/chronic inflammation, the balance between genes for inflammatory mediators and antioxidant/phase II enzymes may be tipped in favor of proinflammatory mediators (Fig. 6.4).

6.11 Chromatin Remodeling (Histone Acetylation and Deacetylation) and Glucocorticoid Inefficacy in Response to Smoking and in Patients with COPD

Tightly bound DNA around a nucleosome core (histone proteins) suppresses gene transcription by decreasing the accessibility of transcription factors, such as NF-κB and AP-1, to the transcriptional complex. A key regulator of gene transcription and expression is the balance of histone acetylases (or histone acetyltransferase [HAT]) and histone deacetylases (HDAC) (Rahman et al. 2004). The activity/expression of the two enzymes controls the access of the transcriptional machinery to bind to regulatory sites on DNA. Acetylation of core histones by HAT leads to a modification of chromatin structure

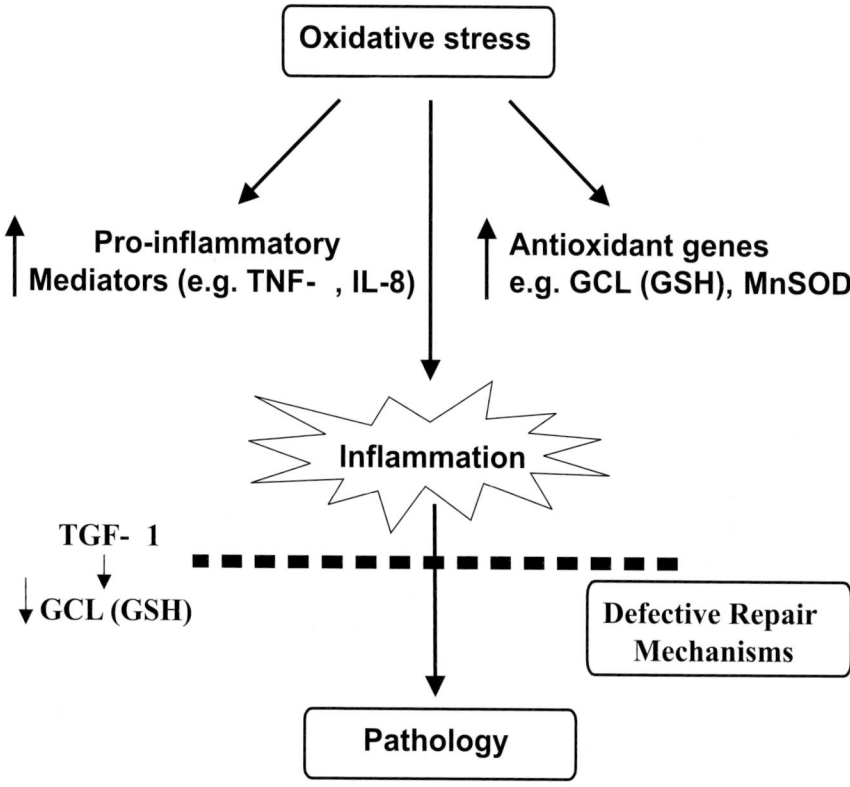

Fig. 6.4 Oxidative stress/cigarette smoke can cause increased gene expression of proinflammatory genes and also activation of protective genes, such as γ-glutamylcysteine synthetase/glutamate cysteine ligase. During sustained/chronic inflammation, the balance between genes for inflammatory mediators and antioxidant/phase II enzymes may be tipped in favor of proinflammatory mediators. It is possible that oxidative stress is enhanced during repair process by decreasing the glutathione (*GSH*) levels, leading to pathology

that affects transcription. Acetylation of lysine residues in the N-terminal tails of the core histone proteins results in uncoiling of the DNA, allowing increased accessibility for transcription factor binding. The acetylation status in turn depends on a balance of both HAT and HDAC. Exposure to cigarette smoke has been reported to alter chromatin remodeling by decreasing HDAC activity, resulting in increased transcription of proinflammatory genes in lungs of rats (Marwick et al. 2004). The above phenomena was linked to an increase in phosphorylated p38 MAPK in the lung concomitant with increased histone 3 phosphoacetylation, histone 4 acetylation, and elevated binding of NF-κB to the DNA, and AP-1. In addition, oxidative stress has also been shown to enhance acetylation of histone proteins and decrease histone deacetylase activity, leading to modulation of NF-κB activation, similar to the effect recorded with cigarette smoke (Moodie et al. 2004).

Ito and coworkers (2001) have shown a role for histone acetylation and deacetylation in IL-1β-induced TNF-α release in alveolar macrophages derived from cigarette smokers. They have also suggested that oxidants may play an important role in the modulation of HDAC and inflammatory cytokine gene transcription. Furthermore, we have shown that both cigarette smoke/H_2O_2 and TNF-α caused an increase in histone acetylation (HAT activity), leading to IL-8 expression in monocytes and alveolar epithelial cells (Rahman et al. 2002, 2004).

It has been suggested that oxidative stress may have a role in the poor efficacy of corticosteroids in COPD. Glucocorticoid suppression of inflammatory genes requires recruitment of HDAC-2 to the transcription activation complex by the glucocorticoid receptor (Ito et al. 2001). This results in deacetylation of histones and a decrease in inflammatory gene transcription. A reduced level of HDAC-2 was associated with increased proinflammatory response and reduced responsiveness to glucocorticoids in alveolar macrophages obtained from smokers (Ito et al. 2001). HDAC-2 has been shown to be modified posttranslationally by 4-HNE and NO/OONO$^-$ (Yang et al. 2006; Rahman et al. 2004). Culpitt and coworkers (2002) have shown that cigarette smoke solution stimulated release of IL-8 and granulocyte-macrophage colony-stimulating factor (GM-CSF), which was not inhibited by dexamethasone, in alveolar macrophages obtained from patients with COPD, compared with that of smokers. They suggested that the lack of efficacy of corticosteroids in COPD might be because of steroid insensitivity of macrophages in the respiratory tract. Thus, cigarette smoke/oxidant-mediated reduction in HDAC-2 levels in alveolar epithelial cells and macrophages will not only lead to an increase in inflammatory gene expression, but will also cause a decrease in glucocorticoid function in pa-

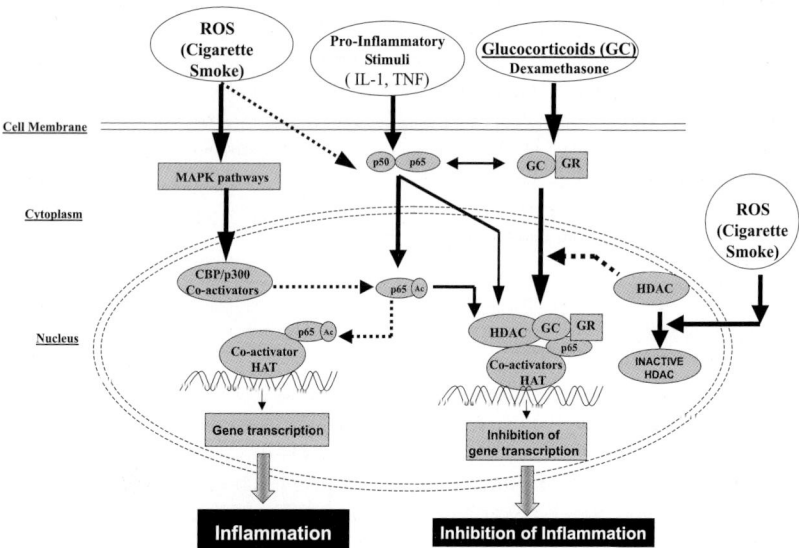

Fig. 6.5 Model illustrating the mechanism of corticosteroid (*GC*) action in suppressing proinflammatory gene expression and its impairment by oxidants. Direct interaction between coactivators histone acetyltransferase (HAT), histone deacetylase (*HDAC*), and the glucocorticoid receptor (*GR*), results in repression of proinflammatory gene expression. HDAC forms a bridge with HAT to inhibit gene transcription. The mitogen-activated protein kinase (*MAPK*) signaling pathways activated by oxidative stress can lead to p65 nuclear factor-kappaB (NF-κB) subunit and histone acetylation. Moreover, when HDAC is inhibited by oxidants/cigarette smoke or the p65 NF-κB subunit is acetylated, steroids may not be able to recruit HDACs into the transcriptional complex to inhibit proinflammatory gene expression

tients with COPD. (Yang et al. 2006) This may be one of the potential reasons for lack of effect of glucocorticoids in COPD (Fig. 6.5).

6.12 Genetic Polymorphisms as Markers of COPD

A genetic predisposition hypothesis has been suggested for COPD in view of the observations that approximately only 15–20% of smokers develop symptoms, and COPD is known to cluster in families. Although several candidate genes have been assessed, the data, however, often do not correlate, and more systematic studies are required to identify disease-associated genes. Understanding the genetic polymorphisms/mechanisms of susceptibility would provide an important insight into the pathogenesis of COPD (Sandford et al. 1997; Silverman and Speizer 1996). α1-AT deficiency has been widely studied as a genetic marker for COPD. Polymorphisms of various genes have been shown to be more prevalent in smokers who develop COPD (Barnes 1999). A number of these polymorphisms may have functional significance, such as the association between the TNF-α (*TNF2*) gene polymorphism, which is associated with increased TNF levels in response to inflammation, and the development of chronic bronchitis (Huang et al. 1997). Relevant to the effects of cigarette smoke is a polymorphism in the gene for microsomal epoxide hydrolase, an enzyme involved in the metabolism of highly reactive epoxide intermediates that are present in cigarette smoke (Smith and Harrison 1997). The proportion of individuals with slow microsomal epoxide hydrolase activity (homozygotes) was significantly higher in patients with COPD and a subgroup of patients shown pathologically to have emphysema (COPD 22%, emphysema 19%), compared with control subjects (6%) (Smith and Harrison 1997). These data have, however, not been reproduced in other patient populations (Yim et al. 2000). Genetic polymorphisms in matrix metalloproteinase genes *MMP1*, *MMP9*, and *MMP12* may also be important in the development of COPD. However, polymorphisms in the *MMP1* and *MMP12* genes, but not *MMP9*, appear to be related to smoking-related lung injury (Joos et al. 2002). They may also be in linkage disequilibrium with other causative polymorphisms (Sandford and Silverman 2002). An association between an *MMP9* polymorphism and the development of smoking-induced pulmonary emphysema was also reported in a population of Japanese smokers (Minematsu et al. 2001). Genetic polymorphism of antioxidant phase II detoxifying gene GSH *S*-transferase is associated with a decline in lung function in smokers (He et al. 2002). Variations in the levels of GSH and the genetic polymorphism of its synthesizing gene, *GCL*, and *HO-1* may represent new oxidative stress susceptibility factor in the pathogenesis in COPD (Cheng et al. 2004). It may be that a panel of "susceptibility" polymorphisms of functional significance in enzymes involved in xenobiotic metabolism or antioxidant enzyme genes may allow individuals to be identified as being susceptible to the effects of cigarette smoke. Nuclear factor erythroid 2-related factor 2 (Nrf2) is essential for the antioxidant-responsive element (ARE)-mediated induction of phase II detoxifying, *GCL* and *HO-1* genes in response to electrophiles present in cigarette smoke. Polymorphisms of GSH *S*-transferases (GSTs), *GCL*, and *HO-1* have been shown in smokers/patients with COPD. Recently, a genetic study has shown that *Nrf2*$^{-/-}$ mice were extremely susceptible to cigarette smoke and developed emphysema (Rangasamy et al. 2004). Hence, polymorphism of *Nrf2* may be present in susceptible smokers. Polymorphisms in the genes encoding for IL-11 (Klein et al. 2004), TGF-β1 (Wu et al. 2004), and the group-specific component of serum globulin (Ito et al. 2004) have been associated with genetic predisposition for COPD. However, some of the gene polymorphism studies could not be replicated among different populations, thus warranting future studies. In the present context and with the availability of the human genome sequence, whole genome screening in patients and unaffected siblings by single-nucleotide polymorphisms (SNPs) might prove to be a promising genetic approach to identify genes associated with COPD.

6.13 Models for Studying COPD

COPD is a complex disease involving several biomolecular, histological, and molecular abnormalities. A systematic approach to the understanding of these aspects is therefore essential to have in-depth knowledge of the disease. To date, three major experimental approaches have been adopted for the study of COPD. COPD was either induced by inhalation of cigarette smoke, noxious stimuli, tracheal instillation of tissue-degrading enzymes to induce emphysema-like lesions, or gene-modifications leading to a COPD-like phenotype (Gorenberg and Chung 2004). These approaches in isolation or in combination may also be applied. Ideally, a number of potential markers for COPD as identified by the GOLD guidelines should be present in animal models of COPD. Because the definition of COPD still relies on lung function measures, ideally, it would be prudent to have reproducible lung function measurements in experimental models (Kips et al. 2003). Measurement of lung function in very small mammals such as mice is difficult, and the use of enhanced pause (Penh) in conscious mice as an indicator of airflow obstruction is not ideal. Therefore, invasive methods remain the method of choice and should be correlated with inflammatory markers and cellular remodeling.

Tobacco smoke has been routinely used as a noxious stimulant to induce COPD in a wide variety of animals. In addition to rabbits, mice, dogs, and rats, guinea pigs—being very susceptible species—were therefore an animal of choice. Within a few months of exposure to active tobacco smoke, guinea pigs develop COPD-like lesions and emphysema-like airspace enlargement (Wright and Churg 1990). In contrast, rats seem to be more resistant to the induction of emphysema-like lesions.

The most favored laboratory animal species with regard to the study of inflammatory and immune mechanisms are mice. This preference is because of the ease of manipulation of gene expression. However, it is more difficult to assess lung function in these animals, and moreover, rodents (including rats) do not have well-developed small airways. Mice are known to tolerate at least two cigarettes daily for a year with minimal alterations in body weight and carboxyhemoglobin levels. Mice differ considerably in respiratory tract functions and anatomy from to humans. They are obligate nose breathers and have lower numbers of cilia, fewer Clara cells, and the submucosal glands are restricted to the trachea. However, emphysema (increased mean linear intercept) is seen in mice after 4 to 6 months of chronic cigarette smoke exposure (≥ 300 mg/m^3 total particulate matter). Mice exhibit lesser pulmonary filteration of tobacco smoke and cough reflex. Mice also respond differently to histamine or tachykinins. The development of emphysema-like lesions in mice is strain dependent (Guerassimove et al. 2004). Another widely employed model of COPD is rats. However, they appear to be relatively resistant to the induction of emphysema-like lesions. Morphometry and histopathologic studies show significant differences in development of emphysema in mice and rats (March et al. 1999). Studies on rats exposed to cigarette smoke have revealed resistance to corticosteroids (Marvick et al. 2004), akin to that in patients with COPD (Culpitt and Rogers 2000; Pauwels et al. 1999).

Tobacco smoke exposure has been generally used to induce COPD and features such as emphysema, airway remodeling, and chronic inflammation. The alterations still differ from the human situation. Many mediators involved in the pathology may have different functional effects, especially in the murine respiratory tract. However, these models still provide useful approaches to investigate cellular and molecular mechanisms underlying the pathogenesis of COPD. In view of the considerable interstrain and interspecies variations found in the models used so far, selection of a strain needs great caution. Animal models of COPD still need to be precisely evaluated as to their ability to mimic features of human COPD, and their limitations must be appreciated. Observations recorded from one or a combination of models may provide in-depth understanding of novel mechanisms involved in COPD.

6.14 Conclusions

Oxidative stress has important implications in several events of lung physiology and for the pathogenesis and progression of COPD. There is now a spate of evidence supporting the notion that increased generation of ROS in COPD is an important factor determining the onset of pathogenesis and severity of this condition. ROS may be critical in amplifying the normal inflammatory response to cigarette smoke/environmental oxidants (noxious agents), through upregulation of redox-sensitive transcription factors and hence, proinflammatory gene expression. They also exert protection against the effects of cigarette smoke via induction of antioxidant genes. Several markers of COPD like 4-HNE, MDA, TBARS, H_2O_2 and isoprostanes, have been identified for diagnosis and prognosis of the disease. The variation in their levels because of several factors has warranted more caution in their interpretation and therefore requires an in depth study. ROS can influence the response at many levels through its impact on signal transduction mechanisms, activation of redox-sensitive transcriptions factors, and chromatin regulation resulting in pro-inflammatory gene expression. It is this impact of ROS on chromatin regulation by reducing the activity of the transcriptional co-repressor, histone deacetylase-2 (HDAC-2), that leads to the poor efficacy of corticosteroids in COPD. Polymorphisms in genes such as *TNF-α, MMP-1, MMP-9, MMP-12, IL-11, GSTs*, GCL, *HO-1*, and microsomal epoxide hydrolase have been identified in COPD and other related conditions. However, vast variations in results obtained from population studies have hindered favorable attention for their use as genetic markers of COPD. Animal models of COPD still need to be precisely evaluated as to their ability to mimic features of human COPD, and their limitations must be appreciated. Various models such as rats, mice, guinea pigs, cell lines that are in vogue, and various agents such as gases, cigarette smoke, tracheal instillation, and proteases have been used to induce emphysema and COPD. The variations in susceptibility to different agents by different animals and cells have produced conflicting results. Therefore, observations recorded from one or a combination of models may provide in-depth understanding of novel mechanisms involved in COPD. Further understanding of the role of ROS in basic cellular functions and molecular mechanisms such as amplification of proinflammatory and immunological responses, defective repair mechanism, signaling pathways and apoptotic mechanisms will provide important information regarding basic pathological processes contributing to COPD.

Acknowledgements

This study was supported by the Environmental Health Sciences Center Support ES01247 and Philip Morris External Research Program, USA. The authors would like to thank Dr. Saibal Biswas and Dr. Aruna Kode for their help in preparing the manuscript.

References

Agusti AG, Sauleda J, Miralles C, Gomez C, Togores B, Sala E, Batle S, Busquets X (2002) Skeletal muscle apoptosis and weight loss in chronic obstructive pulmonary disease. Am J Respir Crit Care Med 166:485–489

Antonicelli F, Parmentier M, Rahman I, Drost E, Hirani N, Donaldson K, MacNee W (2002) Nacystelyn inhibits hydrogen peroxide mediated interleukin-8 expression in human alveolar epithelial cells. Free Radic Biol Med 32:492–502

Aoshiba K, Koinuma M, Yokohori N, Nagai A (2003a) Immunohistochemical evaluation of oxidative stress in murine lungs after cigarette smoke exposure. Inhal Toxicol 15:1029–1038

Aoshiba K, Yokohori N, Nagai A (2003b) Alveolar wall apoptosis causes lung destruction and emphysematous changes. Am J Respir Cell Mol Biol 28:555–562

Avissar N, Finkelstein JN, Horowitz S, Willey JC, Coy E, Frampton MW, Watkins RH, Khullar P, Xu YL, Cohen HJ (1996) Extracellular glutathione peroxidase in human lung epithelial lining fluid and in lung cells. Am J Physiol 270:L173–L182

Barnes PJ (1999) Genetics and pulmonary medicine. 9. Molecular genetics of chronic obstructive pulmonary disease. Thorax 54:245–252

Barnes PJ, Shapiro SD, Pauwels RA (2003) Chronic obstructive pulmonary disease: molecular and cellular mechanisms. Eur Respir J 22:672–688

Beeh KM, Beier J, Koppenhoefer N, Buhl R (2004) Increased glutathione disulfide and nitrosothiols in sputum supernatant of patients with stable COPD. Chest 126:1116–1122

Britton JR, Pavord ID, Richards KA, Knox AJ, Wisniewski AF, Lewis SA, Tattersfield AE, Weiss ST (1995) Dietary antioxidant vitamin intake and lung function in the general population. Am J Respir Crit Care Med 151:1383–1387

Cantin AM, North SL, Hubbard RC, Crystal RG (1987) Normal alveolar epithelial lung fluid contains high levels of glutathione. J Appl Physiol 63:152–157

Caramori G, Romagnoli M, Casolari P, Bellettato C, Casoni G, Boschetto P, Fan Chung K, Barnes PJ, Adcock IM, Ciaccia A, Fabbri LM, Papi A (2003) Nuclear localization of p65 in sputum macrophages but not in sputum neutrophils during COPD exacerbations. Thorax 58:348–351

Carnevali S, Petruzzelli S, Longoni B, Vanacore R, Barale R, Cipollini M, Scatena F, Paggiaro P, Celi A, Giuntini C (2003) Cigarette smoke extract induces oxidative stress and apoptosis in human lung fibroblasts. Am J Physiol 284:L955–L963

Carp H, Miller F, Hoidal JR, Janoff A (1982) Potential mechanisms of emphysema: ∞1-proteinase inhibitor recovered from lungs of cigarette smokers contains oxidised methionine and has decreased elastase inhibitory capacity. Proc Natl Acad Sci U S A 79:2041–2045

Celli BR, Cote CG, Marin JM, Casanova C, Montes de Oca M, Mendez RA, Pinto Plata V, Cabral HJ (2004) The body-mass index, airflow obstruction, dyspnea, and exercise capacity index in chronic obstructive pulmonary disease. N Engl J Med 350:1005–1012

Cheng SL, Yu CJ, Chen CJ, Yang PC (2004) Genetic polymorphism of epoxide hydrolase and glutathione S-transferase in COPD. Eur Respir J 23:818–824

Choi AM, Elbon CL, Bruce SA, Bassett DJ (1994) Messenger RNA levels of lung extracellular matrix proteins during ozone exposure. Lung 172:15–30

Chung KF (2001) Cytokines in chronic obstructive pulmonary disease. Eur Respir J 34:S50–S59

Church T, Pryor WA (1985) Free radical chemistry of cigarette smoke and its toxicological implications. Environ Health Perspect 64:111–126

Corradi M, Rubinstein I, Andreoli Rl, Manini P, Caglieri A, Poli D, Alinovi R, Mutti A (2003) Aldehydes in exhaled breath condensate of patients with chronic obstructive pulmonary disease. Am J Respir Crit Care Med 1671380–1386

Cross CE, van der Vliet A, O'Neill CA, Louie S, Halliwell B (1994) Oxidants, antioxidants, and respiratory tract lining fluids. Environ Health Perspect 102:185–191

Culpitt SV, Rogers DF (2000) Evaluation of current pharmacotherapy of chronic obstructive pulmonary disease. Expert Opin Pharmacother 1:1007–1020

Culpitt SV, Rogers DF, Shah P, De Matos C, Russel RE, Donnelly LE, Barnes PJ (2002) Impaired inhibition by dexamethasone of cytokine release by alveolar macrophages from COPD patients. Am J Respir Crit Care Med 167:24–31

Dentener MA, Vernooy JH, Hendriks S, Wouters EF (2005) Enhanced levels of hyaluronan in lungs patients with COPD: relationship with lung function and local inflammation. Thorax 60:114–119

Di Stefano A, Caramori G, Oates T, Capelli A, Lusuardi M, Gnemmi I, Ioli F, Chung KF, Donner CF, Barnes PJ, Adcock IM (2002) Increased expression of nuclear factor-κB in bronchial biopsies from smokers and patients with COPD. Eur Respir J 20:556–563

Eiserich JP, van der Vliet A, Handelman GJ, Halliwell B, Cross CE (1995) Dietary antioxidants and cigarette smoke-induced biomolecular damage: a complex interaction. Am J Clin Nutr 62: S1490–S1500

Engelen MP, Schols AM, Does JD, Deutz NE, Wouters EF (2000) Altered glutamate metabolism is associated with reduced muscle glutathione levels in patients with emphysema. Am J Respir Crit Care Med 161:98–103

Fahn H, Wang L, Kao S, Chang S, Huang M, Wei Y (1998) Smoking-associated mitochondrial DNA mutation and lipid peroxidation in human lung tissue. Am J Respir Cell Mol Biol 19:901–909

Fischer BM, Voynow JA (2002) Neutrophil elastase induces *MUC5AC* gene expression in airway epithelium via a pathway involving reactive oxygen species. Am J Respir Cell Mol Biol 26:447–452

Gadek J, Fells GA, Crystal RG (1979) Cigarette smoking induces functional antiprotease deficiency in the lower respiratory tract of humans. Science 206:1315–1316

Gensch E, Gallup M, Sucher A, Li D, Gebremichael A, Lemjabbar H, Mengistab A, Dasari V, Hotchkiss J, Harkema J, Basbaum C (2004) Tobacco smoke control of mucin production in lung cells requires oxygen radicals AP-1 and JNK. J Biol Chem 279:39085–39093

Gerritsen WB, Asin J, Zanen P, van den Bosch JM, Haas FJ (2005) Markers of inflammation and oxidative stress in exacerbated chronic obstructive pulmonary disease patients. Respir Med 99:84–90

Gompertz S, Bayley DL, Hill SL, Stockley RA (2001) Relationship between airway inflammation and the frequency of exacerbations in patients with smoking related COPD. Thorax 56:36–41

Grievink L, Smit HA, Ocke MC, van't Veer P, Kromhout D (1998) Dietary intake of antioxidant (pro)-vitamins, respiratory symptoms and pulmonary function: the MORGEN study. Thorax 53:166–171

Groneberg DA, Chung KF (2004) Models of chronic obstructive pulmonary disease. BMC Respir Res 5:18

Guerassimov A, Hoshino Y, Takubo Y, Turcotte A, Yamamoto M, Ghezzo H, Triantafillopoulos A, Whittaker K, Hoidal JR, Cosio MG (2004) The development of emphysema in cigarette smoke-exposed mice is strain dependent. Am J Respir Crit Care Med 170:974–980

Harju T, Kaarteenaho-Wiik R, Soini Y, Sormunen R, Kunnula VL (2002) Diminished immunoreactivity of gamma-glutamylcysteine synthetase in the airways of smokers' lungs. Am J Respir Crit Care Med 166:754–759

Hautamaki RD, Kobayashi DK, Senior RM, Shapiro SD (1997) Requirement for macrophage elastase for cigarette smoke-induced emphysema in mice. Science 277:2002–2004

He JQ, Juan J, Connett JE, Anthonisen NR, Pare PD, Sandford AJ (2002). Antioxidant gene polymorphisms and susceptibility to a rapid decline in lung function smokers. Am J Respir Crit Care Med 166:323–328

Heunks LM, Dekhuijzen PN (2000) Respiratory muscle function and free radicals: from cell to COPD. Thorax 55:704–716

Hogg JC, Chu F, Utokaparch S, Woods R, Elliott WM, Buzatu L, Cherniack RM, Rogers RM, Sciurba FC, Coxson HO, Pare PD (2004) The nature of small-airway obstruction in chronic obstructive pulmonary disease. N Engl J Med 350:2645–2653

Hoshino S, Yoshida M, Inoue K, Yano Y, Yanagita M, Mawatari H, Yamane H, Kijima T, Kumagai T, Osaki T, Tachiba I, Kawase I (2005) Cigarette smoke extract induces endothelial cell injury via JNK pathway. Biochem Biophys Res Commun 329:58–63

Hoshino Y, Mio T, Nagai S, Miki H, Ito I, Izumi T (2001) Cytotoxic effects of cigarette smoke extract on an alveolar type II cell-derived cell line. Am J Physiol 281:L509–L516

Huang S-L, Su C-H, Chang S-C (1997) Tumour necrosis factor-α gene polymorphism in chronic bronchitis. Am J Respir Crit Care Med 156:1436–1439

Hunninghake GW, Crystal RG (1983) Cigarette smoking and lung destruction. Accumulation of neutrophils in the lungs of cigarette smokers. Am Rev Respir Dis 128:833–838

Ichinose M, Sugiura H, Yamagata S, Koarai A, Shirato K (2000) Increase in reactive nitrogen species production in chronic obstructive pulmonary disease airways. Am J Respir Crit Care Med 162:701–706

Ishii T, Matsuse T, Igarashi H, Masuda M, Teramoto S, Ouchi Y (2001) Tobacco smoke reduces viability in human lung fibroblasts: protective effect of glutathione S-transferase P1. Am J Physiol 280:L1189–L1195

Ito I, Nagai S, Hoshino Y, Muro S, Hirai T, Tsukino M, Mishima M (2004) Risk and severity of COPD is associated with the group-specific component of serum globulin 1F allele. Chest 125:63–70

Ito K, Lim G, Caramori G, Chung KF, Barnes PJ and Adcock IM (2001) Cigarette smoking reduces histone deacetylase 2 expression, enhances cytokine expression, and inhibits glucocorticoid actions in alveolar macrophages. FASEB J 15:1110–1112

Jardine H, MacNee W, Donaldson K, Rahman I (2002) Molecular mechanism of TGF-β_1-induced glutathione depletion in alveolar epithelial cells involvement of AP-1/ARE and Fra-1. J Biol Chem 277:21158–21166

Joos L, He JQ, Shepherdson MB, Connette JE, Nichonson R, Anothonisen P, Pare PD, Sandford AJ (2002) The role of matrix metalloproteinase polymorphisms in the rate of decline in lung function. Human Mol Genetics 211:569–678

Kanazawa H, Shiraishi S, Hirata K, Yoshikawa J (2003) Imbalance between levels of nitrogen oxides and peroxynitrite inihibitory activity in chronic obstructive pulmonary disease. Thorax 58:106–109

Karnenburg AR, de Boer WI, Alagappan VK, Sterk PJ, Sharma HS (2005) Enhanced bronchial expression of vascular endothelial growth factors and receptors (Flk-1 and Flt-1) in patients with chronic obstructive pulmonary disease. Thorax 60:106–113

Kasahara Y, Tuder RM, Cool CD, Lynch DA, Flores SC, Voelkel NF (2001) Endothelial cell death and decreased expression of vascular endothelial growth factor and vascular endothelial growth factor receptor 2 in emphysema. Am J Respir Crit Care Med 163:737–744

Kasahara Y, Tuder RM, Taraseviciene-Stewart L, Le Cras TD, Abman S, Hirth PK, Waltenberger J, Voelkel NF (2000) Inhibition of VEGF receptors causes lung cell apoptosis and emphysema. J Clin Invest 106:1311–1319

Keatings VM, Collins PD, Scott DM, Barnes PJ (1996) Differences in interleukin-8 and tumor necrosis factor-alpha in induced sputum from patients with chronic obstructive pulmonary disease or asthma. Am J Respir Crit Care Med 153:530–534

Kharitonov SA, Barnes PJ (2001) Exhaled markers of pulmonary disease. Am J Respir Crit Care Med 163:1693–1722

Kips JC, Anderson GP, Fredberg JJ, Herz U, Inman MD, Jordana M, Kemeny DM, Lotvall J, Pauwels RA, Plopper CG, Schmidt D, Sterk PJ, Van Oosterhout AJ, Vargaftig BB, Chung KF (2003) Murine models of asthma. Eur Respir J 22:374–382

Kirkham PA, Spooner G, Foulkes-Jones C, Calvez, R (2003) Cigarette smoke triggers macrophage adhesion and activation: role of lipid peroxidation products and scavenger receptor. Free Radic Biol Med 35:697–710

Kirkham PA, Spooner G, Rahman I, Rossi AG (2004) Macrophage phagocytosis of apoptotic neutrophils is compromised by matrix proteins modified by cigarette smoke and lipid peroxidation products. Biochem Biophys Res Commun 318:32–37

Klein W, Rohde G, Arinir U, Hagedorn M, Durig N, Schultze-Werninghaus G, Epplen JT (2004) A promotor polymorphism in the Interleukin 11 gene is associated with chronic obstructive pulmonary disease. Electrophoresis 25:804–808

Lapenna, D, Gioia SD, Mezzetti A, Ciofani G, Consoli A, Marzio L, Cuccurullo F (1995) Cigarette smoke, ferritin, and lipid peroxidation. Am J Respir Crit Care Med 151:431–435

Maestrelli P, Messlemani AHE, Fina OD, Nowicki Y, Saetta M, Mapp C, Fabbri LM (2001) Increased expression of heme oxygenase (HO)-1 in alveolar spaces and HO-2 in alveolar walls of smokers. Am J Respir Crit Care Med 164:1508–1513

March TH, Barr EB, Finch GL, Hahn FF, Hobbs CH, Menache MG, Nikula KJ (1999) Cigarette smoke exposure produces more evidence of emphysema in B6C3F1 mice than in F344 rats. Toxicol Sci 51:289–299

Marwick JA, Kirkham PA, Stevenson CS, Danahay H, Giddings J, Butler K, Donaldson K, MacNee W, Rahman I (2004) Cigarette smoke alters chromatin remodelling and induces pro-inflammatory genes in rat lungs. Am J Respir Cell Mol Biol 31:633–642

Marwick JA, Giddings J, Butler K, MacNee W, Rahman I, Kirkham P (2006) Cigarette smoke disrupts the $VEGF_{165}$-KDR receptor signalling complex in rat lungs and patients with COPD: morphological impact of specific KDR inhibition. Am. J. Physiology: Lung Cell Mol Physiol 290:L897–908.

Mezzetti A, Lapenna D, Pierdomenico SD, Calafiore AM, Costantini F, Riario-Sforza G, Imbastaro T, Neri M, Cuccurullo F (1995) Vitamins E, C and lipid peroxidation in plasma and arterial tissue of smokers and non-smokers. Atherosclerosis 112:91–99

Minematsu N, Nakamura H, Tateno H, Nakajima T, Yamaguchi K (2001) Genetic polymorphism in matrix metalloproteinase-9 and pulmonary emphysema. Biochem Biophys Res Commun 289:116–119

Mio T, Romberger DJ, Thompson AB, Robbins RA, Heires A, Rennard SI (1997) Cigarette smoke induces interleukin-8 release from human bronchial epithelial cells. Am J Respir Crit Care Med 155:1770–1776

Mochida-Nishimura K, Sureweicz K, Cross JV, Hejal R, Templeton D, Rich EA, Toossi Z (2001) Differential activation of MAP kinase signaling pathways and nuclear factor-kappaB in bronchoalveolar cells of smokers and non-smokers. Mol Med 7:177–185

Montuschi P, Collins JV, Ciabattoni G, Lazzeri N, Corradi M, Kharitonov SA, Barnes PJ (2000) Exhaled 8-isoprostane as an in vivo biomarker of lung oxidative stress in patients with COPD and healthy smokers. Am J Respir Crit Care Med 162:1175–1177

Moodie FM, Marwick JA, Anderson CS, Szulakowski P, Biswas SK, Bauter MR, Kilty I, Rahman I (2004) Oxidative stress and cigarette smoke alter chromatin remodeling but differentially regulate NF-kappaB activation and proinflammatory cytokine release in alveolar epithelial cells. FASEB J 18:1897–1899

Morrison D, Rahman I, Lannan S, MacNee W (1999) Epithelial permeability, inflammation and oxidant stress in the airspaces of smokers. Am J Respir Crit Care Med 15473–479

Mullick AE, McDonald JM, Melkonian G, Talbot P, Pinkerton KE and Rutledge JC (2002) Reactive carbonyls from tobacco smoke increase arterial endothelial layer injury. Am J Physiol 283:H591–H597

Nakayama T, Church DF, Pryor WA (1989) Quantitative analysis of the hydrogen peroxide formed in aqueous cigarette tar extracts. Free Radical Biol Med 7:9–15

Neurohr C, Lenz A-G, Ding I, Leuchte H, Kolbe T, Behr J (2003) Glutamate-cysteine ligase modulatory subunit in BAL alveolar macrophages of healthy smokers. Eur Respir J 22:82–87

Noguera A, Busquets X, Sauleda J, Villaverde JM, MacNee W, Agusti AG (1998) Expression of adhesion molecules and G-proteins in circulating neutrophils in COPD. Am J Respir Crit Care Med 158:1664–1668

Nowak D, Kasielski M, Antczak A, Pietras T, Bialasiewicz P (1999) Increased content of thiobarbituric acid reactive substances in hydrogen peroxide in the expired breath condensate of patients with stable chronic obstructive pulmonary disease: no significant effect of cigarette smoking. Respir Med 93:389–396

Parfrey H, Mahadeva R, Lomas DA (2003) Alpha(1)-antitrypsin deficiency, liver disease and emphysema. Int J Biochem Cell Biol 351009–1014

Parmentier M, Hirani N, Rahman I, Donaldson K, Antonicelli F (2000) Regulation of lipopolysaccharide-mediated interleukin-1beta release by N-acetylcysteine in THP-1 cells. Eur Respir J 16:933–939

Patel IS, Roberts NJ, Lloyd-Owen SJ, Sapsford RJ, Wedzicha JA (2003) Airway epithelial inflammatory responses and clinical parameters in COPD. Eur Respir J 22:94–99

Pauwels RA, Buist S, Claverley PMA, Jenkins CR, Hurd SS (2001) Global strategy for the diagnosis, management and prevention of chronic obstructive pulmonary disease. Am J Respir Crit Care Med 163:1256–1276

Pauwels RA, Lofdahl CG, Laitinen LA, Schouten JP, Postma DS, Pride NB, Ohlsson SV (1999) Long-term treatment with inhaled budesonide in persons with mild chronic obstructive pulmonary disease who continue smoking. N Engl J Med 340:1948–1953

Petruzzelli S, Puntoni R, Mimotti P, Pulera N, Baliva F, Fornai E, Giuntini C (1997) Plasma 3-nitrotyrosine in cigarette smokers. Am J Respir Crit Care Med 156:1902–1907

Pinamonti S, Leis M, Barbieri A, Leoni D, Muzzoli M, Sostero S, Chicca MC, Carrieri A, Ravenna F, Fabbri LM, Ciaccia A (1998) Detection of xanthine oxidase activity products by EPR and HPLC in bronchoalveolar lavage fluid from patients with chronic obstructive pulmonary disease. Free Radic Biol Med 25:771–779

Prause O, Bozinovski S, Anderson GA, Linden A (2004) Increased matrix metalloproteinase-9 concentration and activity after stimulation with interleukin-17 in mouse airways. Thorax 59:313–317

Rabinovich RA, Ardite E, Trooster T, Carbo N, Alonso J, Gonzalex de Suso JM, Vilaro J, Barbera JA, Polo MF, Argiles JM, Fernandez-Checa JC, Roca J (2001) Reduced muscle redox capacity after endurance training in patients with chronic obstructive pulmonary disease. Am J Respir Crit Care Med 164:1114–1118

Rahman I (2004) Reproducibility of oxidative stress biomarkers in breath condensate: are they reliable? Eur Respir J 23:183–184

Rahman I, Kelly F (2003) Biomarkers in breath condensate: a promising new non-invasive technique in free radical research. Free Radic Res 37:1253–1266

Rahman I, Antonicelli F, MacNee W (1999) Molecular mechanisms of the regulation of glutathione synthesis by tumour necrosis factor-α and dexamethasone in human alveolar epithelial cells. J Biol Chem 274:5088–5096

Rahman I, Biswas SK (2004) Non-invasive breath condensate biomarkers of oxidative stress: reproducibility and methological issues. Redox Report 9:125–143

Rahman I, Biswas SK, Jimenez LA, Torres M, Forman HJ (2005) Glutathione, stress responses and redox signaling in lung inflammation. Antioxid Redox Signal 7:42–59

Rahman I, Gilmour PS, Jimenez LA, MacNee W (2002) Oxidative stress and TNF-alpha induce histone acetylation and NF-kappaB/AP-1 activation in alveolar epithelial cells: potential mechanism in gene transcription in lung inflammation. Mol Cell Biochem 234/235:239–248

Rahman I, Li XY, Donaldson K, Harrison DJ, MacNee W (1995) Glutathione homeostasis in alveolar epithelial cells in vitro and lung in vivo under oxidative stress. Am J Physiol 269:L285–L292

Rahman I, MacNee W (1996) Role of oxidants/antioxidants in smoking-induced airways diseases. Free Radic Biol Med 21:669–681

Rahman I, MacNee W (1998) Role of transcription factors in inflammatory lung diseases. Thorax 53:601–612

Rahman I, MacNee W (1999) Lung glutathione and oxidative stress: Implications in cigarette smoke-induced airways disease. Am J Physiol 277:L1067–L1088

Rahman I, MacNee W (2000) Oxidative stress and regulation of glutathione synthesis in lung inflammation. Eur Respir J 16:534–554

Rahman I, Marwick JA, Kirkham PA (2004) Redox modulation of chromatin remodeling: impact on histone acetylation and deacetylation, NF-kappaB and pro-inflammatory gene expression. Biochem Pharmacol 68:1255–1267

Rahman I, Morrison D, Donaldson K, MacNee W (1996) Systemic oxidative stress in asthma, COPD, and smokers. Am J Respir Crit Care Med 154:1055–1060

Rahman I, Skwarska E, MacNee W (1997) Attenuation of oxidant/antioxidant imbalance during treatment of exacerbations of chronic obstructive pulmonary disease. Thorax 52:565–568

Rahman I, Van Schadewijk AA, Crowther A, Hiemstra PS, Stolk J, MacNee W, De Boer WI (2002) 4-Hydroxy-2-nonenal, a specific lipid peroxidation product, is elevated in lungs of patients with chronic obstructive pulmonary disease (COPD). Am J Respir Crit Care Med 166:490–495

Rangasamy T, Cho CY, Thimmulappa RK, Zhen L, Srisuma SS, Kensler TW, Yamamoto M, Petrache I, Tuder RM, Biswal S (2004) Genetic ablation of Nrf2 enhances susceptibility to cigarette smoke-induced emphysema in mice. J Clin Invest 114:1248–259

Ribera F, N'Guessan B, Zoll J, Fortin D, Serrurier B, Mettauer B, Bigard X, Ventura-Clapier R, Lampert E (2003) Mitochondrial electron transport chain function is enhanced in inspiratory muscles of patients with chronic obstructive pulmonary disease. Am J Respir Crit Care Med 167:873–879

Russell REK, Culpitt SV, DeMatos C, Donnelly L, Smith M, Wiggins J, Barnes PJ (2002) Release and activity of matrix metalloproteinase-9 and tissue inhibitor of matalloproteinase-2 by alveolar macrophages from patients with COPD. Am J Respir Cell Mol Biol 26:602–609

Rusznak C, Mills PR, Devalia JL, Sapsford RJ, Davies RJ, Lozewicz S (2000) Effect of cigarette smoke on the permeability and IL-1beta and sICAM-1 release from cultured human bronchial epithelial cells of never-smokers, smokers, and patients with chronic obstructive pulmonary disease. Am J Respir Cell Mol Biol 23:530–536

Sadowska AM, van Overveld FJ, Gorecka D, Zdral A, Filewska M, Demkow UA, Luyten C, Saenen E, Zielinski J, De Backer WA (2005) The interrelationship between markers of inflammation and oxidative stress in chronic obstructive pulmonary disease: modulation by inhaled steroids and antioxidant. Respir Med 99:241–249

Saitoh M, Nishitoh H, Fujii M, Takeda K, Tobiume K, Sawada Y, Kawabata M, Miyazono K, Ichijo H (1998) Mammalian thioredoxin is a direct inhibitor of apoptosis signal-regulating kinase (ASK) 1. EMBO J 17:2596–2606

Sandford AJ, Silverman EK (2002) Chronic obstructive pulmonary disease. 1: Susceptibility factors for COPD the genotype-environment interaction. Thorax 57:736–741

Sandford AJ, Weir TD, Pare PD (1997) Genetic risk factors for chronic obstructive pulmonary disease. Eur Respir J 10:1380–1391

Santus P, Sola A, Carlucci P, Fumagalli F, Di Gennaro A, Mondoni M, Carnini C, Centanni S, Sala (2004) Lipid peroxidation and 5-lipoxygenase activity in chronic obstructive pulmonary disease subjects. Am J Respir Crit Care Med 171:838–843

Sargeant LA, Jaeckel A, Wareham NJ (2000) Interaction of vitamin C with the relation between smoking and obstructive airways disease in EPIC Norfolk. European Prospective Investigation into Cancer and Nutrition. Eur Respir J 16:397–403

Schunemann HJ, Muti P, Freudenheim JL, Armstrong D, Browne R, Klocke RA, Trevisan M (1997) Oxidative stress and lung function. Am J Epidemiol 146:939–948

Shahar E, Boland LL, Folsom AR, Tockman MS, McGovern PG, Eckfeldt JH (1999) Docosahexaenoic acid and smoking related chronic obstructive pulmonary disease. Atherosclerosis Risk in Communities Study Investigators. Am J Respir Crit Care Med 159:1780–1785

Shapiro SD (2003) Proteolysis in the lung. Eur Respir J 44:S30–S32

Shapiro SD, Goldstein NM, Houghton AMG, Kobayashi DK, Kelley D, Belaaouaj A (2003) Neutrophil elastase contributes to cigarette smoke-induced emphysema in mice. Am J Pathol 163:2329–2335

Shen Y, Rattan V, Sultana C, Kalra VK (1996) Cigarette smoke condensate-induced adhesion molecule expression and transendothelial migration of monocytes. Am J Physiol 39:H1624–H1633

Silverman EK, Speizer FE (1996) Risk factors for the development of chronic obstructive pulmonary disease. Med Clin North Am 80:501–522

Smith CAD, Harrison DJ (1997) Association between polymorphism in gene for microsomal epoxide hydrolase and susceptibility to emphysema. Lancet 350:630–633

Stanescu D, Sanna A, Veriter C, Kostianev S, Calcagni PG, Fabbri LM, Maestrelli P (1996) Airways obstruction, chronic expectoration, and rapid decline of FEV1 in smokers are associated with increased levels of sputum neutrophils. Thorax 51:267–271

Stockley RA (2002) Neutrophils and the pathogenesis of COPD. Chest 121:S151-S155

Takeyama K, Jung B, Shim JJ, Burgel PR, Dao-Pick T, Ueki IF, Protin U, Kroschel P, Nadel JA (2001) Activation of epidermal growth factor receptors is responsible for mucin synthesis induced by cigarette smoke. Am J Physiol 280:L165–L172

Tsuji T, Aoshiba K, Nagai A (2004) Cigarette smoke induces senescence in alveolar epithelial cells. Am J Respir Cell Mol Biol 31:643–649

Tsukagoshi H, Kawata T, Shimizu Y, Ishizuka T, Dobashi K, Mori M (2002) 4-Hydroxy-2-nonenal enhances fibronectin production by IMR-90 human lung fibroblast party via activation of epidermal growth factor receptor-linked extracellular signal-regulated kinase p44/42 pathway. Toxicol Appl Pharmacol 184:127–135

Tuder RM, Zhen L, Cho CY, Taraseviciene-Stewart L, Kasahara Y, Salvemini D, Voelkel NF, Flores SC (2003) Oxidative stress and apoptosis interact and cause emphysema due to vascular endothelial growth factor receptor blockade. Am J Respir Cell Mol Biol 29:88–97

Uchida K, Shiraishi M, Naito Y, Torii N, Nakamura Y, Osawa T (1999) Activation of stress signaling pathways by the end product of lipid peroxidation. J Biol Chem 274:2234–2242

Vayssier M, Favatier F, Pinot F, Bachelet M, Poll BS (1998) Tobacco smoke induces coordinate activation of HSF and inhibition of NFkappaB in human monocytes: effects on TNFalpha release. Biochem Biophys Res Commun 252:249–256

Wang J, Wilcken DE, Wang X L (2001) Cigarette smoke activates caspase-3 to induce apoptosis of human umbilical venous endothelial cells. Mol Genet Metab 72:82–88

Wang RD, Tai H, Xie C, Wang X, Wright JL and Churg A (2003) Cigarette smoke produces airway wall remodelling in rat tracheal explants. Am J Respir Cell Mol Biol 168:1232–1236

Wickenden JA, Clarke MC, Rossi AG, Rahman I, Faux SP, Donaldson K, MacNee W (2003) Cigarette smoke prevents apoptosis through inhibition of caspase activation and induces necrosis. Am J Respir Cell Mol Biol 29:562–570

Witherden IR, Bon EJV, Goldstraw P, Ratcliffe C, Pastorino U, Tetley TD (2004) Primary human alveolar type II epithelial cell chemokine release: Effects of cigarette smoke and neutrophil elastase. Am J Respir Cell Mol Biol 30:500–509

Wright JL, Churg A (1990) Cigarette smoke causes physiologic and morphologic changes of emphysema in the guinea pig. Am Rev Respir Dis 142:1422–1428

Wu L, Chau J, Young RP, Pokorny V, Mills GD, Hopkins R, McLean L, Black PN (2004) Transforming growth factor-beta1 genotype and susceptibility to chronic obstructive pulmonary disease. Thorax 59:126–129

Yang SR, Chida AS, Bauter MR, Shafiq S, Seweryniak K, Maggirwar SB, Kilty I, Rahman (2006) Cigarette smoke induces pro-inflammatory cytokine realease by activation of NF-κB and post-translational modifications of histone deacetylase in macrophages. Am. J. Physiology: Lung Cell Mol Biol. (Epubmed ahead of print).

Yim JJ, Park GY, Lee CT, Kim YW, Han Sk, Shim YS, Yoo CG (2000) Genetic susceptibility to chronic obstructive pulmonary disease in Koreans: combined analysis of polymorphic genotypes for microsomal epoxide hydrolase and glutathione S-transferase M1 and T1. Thorax 55:121125

Chapter 7

Modulation of Cigarette Smoke Effects by Diet and Antioxidants

Marion Dietrich and Gladys Block

Contents

7.1	Introduction	200
7.2	Observational Studies: Modulation of Cigarette Smoking-Related Chronic Diseases by Dietary Antioxidants	201
7.2.1	Lung Cancer	201
7.2.2	Cardiovascular Diseases	202
7.3	Primary Prevention Studies: Modulation of Cigarette Smoking-Related Chronic Diseases by Antioxidant Supplements	203
7.3.1	Lung Cancer and Cardiovascular Diseases	203
7.4	Biomarker Studies: Modulation of Cigarette Smoking-Related Oxidative Stress by Antioxidant Supplements	204
7.4.1	Vitamin C	204
7.4.2.	Vitamin E	207
7.4.3	Combinations of Antioxidants	207
7.5	Summary	208
7.6	Conclusion	209
	References	209

7.1 Introduction

Cigarette smokers as well as passive smokers are exposed to reactive free radicals present in cigarette smoke (Bermudez et al. 1994; Pryor and Stone 1993). Free radicals can cause oxidative damage to DNA, proteins, and lipids and may be involved in the development of chronic diseases like atherosclerosis and cancer (Diplock et al. 1998; Frei et al. 1991; Pryor 1986, 1987). In vitro studies have shown that antioxidants (AO) such as vitamin C, vitamin E, carotenoids, and thiols ameliorate free radical-induced oxidative damage (Burton et al. 1983; Frei et al. 1989, 1991; Pryor 1984; Khanna et al. 1999; Lykkesfeldt et al. 2000). There is evidence from epidemiological studies that persons who consume a diet rich in fruits and vegetables have a lower risk of cancer, cardiovascular diseases, and other diseases (Block et al. 1991, 1992). Because fruits and vegetables are major sources of antioxidants (as well as other factors), it has been hypothesized that antioxidants in fruits and vegetables are the protective compounds or major components of the protective effect (Diplock et al. 1998).

In vitro studies have shown that free radicals in cigarette smoke (CS) deplete certain plasma antioxidants (Frei et al. 1991; Eiserich et al. 1995). A number of studies have found lower plasma antioxidant levels in smokers in vivo (Jarvinen et al. 1994; Lykkesfeldt et al. 2000; Marangon et al. 1998; Norkus et al. 1987; Ross et al. 1995; Schectman et al. 1989; Stryker et al. 1988). Some information is available on the effect of CS exposure on plasma antioxidant concentrations in passive smokers (Alberg et al. 2000; Ayaori et al. 2000; Farchi et al. 2001; Tribble et al. 1993; Valkonen and Kuusi 1998; Dietrich et al. 2003b).

Antioxidant intervention trials in smokers and passive smokers have been conducted to investigate whether antioxidant supplementation can decrease biomarkers of oxidative stress (Davi et al. 1997, 1997; Gokce et al. 1999; Patrignani et al. 2000; Reilly et al. 1996; Dietrich et al. 2002; Dietrich et al. 2003a). Numerous biomarkers for oxidative damage have been used, including biomarkers for DNA damage and for alterations in proteins and lipids (Dean et al. 1997; Roberts and Morrow 2000; Shigenaga et al. 1989). One such biomarker is the F_2-isoprostanes (F_2-IsoPs), which are products of free radical-catalyzed lipid peroxidation of arachidonic acid (Morrow et al. 1990). They are formed in situ, esterified to phospholipids, and subsequently released by phospholipases into the plasma where they can be measured (Morrow et al. 1992). They can also be measured in urine. Increased F_2-IsoP levels in urine or plasma have been found in patients with atherosclerosis (Belton et al. 2000), severe heart failure (Cracowski et al. 2000), diabetes (Mezzetti et al. 2000), Alzheimer's disease (Pratico et al. 2000), as well as in smokers (Morrow et al. 1995; Obata et al. 2000).

This chapter reviews literature on the association between dietary antioxidant intake and chronic disease risks, as well as literature on antioxidant supplementation studies using lipid peroxidation biomarkers as indices for oxidative stress, in smokers, and if available, also in passive smokers.

7.2 Observational Studies: Modulation of Cigarette Smoking-Related Chronic Diseases by Dietary Antioxidants

7.2.1 Lung Cancer

Cigarette smoking is the primary cause of lung cancer. Observational studies have consistently shown an inverse association between fruit and vegetable intake and lung cancer risk (Ziegler et al. 1996). A large review of approximately 200 epidemiological case-control and prospective studies on fruit and vegetable intake and cancer prevention that included studies on lung cancer found significant protection of fruit and vegetable consumption in 24 of 25 studies after controlling for smoking (Block et al. 1992). In 1998, the International Agency of Research on Cancer (IARC) reviewed more than 20 case-control studies and reported that the majority of these studies found strong inverse trends in lung cancer risk with high fruit and vegetable intake (Vainio and Rautalahti 1998). Findings from the European Prospective Investigation into Cancer and Nutrition Study (EPIC Study) on the association of fruit and vegetable intake and lung cancer risk have recently been published (Miller et al. 2004). More than 500,000 individuals from ten European countries participated in the EPIC Study, and 478,021 were included in the analysis on fruit and vegetable intake and lung cancer risk. After adjustment for age, smoking, height, weight, and gender, there was a significant inverse association between fruit consumption and lung cancer risk (hazard ratio for the highest quintile of consumption relative to the lowest 0.60 [95% confidence interval {CI} = 0.46–0.78], p-value for trend = 0.0099). No association between vegetable consumption and lung cancer risk was observed.

Analyses from two reports on pooled analyses of seven or eight large prospective cohort studies including never, past, and current smokers, carried out in North America and Europe have recently been published. One of the analyses focused on fruit and vegetable intake and lung cancer risk (Smith-Warner et al. 2003); the other analysis focused on dietary carotenoid intake and lung cancer risk (Mannistoe et al. 2004). The results from the first study conducted by Smith-Warner et al. suggest that elevated fruit and vegetable consumption is associated with a modest reduction in lung cancer risk, mostly attributable to fruit, not vegetable, intake. When adjusted for smoking status and other lung cancer risk factors, a 21% lower risk of lung cancer was observed among men and women with higher intakes of total fruits and vegetables. Pooling these large cohort studies allowed the authors to analyze the data by smoking status. Among current smokers, a significant 16% lower risk was observed for comparison of the highest versus the lowest quartile of total fruit and vegetable consumption (0.84 [0.71–0.98, relative risk {RR} {95% CI}]; p-value = 0.03 [test for trend]).

The second study analyzing the same prospective cohort studies (Mannistoe et al. 2004) focused on dietary carotenoid intake and lung cancer risk. Carotenoids are fat-soluble compounds abundant in many fruits and vegetables and are hypothesized to be protective compounds against oxidative stress in vivo. Among current smokers, a significant trend for an inverse association between β-cryptoxanthin intake and lung cancer risk was observed (p-value, test for trend <0.001). β-Cryptoxanthin is one of the main carotenoids in citrus fruits, which also contain high amounts of vitamin C and other compounds that may decrease cancer risk. The authors therefore also adjusted the analysis for vitamin C, folate, other carotenoids, and multivitamin use. These adjustments did not alter the inverse association between β-cryptoxanthin and lung cancer risk much, but the authors note that it is possible that other substances than β-cryptoxanthin in fruits and vegetables, particularly in citrus fruit, are primarily responsible for the inverse association observed. High lycopene intake was marginally associated with a lower risk of lung cancer (p-value, test for trend = 0.06). Significantly β-carotene intake was not associated with lung cancer risk (p-value, test for trend = 0.62).

The association of passive smoking with fruit and vegetable consumption, or with specific carotenoids, and lung cancer could not be investigated in these pooled analyses of prospective studies because most studies did not collect information on environmental tobacco smoke exposure.

A cohort study that was included in the two pooled analyses described above also analyzed the role of folate and vitamin C in the association of fruit and vegetable consumption and lung cancer risk (Voorrips et al. 2000). Results from that study showed highly significant inverse associations for vitamin C and folate with lung cancer risk (p-value, tests for trend <0.0001 for both micronutrients). The authors concluded that high folate and vitamin C intakes might be better protective compounds than the carotenoids. Several epidemiological studies have investigated whether dietary vitamin C intake is protective against lung cancer. A case-control study including smokers, past smokers, and nonsmokers conducted by Fontham et al. (1988) found a strong protective effect of vitamin C for lung cancer among men and women in Louisiana (odds ratio = 0.65, 0.50–0.87, high intake). This association was significantly stronger than the inverse association the authors observed for carotene (odds ratio = 0.84, 95% CI = 0.64–1.09). A more recent prospective study by Yong et al. (Yong et al. 1997) also found a significant inverse association between dietary vitamin C intake and risk of lung cancer in data from the First National Health and Nutrition Examination Survey Epidemiologic follow-up study. In a multivariate analysis adjusted for smoking status, the RR of lung cancer for subjects in the highest quartile of dietary vitamin C intake, compared with those in the lowest quartile was 0.66 (95% CI = 0.45–0.96). The authors also investigated the effect of supplement use but did not find additional protective effects of vitamin C supplements beyond that provided through dietary intake. Several other cohort studies observed inverse relationships between vitamin C intake and risk of lung cancer. For example, in the New York State Cohort Study, a prospective study including 48,000 male and female smokers and nonsmokers, an inverse dose–response relationship was observed in men. In males, the adjusted RRs for the medium and highest level of consumption, compared with the lowest one were 0.78 (CI = 0.62–0.98) and 0.63 (CI = 0.53–0.88), respectively. A similar protective relationship was observed for folate and carotenoids. In women, weaker, nonsignificant inverse relationships were observed for all of the investigated micronutrients. The authors also investigated the role of vitamin supplementation by adjustment for the corresponding supplement. Results were essentially the same (Bandera et al. 1997). Two large case-control studies conducted by Hinds et al. (1984) and Le Merchand et al. (1989) in Hawaii found an inverse association with lung cancer for total vitamin C (diet plus supplements) in men, but not in women.

7.2.2 Cardiovascular Diseases

Smoking and exposure to environmental tobacco smoke are associated with oxidative stress and with increased risk of atherosclerosis and cardiovascular diseases (Glantz and Parmley 1995; Wells 1994). Oxidative stress can lead to the oxidative modification of low-density lipoprotein (LDL), a process that has been strongly hypothesized to be involved in the initiation of atherosclerosis. Antioxidants may ameliorate these effects. Epidemiologic studies have been conducted in order to investigate if dietary intake of antioxidants is associated with the reduction of cardiovascular and cerebrovascular events, such as stroke. In the Rotterdam Study, for example, Voko et al. (2003) investigated whether high intake of antioxidants from food is associated with the risk of ischemic stroke. A higher intake of antioxidants was associated with a lower risk of ischemic stroke among approximately 6,000 participants of this prospective study. The relationship was significant for vitamin C and most pronounced in smokers. These results indicate that a high dietary intake of vitamin C in smokers may reduce the risk of coronary artery diseases. Hirvonen et al. (2000) investigated the association between dietary antioxidants and risk of stroke in participants of the Alpha-Tocopherol, Beta-Carotene Cancer Prevention Study (ATBC Study) during a 6.1-year follow-up using dietary baseline data. More than 26,000 male smokers, aged 50–69 years, were included in that analysis. Dietary intake of β-carotene was significantly inversely associated with the risk for cerebral infarction (relative risk [RR] of highest vs lowest quartile = 0.74, 95% CI = 0.60–0.91). No association was detected between other dietary antioxidants and risk for stroke. Results from these studies suggest that high dietary antioxidant intakes, especially of vitamin C and β-carotene, may have protective effects against stroke in smokers.

7.3 Primary Prevention Studies: Modulation of Cigarette Smoking-Related Chronic Diseases by Antioxidant Supplements

7.3.1 Lung Cancer and Cardiovascular Diseases

Two large primary prevention trials have been conducted with antioxidants specifically in smokers, the ATBC Study (The ATBC Cancer Prevention Study Group 1994) including more than 29,000 male smokers and the Beta-Carotene and Retinol Efficacy Trial (CARET study), which included more than 14,000 male and female heavy current and former smokers (Omenn et al. 1996). The antioxidants administered were α-tocopherol and/or β-carotene in the ATBC Study and β-carotene combined with retinol (vitamin A) in the CARET study. These intervention studies were initiated after epidemiologic studies linked vegetables high in carotenoids with lower lung cancer risk (National Research Council 1982; Peto et al. 1981). In the ATBC Study, after 5–8 years of treatment, no reduction in incidence of lung cancer was observed among men who were supplemented with α-tocopherol. A higher incidence of lung cancer was observed among subjects who received β-carotene. In the CARET study, after 4 years of supplementation, subjects in the β-carotene/vitamin A treatment group had a significantly higher relative risk of lung cancer of 28% when compared to the placebo group.

Toernwall et al. (2004) very recently published results from an evaluation of the 6-year posttrial effects of α-tocopherol and β-carotene supplementation on coronary heart disease in the ATBC Study. The authors report that β-carotene seemed to increase the posttrial risk of first-ever nonfatal myocardial infarction in male smokers, and state that their findings do not support the use of β-carotene or α-tocopherol supplements in the prevention of coronary heart disease among male smokers.

Another large randomized β-carotene intervention study on cancer and cardiovascular disease is the Physicians' Health Study (Hennekens et al. 1996). That cohort of male subjects included 11% of current smokers and 39% former smokers. After a follow-up of 12.5 years, no effect of β-carotene supplementation on cancer or heart disease was observed, indicating that β-carotene supplementation had neither beneficial nor harmful effects with regard to cancer or cardiovascular disease. However, only a small proportion of the subjects were smokers and low numbers of lung cancer cases could have decreased the statistical power necessary to detect treatment effects.

7.4 Biomarker Studies: Modulation of Cigarette Smoking-Related Oxidative Stress by Antioxidant Supplements

As mentioned in the Introduction, a range of oxidative damage biomarkers can be applied to measure smoking-associated oxidative stress and the effects of antioxidants on those biomarkers. However, in this chapter, we focus mainly on biomarkers for lipid peroxidation because this is the research field where most of the work in our group has been conducted.

7.4.1 Vitamin C

Several studies investigated the effect of vitamin C in smokers, using a variety of lipid peroxidation biomarkers. We reviewed eight studies that investigated the effects of vitamin C on lipid peroxidation biomarkers in smokers (see Table 7.1 for details). Four of these eight studies found statistically significant protective effects, two observed no effects. One small study on eight subjects found a nonsignificant 26% reduction in malondialdehyde (MDA) in the vitamin C group, compared with a 9% reduction in the placebo group. One study that measured two different biomarkers found no effect on one biomarker but an increasing effect on the other biomarker (Nyyssoenen et al. 1997).

A relatively small study by Harats et al. (1990) investigated the acute effect of smoking on plasma lipoproteins in 17 smokers after vitamin C supplementation with 1,000 or 1,500 mg daily for 2 or 4 weeks. The authors found that vitamin C significantly decreased oxidation of plasma LDL measured by thiobarbituric acid-reactive substances (TBARS). A similar-sized study by Fuller et al. (1996) in which 19 healthy smokers were supplemented with 1,000 mg of vitamin C for 4 weeks found that the vitamin C supplementation led to a significant reduction in plasma LDL oxidative susceptibility as measured by TBARS. A study in smokers that used F_2-IsoPs as the marker for lipid peroxidation is the study by Reilly et al. (1996). These authors reported that a 5-day supplementation of smokers with 2,000 mg vitamin C significantly reduced their urinary excretion of F_2-IsoPs. We conducted a large double-blind, placebo-controlled vitamin C intervention study in 81 smokers, measuring plasma F_2-IsoPs (Dietrich et al. 2002). We also found a significant decrease in this biomarker by vitamin C, but only in smokers with a body mass index (BMI) above the median. Overweight/obesity is associated with elevated oxidative stress. Our finding of only a protective effect of vitamin C in overweight smokers might indicate that a certain threshold level of oxidative stress is necessary to see a treatment effect with antioxidants. Three studies did not observe statistically significant protective effects (Mulholland et al. 1996; Nyyssoenen et al. 1997; Samman et al. 1997). Two of these studies were very small, and their intervention period was shorter than that

Table 7.1 Antioxidant supplementation studies in smokers and passive smokers using biomarkers for lipid peroxidation

Reference	Subjects	Type and dose of antioxidant	Duration	Body fluid	Biomarker used and results
Smokers					
Harats et al. 1990	17 smokers	-Vitamin C (1,000 + 1,500 mg/day)	2 + 4 weeks	Plasma, in vitro	LDL TBARS: significantly decreased
Fuller et al. 1996	19 smokers	-Vitamin C (1,000 mg/day)	4 weeks	Plasma, in vitro	LDL oxidizability: significantly decreased (measured by TBARS)
Reilly et al. 1996	16 heavy smokers	-Vitamin C (2,000 mg/d, $n=5$) -Vitamin E (800 IU/d, $n=7$) -Vitamin C (2,000 mg/day) and vitamin E (800 IU/day) in combination ($n=4$)	5 days	Urine	F_2-IsoPs: -Vitamin C alone: significantly decreased F_2-IsoPs -Vitamin E alone: no effect -Vitamin C plus vitamin E combination: significantly decreased F_2-IsoPs
Mulholland et al. 1996	8 smokers (8 placebo)	-Vitamin C (1,000 mg/day)	2 weeks	Serum	TBARS: vitamin C group decreased TBARS 26%, placebo 9%, not statistically significant
Nyyssoenen et al. 1997	59 smokers (19 placebo, 19 plain vitamin C, 20 slow-release vitamin C)	-Vitamin C (500 mg/day)	8 weeks	Plasma, in vitro and in vivo	LDL oxidizability (measured by CD): no change when compared with placebo group Plasma MDA: increased significantly when compared with placebo group
Samman et al. 1997	8 smokers crossover, 8 day washout between periods	-Vitamin C (1,000 mg/day)	2 weeks	Plasma, in vitro	LDL oxidizability (measured by CD): declined, not statistically significant
Steinberg and Chait 1998	20 smokers (19 placebo)	-Vitamin C (600 mg/day), vitamin E (400 IU/day), and β-carotene (30 mg/day) in combination, in tomato juice	4 weeks	Plasma, in vitro	LDL oxidizability (measured by CD): combination of AO significantly decreased when compared with placebo group
Patrignani et al. 2000	34 smokers (12 placebo)	-Vitamin E (300 mg/day, $n=11$) -Vitamin E (600 mg/day, $n=12$) -Vitamin E (1,200 mg/day, $n=11$)	3 weeks	Urine	F_2-IsoPs: no significant effect on F_2IsoPs of either dose

Reference	Subjects	Type and dose of antioxidant	Duration	Body fluid	Biomarker used and results
Fuller et al. 2000	22 smokers (8 placebo)	-Vitamin C (1,000 mg/day, $n=6$) -Vitamin E (400 IU/day, $n=8$) -Vitamin C (1,000 mg/day) and vitamin E (400 IU/day) in combination ($n=8$)	8 weeks	Plasma, in vitro	LDL oxidizability (measured by CD): -Vitamin C alone: no changes -Vitamin E alone: significantly decreased LDL oxidizability -Vitamin C plus vitamin E combination: significantly decreased LDL oxidizability
Dietrich et al. 2002	81 smokers (45 placebo)	-Vitamin C (500 mg/day) ($n=42$) -AO cocktail containing vitamin C, vitamin E, and α-lipoic acid[a] ($n=39$)	8 weeks	Plasma	F_2-IsoPs: -Vitamin C alone: significantly decreased F_2-IsoPs[b] when compared with change in placebo -AO cocktail: no effect when compared with change in placebo
Passive smokers					
Howard et al. 1998	36 passive smokers	-AO mixture containing vitamin C, vitamin E, β-carotene, and minerals[c]	8 weeks	Plasma	TBARS: 7% decrease, statistical significance not provided
Valkonen and Kuusi 2000	10 passive smokers	-Vitamin C (3,000 mg/day)	Single dose	Plasma, in vitro	TRAP, LDL oxidizability, TBARS: significant protective effect of vitamin C on all of these measures
Dietrich et al. 2003	43 passive smokers (24 placebo)	-Vitamin C (500 mg/day, $n=22$) -AO cocktail containing vitamin C, vitamin E, and α-lipoic acid[a] ($n=21$)	8 weeks	Plasma	F_2-IsoPs: -Vitamin C alone: significantly decreased F_2-IsoPs when compared with change in placebo -AO cocktail: significantly decreased F_2-IsoPs when compared with change in placebo

LDL low-density lipoprotein, *TBARS* thiobarbituric acid reactive substances, F_2-*IsoPs* F_2-isoprostanes, *CD* conjugated dienes, *MDA* malondialdehyde, *AO* antioxidants, *TRAP* total peroxyl radical trapping potential of serum

[a]AO cocktail: 500 mg vitamin C, 371 mg α-tocopherol, 171 mg γ-tocopherol, 50 mg α-tocotrienol, 184 mg γ-tocotrienol, 18 mg δ-tocotrienol, 95 mg α-lipoic acid

[b]Only in smokers with body mass index above median

[c]3,000 μg β-carotene, 60 mg vitamin C, 30 IU α-tocopherol, 40 mg zinc, 40 μg selenium, 2 mg copper

of most of the other studies, which could have led to the negative result. However, the study by Nyyssoenen et al. (1997), which also did not observe a protective effect, was rather large with 59 subjects, and the intervention period was as long as other studies that did observe protective effects. In fact, Nyyssoenen et al. observed increased plasma MDA levels in the group of subjects taking ascorbic acid, compared with subjects in the placebo group. The authors note that this was an unexpected result and could not be explained by artificial formation of lipid peroxides during sample preparation or by interday laboratory variability. The authors conclude that long-term ascorbic acid supplementation alone without any other antioxidant might promote the formation of MDA. However, in our large intervention study of the same duration, we found a significant reduction in MDA in the vitamin C treatment group (unpublished data).

With regard to vitamin C supplementation and lipid peroxidation in passive smokers, only two studies have been published to date, and both showed protective effects of vitamin C. Valkonen and Kuusi (2000) conducted a small study with ten nonsmokers who were exposed to environmental tobacco smoke for 30 min on 2 consecutive days. Vitamin C significantly prevented the formation of serum TBARS. The other study was a randomized double-blind placebo controlled study including 67 healthy passive smokers and was conducted by our group (Dietrich et al. 2003). We found that vitamin C significantly decreased plasma F_2-IsoPs in passive smokers.

7.4.2. Vitamin E

Three studies reviewed here investigated the effect of vitamin E in smokers. One found a lipid peroxidation-lowering effect; two found no statistically significant effects. The study by Reilly et al. (1996), which did not find a protective effect of vitamin E alone, was a very short-term study of only 5 days. This might have not a long enough time to see any effects of vitamin E. However, they did find a positive effect when vitamin E was administered in combination with vitamin C, which suggests that vitamin C and vitamin E act in combination. On the other hand, Fuller et al. (2000) observed lipid peroxidation decreasing effects of vitamin E given alone or in combination with vitamin C, but no decreasing effects of vitamin C alone. Patrignani et al. (2000) conducted a study administering three different doses of vitamin E to a total of 34 subjects and measured lipid peroxidation in form of urinary F_2-IsoPs. The authors observed no effect of any of the given vitamin E doses.

7.4.3 Combinations of Antioxidants

Five studies investigated the effect of combinations of antioxidants on lipid peroxidation markers in smokers and passive smokers (Reilly et al. 1996, Steinberg and Chait 1998, Fuller et al. 1998, Dietrich et al. 2002, Dietrich et al. 2003). The combinations were either vitamin C and vitamin E combined, or these two vitamins combined in addition with β-carotene, minerals (Howard et al. 1998), or α-lipoic acid. One study administered an antioxidant combination in tomato juice (Steinberg and Chait 1998). Most of the studies observed lipid peroxidation-lowering effects in smokers and passive smokers (see Table 7.1 for details). However, in our intervention study, which was done in smokers and in passive smokers, the antioxidant combination lowered F_2-IsoP in passive smokers (Dietrich et al. 2003), but not in smokers (Dietrich et al. 2002). This result was unexpected and is difficult to explain. It might be possible that components of the combination counteracted the effect of vitamin C on F_2-IsoPs, because, as mentioned above, significant treatment effects by the same dose of vitamin C were observed in the vitamin C treatment group.

7.5 Summary

In summary, epidemiologic studies consistently showed significant, though modest, inverse associations of high fruit and vegetable intake with lung cancer risk. Carotenoids found in fruits and vegetables have been significantly associated with lower lung cancer risks, such as, for example, β-cryptoxanthin. However, it cannot be ruled out that the protective effects seen for this specific carotenoid are indicative of other protective compounds abundant in fruits and vegetables, such as vitamin C or folate, or by a combination of those. Most of the studies that investigated dietary vitamin C and lung cancer risk found significant inverse associations.

Interestingly, two large cohort studies, the EPIC Study and the pooled analysis study by Smith-Warner et al. (Smith-Warner et al. 2003), observed stronger protective effects against lung cancer for high fruit intake than for high vegetable intake. This might indicate that micronutrients that are abundant in higher concentrations in fruits, compared with in vegetables might be responsible for that effect. However, the authors of the EPIC Study hypothesize that smoking as a high risk factor for lung cancer has overhelmed any protective associations of vegetable consumption (Miller et al. 2004).

It is notable that with respect to antioxidant nutrients, current smoking is an effect modifier of the role of nutrients on disease, rather than a confounder. That is, the effect of a given level of intake is likely to be different in current smokers versus nonsmokers, based on the fact that the blood antioxidant levels obtained on the same antioxidant intake are lower in smokers than in nonsmokers. Unfortunately most of the observational studies did not examine the relationships in this way, and few stratified on current smoking status.

Most of these cohort studies did not estimate the possible protective effect of total antioxidant intake, wich consists of intake from both food and supplements. This could underestimate the nutrient effect. Similarly, most studies did not stratify by antioxidant supplement use when examining the fruit and vegetable effect, which could lead to underestimations of the risk reduction by fruit and vegetable intake.

The discrepancy between the observational studies, which suggested a protective role for fruits and vegetables, and the ATBC and other randomized trials, which found null or even harmful effects, is troubling. The issues have been discussed elsewhere (Blumberg and Block 1994). However, the discrepancy does not necessarily invalidate the findings of the observational studies, for several reasons. The primary reason is that the randomized trial tested whether beginning high-dose treatment after smokers had been smoking for an average of 36 years could prevent progression to lung cancer. It does not provide any evidence regarding whether a diet rich in antioxidants throughout those 36 years might have prevented, or reduced the risk of, lung cancer. Furthermore, the dose of β-carotene used in the trials is at least five times higher than what is commonly achieved through diet.

With regard to the effects of antioxidants on oxidative stress biomarkers, the majority of intervention studies administering vitamin C found lipid peroxidation-lowering effects in both smokers and passive smokers. These results indicate that vitamin C ameliorates smoking-related oxidative stress. Results from studies that administered vitamin E were less consistent. However, most studies that administered combinations of antioxidants found lipid peroxidation-preventing effects.

7.6 Conclusion

In conclusion, despite the observed small to modest cancer risk reduction by high fruit and vegetable intake in smokers, and the lipid peroxidation lowering effect of supplemental vitamin C in smokers and passive smokers, the most efficient way of preventing smoking-related oxidative stress and diseases is smoking cessation. Therefore, smoking prevention and cessation should be the primary focus in public health for the prevention of lung cancer incidences.

References

Alberg AJ, Chen JC, Zhao H, Hoffman SC, Comstock GW, Helzlsouer KJ (2000) Household exposure to passive cigarette smoking and serum micronutrient concentrations. Am J Clin Nutr 72:1576–1582

Ayaori M, Hisada T, Suzukawa M, Yoshida H, Nishiwaki M, Ito T, Nakajima K, Higashi K, Yonemura A, Ishikawa T, Ohsuzu F, Nakamura H (2000) Plasma levels and redox status of ascorbic acid and levels of lipid peroxidation products in active and passive smokers. Environ Health Perspect 108:105–108

Bandera EV, Freudenheim JL, Marshall JR, Zielezny M, Priore RL, Brasure J, Baptiste M, Graham S (1997) Diet and alcohol consumption and lung cancer risk in the New York State Cohort. Cancer Causes Control 8:828–840

Belton O, Byrne D, Kearney D, Leathy A, Fitzgerald DJ (2000) Cyclooxygenase-1 and-2-dependent prostacyclin formation in patients with atherosclerosis. Circulation 102:840–845

Bermudez E, Stone K, Carter KM, Pryor WA (1994) Environment tobacco smoke is just as damaging to DNA as mainstream smoke. Environ Health Perspect 102:870–874

Block G (1991) Vitamin C and cancer prevention: the epidemiologic evidence. Am J Clin Nutr 53: S270–S282

Block G, Patterson B, Subar A (1992) Fruit, vegetables, and cancer prevention: a review of the epidemiologic evidence. Nutr Cancer 18:1–29

Blumberg J, Block G (1994) The alpha-tocopherol,beta-carotene cancer prevention study in Finland. Nutr Rev 52:242–250

Burton GW, Joyce A, Ingold KU (1983) Is vitamin E the only lipid-soluble, chain-breaking antioxidant in human blood plasma and erythrocyte membranes? Arch Biochem Biophys 221:281–290

Cracowski JL, Tremel F, Marpeau C, Baguet JP, Stanke-Labesque F, Mallion JM, Bessard G (2000) Increased formation of F_2-isoprostanes in patients with severe heart failure. Heart 84:439–440

Davi G, Allessandrini P, Mezzetti A, Minotti G, Bucciarelli T, Costantini F, Cipollone F, Bon GB, Ciabattoni G, Patrono C (1997) In vivo formation of 8-epi-prostaglandin $F_{2\alpha}$ is increased in hypercholesterolemia. Arterioscler Thromb Vasc Biol 17:3230–3235

Davi G, Ciabattoni G, Consoli A, Mezzetti A, Falco A, Santarone S, Pennese E, Vitacolonna E, Bucciarelli T, Costantini F, Capani F, Patrono C (1999) In vivo formation of 8-iso-prostaglandin $F_{2\alpha}$ and platelet activation in diabetes mellitus. Effects of improved metabolic control and vitamin E supplementation. Circulation 99:224–229

Dean RT, Fu S, Stocker R, Davies MJ (1997) Biochemistry and pathology of radical-mediated protein oxidation. Biochem J 324:1–18

Dietrich M, Block G, Benowitz NL, Morrow JD, Hudes M, Jacob PI, Norkus EP, Packer L (2003a) Vitamin C supplementation decreases oxidative stress biomarker F_2-isoprostanes in plasma of nonsmokers exposed to environmental tobacco smoke. Nutr Cancer 45:176–184

Dietrich M, Block G, Norkus EP, Hudes M, Traber MG, Cross CE, Packer L. (2003b) Smoking and exposure to environmental tobacco smoke decrease some plasma antioxidants and increase gamma-tocopherol in vivo after adjustment for dietary antioxidant intakes. Am J Clin Nutr. 2003 Jan;77(1):160-6.

Dietrich M, Block G, Hudes M, Morrow JD, Norkus EP, Traber MG, Cross CE, Packer L (2002) Antioxidant supplementation decreases lipid peroxidation biomarker F_2-isoprostanes in plasma of smokers. Cancer Epidemiol Biomarkers Prev 11:7–13

Diplock AT, Charleux JL, Crozier-Willi G, Kok FJ, Rice-Evans CA, Roberfroid M, Stahl W, Vina-Ribes J (1998) Functional food science and defence against reactive oxidative species. Br J Nutr 80:S77–S112

Eiserich JP, van der Vliet A, Handelman GJ, Halliwell B, Cross CE (1995) Dietary antioxidants and cigarette smoke-induced biomolecular damage: a complex interaction. Am J Clin Nutr 62:S1490–S1500

Farchi S, Forastiere F, Pistelli R, Baldacci S, Simoni M, Perucci CA, Viegi G (2001) Exposure to environmental tobacco smoke is associated with lower plasma beta-carotene levels among nonsmoking women married to a smoker. Cancer Epidemiol Biomarkers Prev 10:907–909

Fontham ETH, Pickle LW, Haenszel W, Correa P, Lin Y, Falk RT (1988) Dietary vitamins A and C and lung cancer risk in Louisiana. Cancer 62:2267–2273

Frei B (1991) Ascorbic acid protects lipids in human plasma and low-density lipoprotein against oxidative damage. Am J Clin Nutr 54:S1113–S1118

Frei B, England L, Ames BN (1989) Ascorbate is an outstanding antioxidant in human blood plasma. Proc Natl Acad Sci U S A 86:6377–6381

Frei B, Forte TM, Ames BN, Cross CE (1991) Gas phase oxidants of cigarette smoke induce lipid peroxidation and changes in lipoprotein properties in human blood plasma. Biochem J 277:133–138

Fuller CJ, Grundy SM, Norkus EP, Jialal I (1996) Effect of ascorbate supplementation on low density lipoprotein oxidation in smokers. Atherosclerosis 119:139–150

Fuller CJ, May MA, Marin KJ (2000) The effect of vitamin E and vitamin C supplementation on LDL oxidizability and neutrophil respiratory burst in young smokers. J Am Coll Nutr 19:361–369

Glantz SA, Parmley WW (1995) Passive smoking and heart disease: mechanisms and risk. JAMA 273:1047–1053

Gokce N, Keaney JF, Frei B, Holbrook M, Olesiak M, Zachariah BJ, Leeuwenburgh C, Heinecke JW, Vita JA (1999) Long-term ascorbic acid administration reverses endothelial vasomotor dysfunction in patients with coronary artery disease. Circulation 99:3234–3240

Harats D, Ben-Naim M, Dabach Y, Hollander G, Havivi E, Stein O, Stein Y (1990) Effect of vitamin C and E supplementation on susceptibility of plasma lipoproteins to peroxidation induced by acute smoking. Atherosclerosis 85:47–54

Hennekens CH, Buring JE, Manson JE, Stampfer M, Rosner B, Cook NR, Belanger C, Lamotte F, Gaziano JM, Ridker PM, Willett W, Peto R (1996) Lack of effect of long-term supplementation with beta carotene on the incidence of malignant neoplasms and cardiovascular disease. N Engl J Med 334:1145–1149

Hinds MW, Kolonel LN, Hankin JH, Lee J (1984) Dietary vitamin A, carotene, vitamin C and risk of lung cancer in Hawaii. Am J Epidemiol 119:227–237

Hirvonen T, Virtamo J, Korhonen P, Albanes D, Pietinen P (2000) Intake of flavonoids, carotenoids, vitamins C and E, and risk of stroke in male smokers. Stroke 31:2301–2306

Howard DJ, Ota RB, Briggs LA, Hampton M, Pritsos CA (1998) Oxidative stress induced by enviromental tobacco smoke in the workplace is mitigated by antioxidant supplementation. Cancer Epidemiol Biomarkers Prev 7:981–988

Jarvinen R, Knekt P, Seppanen R, Reunanen A, Heliovaara M, Maatela J, Aromaa A (1994) Antioxidant vitamins in the diet: Relationships with other personal characteristics in Finland. J Epidemiol Community Health 48:549–554

Khanna S, Atalay M, Laaksonen DE, Gul M, Roy S, Sen CK (1999) α-Lipoic acid supplementation: tissue glutathione homeostasis at rest and after exercise. J Appl Physiol 86:1191–1196

Le Marchand L, Yoshizawa CN, Kolonel LN, Hankin JH, Goodman MT (1989) Vegetable consumption and lung cancer risk: a population-based case-control study in Hawaii. J Natl Cancer Inst 81:1158–1164

Lykkesfeldt J, Christen S, Wallock LM, Chang HH, Jacob RA, Ames BN (2000) Ascorbate is depleted by smoking and repleted by moderate supplementation: a study in male smokers and nonsmokers with matched dietary antioxidant intakes. Am J Clin Nutr 71:530–536

Mannistoe S, Smith-Warner SA, Spiegelman D, Albanes D, Anderson K, Van den Brandt PA, Cerhan JR, Colditz G, Feskanich D, Freudenheim JL, Giovannucci E, Goldbohm RA, Graham S, Miller AB, Rohan TE, Virtamo J, Willett WC, Hunter DJ (2004) Dietary carotenoids and risk of lung cancer in a pooled analysis of seven cohort studies. Cancer Epidemiol Biomarkers Prev 13:40–48

Marangon K, Herbeth B, Lecomte E, Paul-Dauphin A, Grolier P, Chancerelle Y, Artur Y, Siest G (1998) Diet, antioxidant status, and smoking in French men. Am J Clin Nutr 67:231–239

Mezzetti A, Cipollone F, Cuccurullo F (2000) Oxidative stress and cardiovascular complications in diabetes: isoprostanes as new markers on an old paradigm. Cardiovasc Res 47:475–488

Miller AB, Altenburg HP, Bueno-de-Mesquita B, Boshuizen HC, Agudo A, Berrino F, Gram IT, Janson L, Linseisen J, Overvad K, Rasmuson T, Vineis P, Lukanova A, Allen N, Amiano P, Barricarte A, Berglund G, Boeing H, Clavel-Chapelon F, Day NE, Hallmans G, Lund E, Martinez C, Navarro C, Palli D, Panico S, Peeters PH, Quiros JR, Tjonneland A, Tumino R, Trichopoulou A, Trichopoulos D, Slimani N, Riboli E, Palli D (2004) Fruits and vegetables and lung cancer: findings from the European Prospective Investigation into Cancer and Nutrition. Int J Cancer 108:269–276

Morrow JD, Awad JA, Boss HJ, Blair IA, Roberts LJ (1992) Non-cyclooxygenase-derived prostanoids (F_2-isoprostanes) are formed in situ on phospholipids. Proc Nat Acad Sci U S A 89:10721–10725

Morrow JD, Frei B, Longmire AW, Gaziano JM, Lynch SM, Shyr Y, Strauss WE, Oates JA, Roberts LJ (1995) Increase in circulating products of lipid peroxidation (F_2-isoprostanes) in smokers—smoking as a cause of oxidative damage. N Engl J Med 332:1198–1203

Morrow JD, Hill KE, Burk RF, Nammour TM, Badr KF, Roberts LJ (1990) A series of prostaglandin F_2-like compounds are produced in vivo in humans by a non-cyclooxygenase, free radical-catalyzed mechanism. Proc Nat Acad Sci U S A 87:9383–9387

Mulholland CW, Strain JJ, Trinick TR (1996) Serum antioxidant potential, and lipoprotein oxidation in female smokers following vitamin C supplementation. Int J Food Sci Nutr 47.227–231

National Research Council (1982) Diet, nutrition, and cancer. National Academy Press, Washington, D.C.

Norkus EP, Hsu H, Cehelsky MR (1987) Effect of cigarette smoking on the vitamin C status of pregnant women and their offspring. Ann N Y Acad Sci 498:500–501

Nyyssoenen K, Poulsen HE, Hayn M, Agerbo P, Porkkala-Sarataho E, Kaikkonen J, Salonen R, Salonen JT (1997) Effect of supplementation of smoking men with plain or slow release ascorbic acid on lipoprotein oxidation. Eur J Clin Nutr 51:154–163

Obata T, Tomaru K, Nagakura T, Izumi Y, Kawamoto T (2000) Smoking and antioxidant stress: essay of isoprostane in human urine by gas chromatography-mass spectrometry. J Chromatogr B Biomed Sci Appl 746:11–15

Omenn GS, Goodman GE, Thornquist MD, Balmes J, Cullen MR, Glass A, Keogh JP, Meyskens JFL, Valanis B, Williams JJH, Barnhart S, Hammar S (1996) Effects of a combination of beta carotene and vitamin A on lung cancer and cardiovascular disease. N Engl J Med 334:1150–1155

Patrignani P, Panara MR, Tacconelli S, Seta F, Bucciarelli T, Ciabattoni G, Alessandrini P, Mezzetti A, Santini G, Sciulli MG, Cipollone F, Davi G, Gallina P, Bon GB, Patrono C (2000) Effects of vitamin E supplementation on F_2-isoprostane and thromboxane biosynthesis in healthy cigarette smokers. Circulation 102:539–545

Peto R, Doll R, Buckley JD, Sporn MB (1981) Can dietary beta-carotene materially reduce human cancer rates? Nature 290:201–208

Pratico D, Clark CM, Lee VMY, Trojanowski JQ, Rokach J, FitzGerald GA (2000) Increased 8,12-iso-iPF(2 alpha)-VI in Alzheimer's disease: correlation of a noninvasive index of lipid peroxidation with disease severity. Ann Neurol 48:809–812

Pryor WA (1984) Free radicals in autoxidation and in aging. In: Armstrong D, Sohal RS, Cutler RG, Slater TF (eds) Free radicals in molecular biology, aging and disease. Raven, New York, pp 13–41

Pryor WA (1986) Cancer and free radicals. In: Shankel DM (ed) Antimutagenesis and anticarcinogenesis: mechanisms. Plenum, New York, pp 45–59

Pryor WA (1987) Cigarette smoke and the involvement of free radical reactions in chemical carcinogenesis. Br J Cancer 55:19–23

Pryor WA, Stone K (1993) Oxidants in cigarette smoke. Radicals, hydrogen peroxide, peroxynitrate, and peroxynitrite. Ann N Y Acad Sci 686:12–28

Reilly M, Delanty N, Lawson JA, FitzGerald GA (1996) Modulation of oxidant stress in vivo in chronic cigarette smokers. Circulation 94:19–25

Roberts LJ, Morrow JD (2000) Measurement of F_2-isoprostanes as an index of oxidative stress in vivo. Free Radic Biol Med 28:505–513

Ross MA, Crosley LK, Brown KM, Duthie SJ, Collins AC, Arthur JR, Duthie GG (1995) Plasma concentrations of carotenoids and antioxidant vitamins in Scottish males: influences of smoking. EJCN 49:861–865

Samman S, Brown AJ, Beltran C, Singh S (1997) The effect of ascorbic acid on plasma lipids and oxidisability of LDL in male smokers. Eur J Clin Nutr 51:472–477

Schectman G, Byrd JC, Gruchow HW (1989) The influence of smoking on vitamin C status in adults. Am J Public Health 79:158–162

Shigenaga MK, Gimeno CJ, Ames BN (1989) Urinary 8-hydroxy-2'-deoxyguanosine as a biomarker of in vivo oxidative DNA damage. Proc Natl Acad Sci U S A 96:9697–9701

Smith-Warner SA, Spiegelman D, Yaun S-S, Albanes D, Beeson WL, Van den Brandt PA, Feskanich D, Folsom AR, Fraser GE, Freudenheim JL, Giovannucci E, Goldbohm RA, Graham S, Kushi LH, Miller AB, Pietinen P, Rohan TE, Speizer FE, Willett WC, Hunter DJ (2003) Fruits, vegetables and lung cancer: a pooled analysis of cohort studies. Int J Cancer 107:1001–1011

Steinberg FM, Chait A (1998) Antioxidant vitamin supplementation and lipid peroxidation in smokers. Am J Clin Nutr 68:319–327

Stryker WS, Kaplan LA, Stein EA, Stampfer MJ, Sober A, Willett WC (1988) The relation of diet, cigarette smoking, and alcohol consumption to plasma β-carotene and α-tocopherol levels. Am J Epidemiol 127:283–296

The Alpha-Tocopherol, Beta-Carotene Cancer Prevention Study Group (1994) The effect of vitamin E and beta carotene on the incidence of lung cancer and other cancers in male smokers. N Engl J Med 330:1029–1035

Tornwall ME, Virtamo J, Korhonen PA, Virtanen MJ, Taylor PR, Albanes D, Huttunen JK (2004) Effect of α-tocopherol and β-carotene supplementation on coronary heart disease during the 6-year post-trial follow-up in the ATBC study. Eur Heart J 25:1171–1178

Tribble DL, Giuliano LJ, Fortmann SP (1993) Reduced plasma ascorbic acid concentrations in nonsmokers regularly exposed to environmental tobacco smoke. Am J Clin Nutr 58:886–890

Vainio H, Rautalahti M (1998) An international evaluation of the cancer preventive potential of carotenoids. Cancer Epidemiol Biomarkers Prev 7:725–728

Valkonen M, Kuusi T (1998) Passive smoking induces atherogenic changes in low-density lipoprotein. Circulation 97:2012–2016

Valkonen MM, Kuusi T (2000) Vitamin C prevents the acute atherogenic effects of passive smoking. Free Radic Biol Med 28:428–436

Voko Z, Hollander M, Hofman A, Koudstaal PJ, Breteler MM (2003) Dietary antioxidant and the risk of ischemic stroke: the Rotterdam study. Neurology 61:1273–1275

Voorrips LE, Goldbohm RA, Brants HAM, Van Poppel GAFC, Sturmans F, Hermus RJJ, Van den Brandt PA (2000) A perspective cohort study on antioxidant and folate intake and male lung cancer risk. Cancer Epidemiol Biomarkers Prev 9:357–365

Wells AJ (1994) Passive smoking as a cause of heart disease. J Am Coll Cardiol 24:546–554

Yong L-C, Brown CC, Schatzkin A, Dresser CM, Slesinski MJ, Cox CS, Taylor PR (1997) Intake of vitamins E, C, and A and risk of lung cancer. The NHANES I epidemiologic followup study. Am J Epidemiol 146:231–243

Ziegler RG, Mayne ST, Swanson CA (1996) Nutrition and lung cancer. Cancer Causes Control 7:157–177

Chapter 8

Modulation of Cigarette Smoke Effects by Antioxidants: Oxidative Stress and Degenerative Diseases

Jari Kaikkonen and Jukka T. Salonen

Contents

8.1	Introduction	216
8.2	Oxidative Stress and Lipid Peroxidation	216
8.2.1	Effects of Smoking on Lipid Peroxidation	216
8.2.2	Effects of General Factors on Lipid Peroxidation	217
8.2.3	Assessment of Lipid Peroxidation and DNA Oxidation	217
8.3	Antioxidants and Their Mechanisms of Action	218
8.3.1	Adaptive Mechanisms of Antioxidants in Smokers	218
8.3.2	Prooxidant Effects of Antioxidants	219
8.4	Effects of Smoking and Quitting Smoking on the Plasma Levels of Antioxidants	219
8.5	Effects of Antioxidant Supplementation on Lipid Peroxidation and DNA Damage in Smokers	220
8.5.1	Vitamin C	220
8.5.2	Vitamin E	220
8.5.3	β-Carotene	221
8.5.4	Antioxidant Cocktails and Polyphenols	221
8.5.4.1	Antioxidant Cocktails	221
8.5.4.2	Polyphenols	223
8.5.4.3	Fruit-and-Vegetable-Rich Diet and Oxidative Stress in Smokers	224
8.6	Antioxidants and the Risk of Degenerative Diseases in Smokers	224
8.6.1	Clinical Outcome Studies with Antioxidant Supplements	224
8.6.1.1	Alpha-Tocopherol, Beta-Carotene Study	225
8.6.1.2	Carotene and Retinol Efficacy Trial	225

Contents

8.6.1.3	Physicians' Health Study	225
8.6.1.4	Women's Health Study	226
8.6.1.5	Antioxidant Polyp Prevention Studies	226
8.6.1.6	Summary and Discussion of Clinical Outcome Studies	227
8.6.2	Dietary Intake of Polyphenols and the Disease Risk	228
8.7	Conclusion	228
	References	230

8.1 Introduction

Smoking is an important risk factor in many diseases and disease states, for example, lung diseases. These include asthma, chronic obstructive pulmonary diseases (COPD), chronic bronchitis and emphysema, and lung cancer (Eiserich et al. 1995; Virtamo 1999). Smoking is also associated with some other cancers, such as cancers of the head and neck, bladder, esophagus, pancreas, stomach, and kidney (Kuper et al. 2002), and smoking elevates the risk of cardiovascular diseases (Ambrose and Barua 2004). There is an accumulating body of evidence demonstrating that smokers have a lower intake of fruits and vegetables, lower plasma antioxidant levels, and they are more susceptible to lipid and DNA oxidation, as compared with former smokers or nonsmokers (Alberg 2002; Morrow et al. 1995; Prieme et al. 1998).

In the above-mentioned degenerative diseases, oxidative stress/lipid peroxidation seems to play a vital role (Mayne 2003). The harmful effects of cigarette smoking are mediated via the carcinogens present in the smoke, such as polycyclic aromatic hydrocarbons (PAH compounds) (Pfeifer et al. 2002), but also via its prooxidant, lipid peroxidation-increasing effects.

Even though smokers are encouraged to break their habit, which is undoubtedly the best way to minimize the harmful effects of smoking, many smokers fail to refrain from smoking. It has been proposed that some of the harmful effects of the cigarette smoking could be reduced by antioxidant supplementation. To answer this question, we have reviewed the current literature concerning antioxidants, oxidative stress, and their interaction with smoking in different case-control, cross-sectional, intervention, and follow-up studies in smokers, somewhat emphasizing the research related to carotenoids and polyphenols.

8.2 Oxidative Stress and Lipid Peroxidation

8.2.1 Effects of Smoking on Lipid Peroxidation

It has been estimated that cigarette smoke contains 10^{14} free radicals per inhalation (Church and Pryor 1985). Hydroxyl radicals, aldehydes, and nitrogen oxides in cigarette smoke are thought to be significant contributors to biomolecular damage (Eiserich et al. 1995; Spencer et al. 1995). Cigarette smoking also increases the numbers of alveolar neutrophils and macrophages, which once activated, can produce strong oxidizing agents, such as superoxide radicals (Halliwell and Gutteridge 1989). Thus, inflammation, as reflected in the elevated C-reactive protein (CRP) levels (Block et al. 2004), may be an important further mechanism increasing free radical stress in smokers. Dietary habits are less healthy in smokers, which means they have a lower intake of fruits and vegetables, and consequently, of antioxidants (Dyer et al. 2003; Walmsley et al. 1999). In addition, there are several studies that have reported that smoking itself can directly decrease antioxidant levels (Eiserich et al. 1995; Handelman et al. 1996). The in vivo mechanism is unclear, but it may involve increased consumption/cycling, lowered absorption, or increased elimination rate of the antioxidants. In in vitro models, the exposure of plasma to gas-phase cigarette smoke has evoked depletion of urate, ascorbate, ubiquinol 10, α-tocopherol, and a variety of carotenoids (Eiserich et al. 1995; Handelman et al. 1996). Lipid peroxidation end products can further mediate the harmful effects of free radicals. For example, there is some evidence that $F_{2\alpha}$-isoprostanes possess bioactive pulmonary and vasoconstrictive effects (Basu 2004).

8.2.2 Effects of General Factors on Lipid Peroxidation

There are several factors that can modulate the effects of cigarette smoking. The most recent evidence has dealt with genetic factors. Genotype variations between subjects in their antioxidant enzymes can confound the findings of population-based studies, i.e., individuals with certain genotypes may be more prone to the harmful effects of cigarette smoke. Polymorphism in the paraoxonase (*PON2*) gene in smokers is one example of such a phenomenon (Martinelli et al. 2004). Other general factors increasing lipid peroxidation include male gender, inflammation, high cholesterol levels, low plasma levels of different dietary antioxidants, such as vitamin C and β-carotene (Block et al. 2002), and recently performed exhaustive exercise (Kaikkonen et al. 1998), which is nevertheless quite an unusual event in smokers. It is still not clear whether age is a major primary factor associated with the status of lipid peroxidation, and the so-called free radical theory, which claims that as an individual ages, the radical burden increases still need to be confirmed (Wickens 2001). Also, the content of the ingested fatty acids may modify the findings. There are many studies showing that providing individuals with vitamin E supplements can lower plasma lipid peroxidation. However, Weinberg and coworkers (2001) found that smoking subjects supplemented with vitamin E and consuming a high-polyunsaturated fat diet were more prone to oxidation as measured by increased total F_2-isoprostane and prostaglandin (PG)$F_{2\alpha}$ levels, as compared with subjects receiving no vitamin E. Thus, studies investigating the effects of antioxidants in smokers should take these confounding factors into consideration, especially in epidemiological studies. Naturally, the randomization and the group size need to be sufficiently large to correct for these interfering factors in intervention studies.

8.2.3 Assessment of Lipid Peroxidation and DNA Oxidation

In general, it is quite difficult to assess oxidative stress in humans, partly because no standardized methods are available in this area. For example, it has been observed that several simultaneously performed measurements can give conflicting, even opposite, findings.

There are several approaches that can be used to assess lipid peroxidation and oxidative stress. First, the oxidation susceptibility of lipid-containing body liquids and liquid fractions can be assessed in test tubes ex vivo by using oxidizing agents, such as transition metals or azo-compounds, which act as initiators of lipid peroxidation. Copper ions, iron ions, 2,2′-azobis(2-amidinopropane) hydrochloride (AAPH) and 2,2′-azobis(2,4-dimethylvaleronitrile) (AMVN) have been the most commonly used initiators. Accumulation of different propagation- and termination-phase products, such as conjugated dienes and lipid hydroperoxides, have been quantified in these induction experiments (Corongiu et al. 1989; Esterbauer et al. 1992; Neuzil et al. 1997; Rice-Evans and Miller 1994). Second, oxidation products formed in vivo in the human body can be determined. Thiobarbituric acid reactive substances (TBARS) have been measured either in vivo or after in vitro oxidation of lipoproteins (Esterbauer et al. 1984; Richard et al. 1992). One clear shortcoming of this method is that a part of the TBARS might be formed during the assay itself. Breath alkane excretion has been used as a marker of in vivo fatty acid peroxidation in lungs, but unfortunately, this marker is considered to be quite unspecific. Products of polyunsaturated fatty acid (PUFA) and monounsaturated fatty acid (MUFA) oxidation, i.e., hydroxy fatty acids, oxysterols, and total F_2-isoprostanes, or more specific $F_{2\alpha}$-isoprostanes (8-iso-PGF$_{2\alpha}$, PGF$_{2\alpha}$), have been mainly determined by gas or liquid chromatography/mass spectrometry (GC/MS or LC/MS) or by immunoassay. $F_{2\alpha}$-isoprostanes are considered as one of the most reliable and specific markers of in vivo lipid peroxidation (Basu 2004, Salonen 2000; Kaikkonen et al. 2004). Third, the activities of different antioxidant enzymes, such as blood/plasma glutathione peroxidase (GPx), superoxide dismutase (SOD), or catalase (CAT) can be measured, and antioxidants and their redox pairs assessed (Kaikkonen et al. 2004; Salonen 2000).

Because lipid peroxidation is thought to be high in smokers, it is plausible that the effects of antioxidant supplementation would be easier to identify in such subjects. For this reason, numerous supplementation trials have been carried out in smokers. Because $F_{2\alpha}$-isoprostanes are known to be one of the most reliable indicators of lipid peroxidation, we have mainly focused on studies that have concentrated on this compound, though other in vivo measurements of lipid and DNA oxidation have also been considered.

8.3 Antioxidants and Their Mechanisms of Action

8.3.1 Adaptive Mechanisms of Antioxidants in Smokers

There is some evidence that the human body can adapt to the cigarette smoke by increasing the recycling of the consumed antioxidants back to their active forms, e.g., ascorbic acid. Ascorbic acid recycling describes the process in which ascorbic acid is oxidized to dehydroascorbic acid by various pathways, and subsequently reduced back to ascorbic acid intracellularly, thereby preserving the ascorbic acid pool (Lykkesfeld et al. 2003). The kinetics of deuterium-labeled tocopheryl acetate has also been compared between smokers and nonsmokers. Traber and coworkers (2001) found that smoking appeared to increase the plasma vitamin E disappearance rate. Glutathione (GSH) is an endogenous water-soluble antioxidant, and it is unclear how it reacts to cigarette smoke. Hininger and colleagues (1997) noted that the whole-blood concentrations of reduced GSH were higher in smokers than in nonsmokers, and decreased to the levels measured from nonsmokers during a 2-week supplementation with fruits and vegetables. Recently, Moriarty and coworkers (2003) have reported that GSH levels were significantly lower in smokers

(n=43), compared with nonsmokers (n=78). Correspondingly, it is also unclear whether the expression/activities of antioxidant enzymes are lowered or increased as a result of smoking. Boemi and coworkers (2004) found that paraoxonase (PON1) mass and activity were lower in smokers, and smoking was an independent determinant of PON1 status. In another study, the expression of manganese SOD, copper zinc SOD, and extracellular SOD were investigated by immunohistochemistry in the airways of nonsmokers (n=13), smokers (n=20), and COPD patients (n=22). The expression of manganese SOD was higher in the central bronchial and alveolar epithelium among smokers, and in addition, the activity of the enzyme was higher in smokers than in nonsmokers (Harju et al. 2004).

8.3.2 Prooxidant Effects of Antioxidants

Both vitamin C and E possess prooxidant properties, at least in vitro, depending on their concentration, and the existence of regenerating coantioxidants, plus, for example, on the amount of polyunsaturated fatty acids. Carotenoids may act as prooxidants if the partial pressure of oxygen is above the oxygen pressure in the air (Burton and Ingold 1984; Chen and Djuric 2001; El-Agamey et al. 2004). Thus, exposure of lungs to elevated oxygen concentrations (Halliwell and Gutteridge 1989) might explain, at least partly, the harmful findings of long-term β-carotene supplementations in smokers. Most tissues, however, are exposed to normal oxygen pressure under physiological conditions (Burton and Ingold 1984; Krinsky 2001). The prooxidative effects of β-carotene may also be mediated via changes in the enzyme activity of cytochrome P450 (CYP) isoforms. In an animal model, β-carotene caused a booster effect on phase I enzymes, which are enzymes that can activate the formation of carcinogens in lungs (Paolini et al. 2003). In rat fibroblasts, tobacco smoke condensate increased significantly the production of 8-OHdG at physiological concentrations (0.75–4.0 μM) of β-carotene. This effect of β-carotene on 8-OHdG production was dose and time dependent (Palozza et al. 2004). The role of carotenoid cleavage products might also be important as an inducer of these oxidative reactions (Siems et al. 2003).

8.4 Effects of Smoking and Quitting Smoking on the Plasma Levels of Antioxidants

There is a large body of evidence showing that smoking decreases the plasma levels of different antioxidants (Alberg 2002; Kaikkonen et al. 2001). A recent review evaluated antioxidant concentrations in smokers and former smokers in comparison with nonsmokers and never smokers. In general, smokers and former smokers have lower plasma concentrations of vitamin C and carotenoids, in particular β-carotene, but vitamin E concentrations do not usually differ significantly (Alberg 2002). Plasma γ-tocopherol levels have even been reported to be higher in active or passive smokers, as compared with nonsmokers (Dietrich et al. 2003a). Likewise, some studies have also noted that there are higher plasma concentrations of some individual carotenoids, such as lutein, zeaxanthine, lycopene, or β-carotene, in former smokers than in nonsmokers (Brady et al. 1996; Marangon et al. 1998; Theron et al. 1994).

It seems on average that the circulating levels of β-carotene are 34% lower in smokers than in nonsmokers, whereas in former smokers, the concentration of β-carotene is 22% lower in contrast to never smokers. The corresponding values for vitamin C concentrations are −27% and −6%. Clear dose–response trends have been observed between decreased plasma concentrations of β-carotene and vitamin C, and the increased number of cigarettes smoked per day. Also, passive smoking seems to have a similar effect, indicating that already low-dose exposure to cigarette smoke has clear unfavorable effects (Alberg 2002; Alberg et al. 2000; Dietrich et al. 2003a; Farchi et al. 2001; Marangon et al. 1998; Polidori et al. 2003; Tröbs et al. 2002). In an experimental study ($n=15$, ≥7 cigarettes per day) quitting smoking seemed to elevate the vitamin levels by 4 weeks at near or equal to those found in nonsmokers, resulting in plasma that was less susceptible to oxidation (Polidori et al. 2003). In addition, in vivo markers of oxidative stress, i.e., 8-epi-PGF$_{2α}$ (Pilz et al. 2000) and urinary 8-OHdG excretion (Prieme et al. 1998) have been noted to decrease as a result of smoking cessation.

Although the relation between smoking and plasma concentration of antioxidants seem to be quite clear, different findings have also been observed. The most important predictive factor for plasma/serum carotenoid concentrations in 3,043 European subjects from 16 different regions, including nine different European countries, was simply the region in which they lived, not the smoking status (Al-Delaimy et al. 2004). In Japanese men, the alcohol consumption exhibited an inverse association with serum carotenoid levels, and the levels were independent on the smoking status or on the number of smoked cigarettes per day (Fukao et al. 1996). Despite of these opposite findings, major part of the studies have reported dose–response-related strong associations between low circulating levels of antioxidants and smoking status or passive smoking.

8.5 Effects of Antioxidant Supplementation on Lipid Peroxidation and DNA Damage in Smokers

8.5.1 Vitamin C

The effects of vitamin C have been tested in smokers by using several different ex vivo analyses of lipid peroxidation, such as low-density lipoprotein (LDL) susceptibility to oxidation and unspecific TBARS/malondialdehyde (MDA). Findings from these studies suggest that vitamin C supplementation seems to be unable to increase oxidation resistance of isolated LDL or to result in lower TBARS/MDA levels in smokers (Kelly 2003). In addition to these studies, numerous antioxidant cocktail and disease association studies have been published related to vitamin C (see below).

8.5.2 Vitamin E

Patrignani and coworkers (2000) performed a randomized double-blind, placebo-controlled study of the effects of vitamin E (300, 600, and 1,200 mg of DL-α-tocopheryl acetate daily, each dose for 3 consecutive weeks) on 8-iso-PGF$_{2α}$ in 48 moderate cigarette smokers (30 male and 18 female volunteers, aged 20–47 years, smoking 15–30 cigarettes per day). Vitamin E supplementation caused a dose-dependent increase in its plasma levels that reached a plateau at 600 mg ($42±11$ μmol/l, $p<0.001$). This increase was not associated with any statistically significant change in urinary immunoreactive 8-iso-PGF$_{2\alpha}$.

Weinberg and coworkers (2001) reported in their crossover study that supplemented vitamin E (400 IU DL-α-tocopheryl acetate daily) could function as a prooxidant in ten smokers (seven female, three male, >20 cigarettes per day, aged 37 ± 1 years, [mean ± SE]), who consumed a high-polyunsaturated fat diet containing linoleic safflower oil. A diet of olive oil for 3 weeks was used as the control diet, following 3-week safflower oil and safflower plus vitamin E diets. In their study, the safflower oil diet increased total F$_2$-isoprostanes from 53.0±7.2 to 116.2±11.2 nmol/l and PGF$_{2\alpha}$ from 3.5±0.2 to 5.5±0.5 nmol/l, without changing LDL oxidation parameters. Addition of vitamin E further increased the total F$_2$-isoprostanes to 188.2±10.9 nmol/l and PGF$_{2\alpha}$ to 7.8±0.4 nmol/l.

In addition, the effect of vitamin E supplementation (600 IU/day for 4 weeks) on plasma total oxysterol levels have been investigated in 12 smokers (≥15 cigarettes per day, four males, eight females) and 14 controls (eight males, six females), aged 18–70 years. The levels of oxysterols were higher in smokers versus controls (354 ± 104 vs 265 ± 66 nmol/l, $p<0.05$), but vitamin E supplementation did not affect the plasma oxysterol levels (Mol et al. 1997).

8.5.3 β-Carotene

As far as we are aware, only one pure β-carotene supplementation study has been carried out using F$_2$-isoprostanes as the marker of lipid peroxidation. Mayne and coworkers (2004) studied the possible prooxidant effects of a high dose of β-carotene (50 mg/day) in a subpopulation ($n=55$) of a multiyear (median, 4.0 years) randomized placebo-controlled chemoprevention trial with supplemental β-carotene. The effects of β-carotene in smokers and former/never smokers were monitored with creatinine adjusted spot urine total and 8-iso-PGF$_{2\alpha}$ isoprostanes, which decreased during the supplementation period both in smokers ($n=12$) and former ($n=36$)/never ($n=2$) smokers, though not significantly. The number of the subjects in different groups was quite small, and therefore, it is difficult to draw any clear conclusions from these results.

Block and coworkers (2002) studied the associations between plasma antioxidants and biomarkers of lipid peroxidation in 298 healthy adults aged 19–78 years. The study subjects were smokers (>15 cigarettes per day), passive smokers, or nonsmokers. An inverse association was observed between plasma diet-derived β-carotene and plasma F$_{2\alpha}$-isoprostane levels. The contribution of β-carotene concentrations to the prediction of F$_{2\alpha}$-isoprostane levels was stronger than were current smoking status and age, but lower than were sex, race, body mass index (BMI) or plasma ascorbic acid.

8.5.4 Antioxidant Cocktails and Polyphenols

8.5.4.1 Antioxidant Cocktails

Reilly and coworkers (1996) studied in a crossover study the effects of 5-day dosing with vitamin E (800 IU per day), vitamin C (2 g per day), and their combination on urinary F$_{2\alpha}$-isoprostane levels in four to seven heavy-smoking subjects, aged 20–47 years, smoking a mean of 38 cigarettes per day. There was a 2-week washout period between the treatments. Vitamin C ($p<0.05$) and the combination of vitamin C and E ($p<0.05$) suppressed significantly urinary excretion of 8-epi-PGF$_{2\alpha}$, whereas vitamin E alone had no effect (Reilly et al. 1996).

In a 2-month, randomized double-blind, placebo-controlled trial, Dietrich and coworkers (2003b) investigated whether supplementation with vitamin C (500 mg) or an antioxidant mixture containing vitamin C (500 mg), α-lipoic acid (95 mg), and vitamin E (371 mg of *RRR*-α-tocopherol, 171 mg of *RRR*-γ-tocopherol, 50 mg of α-tocotrienol, 184 mg of γ-tocotrienol, 18 mg of δ-tocotrienol) daily for 2 months could decrease plasma F$_{2\alpha}$-isoprostane levels in 126 smokers, aged 20–78 years, mean age of 46 years, smoking at least 15 cigarettes per day. In smokers with a BMI above the median, the vitamin C supplement did decrease plasma F$_{2\alpha}$-isoprostane levels by 28.8 pmol/l when compared with the placebo group ($p=0.001$). In subjects with BMI below the median, no effect was observed. This group restudied the effect of the antioxidant supplementation in nonsmokers exposed to environmental tobacco smoke and found changes in the same direction.

Kaikkonen and colleagues (2001) studied the effect of vitamin C (500 mg of slow-release ascorbate daily), vitamin E (200 mg of d-α-tocopheryl acetate daily), their combination and placebo on the plasma F$_{2\alpha}$-isoprostane levels in 100 men, aged 45–70 years. Half of the men were smokers (≥5 cigarettes per day). Only vitamin E lowered this index of lipid peroxidation. There was a tendency that the treatment effect was stronger in smokers as compared with nonsmokers. The increase in lipid-standardized vitamin E was associated with the decrease in F$_{2\alpha}$-isoprostanes, both in smokers and nonsmokers.

Jacob and coworkers (2003) tested whether moderate antioxidant supplementation with vitamin C (272 mg), *all-rac*-α-tocopherol (31 mg), and folic acid (400 mg) daily for 3 months could decrease lipid peroxidation in vivo in 38 male smokers (≥10 cigarettes per day) and in 39 nonsmokers, aged 20–51 years. The supplementation used did not lower the oxidative stress in either smokers or nonsmokers. There were several indicators of oxidative stress examined, e.g., F$_2$-isoprostanes, both total and 8-isoprostanes, TBARS, and protein carbonyls.

The effects of different vitamins on the oxidative DNA damage in smokers have been studied in small clinical trials. Fifteen smokers were divided into the following supplementation groups: vitamin E (200 IU/day), β-carotene (9 mg/day), vitamin C (500 mg/day), red ginseng (1.8 g/day), and placebo. Supplementation was given to smokers for 4 weeks. The carbonyl content of the proteins and 8-OHdG excretion were used to assess the effects of supplemented antioxidants on the oxidative damage of DNA in smokers. No effects in β-carotene or vitamin C group were observed, whereas vitamin E and ginseng extracts were effective in lowering both markers (Lee et al. 1998). Welch and colleagues (1999) studied the effects of ascorbic acid (350 mg/day), *RRR*-α-tocopherol (250 mg/day), β-carotene (60 mg/day), selenium (80 μg/day of sodium selenite), and ascorbic acid plus *RRR*-α-tocopherol (350+250 mg/day) supplementation on DNA damage in smokers ($n=9$) and nonsmokers ($n=12$). Supplementation with β-carotene for 4 weeks decreased the level of 8-OHdG in leukocytes of nonsmokers, but conversely increased its concentrations in smokers, whereas the other antioxidants had no effects.

The effects have also been investigated of combination of vitamin E (1,200 IU/day), C (1,500 mg/day) and β-carotene (22.5 mg/day) supplementation on the intracellular activities of different antioxidant enzymes, such as superoxide dismutase, GPx and catalase. Six-week supplementation increased the plasma levels of all of the ingested vitamins in 14 smokers and in 8 nonsmokers. The concentrations of all vitamins were much higher in lung lavage cells of the smokers in contrast to nonsmokers, but no significant downregulation of the antioxidant enzymes was observed (Hilbert and Mohsenin 1996). Tomato oleoresin capsules, which contained lycopene (4.9 mg), α-tocopherol (1.2 mg), phytoene (0.5 mg), and phytofluene (0.4 mg), were given three per day for 2 weeks to 12 smokers and 15 nonsmokers, with the control groups receiving placebo capsules. The tomato oleoresin capsules were ineffective in protecting the smokers against the oxidative damage of DNA, which was determined by the number of DNA strand breaks, but in nonsmokers the amount of undamaged DNA was higher after the supplementation period (Briviba et al. 2004).

8.5.4.2 Polyphenols

Similar to the situation with epidemiological studies, there are only a few clinical trials that have examined the effects of polyphenol supplementation on the oxidative damage in smokers, and only one of these studies has utilized in vivo markers of lipid peroxidation (Caccetta et al. 2001), the other studies having resorted to the markers of antioxidant capacity (Young et al. 2002), the oxidation susceptibility of LDL (Princen et al. 1998, Vigna et al. 2003), and the markers of oxidative damage of DNA (Hakim et al. 2003).

Caccetta and coworkers (2001) studied the effects of consumption of red wine (375 ml, 450 mg of polyphenols), white wine (375 ml, 130 mg of polyphenols), and dealcoholized red wine (500 ml, 450 mg of polyphenols) on the production of F_2-isoprostanes in smoking men ($n=18$, aged 25–71 years). In their randomized trial, plasma free plus esterified F_2-isoprostanes decreased significantly (from 882.5 to 703.4 pmol/l) after 2-week consumption of dealcoholized red wine, but not after the consumption of red or white wine as such.

Vigna and coworkers (2003) studied the effects of grape polyphenol supplementation (300 mg of procyanidin extract) on TBARS and LDL susceptibility to oxidation in a randomized double-blind, crossover study in heavily smoking men ($n=24$, >50 years of age). Four-week polyphenol supplementation decreased the concentration of TBARS and prolonged the lag phase.

The effects of green tea extract on the markers of oxidative status were studied in a blind, crossover intervention study with nonsmokers ($n=8$) and smokers ($n=8$, 10–15 cigarettes per day), aged 20–31 years. Three-week consumption of green tea extract (18.6 mg of catechins/day, equivalent to one to two cups of green tea) did not have any effect on the markers of oxidative stress measured from fasting blood samples. However, green tea extract did increase the plasma antioxidant capacity in postprandial plasma, with this increase being most prominent in smokers (Young et al. 2002).

Princen and coworkers (1998) studied the effects of consumption of green tea (equivalent to 6 cups per day), black tea (equivalent to 6 cups per day), or high amount of isolated green tea polyphenols (3.6 g of tea polypheols, equivalent to 18 cups per day) on oxidative stress in male ($n=32$) and female ($n=32$) smokers (aged 34±12 years, at least 10 cigarettes per day) in a randomized placebo-controlled study. No differences in the concentration of plasma antioxidants or parameters of LDL oxidation were detected after 4 weeks of the intervention.

Hakim and coworkers (2003) tested the effects of 4 months' consumption of either black (four cups, 450 mg of polyphenols) or green tea (four cups, 580 mg of polyphenols) on the oxidative damage of DNA in female ($n=100$) and male ($n=33$) smokers

(>10 cigarettes per day), who were 18–79 years of age, in a randomized controlled study. Urinary excretion of 8-OHdG decreased (−31%) after 4 months of drinking decaffeinated green tea, whereas no effect was seen after the consumption of black tea.

The number of polyphenol supplementation studies in smokers is limited, and so far, only one study has reported results using F_2-isoprostanes as a marker of oxidative stress. Studies that have utilized ex vivo methodology have led to inconsistent findings. Therefore, no conclusions can be drawn about the effects of polyphenol supplementation on oxidative stress in smokers.

8.5.4.3 Fruit-and-Vegetable-Rich Diet and Oxidative Stress in Smokers

A diet supplemented with fruits and vegetables contains a great many potentially beneficial components, which is not the case when vitamin supplements are ingested. Thus, changes in the diet can affect the intake of several vitamins and polyphenols, which may cause problems in interpretation of the results.

The effects of the increased intake of vegetables and fruits on activities of various antioxidant enzymes in smokers have been determined (Hininger et al. 1997; van den Berg et al. 2001). Diet rich in fruits and vegetables provided 30 mg/day of carotenoids, which increased the plasma concentrations of carotenoids by 23% in smokers and by 11% in nonsmokers. The resistance of LDL to oxidation increased by 14% within 2 weeks in smokers, and by 28% in nonsmokers. However, no effect was observed on the activity of antioxidant enzymes (SOD and GPx) (Hininger et al. 1997).

The effects of vegetable burgers and fruit drinks on antioxidant enzymes and markers of lipid peroxidation were studied in 24 smoking men using a 3-week crossover design with a 2-week washout between the supplementation and control periods. The vegetable burger-and-fruit drink diet provided 18 mg/day of carotenoids, 118 mg/day of vitamin C, 13 mg/day of vitamin E and 28.5 mg/day of flavonoids. No effects were observed on any of the markers of lipid oxidation (TBARS/MDA and plasma 8-epi-PGF$_{2\alpha}$) protein and DNA oxidation (carbonyls and Comet assay), or antioxidant enzymes (GSH-S-transferase-α and -π), but the plasma concentrations of antioxidants did increase (van den Berg et al. 2001).

According to these results, dietary changes did affect the plasma concentration of vitamins and flavonoids in smokers, but altered poorly to the markers of lipid peroxidation or DNA damage.

8.6 Antioxidants and the Risk of Degenerative Diseases in Smokers

8.6.1 Clinical Outcome Studies with Antioxidant Supplements

Randomized placebo-controlled studies, which have evaluated the incidence of cardiovascular disease (CVD) and cancer and mortality from these diseases, have provided the strongest evidence for beneficial health effects of antioxidants. To date, several large-scale controlled clinical trials evaluating the effects of vitamin supplementation on the prevention of cardiovascular diseases or cancer have been conducted. In this chapter, we concentrate on studies that have been conducted in smokers, or studies in which the findings concerning the subgroup of smokers have been presented separately. Four large antioxidant primary prevention supplementation trials have now been completed, and two trials have evaluated the effect on secondary prevention of cancer in smokers.

8.6.1.1 Alpha-Tocopherol, Beta-Carotene Study

The first study, the Alpha-Tocopherol, Beta-Carotene Study (ATBC Study), was a randomized double-blind, placebo-controlled supplementation trial designed to study whether supplementation of α-tocopherol (50 mg/day), β-carotene (20 mg/day), or their combination would reduce the incidence of different cancers in smokers (ATBC Study Group 1994). A total of 29,133 Finnish male smokers, aged from 50 to 69 (a mean age of 57 years) were recruited for the study. The average amount of cigarettes smoked per day was 20.4, and the average smoking history was 35.9 years. The follow-up time varied from 5 to 8 years (a median of 6.1 years), and during this time 876 new cases of lung cancer were diagnosed. The main finding of the study was that β-carotene supplementation increased the incidence of lung cancer by 16% (95% confidence interval [CI] = 2–33%), and also the total mortality was 8% (95% CI = 1–16%) higher in the β-carotene group (Albanes et al. 1996), but no separate effect on the primary coronary heart disease outcomes was observed (Virtamo et al. 1998). Vitamin E (α-tocopherol) supplementation had no significant effect on either the incidence of lung cancer or on the primary coronary heart disease outcomes (Virtamo et al. 1998). However, vitamin E (α-tocopherol) supplementation decreased the incidence of prostate cancer and mortality from that disease (ATBC Study Group 1994).

8.6.1.2 Carotene and Retinol Efficacy Trial

The Carotene and Retinol Efficacy Trial (CARET) was a randomized multicenter, placebo-controlled trial designed to study the effects of β-carotene (30 mg/day) and retinol (25,000 IU/day) on the incidence of lung cancer in smokers and/or workers with an occupational history of asbestos exposure in the United States. A total of 18,314 smokers (60%) and former smokers (39%), aged from 45 to 74 years, were recruited. The CARET study was stopped prematurely after a mean follow up time of 4.0 years because of the significant 28% (95% CI = 4–57%) increase in the lung cancer incidence. Also, the deaths from lung cancer (relative risk [RR]=1.46, 95% CI = 1.07–2.00), CVD (RR = 1.26, 95% CI = 0.99–1.61), and any reason mortality (RR = 1.17, 95% CI = 1.03 = 1.33) increased (Omenn et al. 1996).

8.6.1.3 Physicians' Health Study

The Physicians' Health Study (PHS) was a long-term randomized double-blind, placebo-controlled trial designed to study the effects of aspirin (325 mg/every other day), β-carotene (50 mg/every other day), or their combination on the incidence of cancer, CVD, and mortality from those diseases. The study population consisted of a total of 22,071 male physicians, aged 40–84 years, of whom 11% were classified as being current smokers and 39% as former smokers. During the 12-year follow-up time, 125 lung cancer deaths occurred. β-Carotene had no significant treatment effect on the endpoints investigated. The results were similar in the subgroups of current and former smokers (Hennekens et al. 1996).

8.6.1.4 Women's Health Study

Lee and colleagues (1999) studied the effects of β-carotene (50 mg/every other day), aspirin (100 mg/day), and vitamin E (600 IU/day) supplementation in women in a randomized double-blind, placebo-controlled trial. Out of a total amount of 39,876 participants, 13% were classified as current smokers. Neither vitamin E nor β-carotene supplementation affected the incidence of cancer or cardiovascular disease in smokers or in nonsmokers. The median follow-up time was 4.1 years (Lee et al. 1999).

8.6.1.5 Antioxidant Polyp Prevention Studies

In addition to primary prevention supplementation studies, several secondary prevention studies have been conducted to evaluate whether the recurrence of different cancers can be prevented by vitamin supplementation, but as far as we are aware, only two of these studies have been conducted with smokers.

Baron and colleagues (2003) studied the effect of β-carotene (25 mg/day), vitamin C, and α-tocopherol (1,000 and 400 mg) supplementation on colorectal adenoma recurrence. A total of 864 subjects who had an adenoma removed participated in this double-blind, placebo-controlled clinical trial. Among the subjects who neither smoked nor drank alcohol, the β-carotene supplementation was associated with a decreased risk of recurrent adenomas (RR = 0.56, 95% CI = 0.35–0.89). However, in smokers, the supplementation was associated with a modest, but a nonsignificant increase in the risk of recurrence (RR = 1.36, 95% CI = 0.70–2.62). Similar findings were reported in the subjects who drank more than one serving of alcohol per day (RR = 1.13, 95% CI = 0.89–1.43). Among those participants, who both smoked and drank alcohol, the risk was almost doubled (RR = 2.07, 95% CI = 1.39–3.08). According to these results, alcohol intake and cigarette smoking appeared to modify the effects of β-carotene on colorectal adenoma recurrence. Vitamin C or E supplementation did not have any effects, positive or negative (Greenberg et al. 1994).

Mayne and colleagues (2001) studied the effects of β-carotene (50 mg/day) on the recurrence of head and neck cancers. The participants consisted of 264 patients who had been curatively treated for cancer of the oral cavity, pharynx, or larynx. At baseline, 48% of the participants receiving β-carotene were classified as current smokers and 45% as former smokers. After a median follow-up time of 51 months, β-carotene supplementation did not have any effect on the recurrence of cancers of the head and neck. The cumulative probability of survival was nonsignificantly better for both smokers and nonsmokers in the β-carotene supplemented group.

8.6.1.6 Summary and Discussion of Clinical Outcome Studies

The results of the randomized primary prevention trials have not supported the view that prolonged high dose of antioxidant supplementation would decrease the risk of lung cancer or cardiovascular diseases. In fact, the results in two of these studies (ATBC, CARET) pointed to potentially adverse effects of β-carotene supplementation in smokers, and this led to the premature termination of these studies. However, in both of these studies the supplementation of β-carotene did not seem to increase the risk of lung cancer in general. In the ATBC Study, the RR for lung cancer was 0.93 (95% CI = 0.65–1.33) for nondrinkers in the β-carotene supplemented group, but was 1.35 (95% CI = 1.01–1.81) among those who reported consuming one or more alcohol containing drinks per day (Albanes et al. 1996). The incidence of lung cancer was higher also among those subjects who smoked at least 20 cigarettes daily when compared with those who smoked 5–19 cigarettes per day. A similar trend was seen also in the CARET study in which the RR for nondrinkers was 1.07 (95% CI = 0.76–1.51), but 1.99 (95% CI = 1.28–3.09) among subjects in the highest quartile of alcohol intake (Omenn et al. 1996). These observations suggest that β-carotene may be detrimental only to those who are heavy smokers and/or regular consumers of alcohol (Mayne et al. 1996). The results of the PHS did not confirm these findings (Cook et al. 2000). The relative risk for lung cancer was 0.8 (95% CI = 0.5–1.2) among the daily consumers of alcohol. Several explanations have been proposed for the discrepancy between the results, e.g., simply because of chance, differences in the study populations, the dose (PHS: 50 mg in every other day, ATBC: 50 mg/day, and CARET: 30 mg/day), differences in the serum concentrations, or the duration of the supplementation (PHS, 13 years; ATBC, 6 years; and CARET, 4 years) (Cook et al. 2000).

There are several possible reasons why β-carotene has not been able to protect against chronic diseases, such as cancer, in large-scale supplementation studies (Omaye et al. 1997). It has been suggested that (1) β-carotene may not be the crucial protecting factor present in fruits and vegetables, (2) β-carotene has to interact with other nutrients in food, (3) β-carotene only has efficacy against precancerous lesions, (4) the dose used in the studies was too high or low, and/or (5) the populations may have had sufficient β-carotene status and additional supplementation would thus provide no further benefit. In addition, even though there are over 600 identified carotenoids, the studies have concentrated mainly on β-carotene. Other carotenoids present in fruits and vegetables may have an effect on the risk of chronic diseases.

The mechanism by which β-carotene supplementation could increase the lung cancer risk has not yet been firmly elucidated. The local concentrated oxygen concentration (Burton and Ingold 1984; Chen and Djuric 2001; El-Agamey et al. 2004) or a variation in the activity of CYP enzyme isoforms may play some role (Paolini et al. 2003). It has also been suggested that components of cigarette smoke may induce oxidation of β-carotene, resulting in the formation of oxidized metabolites or cleavage products with prooxidant capabilities (Mayne et al. 1996, Siems et al. 2003). This has been studied in vitro with human bronchial epithelial cells, where tobacco smoke did not have any prooxidant effects on β-carotene (Arora et al. 2001). On the other hand, in recent in vitro studies, some evidence for prooxidation has been demonstrated (Palozza et al. 2004; Paolini et al. 2003). It is obvious that further studies are needed to clarify the role of β-carotene in the etiology of lung cancer.

8.6.2 Dietary Intake of Polyphenols and the Disease Risk

There are several studies that have evaluated the association between flavonoid intake and the risk of chronic diseases, but only one prospective study (ATBC Study) has concentrated solely on smokers, whereas other studies have included both smokers and nonsmokers. In the ATBC Study, a moderate inverse association was found between the intake of flavanols and flavones and the risk of nonfatal myocardial infarctions (MI) in male smokers. The relative risk for nonfatal MI was 0.77 (95% CI = 0.64–0.93) for the men in the highest (18 mg/day) versus the lowest quintile (4 mg/day) of intake (Hirvonen et al. 2001a). No significant associations with the other cardiovascular disease endpoints were observed. A high intake of flavonoids was also associated with a decreased risk of lung cancer (RR = 0.56, 95% CI = 0.45–0.69), whereas no evident association with the risk of other cancers was found (Hirvonen et al. 2001b). In the Finnish Mobile Clinic Health Examination Survey, Knekt and colleagues (1997, 2002) found that a high intake of one flavonoid, quercetin, was associated with a reduced risk of lung cancer in smokers (RR = 0.49, 95% CI = 0.28–0.86), even though the association was stronger in nonsmokers (RR = 0.13, 95% CI = 0.03–0.57).

A number of case-control studies have also evaluated the effects of flavonoids and the risk of lung cancer in smokers. Many of these studies have reported some association between the high flavonoid or tea intake and decreased risk of lung cancer in smokers (Le Marchand et al. 2000; Mendilaharsu et al. 1998). These results have not been confirmed in other trials (Garcia-Closas et al. 1998; Zhong et al. 2001).

The results of the two prospective cohort studies suggest that a high-flavonoid intake may decrease the risk of lung cancer in smokers. However, the role of flavonoids in lung cancer or in the other chronic diseases cannot be adequately evaluated, because of the limited number of existing studies and partly because the intake of flavonoids depends clearly on the quality of the diet, e.g., a diet rich in flavonoids is usually rich in other antioxidants.

8.7 Conclusion

In this chapter, we have examined the effect of smoking on plasma vitamin levels, the capability of vitamin supplementation to attenuate oxidative stress, and the risk of degenerative diseases in smokers. Furthermore, analytical methods used for assessing lipid peroxidation/oxidative stress have been briefly reviewed.

In smokers, the plasma levels of all of the most important nutritional antioxidants are lower than in nonsmokers, though vitamin E represents an exception, revealing no difference between smokers and nonsmokers. It is evident that smoking itself is at least partly responsible for this decrease in antioxidant levels, and it cannot simply be attributed to the poorer dietary habits of smokers. Also, in passive smokers, one can observe a similar trend. One possible explanation for this finding could be that passive smokers belong to the same social class, family, or working environment as the smokers, and have therefore similar dietary habits. For these reason, it has been recommended that smokers should use antioxidant supplements to achieve the same plasma levels of vitamins as nonsmokers. In fact, daily recommendations have even been calculated for smokers, e.g., the daily dose of vitamin C should be as high as 124–200 mg to achieve the levels of non-smokers (Kelly 2003). The most frequently studied antioxidants are vitamin C and vitamin E, even though it seems that smoking does not decrease the plasma vitamin E levels. The results found are somewhat conflicting, with some groups claiming that vitamin C is capable of lowering oxidative stress in smokers, but some others attributing this effect to vitamin E. Similar conflicting results have also been found with carotenoids, such as β-carotene, but also with polyphenols. In fact, for the polyphenols, there is even more complexity as there is extensive structural variation because these compounds can exist as both free and conjugated forms and give rise to a variety of different metabolites.

When results of antioxidant cocktail studies are evaluated, one can quite clearly conclude that the tested antioxidant mixtures do not possess cumulative or interacting effects, as compared with single substances. Also, many of the tested antioxidants seem to possess prooxidant properties under certain circumstances. Markers of lipid peroxidation have been mainly used in small supplementation studies, whereas in larger clinical studies, only the disease endpoints have been assessed. β-Carotene has been a focus of interest since the Finnish finding (ATBC Study) that β-carotene supplementation in smokers tended to increase rather than decrease the risk of lung cancer (ATBC Study Group 1994). However, the pooled analysis of seven cohort studies assessing the dietary intake of β-carotene does not support this finding (Männistö et al. 2004).

It is difficult to compare different supplementation studies, as (1) the definition for a smoker differs between the studies, i.e., in some studies an individual smoking 5 or more cigarettes a day is a smoker, but in others, more than 20 cigarettes need to be inhaled; (2) there are differences in the structure of the supplements (for example slow-release and "normal" vitamin C) and in their doses; (3) there have been a variety of different supplement cocktails examined; and (4) there are a variety of analytical methods used to assess lipid peroxidation. For example, even though $F_{2\alpha}$-isoprostanes are considered as one of the most reliable indicators of lipid peroxidation, there are several modifications also from this single measurement, including enzyme-linked immunosorbent assays and gas and liquid chromatographic mass spectrometric methods. In addition, the forms of F_2-isoprostanes measured vary between studies, i.e., from free to esterified forms and from total concentration to specific 8-epi-$PGF_{2\alpha}$. In other analyses, such as in in vitro oxidation experiments, the variation is even higher. The possible publication bias can also lead to an underestimation of the real number of negative findings. In smokers, the role of the studied antioxidants is still unclear both in the inhibition of oxidative stress and in the etiology of degenerative diseases. Prooxidant or antioxidant, this is the dilemma, at least with respect to β-carotene.

As the findings concerning the effects of antioxidant supplementation in smokers are conflicting, it does seem that the best advice one can give to smokers if they wish to minimize the harmful prooxidant effects of smoking is that they should give up smoking.

Acknowledgement

J.K. is a Research Fellow of the Academy of Finland (grant 80624).

References

Albanes D, Heinonen P, Taylor PR, Virtamo J, Edwards BK, Rautalahti M, Hartman AM, Palmgren J, Freedman LS, Haapakoski J, Barrett MJ, Pietinen P, Malila N, Tala E, Liippo K, Salomaa ER, Tangrea JA, Teppo L, Askin FB, Taskinen E, Erozan Y, Greenwald P, Huttunen JK (1996) Alpha-tocopherol and beta-carotene supplements and lung cancer incidence in the alpha-tocopherol, beta-carotene cancer prevention study: effects of baseline characteristics and study compliance. J Natl Cancer I 88:1560–1570

Alberg AJ (2002) The influence of cigarette smoking on circulating concentrations of antioxidant micronutrients. Toxicology 180:121–137

Alberg AJ, Chen JC, Zhao H, Hoffman SC, Comstock GW, Helzlsouer KJ (2000) Household exposure to passive cigarette smoking and serum micronutrient concentrations. Am J Clin Nutr 72:1576–1582

Al-Delaimy WK, Van Kappel AL, Ferrari P, Slimani N, Steghens JP, Bingham S, Johansson I, Wallström P, Overvad K, Tjonneland A, Key TJ, Welch AA, Bas Bueno-De-Mesquita H, Peeters PH, Boeing H, Linseisen J, Clavel-Chapelon F, Guibot C, Navarro C, Quiros JR, Palli D, Celetano E, Trichopoulou A, Benetou V, Kaaks R, Riboli E (2004) Plasma levels of six carotenoids in nine European countries: report from the European Prospective Investigation into Cancer and Nutrition (EPIC). Pub Health Nutr 7:713–722

Ambrose JA, Barua RS (2004) The pathophysiology of cigarette smoking and cardiovascular disease: an update. J Am Coll Cardiol 43:1731–1737

Arora A, Willhite CA, Liebler DC (2001) Interactions of β-carotene and cigarette smoke in human bronchial epithelial cells. Carcinogenesis 22:1173–1178

ATBC Study Group (1994) The effect of vitamin E and β-carotene on the incidence of lung cancer and other cancers in male smokers. The Alpha-Tocopherol, Beta-Carotene Cancer Prevention Study Group. N Engl J Med 330:1029–1035

Baron JA, Cole BF, Mott L, Haile R, Grau M, Church TR, Beck GJ, Greenberg ER (2003) Neoplastic and antineoplastic effects of β-carotene on colorectal adenoma recurrence: results of a randomized trial. J Natl Cancer I 95:717–722

Basu S (2004) Isoprostanes: novel bioactive products of lipid peroxidation. Free Radic Res 38:105–122

Block G, Dietrich M, Norkus EP, Morrow JD, Hudes M, Caan B, Packer L (2002) Factors associated with oxidative stress in human populations. Am J Epidemiol 156:274–285

Block G, Jensen C, Dietrich M, Norkus EP, Hudes M, Packer L (2004) Plasma C-reactive protein concentrations in active and passive smokers: influence of antioxidant supplementation. J Am Coll Nutr 23:141–147

Boemi M, Sirolla C, Testa R, Cenerelli S, Fumelli P, James RW (2004) Smoking is associated with reduced serum levels of the antioxidant enzyme, paraoxonase, in type 2 diabetic patients. Diabet Med 21:423–427

Brady WE, Mares-Perlman JA, Bowen P, Stacewicz-Sapuntzakis M (1996) Human serum carotenoid concentrations are related to physiologic and lifestyle factors. J Nutr 126:129–137

Briviba K, Kulling SE, Möseneder J, Watzl B, Rechkemmer G, Bub A (2004) Effects of supplementing a low-carotenoid diet with a tomato extract for 2 weeks on endogenous levels of DNA single strand breaks and immune functions in healthy non-smokers and smokers. Carcinogenesis 25:2373–2378

Burton GW, Ingold KU (1984) β-Carotene: an unusual type of lipid antioxidant. Science 224:569–573

Caccetta RAA, Burke V, Mori TA, Beilin LJ, Puddey IB, Croft KD (2001) Red wine polyphenols, in the absence of alcohol, reduce lipid peroxidative stress in smoking subjects. Free Radic Biol Med 30:636–642

Chen G, Djuric Z (2001) Carotenoids are degraded by free radicals but not affect lipid peroxidation in unilamellar liposomes under different oxygen tension. FEBS Lett 505:151–154

Church DF, Pryor WA (1985) Free radical chemistry of cigarette smoke and its toxicological implications. Environ Health Perspect 64:111–126

Cook NR, Lee IM, Manson JE, Buring JE, Hennekens CH (2000) Effects of β-carotene supplementation on cancer incidence by baseline characteristics in the Physicians' Health Study (United States). Cancer Cause Control 11:617–626

Corongiu FP, Banni S, Dessi MA (1989) Conjugated dienes detected in tissue lipid extracts by second derivative spectroscopy. Free Radic Biol Med 7:183–186

Dietrich M, Block G, Hudes M, Morrow JD, Norkus EP, Traber MG, Cross CE, Packer L (2002) Antioxidant supplementation decreases lipid peroxidation biomarker F_2-isoprostanes in plasma of smokers. Cancer Epidemiol Biomarkers Prev 11:7–13

Dietrich M, Block G, Benowitz NL, Morrow JD, Hudes M, Jacob P 3rd, Norkus EP, Packer L (2003a) Vitamin C supplementation decreases oxidative stress biomarker F2-isoprostanes in plasma of non-smokers exposed to environmental tobacco smoke. Nutr Cancer 45:176–184

Dietrich M, Block G, Norkus EP, Hudes M, Traber MG, Cross CE, Packer L (2003b) Smoking and exposure to environmental tobacco smoke decrease some plasma antioxidants and increase γ-tocopherol in vivo after adjustment for dietary antioxidant intakes. Am J Clin Nutr 77:160–166

Dyer AR, Elliot P, Stamler J, Chan Q, Usehima H, Zhou BF, Group IR (2003) Dietary intake in male and female smokers, ex-smokers, and never-smokers: the INTERMAP study. J Hum Hypertens 17:641–654

Eiserich JP, van der Vliet A, Handelman GJ, Halliwell B, Cross CE (1995) Dietary antioxidants and cigarette smoke-induced biomolecular damage: a complex interaction. Am J Clin Nutr 62: S1490–S1500

El-Agamey A, Lowe GM, McGarvey DJ, Mortensen A, Phillip DM, Truscott TG, Young AJ (2004) Carotenoid radical chemistry and antioxidant/pro-oxidant properties. Arch Biochem Biophys 430:37–48

Esterbauer H, Lang J, Zadravec S, Slater TF (1984) Detection of malonaldehyde by high-performance liquid chromatography. Method Enzymol 105:319–328

Esterbauer H, Gebicki J, Puhl H, Jurgens G (1992) The role of lipid peroxidation and antioxidants in oxidative modification of LDL. Free Radic Biol Med 13:341390

Farchi S, Forastiere F, Pistelli R, Baldacci S, Simoni M, Perucci CA, Viegi G (2001) Exposure to environmental tobacco smoke is associated with lower plasma β-carotene levels among non-smoking women married to smokers. Cancer Epidemiol Biomarkers Prev 10:907–909

Fukao A, Tsubono Y, Kawamura M, Ido T, Akazawa N, Tsuji I, Komatsu S, Minami Y, Hisamichi S (1996) The independent association of smoking and drinking with serum beta-carotene levels among males in Miyagi, Japan. Int J Epidemiol 25:300–306

Garcia-Closas R, Agudo A, Gonzalez CA, Riboli E (1998) Intake of specific carotenoids and flavonoids and the risk of lung cancer in women in Barcelona, Spain. Nutr Cancer 32:154–158

Greenberg ER, Baron JA, Tosteson TD, Freeman DHJ, Beck GJ, Bond JH, Colacchio TA, Coller JA, Frankl HD, Haile RW (1994) A clinical trial of antioxidant vitamins to prevent colorectal adenoma. N Engl J Med 331:141–147

Hakim IA, Harris RB, Brown S, Chow HH, Wiseman S, Agarwal S, Talbot W (2003) Effect of increased tea consumption on oxidative DNA damage among smokers: a randomized controlled study. J Nutr 133:S3303–S3309

Halliwell B, Gutteridge JMC (1989) Free radicals in biology and medicine. Clarendon Press, Oxford

Handelman GJ, Packer L, Cross CE (1996) Destruction of tocopherols, carotenoids, and retinol in human plasma by cigarette smoke. Am J Clin Nutr 63:559–565

Harju T, Kaarteenaho-Wiik R, Sirviö R, Paakko P, Crapo JD, Oury TD, Soini Y, Kinnula VL (2004) Manganese superoxide dismutase is increased in the airways of smokers' lungs. Eur Respir J 24:765–771

Hennekens CH, Buring JE, Manson JE, Stampfer M, Rosner B, Cook NR, Belanger C, LaMotte F, Gaziano JM, Ridker PM, Willet W, Peto R (1996) Lack of effect of long-term supplementation with β-carotene on the incidence of malignant neoplasms and cardiovascular disease. N Engl J Med 334:1145–1149

Hilbert J, Mohsenin V (1996) Adaptation of lung antioxidants to cigarette smoking in humans. Chest 110:916–920

Hininger I, Chopra M, Thurnham DI, Laporte F, Richard MJ, Favier A, Roussel AM (1997) Effect of increased fruit and vegetable intake on the susceptibility of lipoprotein to oxidation in smokers. Eur J Clin Nutr 51:601–606

Hirvonen T, Pietinen P, Virtanen M, Ovaskainen ML, Hakkinen S, Albanes D, Virtamo J (2001a) Intake of flavonols and flavones and risk of coronary heart disease in male smokers. Epidemiology 12:62–67

Hirvonen T, Virtamo J, Korhonen P, Albanes D, Pietinen P (2001b) Flavonol and flavone intake and the risk of cancer in male smokers (Finland). Cancer Causes Control 12:789–796

Jacob RA, Aiello GM, Stephensen CB, Blumberg JB, Milbury PE, Wallock LM, Ames BN (2003) Moderate antioxidant supplementation has no effect on biomarkers of oxidant damage in healthy men with low fruit and vegetable intakes. J Nutr 133:740–743

Kaikkonen J, Kosonen L, Nyyssönen K, Porkkala-Sarataho E, Salonen R, Korpela H, Salonen JT (1998) Effect of combined coenzyme Q10 and δ-α-tocopherol acetate supplementation on exercise induced lipid peroxidation and muscular damage: a placebo-controlled double-blind study in marathon runners. Free Radic Res 29:85–92

Kaikkonen J, Porkkala-Sarataho E, Morrow JD, Roberts LJ II, Nyyssönen K, Salonen R, Tuomainen TP, Ristonmaa U, Poulsen HE, Salonen JT (2001) Supplementation with vitamin E but not with vitamin C lowers lipid peroxidation in vivo in mildly hypercholesterolemic men. Free Radic Res 35:967–978

Kaikkonen J, Tuomainen TP, Nyyssönen K, Morrow JD, Salonen JT (2004) C18 hydroxy fatty acids as markers of lipid peroxidation ex vivo and in vivo. Scand J Clin Lab Invest 64:457–468

Kelly G (2003) The interaction of cigarette smoking and antioxidants. Part III: ascorbic acid. Altern Med Rev 8:43–45

Knekt P, Järvinen R, Seppänen R, Heliövaara M, Teppo L, Pukkala E, Aromaa A (1997) Dietary flavonoids and the risk of lung cancer and other malignant neoplasms. Am J Epidemiol 146:223–230

Knekt P, Kumpulainen J, Järvinen R, Rissanen H, Heliövaara M, Reunanen A, Hakulinen T, Aromaa A (2002) Flavonoid intake and risk of chronic diseases. Am J Clin Nutr 76:560–568

Krinsky NI (2001) Carotenoids as antioxidants. Nutrition 17:815–817

Kuper H, Boffetta P, Adami HO (2002) Tobacco use and cancer causation: association by tumour type. J Intern Med 252:206–224

Le Marchand L, Murphy SP, Hankin JH, Wilkens LR, Kolonel LN (2000) Intake of flavonoids and lung cancer. J Natl Cancer I 92:154–160

Lee BM, Lee SK, Kim HS (1998) Inhibition of oxidative DNA damage, 8-OHdG, and carbonyl contents in smokers treated with antioxidants (vitamin E, vitamin C, β-carotene and red ginseng). Cancer Lett 132:219–227

Lee IM, Cook NR, Manson JE, Buring JE, Hennekens CH (1999) β-Carotene supplementation and incidence of cancer and cardiovascular disease: the Women's Health Study. J Natl Cancer I 91:2102–2106

Lykkesfeld J, Viscovich M, Poulsen HE (2003) Ascorbic acid recycling in human erythrocytes is induced by smoking in vivo. Free Radic Biol Med 35:1439–1447

Marangon K, Herbeth B, Lecomte E, Paul-Dauphin A, Grolier P, Chancerelle Y, Artur Y, Siest G (1998) Diet, antioxidant status, and smoking habits in French men. Am J Clin Nutr 67:231–239

Martinelli N, Girelli D, Olivieri O, Stranieri C, Trabetti E, Pizzolo F, Friso S, Tenuti I, Cheng S, Grow MA, Pignatti PF, Corrocher R (2004) Interaction between smoking and PON2 Ser311Cys polymorphism as a determinant of the risk of myocardial infarction. Eur J Clin Invest 34:14–20

Mayne ST (2003) Antioxidant nutrients and chronic disease: use of biomarkers of exposure and oxidative stress status in epidemiologic research. J Nutr 133:S933–S940

Mayne ST, Handelman GJ, Beecher G (1996) β-Carotene and lung cancer promotion in heavy smokers—a plausible relationship? J Natl Cancer I 88:1513–1515

Mayne ST, Cartmel B, Baum M, Shor-Posner G, Fallon BG, Briskin K, Bean J, Zheng T, Cooper D, Friedman C, Goodwin WJJ (2001) Randomized trial of supplemental β-carotene to prevent second head and neck cancer. Cancer Res 61:1457–1463

Mayne ST, Walter M, Cartmel B, Goodwin WJJ, Blumberg J (2004) Supplemental β-carotene, smoking, and urinary F_2-isoprostane excretion in patients with prior early stage head and neck cancer. Nutr Cancer 49:1–6

Mendilaharsu M, De Stefani E, Deneo-Pellegrini H, Carzoglio JC, Ronco A (1998) Consumption of tea and coffee and the risk of lung cancer in cigarette-smoking men: a case-control study in Uruguay. Lung Cancer 19:101–107

Mol MJ, de Rijke YB, Stalenhoef AF (1997) Plasma levels lipid and cholesterol oxidation products and cytokines in diabetes mellitus and cigarette smoking: effects of vitamin E treatment. Atherosclerosis 129:169–176

Moriarty SE, Shah JH, Lynn M, Jiang S, Openo K, Jones DP, Sternberg PJ (2003) Oxidation of gluthathione and cysteine in human plasma associated with smoking. Free Radic Biol Med 35:1582–1588

Morrow JD, Frei B, Longmire AW, Gaziano JM, Lynch SM, Shyr Y, Strauss WE, Oates JA, Roberts LJ (1995) Increase in circulating products of lipid peroxidation (F_2-isoprostanes) in smokers. N Engl J Med 332:1198–1203

Männistö S, Smith-Warner SA, Spiegelman D, Albanes D, Anderson K, van Der Brandt PA, Cerhan JR, Colditz GA, Feskanich D, Freudenheim JL, Giovannucci E, Goldbohm RA, Graham S, Miller AB, Rohan TE, Virtamo J, Willet WC, Hunter DJ (2004) Dietary carotenoids and risk of lung cancer in a pooled analysis of seven cohort studies. Cancer Epidemiol Biomarkers Prev 13:40–48

Neuzil J, Thomas SR, Stocker R (1997) Requirement for, promotion, or inhibition by alpha-tocopherol of radical-induced initiation of plasma lipoproteins and lipid peroxidation. Free Radic Biol Med 22:57–71

Omaye ST, Krinsky NI, Kagan VE, Mayne ST, Liebler DC, Bidlack WR (1997) β-Carotene: friend or foe? Fundam Appl Toxicol 46:163–174

Omenn GS, Goodman GE, Thornquist MD, Balmes J, Cullen MR, Glass A, Keogh JP, Meyskens FL, Valanis B, Williams JH, Barnhart S, Hammar S (1996) Effects of combination of β-carotene and vitamin A on lung cancer and cardiovascular disease. N Engl J Med 334:1150–1155

Palozza P, Serini S, Di Nicuolo F, Boninsegna A, Torsello A, Maggiano N, Ranelletti FO, Wolf FI, Calviello G, Cittadini A (2004) β-Carotene exacerbates DNA oxidative damage and modifies p53-related pathways of cell proliferation and apoptosis in cultured cells exposed to tobacco smoke condensate. Carcinogenesis 25:1315–1325

Paolini M, Abdel-Rahman SZ, Sapone A, Pedulli GF, Perocco P, Cantelli-Forti G, Legator MS (2003) β-Carotene: a cancer chemopreventive agent of a co-carcinogen? Mutat Res 543:195–200

Patrignani P, Panara MR, Tacconelli S, Seta F, Bucciarelli T, Ciabattoni G, Alessandrini P, Mezzetti A, Santini G, Sciulli MG, Cipollone F, Davi G, Gallina P, Bon GB, Patrono C (2000) Effects of vitamin E supplementation of F_2-isoprostane and thromboxane biosynthesis in healthy cigarette smokers. Circulation 102:539–545

Pfeifer GP, Denissenko MF, Olivier M, Tretyakova N, Hecht SS, Hainaut P (2002) Tobacco smoke, DNA damage and *p53* mutations in smoking-associated cancers. Oncogene 21:7435–7451

Pilz H, Oguogho A, Chehne F, Lupattelli G, Palumbo B, Sinzinger H (2000) Quitting cigarette smoking results in a fast improvement of in vivo oxidation injury (determined via plasma, serum and urinary isoprostane). Thromb Res 99:209–221

Polidori MC, Mecocci P, Stahl W, Sies H (2003) Cigarette smoking cessation increases plasma levels of several antioxidant micronutrients and improves resistance towards oxidative challenge. Br J Nutr 90:147–150

Prieme H, Loft S, Klarlund M, Gronbaek K, Tonnesen P, Poulsen HE (1998) Effect of smoking cessation on oxidative DNA modification estimated by 8-oxo-7,8-dihydro-2'-deoxyguanosine excretion. Carcinogenesis 19:347–351

Princen HM, van Duyvenvoorde W, Buytenhek R, Blonk C, Tijburg LB, Langius JA, Meinders AE, Pijl H (1998) No effect of consumption of green and black tea on plasma lipid antioxidant level and on LDL oxidation in smokers. Arterioscl Throm Vas 18:833–841

Reilly M, Delanty N, Lawson JA, FitzGerald GA (1996) Modulation of oxidant stress in vivo in chronic cigarette smokers. Circulation 94:19–25

Rice-Evans C, Miller NJ (1994) Total antioxidant status in plasma and body fluids. Methods Enzymol 234:279–293

Richard MJ, Portal B, Meo J, Coudray C, Hadjian A, Favier A (1992) Malondialdehyde kit evaluated for determining plasma and lipoprotein fractions that react with thiobarbituric acid. Clin Chem 38:704–709

Salonen JT (2000) Markers of oxidative damage and antioxidant protection: assessment of LDL oxidation. Free Radic Res 33:41–46

Siems W, Capuozzo E, Crifo C, Sommerburg O, Langhans C-D, Schlipalius L, Wiswedel I, Kraemer K, Salerno C (2003) Carotenoid cleavage products modify respiratory burst and induce apoptosis of human neutrophils. Biochim Biophys Acta 1639:27–33

Spencer JP, Jenner A, Chimel K, Aromaa OI, Cross CE, Wu R, Halliwell B (1995) DNA damage in human respiratory tract epithelial cells: damage by gas phase cigarette smoke apparently involves attack by reactive nitrogen species in addition to oxygen radicals. FEBS Lett 375:179–182

Theron AJ, Richard GA, Myer MS, van Antwerpen VL, Sluis-Cremer GK, Wolmarans L, van der Merwe CA, Anderson R (1994) Investigation of the relative contributions of cigarette smoking and mineral dust exposure to activation of circulating phagocytes, alterations in plasma concentrations of vitamin C, vitamin E, and beta-carotene, and pulmonary dysfunction in South African gold miners. Occup Environ Med 51:564–567

Traber MG, Winklhofer-Roob BM, Roob JM, Khoschsorur G, Aigner R, Cross C, Ramakrishnan R, Birgelius-Flohe R (2001) Vitamin E kinetics in smokers and non-smokers. Free Radic Biol Med 31:1368–1374

Tröbs M, Renner T, Scherer G, Heller W-D, Geis HC, Wolfram G, Haas G-M, Schwandt P (2002) Nutrition, antioxidants, and risk factor profile of non-smokers, passive smokers and smokers of the prevention education program (PEP) in Nuremberg, Germany. Prev Med 34:600–607

van den Berg R, van Vliet T, Broekmans WM, Cnubben NH, Vaes WH, Roza L, Haenen GR, Bast A, van den Berg H (2001) A vegetable/fruit concentrate with high antioxidant capacity has no effect on biomarkers of antioxidant status in male smokers. J Nutr 131:1714–1722

Vigna GB, Constantini F, Aldini G, Carini M, Catapano A, Schena F, Tangerini A, Zanca R, Bombardelli E, Morazzoni P, Mezzetti A, Fellin R, Maffei Facino R (2003) Effect of standardized grape seed extract on low-density lipoprotein susceptibility to oxidation in heavy smokers. Metabolism 52:1250–1257

Virtamo J (1999) Vitamins and lung cancer. Proc Nutr Soc 58:329–333

Virtamo J, Rapola JM, Ripatti S, Heinonen OP, Taylor PR, Albanes D, Huttunen JK (1998) Effect of vitamin E and β-carotene on the incidence of primary nonfatal myocardial infarction and fatal coronary heart disease. Arch Intern Med 158:668–675

Walmsley CM, Bates CJ, Prentice A, Cole TJ (1999) Relationship between cigarette smoking and nutrient intakes and blood status indices of older people living in the UK: further analysis of data from the National Diet and Nutrition Survey of people aged 65 years and over, 1994/95. Pub Health Nutr 2:199–208

Weinberg RB, VanderWerken BS, Anderson RA, Stegner JE, Thomas MJ (2001) Pro-oxidant effect of vitamin E in cigarette smokers consuming a high polyunsaturated fat diet. Arterioscl Throm Vas 21:1029–1033

Welch RW, Turley E, Sweetman SF, Kennedy G, Collins AR, Dunne A, Livingstone MB, McKenna PG, McKelvey-Martin VJ, Strain JJ (1999) Dietary antioxidant supplementation and DNA damage in smokers and nonsmokers. Nutr Cancer 34:167–172

Wickens AP (2001) Ageing and the free radical theory. Respir Physiol 128:379–391

Young JF, Dragstedt LO, Haraldsdottir J, Daneshvar B, Kal MA, Loft S, Nilsson L, Nielsen SE, Mayer B, Skibsted LH, Huynh-Ba T, Hermetter A, Sandström B (2002) Green tea extract only affects markers of oxidative status postprandially: lasting antioxidant effect of flavonoid-free diet. Br J Nutr 87:343–355

Zhong L, Goldberg MS, Gao YT, Hanley JA, Parent ME, Jin F (2001) A population-based case-control study of lung cancer and green tea consumption among women living in Shanghai, China. Epidemiology 12:695–700

Chapter 9

Smoking Depletes Vitamin C: Should Smokers Be Recommended to Take Supplements?

Jens Lykkesfeldt

Contents

9.1	Introduction	238
9.2	The Antioxidant Activity of Vitamin C	239
9.3	Vitamin C Homeostasis in Smokers	240
9.3.1	The RDA for Vitamin C in Smokers	241
9.3.2	Repletion of Vitamin C in Smokers	243
9.4	Prevalence and Clinical Significance of Low Vitamin C Status	243
9.4.1	Severe Vitamin C Deficiency	244
9.4.2	Marginal Vitamin C Deficiency	245
9.4.3	Suboptimal Vitamin C Status	246
9.5	The Pros of Vitamin C Supplementation to Smokers	247
9.6	The Cons of Vitamin C Supplementation to Smokers	248
9.7	Conclusion	250
	References	251

9.1 Introduction

Smoking has been identified as one of the major risk factors in human diseases such as atherosclerosis and several cancers (Doll et al. 1994; Mosca et al. 1997; Palmer 1985; Stein et al. 1993), yet approximately one third of the Western World's adult population continues to smoke (WHO Health for All Database 2000). Among other factors, oxidative stress has been suggested to play an important role as initiator of the pathological conditions resulting from tobacco smoking (Colditz et al. 1987; Frei et al. 1991; Genkinger et al. 2004; Gey 1986; Hirvonen et al. 2000; Macfarlane et al. 1995; Poulsen et al. 1998; Pryor and Stone 1993). Because cigarette smoke has been shown to result in increased oxidative stress as measured by a variety of biochemical markers, it has been speculated that increased consumption of fruits and vegetables rich in antioxidants or even specific antioxidant supplements could perhaps be particularly beneficial to smokers (Ames 1998; Ames and Gold 1998; Ames and Wakimoto 2002; Ames et al. 1995;). Indeed, numerous reports have shown that cigarette smokers have lower plasma concentrations of almost all low-molecular-weight antioxidants (Eiserich et al. 1995; Kallner et al. 1981; Lykkesfeldt et al. 1997; Munro et al. 1997). This condition results from at least two factors, one of diet and one of smoking (Dietrich et al. 2003; Lykkesfeldt et al. 1996, 2000; Schectman 1993; Schectman et al. 1991). Thus, because of the consumption of a diet containing more fat and less fruits and vegetables, smokers have a lower intake of a variety of phytonutrients, compared with nonsmokers (Dallongeville et al. 1998; Faruque et al. 1995; Jarvinen et al. 1994; Larkin et al. 1990; Ma et al. 2000; Marangon et al. 1998a; Morabia and Wynder, 1990; Preston, 1991; Serdula et al. 1996; Zondervan et al. 1996). However, in addition to dietary differences, it has been shown in studies correcting for dietary intakes of antioxidants, that in particular, vitamin C is further depleted by the smoke itself (Dietrich et al. 2003; Lykkesfeldt et al. 1996, 2000; Schectman et al. 1991). So the question remains: Should supplementation with vitamin C among smokers be a higher priority for health professionals?

A high intake of fruits and vegetables has long been associated with a reduced risk of developing cardiovascular disease and cancer (Knekt et al. 1991b). A critical evaluation of the cancer-related literature by the International Agency for Research on Cancer under the World Health Organization recently confirmed this and concluded that there was evidence, albeit limited, for a beneficial effect of fruits and vegetables on some types of cancers (mouth, pharynx, esophagus, stomach, colorectal, larynx, lung, ovary, bladder and kidney), but insufficient evidence for a beneficial effect on all other cancer types (International Agency for Research on Cancer WHO 2005). It has been suggested that particularly the antioxidant content of the fruits and vegetables could be responsible for the beneficial effect. In agreement with this notion, longitudinal studies have linked low plasma concentrations of antioxidants to increased risk of developing, e.g., lung and prostate cancer and cardiovascular disease (Eichholzer et al. 1996; Knekt et al. 1991a, 1994).

In contrast, large prospective studies using antioxidant supplements have been less promising. Thus, none of the major clinical studies using mortality or morbidity as end points has found significant positive effects of supplementation with such as vitamin C, vitamin E, or β-carotene (Blot et al. 1993; Heart Protection Study Collaborative Group 2002; Miller III et al. 2005). In contrast to the negative results of these larger studies, many smaller or more specific studies suggest a beneficial role of vitamin C supplementation. For example, the Antioxidant Supplementation in Atherosclerosis Prevention (ASAP) Study found that in male smokers, a combination of vitamins C and E could retard atherosclerotic progression in hypercholesterolemic subjects as measured by carotid intima thickness (Salonen et al. 2000, 2003). Also, high doses of vitamin C given by infusion have been shown to improve the endothelial dysfunction typically observed in smokers (Traber et al. 2000). Moreover, numerous studies using surrogate markers of disease such as, e.g., lipid peroxidation have shown a positive effect of antioxidant supplementation (Carr and Frei 1999b). Finally, most in vitro studies have suggested a positive effect with increasing vitamin C concentrations (Carr and Frei 1999a).

Thus, whereas unequivocal evidence appears to exist supporting the observation that smoking results in lower plasma concentrations of vitamin C, the clinical significance of this depletion—beyond that of scurvy—remains to be clarified. Studies of the possible beneficial effect of antioxidant supplementation to smokers have produced ambiguous data. However, it should not be overlooked that a substantial part of the population in the developed countries apparently suffers from subclinical vitamin C deficiency that may well affect both short- and long-term health, and could easily be cured. This chapter examines the clinical significance of long-term low vitamin C status in smokers and the current pros and cons of supplementing smokers with vitamin C.

9.2 The Antioxidant Activity of Vitamin C

Vitamin C, or ascorbic acid, is a simple, low-molecular-weight carbohydrate, yet its enediol structure provides it with a highly complex chemistry. Of its many chemical properties, the monoanion ascorbate—the predominant form of vitamin C at physiological pH—fulfills the criteria of an effective antioxidant (Halliwell 1996). In fact, the electron donor properties of ascorbate account for all its known functions. It has a complicated redox chemistry that involves comparatively stable radical intermediates and is heavily influenced by the acidic properties of the molecule. It has been known for many years that ascorbate is easily oxidized by molecular oxygen. The two-electron oxidation product in this reaction is dehydroascorbic acid (DHA), which also has antiscorbutic properties and is readily converted back to amino acids in vivo by both chemical and enzymatic means (Poulsen et al. 2004). Further oxidation/hydrolysis renders the vitamin inactive by leading to the irreversible formation of 2,3-diketoglulonate as well as oxalate, threonate, and other products (Poulsen et al. 2004). DHA has a half-life of only a few minutes at physiological pH (Bode et al. 1990). Consequently, highly efficient ways of regenerating ascorbate in vivo have evolved. These processes are of major importance in maintaining ascorbate in its active reduced state—in particular in species that lack the ability to synthesize ascorbate such as humans.

Vitamin C plays a pivotal role in the antioxidant defense. The molecule has been called the most important water-soluble antioxidant in biological fluids (Frei et al. 1989, 1990) and has earned this honor for several reasons. Chemically speaking, both ascorbate and its one-electron oxidation product ascorbate free radical have remarkably low one-electron reduction potentials of +282 and –174 mV, respectively (Buettner 1993), placing ascorbate at the bottom of the antioxidant hierarchy. This means that on top of the ability to reduce virtually all physiologically relevant oxidants, ascorbate is capable of regenerating other antioxidants such as vitamin E from the α-tocopheroxyl radical and glutathione from the glutathiyl radical back into their active states (Buettner and Schafer 2004). Equally importantly, the relative stability of the ascorbate free radical renders it a harmless intermediate incapable of inducing free radical damage itself. Instead, at physiological pH, the ascorbate free radical primarily disproportionates via dimer formation into one molecule of ascorbate and one of DHA (Buettner and Schafer 2004). DHA is subsequently recycled by means of either glutathione- or NADPH-dependent dehydroascorbic acid reductases (Del Bello et al. 1994; May et al. 1997, 2001; Park and Levine 1996; Wells and Xu, 1994; Wells et al. 1990, 1995).

Whereas the more electrochemical evidence outlined above suggests that ascorbate is indeed a unique antioxidant, in vitro experiments have confirmed that ascorbate plays a key role in the antioxidant defense as a whole. For example, Frei and coworkers have shown under a variety of oxidizing conditions—including that of cigarette smoke—that ascorbate is the only antioxidant capable of completely preventing lipid oxidation in plasma and once ascorbate is depleted; lipid hydroperoxides are formed despite the presence of other plasma antioxidants such as α-tocopherol and β-carotene (Frei et al. 1988, 1991; Gokce and Frei 1996; Lynch et al. 1994; McCall and Frei 1999). These and other findings suggest that the presence of adequate amounts of vitamin C in particular could be of major importance for the maintenance of redox homeostasis in vivo.

9.3 Vitamin C Homeostasis in Smokers

It has been known since the 1950s that smoking results in lower vitamin C in plasma (Pelletier 1968, 1970); however, the precise mechanism of this effect has still not been fully characterized.

Several epidemiological studies have demonstrated that smokers have a lower intake of phytonutrients—including antioxidants—compared with nonsmokers (Dallongeville et al. 1998; Faruque et al. 1995; Jarvinen et al. 1994; Larkin et al. 1990; Marangon et al. 1998b; Morabia and Wynder 1990; Preston 1991; Serdula et al. 1996; Zondervan et al. 1996). This has hampered the ability to distinguish between effects of smoking and diet on the depletion of antioxidants consistently observed among smokers. In a large epidemiological study, the National Health and Nutrition Examination Survey (NHANES), Schectman et al. compared the vitamin C intake and plasma vitamin C concentrations of smokers consuming >1, 1, or <1 pack of cigarettes per day, and nonsmokers, who had stopped smoking <1 year ago, >1 year ago, or had never smoked (Schectman et al. 1990). The results showed that smokers and nonsmokers who had stopped smoking within the last year had a markedly lower intake of vitamin C, compared with that of never smokers. However, as the effect of smoking on the plasma concentration of vitamin C persisted even when corrected for dietary intake, they concluded that depletion of vitamin C as a result of smoking presumably occurs predominantly via mechanisms independent of dietary intake (Schectman et al. 1990). In agreement with this conclusion, clinical studies adjusting for differences in vitamin C intake, and those assessing populations with similar fruit and vegetable intake have found that smokers have lower plasma vitamin C concentrations than have nonsmokers (Dietrich et al. 2001; Lykkesfeldt et al. 2000; Marangon et al. 1998a). Moreover, smoking cessation quickly results in a substantial elevation of plasma vitamin C concentrations, apparently independent of dietary changes (Lykkesfeldt et al. 1996). These results all suggest that smoking per se predisposes to lower vitamin C status.

In their latest report, the Food and Nutrition Board (2000) recommended that the RDA for vitamin C for smokers be increased to 125 and 110 mg/day for men and women, respectively, compared with those for nonsmokers of 90 and 75 mg/day. The basis for this recommendation was primarily the study by Kallner and coworkers (1981) showing increased metabolic turnover of vitamin C in smokers, compared with nonsmokers. They found a vitamin C turnover among smokers of 70 mg/day, compared with 36 mg/day in nonsmokers, suggesting that smokers need an additional 34 mg vitamin C per day.

As mentioned above, the actual mechanisms by which the vitamin C status is compromised remains less well characterized. However, many data point toward increased oxidative stress as the mediator of this effect. One puff of cigarette smoke has been estimated to contain as many as 10^{15} of gas-phase radicals and 10^{14} of tar-phase radicals (Pryor and Stone 1993). Evidently, it has been suggested that oxidative stress arising directly from the toxicity of the smoke itself can increase vitamin C turnover (Pryor 1997). Also, smoke-induced inflammatory responses may indirectly increase oxidative stress, thereby contributing to the turnover of vitamin C (Anderson 1991; Elneihoum et al. 1997; Langlois et al. 2001a; Lehr et al. 1997). Whether directly or indirectly, cigarette smoke results in an increase vitamin C oxidation ratio (%DHA of total vitamin C) among smokers (Lykkesfeldt et al. 1997). This suggests that vitamin C acts as a free radical scavenger in smokers but could also be because of an impairment of the enzymatic recycling of vitamin C. However, in a recent report, it was shown that recycling of vitamin C is, in fact, increased in smokers, and that this activity is not related to differences in vitamin C transport, glutathione concentration, or cellular energy status (Lykkesfeldt et al. 2003b). From these results, it may be concluded that the rate of vitamin C oxidation exceeds that of the DHA reductases in smokers (Lykkesfeldt et al. 2003b). Other studies have suggested that differences in vitamin C status between smokers and nonsmokers be unrelated to altered pharmacokinetics, although possible differences in sodium-dependent vitamin C transport has not been accounted for (Lykkesfeldt et al. 2003a; Viscovich et al. 2004). Taken together with the observed increased oxidative damage among smokers as measured by biochemical markers, the evidence is building up for an oxidative stress mediated depletion of vitamin C.

9.3.1 The RDA for Vitamin C in Smokers

In the debate against or in favor of antioxidant supplementation to smokers, one of the major points of discussion has been how to determine the proper RDA for smokers. Although smokers have been shown to have lower plasma concentrations of several antioxidants, only the RDA for vitamin C has so far been increased. Based on the data outlined above, this seems appropriate because the depletion of antioxidants other than vitamin C appears to result primarily from altered dietary habits. However, the question remains: How is the correct RDA for vitamin C in smokers determined?

As mentioned previously, the Food and Nutrition Board (2000) currently recommends an RDA for vitamin C for smokers of 125 and 110 mg/day for men and women, respectively. However, Schectman and coworkers proposed a higher RDA for smokers, based on their comprehensive material from the second NHANES (II) (Schectman 1993; Schectman et al. 1989, 1990, 1991). By simply plotting the serum level of vitamin C on the daily intake of vitamin C for smokers and nonsmokers separately, they were able to show that smokers would require a daily intake of 200 mg vitamin C to achieve the serum concentration of nonsmokers consuming 60 mg vitamin C per day (the previous RDA for vitamin C), i.e., resulting in serum levels around 70 µM (Schectman et al. 1990).

In another approach to this problem, Levine and coworkers (1995, 1996b, 1997) studied vitamin C pharmacokinetics in detail. They found that in nonsmokers, consumption of 60 mg of vitamin C per day resulted in a plasma concentration around 25 µM, i.e., considerably less than the concentration indicated by Schectman's data, whereas ingestion of 200 mg vitamin C per day resulted in a plasma concentration of about 66 µM (Levine et al. 1996b). Higher doses did not increase plasma concentrations considerably, and doses above 500 mg were largely excreted unabsorbed. Based on their studies, Levine et al. concluded that the RDA for vitamin C should be increased to 200 mg per day.

Using DHA as biomarker of smoking-induced oxidative stress added a new way of estimating an increased vitamin C requirement in smokers (Lykkesfeldt et al. 1997). Lykkesfeldt et al. (1997) found no DHA in the plasma of nonsmokers regardless of their vitamin C status, whereas a significant inverse correlation between plasma DHA and plasma vitamin C was observed in smokers. Complete reduction of DHA was maintained and not different from that of nonsmokers for plasma vitamin C concentrations higher than 70 µM. Consequently, the data could be interpreted as supporting an RDA for smokers that result in a plasma concentration of about 70 µM. Based on the data from Schectman et al. (1990) and in agreement with their conclusions, this would require an intake of 200 mg vitamin C per day.

An equally important aspect of an increased RDA for vitamin C for smokers is the possibility of getting the recommended amount of vitamin C through the regular diet. Dietary guidelines currently recommend five to nine servings per day of fruits and vegetables (National Research Council 1990). However, several studies suggest that only a relative small proportion of the US population routinely has an intake in the recommended range (Krebs-Smith et al. 1995; Munoz et al. 1997; Rogers et al. 1995). Moreover, as mentioned previously, considerable evidence has been presented to demonstrate that smokers constitute a relative large part of those having a low intake of fruits and vegetables (Dallongeville et al. 1998; Faruque et al. 1995; Jarvinen et al. 1994; Larkin et al. 1990; Marangon et al. 1998b; Morabia and Wynder 1990; Preston, 1991; Serdula et al. 1996; Zondervan et al. 1996). In contrast to this reality, a daily intake of 200 mg vitamin C has been estimated by the Food and Nutrition Board to require the consumption of a minimum of five servings per day of fruits and vegetables. Thus, conforming to the guidelines for fruit and vegetable consumption will result in nonsmokers getting more than 2-fold their current RDA for vitamin C, whereas smokers would get about 1.5 times their RDA and indeed, the 200 mg per day suggested above. However, a significant dietary modification would be required for most smokers to overcome their increased risk of hypovitaminosis C (Schectman 1993). As this may be practically impossible for many, supplementation with vitamin C may be necessary to reduce the prevalence of low plasma ascorbate concentrations of smokers to rates acceptable for nonsmokers. These considerations have warranted studies to investigate the effects of vitamin C supplementation in smokers in particular.

In the 2000 revision of the RDA for vitamin C from the Food and Nutrition Board (2000), the overwhelming evidence supporting an important role of vitamin C in the defense against oxidative stress was taken into account for the first time. Indeed, the current RDA for vitamin C is primarily based on the intake necessary to achieve about 80% saturation of neutrophils (Levine et al. 2004). In contrast, previous recommendations were based primarily on clinical evidence, i.e., the prevention of scurvy and hypovitaminosis C. This acceptance of biochemical evidence in support of a higher RDA for vitamin C may well result in the RDA for smokers being further increased in the future.

9.3.2 Repletion of Vitamin C in Smokers

Ever since it became clear half a century ago that smoking apparently predisposes to lower vitamin C status, there have been speculations regarding the possible beneficial effect of antioxidant supplementation. Although it would seem very unlikely that antioxidant supplementation alone should be able to prevent the multiple deleterious effects of smoking, there has been an obvious interest in trying to counter the depletion of antioxidants in smokers: (1) it fits the basic theory of smoking-induced oxidative stress and damage, (2) oxidative stress has been suggested to play an important role as initiator of the pathological conditions resulting from smoking, and (3) plasma concentrations of antioxidants are easily elevated by daily administration of a multivitamin pill. However, one adverse effect may be that these studies can unintentionally detract the focus from the only known effective remedy against smoking-related diseases: to stop smoking. In other words, the smokers may be waiting for a miracle.

As pointed out above, some controversy still exists on the proper RDA for vitamin C for smokers. However, the fact that an increased RDA for smokers exists may be interpreted as acceptance of the basic idea that vitamin C supplementation can be a treatment of oxidative stress caused by smoking. Numerous studies of vitamin C intervention in smokers have been published over the past four decades (Carr and Frei 1999b; Traber et al. 2000). Most studies have used doses between 500 mg and 2 g of vitamin C per day, and found plasma levels saturating around 70 µmol/l. Sodium-dependent vitamin-C transporter 1 (SVCT1) activity, responsible for both primary absorption in the intestine and secondary reabsorption in the kidney, is dependent on the concentration of vitamin C, and the kidney threshold for active tubular reabsorption is around 70µmol/l (MacDonald et al. 2002; Oreopoulos et al. 1993). Based on the detailed pharmacokinetics provided by Levine et al. (1996b) as well as what could realistically be obtained from a diet rich in fruits and vegetables, it has been shown that only 250 mg of vitamin C per day can restore plasma vitamin C levels in poorly nourished smokers from an average of only 23 µmol/l to that of near saturation around 70 µmol/l (Lykkesfeldt et al. 2000). These data also provide indirect evidence that intestinal and renal SVCT1 activity is not impaired by smoking, and that decreased SVCT1 capacity cannot explain the depletion of vitamin C among smokers.

9.4 Prevalence and Clinical Significance of Low Vitamin C Status

Although the definition of optimal vitamin C status remains a matter of some controversy, the opinions appear to converge around the level of apparent saturation, i.e., a plasma concentration of approximately 70 µmol/l (Carr and Frei 1999b; Levine et al. 1995, 1996b, 1997, 2004). Defining vitamin C deficiency is equally complex, because considerable individual variation exists regarding the relationship between the plasma concentration of vitamin C and the classical hallmark of severe vitamin C deficiency: scurvy (Newton et al. 1985; Schorah et al. 1979). Moreover, the clinical significance of vitamin C deficiency—beyond that of scurvy—has not been clearly defined. Guidelines developed by the National Survey of Canada suggested categories of "severe vitamin C deficiency" (serum level <11 µmol/l) and "marginal vitamin C deficiency" (serum levels between 11 and 23 µmol/l) (Smith and Hodges 1987). As the RDA for vitamin C has been increased since these categories were put forward in 1987, and considering the believed optimal vitamin C level in plasma of 70 µmol/l, a new category (e.g., for serum levels between 23 and, e.g., 50 µmol/l) should be added and could be termed "suboptimal vitamin C status."

9.4.1 Severe Vitamin C Deficiency

Scurvy is normally the clinical manifestation of prolonged and severe vitamin C deficiency. In nonsmokers, scurvy is prevented by a daily intake of as little as 10 mg of vitamin C (Weber et al. 1996b). Clinical symptoms include follicular hyperkeratosis, petechiae, ecchymoses, coiled hairs, inflamed and bleeding gums, perifollicular hemorrhages, joint effusions, arthralgia, and impaired wound heeling (Chazan and Mistilis 1963). Other symptoms include dyspnea, weakness, fatigue, and depression. Scurvy usually occurs in individuals with plasma concentrations lower than 11 µmol/l, i.e., those diagnosed as having severe vitamin C deficiency. However, far from all individuals with plasma levels <11 µmol/l actually develop clinical scurvy (Newton et al. 1985; Schorah et al. 1979). Thus, the relationship between plasma vitamin C status and scurvy is not entirely clear.

Although the basic symptoms and cure of the disease have been known for centuries, a significant part of the population in developed countries—and the smokers in particular—suffer from severe vitamin C deficiency and thus have increased risk of experiencing scurvy-like symptoms. Data from the NHANES II (11,592 subjects, collected from 1976–1980) show that of all smokers (including those taking vitamin C supplements), 7.4% suffered from severe vitamin C deficiency, compared with 1.9% of the nonsmokers, giving rise to a risk odds ratio relative to smoking of 3.0 after adjusting for vitamin C intake (Schectman et al. 1989). A Swiss study of more than 4,000 employees came to the same conclusion (Ritzel and Bruppacher 1977). More recent data suggest that the incidence of severe vitamin C deficiency in developed countries is not declining, but may actually be increasing, although improved analytical methodology may also account for a more accurate categorization of the population as older methods may have overestimated vitamin C (Lykkesfeldt, 2002; Washko et al. 1992). Regardless, data from NHANES III (15,769 subjects, collected from 1988 to 1994) showed that in the United States, 14% of males and 10% of females suffered from severe vitamin C deficiency (Hampl et al. 2004). Of smokers, the numbers were 31 and 25%, respectively. The third Glasgow Multinational Monitoring of Trends and Determinants in Cardiovascular Disease (MONICA) population survey (1,267 subjects) found 26% of males and 14% of females suffered severe vitamin C deficiency (Wrieden et al. 2000). Among the smokers alone, the numbers were 36 and 23% of men and women, respectively (Wrieden et al. 2000). A French population study (1,039 subjects) found severe vitamin C deficiency in 7 to 12% of men and 3 to 5% of women, depending on age group (Hercberg et al. 1994).

The clinical significance of severe vitamin C deficiency extends beyond that of scurvy. In clinical studies in which subjects were made vitamin C deficient, common complaints as gingival inflammation and fatigue were among the most sensitive markers of deficiency (Leggott et al. 1986, Levine et al. 1996b). In a prospective population study, Nyyssönen et al. (1997) found a higher risk of myocardial infarction (relative risk, 3.5) among men with severe vitamin C deficiency constituting about 6% of their Finnish cohort (1,605 subjects). Moreover, Langlois et al. (2001b) recently showed that 14% of patients with peripheral arterial disease suffered from severe vitamin C deficiency as compared with none of the healthy controls and suggested a relationship between vitamin C status and severity of atherosclerosis. In a study with advanced cancer patients, 30% had severe vitamin C deficiency and these patients had shorter survival (Mayland et al. 2005).

9.4.2 Marginal Vitamin C Deficiency

As defined above, plasma concentrations between 11 and 23 µmol/l constitutes a situation of marginal vitamin C deficiency. Hypovitaminosis C has been characterized as having a plasma concentration of vitamin C <23 µmol/l (Schectman 1993), i.e., encompassing both severe and marginal vitamin C deficiency. As with severe vitamin C deficiency, smokers also have increased risk of marginal vitamin C deficiency. Thus in the NHANES II, 19.7% of the smokers showed marginal vitamin C deficiency, compared with 8.2% of the nonsmokers (Schectman et al. 1989). The Scottish MONICA Study found marginal vitamin C deficiency among 30% of smoking men, compared with 22% of nonsmoking men and 30% of smoking women, compared with 16% of nonsmoking women (Wrieden et al. 2000). In the cohort as a whole, the numbers were 26 and 22% for men and women, respectively (Wrieden et al. 2000). In the NHANES III, marginal vitamin C deficiency was found in 20% of males and 17% of females, the upper limit of the group being set at 28 µmol/l (Hampl et al. 2004). In a Parisian cohort, 10–46% of males and 3–15% of females had plasma vitamin C concentrations between 11 and 19 µmol/l, depending on the age group (Hercberg et al. 1994). These data clearly demonstrate that a substantial part of the populations in the developed countries can be diagnosed with vitamin C deficiency.

The clinical significance of marginal vitamin C deficiency—as isolated from severe vitamin C deficiency—has not been thoroughly investigated. In most studies, upper and lower tertiles, quartiles, or quintiles are compared, making it difficult to compare groups between studies. Consequently, the category of marginal vitamin C deficiency can rarely be singled out from all vitamin C deficiency/hypovitaminosis C. With respect to scurvy, clinical cases among people with marginal vitamin C deficiency are rare, but do occur (Hodges et al. 1971; Reuler et al. 1985). Probably more importantly, considerable epidemiological evidence suggests that there may other clinical consequences of marginal vitamin C deficiency. Thus, in a recent reexamination of the NHANES II data combined with a follow-up on vital status 12–16 years later, Loria et al. (2000) found that men in the lowest (<28.4 µmol/l), compared with the highest (>73.8 µmol/l) serum ascorbate quartile had a 57% higher risk of death from any cause and a 62% higher risk of dying from cancer. A similar conclusion was reached by Simon et al. (2001), who also found that severe or marginal vitamin C deficiency was significantly associated with all-cause mortality while being weakly associated with death from cardiovascular disease.

In a 20-year follow study in Britain (730 subjects), significantly higher risk of mortality from stroke was observed in elderly men and women with severe and marginal vitamin C deficiency separately, compared with those with plasma concentrations of vitamin C >28 μmol/l (Gale et al. 1995). The authors concluded that vitamin C status was as strong a predictor of death from stroke as diastolic blood pressure (Gale et al. 1995). An inverse correlation between vitamin C status and stroke was also reported from a study (2,121 subjects) in a rural Japanese population, aged 40 years or more (Yokoyama et al. 2000). In the 12-year follow-up on the Basel Prospective Study, significantly increased risk of ischemic heart disease and stroke was found in individuals with plasma ascorbate <22.7 μmol/l, corresponding to severe or marginal vitamin C deficiency (Gey et al. 1987, 1993a, b).

9.4.3 Suboptimal Vitamin C Status

Based on the increased RDA for vitamin C as well as the indication that a plasma concentration of vitamin C of about 70 μmol/L is currently considered optimal for health, a new category of suboptimal vitamin C status is reasonable for those individuals with plasma concentrations between 23 and about 50 μmol/l. The obvious rationale for this additional category could be that if 70 μmol/l is optimal, e.g., 35 μmol/l is probably not, and therefore, investigations into the clinical significance of a suboptimal vitamin C status are warranted. However, limited data are available and need to be extracted from the few studies discriminating between the concentrations of suboptimal and optimal vitamin C status.

In the Coronary Artery Risk Development in Young Adults (CARDIA) Study, Simon et al. (2004) divided 2,637 subjects (originally enrolled as young adults, aged 18–30 years) into four groups with respect to plasma vitamin C levels, and their "low normal" group (between 23 and 45 μmol/l) corresponds approximately that of suboptimal vitamin C status. At the 10-year follow-up, 26% of the smokers suffered from severe or marginal vitamin C deficiency, whereas about 40% had suboptimal vitamin C status. Among the never smokers, the numbers were 8 and 33%, respectively (Simon et al. 2004). At a 15-year follow-up, they found that low vitamin C status (as measured at 10 years) was associated with a higher prevalence of coronary artery calcium among men but not women. Statistics was not performed individually on the male low-normal group having an odds ratio of 2.09 to 1, compared with the "saturation" group (plasma vitamin C level >62.5 μmol/l). In a larger population sample of 8,453 subjects, aged 30 years or older from the NHANES II, a similar prevalence for vitamin C deficiency or suboptimal vitamin C status among smokers was observed. Thirty percent of the smokers suffered from severe or marginal vitamin C deficiency, whereas 35% had suboptimal vitamin C status (plasma vitamin C between 23 and 55 μmol/l). Among never smokers, the numbers were 9 and 31%, respectively (Simon et al. 2001).

Several large prospective studies have shown an inverse relationship between plasma vitamin C status and risk of cardiovascular disease and/or all-cause mortality (Eichholzer et al. 1996; Gale et al. 1995; Khaw et al. 2001; Loria et al. 2000; Nyyssonen et al. 1997; Riemersma et al. 1991; Sahyoun et al. 1996; Singh et al. 1995). However, no studies have investigated the specific clinical significance of suboptimal vitamin C status as compared with the optimal. Thus, it remains to be established if the biochemical evidence pointing toward an optimal plasma level around 70 μmol/l can be backed up in larger epidemiological studies or clinical trials. Clearly, the effects of suboptimal, compared with optimal vitamin C status are likely to be at most moderate and presumably relevant only in the long perspective, if at all. Thus, it is debatable if studies aimed at clarifying such a limited risk are feasible bearing the high cost in mind. On the other hand, the problems potentially associated with low vitamin C status affects a large percentage of the population and can be readily and inexpensively cured.

9.5 The Pros of Vitamin C Supplementation to Smokers

As outlined above, it is well established that smoking predisposes to low vitamin C status. However, whereas it is questionable if smokers in general are capable of conforming to such a significant modification of their diet as would be required to comply with the dietary guidelines (Schectman 1993), moderate amounts (250 mg) of vitamin C given as supplement saturates even poorly nourished smokers (Lykkesfeldt et al. 2000). Thus, the inability of most smokers to comply with dietary guidelines indirectly supports the recommendation of supplements. In addition, supplementing smokers with moderate amounts of vitamin C is safe. Moreover, the bioavailability of vitamin C from supplements is not different from that of vitamin C from natural sources (Johnston and Luo 1994; Mangels et al. 1993). The amount needed to supply smokers is far from the tolerable upper intake level (UL) of 2 g/day of the Food and Nutrition Board's most recent reference values (2000). A large body of evidence agrees that ingestion of <500 mg/day poses no significant risk to human health, and even several-fold higher daily doses of vitamin C have indicated low toxicity (Johnston 1999). Unfortunately, those currently eating supplements are the least likely to need them (Kirk et al. 1999; McNaughton et al. 2005; Sinha et al. 1994). One might add that they are also the least likely to benefit from them, as saturation kinetics will result in excretion of surplus amounts. Supplementing smokers with vitamin C will shift this balance toward those most likely to need and benefit from them. In the NHANES II, 63% of those suffering from severe or marginal vitamin C were smokers and in this group; only 1% of both smokers and nonsmokers used vitamin C or multivitamin supplements (Loria et al. 2000). In the NHANES III, only 7% of male and 5% of female users of any supplement suffered from severe vitamin C deficiency (Hampl et al. 2004). Thus, supplementing smokers with vitamin C will substantially lower the risk of smokers suffering from scurvy-like symptoms, including those of weakness, fatigue, and depression.

Another part of the rationale for supplementing smokers with vitamin C is based on the so-called oxidation theory of atherosclerosis in which oxidized low-density lipoprotein (LDL) lipid is thought to play a key role in the initiation and progression of the disease (reviewed recently by Witting and Stocker 2004). Other hallmarks of atherosclerosis include endothelial dysfunction and leukocyte adhesion to the endothelium, both of which are increased in smokers (Kalra et al. 1994; Lehr et al. 1993; Morrow et al. 1995; Vita et al. 1990; Weber et al. 1996a; Zeiher et al. 1991).

As mentioned previously, increased oxidative stress and damage have consistently been observed in smokers. This oxidative stress has been suggested to play an important role as initiator of the pathological conditions resulting from smoking (Colditz et al. 1987; Frei et al. 1991; Genkinger et al. 2004; Gey 1986; Hirvonen et al. 2000; Macfarlane et al. 1995; Poulsen et al. 1998; Pryor and Stone 1993). With respect to atherosclerosis, lipid oxidation has been suggested as an early marker (Steinberg 1997). Consistent with this theory, increasing amounts of F_2-isoprostanes, a marker of lipid oxidation, have been found in smokers (Morrow et al. 1995). Increased amounts of malondialdehyde, another frequently used—albeit more unspecific—marker of lipid peroxidation, has also been found in smokers (Lykkesfeldt et al. 2004). In a recent survey, low vitamin C status was among the strongest predictors of lipid peroxidation (Block et al. 2002). In agreement, vitamin C supplementation has been shown to decrease lipid oxidation in smokers (Dietrich et al. 2002; Helen and Vijayammal, 1997; Motoyama et al. 1997; Nyyssonen et al. 1994; Panda et al. 2000; Valkonen and Kuusi 2000), although not all studies have found an effect (Jacob et al. 2003; Kaikkonen et al. 2001). However, the clinical significance of increased lipid oxidation remains to be further established.

Moving from biomarkers to clinically more relevant studies, vitamin C has been found to improve endothelial dysfunction in smokers, apparently by increasing the bioavailability of nitric oxide (NO) (Antoniades et al. 2003; Carr and Frei 2000; Frei 1999; Heitzer et al. 1996; Kaufmann et al. 2000; Lehr et al. 1997; Levine et al. 1996a; Salonen et al. 1991; Schindler et al. 2000) although conflicting reports also exists (Pellegrini et al. 2004; Raitakari et al. 2000; Scott et al. 2005; Van Hoydonck et al. 2004). The mechanism was initially thought to involve direct scavenging of superoxide radicals (May 2000). However, although intracellular concentrations of ascorbate could potentially be high enough for ascorbate to be able to compete with NO for the reaction with superoxide, the reaction kinetics are unfavorable for ascorbate (Jackson et al. 1998). More recently, it has been shown that vitamin C in physiological amounts can increase the production of NO substantially in human endothelial cell in culture (Heller et al. 1999). The mechanism is believed to involve a vitamin C mediated increase in tetrahydrobiopterin, which increases NO activity via endothelial NO synthase (eNOS) in a dose-dependent manner (Heitzer et al. 2000; Heller et al. 1999; Huang et al. 2000a). High plasma concentrations achieved by infusion have been reported to improve endothelial-dependent vasodilation in, e.g., smokers and patients with type 1 and 2 diabetes and coronary artery disease (Chambers et al. 1999; Gokce et al. 1999; Heitzer et al. 1996; Hornig et al. 1998; Ito et al. 1998; Kugiyama et al. 1998; Levine et al. 1996a; Motoyama et al. 1997; Solzbach et al. 1997; Taddei et al. 1998; Timimi et al. 1998; Ting et al. 1996, 1997). Although unphysiologic levels are achieved, this line of research shows interesting potential—in particular for smokers.

Clinical evidence that vitamin C can actually prevent atherosclerosis is limited, and studies have not been performed in particular with subjects selected for low vitamin C status. In the ASAP Study, the effect of vitamin C, vitamin E, or a combination on carotid intima thickness was studied as a marker of a atherosclerotic progression (Salonen et al. 2000). The authors found that 3 years of supplementation with vitamins C and E in combination—but not vitamin C alone—significantly decreased the intima progression rate in men but not women. Similar results were found at the 6-year follow-up, and the authors concluded that supplementation with vitamins C and E in combination slows down atherosclerotic progression in hypercholesterolemic men (Salonen et al. 2003). Also, another study in women found no effect of vitamins C and E in combination for almost 3 years on the progression of coronary atherosclerosis (Waters et al. 2002).

9.6 The Cons of Vitamin C Supplementation to Smokers

The main problem in recommending vitamin C supplements to smokers can be summarized by looking at two separate observations: (1) smoking predisposes to low vitamin C status and (2) smoking increases the risk of developing chronic diseases such as atherosclerosis and cancer, and every second smoker will die from the habit (Doll et al. 1994; Mosca et al. 1997; Palmer 1985; Stein et al. 1993). The problem is that limited evidence links the two observations, a situation that mainly boils down to the classic issue in epidemiology: Is smoking-induced vitamin C depletion a cause or a consequence of smoking-related diseases?

The few large prospective intervention studies have consistently found no positive effect of vitamin C supplementation on morbidity and mortality (Blot et al. 1993; Greenberg et al. 1994; Heart Protection Study Collaborative Group 2002). However, none of them used vitamin C as a single substance but included β-carotene or vitamin E as well as other antioxidant vitamins and substances. Regardless, the use of vitamin C and other antioxidants for protection against, e.g., cardiovascular disease in high-risk individuals as those in the British Heart Protection Study is difficult to justify (Heart Protection Study Collaborative Group 2002). Notable for the present discussion is that the subjects included in the Heart Protection Study (20,536 subjects) did generally not suffer from severe or marginal vitamin C deficiency, but rather represented the general population in terms of vitamin C status and thus were less likely to benefit from the intervention. In contrast, the subjects included in the vitamin C part of the Linxian (China) Study (about 18,000 subjects) presumably suffered from vitamin C deficiency in general, although this assumption is based on screening of a sample of only 49 individuals showing an average plasma vitamin C concentration of 8.6 µmol/l (Blot et al. 1993). Following 5 years of intervention with 120 mg vitamin C and 30 mg molybdenum per day, the plasma concentration of vitamin C increased to an average of 46.6 µmol/l, i.e., far from saturation. No effect of the intervention was observed on cancer development or mortality while endpoints such as scurvy symptoms were not included. Only 1% of the deaths among the study participants were attributed to ischemic heath disease, thus limiting the evaluation of intervention effects on this endpoint. As pointed out by the authors, the 5-year duration of the study may have been too short to monitor any effects on cancer incidence, but it might be added that the 120 mg of vitamin C was apparently insufficient to saturate the intervention group with vitamin C, and this may also have impacted the results. Moreover, the main causes of death in Linxian differ from those of the developed countries in that the incidence of cardiovascular disease is considerably lower and that of, e.g., epithelial cancers is extraordinarily high presumably because of dietary and lifestyle differences.

With respect to cancer prevention, clinical intervention trials with vitamin C using surrogate endpoints such as oxidative DNA damage have also been unpromising (reviewed recently by Poulsen et al. 2004). Thus, most studies found no effect of vitamin C supplementation on markers of DNA damage, typically in urine or lymphocytes (Anderson et al. 1997; Brennan et al. 2000; Green et al. 1994; Huang et al. 2000b; Jacobson et al. 2000; Lee et al. 1998; Panayiotidis and Collins, 1997; Porkkala-Sarataho et al. 2000; Prieme et al. 1997; Proteggente et al. 2000; Vojdani et al. 2000; Welch et al. 1999; White et al. 2002; Witt et al. 1992), although positive reports also exist (de la Asuncion et al. 1996; Howard et al. 1998; Moller et al. 2004; Rehman et al. 1998; Schneider et al. 2001).

A different aspect of vitamin C supplementation is the actual timing. For example, should the dose be increase in case of disease or should supplementation be discontinued? High plasma concentrations achieved by infusion have been found to improve, e.g., endothelial-dependent vasodilation. However, vitamin C homeostasis is normally under a tight control, maintaining the concentration within a narrow range at steady state (Levine et al. 2004). This could suggest that higher "unphysiologic" levels are potentially either directly toxic perhaps because of the often-discussed prooxidant effect of vitamin C, or indirectly because putative regulatory function could be lost when vitamin C concentrations in general approach regulatory levels. Excess levels of oxidants are important for, e.g., activation of internal cellular cascades of apoptosis that again are involved in the protective mechanisms that kill cancer cells and also critical for effective cancer treatment (Blumenthal et al. 2000; Kuipers and Lafleur 1998; Weijl et al. 1997). As pointed out by Zeisel (2004), indiscriminate use of high-dose antioxidant supplements should probably be avoided, at least until the potential risks and benefits have been more clearly characterized.

A completely different reservation against recommending vitamin C supplementation to smokers may be that such action could be interpreted as a potential "cure" for smoking-related diseases and thereby take the wind out of the long-preferred and simple message to the smokers: The only known effective remedy against smoking-related diseases is to quit in time. If vitamin C supplements are eventually recommended particularly to smokers, it is crucial that the potential perspectives—or lack of—are kept in mind and communicated unambiguously. Clearly, vitamin C supplements only have the potential of relieving a relative small part of the problems associated with smoking.

9.7 Conclusion

Whereas considerable literature has identified an inverse correlation between vitamin C status and mortality, the current evidence is primarily of epidemiological nature and thus lacks the ability to establish causality. None of the large prospective intervention studies with vitamin C have been able to establish this causality, which should be kept in mind regardless of the fact that the studies were not designed to look at poorly nourished people with a Western lifestyle, i.e., the group most likely to immediately benefit from such intervention.

However, the fact that a substantial part of the population of the developed countries are suffering from subclinical vitamin C deficiency taken together with the potential health problems and expenses for society associated with this condition as well as its easy and inexpensive cure, demonstrates that action is urgently needed to establish if vitamin C supplements to this part of the population is associated with improved health.

Those presumably in need of vitamin C supplements are the least likely to ingest them. Smokers that currently do not take supplements constitute the largest subpopulation that would potentially benefit from vitamin C supplements because a major proportion remains at increased risk of vitamin C deficiency because of poor dietary habits and the enormous voluntary oxidant exposure. A likely short-term benefit from such a supplementation may be a substantially decreased risk of suffering from scurvy-like symptoms, including weakness, fatigue, and depression. Whether a long-tern benefit exists in terms of lower incidence of cardiovascular disease and cancers can only be established by large controlled clinical trials. Thus, it is important that future studies focus on individuals with a low daily intake of vitamin C. Controlled studies are needed to clarify further the long-term consequences of low vitamin C status in both smokers and the general population as well as the clinical effects of moderate supplementation with vitamin C to these specific individuals. There appears to be a good chance of a value-for-money health benefit for a considerable part of the population.

References

(2000) Dietary reference intakes for vitamin C, vitamin E, selenium and carotenoids: a report of the Panel on Dietary Antioxidants and Related Compounds, Subcommittees on Upper Reference Levels of Nutrients and of the Interpretation and Use of Dietary Reference Intakes, and the Standing Committee on the Scientific Evaluation of Dietary Reference Intakes, Food and Nutrition Board, Institute of Medicine, National Academy of Sciences. National Academy Press, Washington D.C

(1994) The effect of vitamin E and beta carotene on the incidence of lung cancer and other cancers in male smokers. The Alpha-Tocopherol, Beta Carotene Cancer Prevention Study Group. N Engl J Med 330:1029–1035

(1990) Diet and health: implications for reducing chronic disease risk. National Research Council. National Academy Press, Washington D.C

Ames BN (1998) Micronutrients prevent cancer and delay aging. Toxicol Lett 102–103:5–18

Ames BN, Gold LS (1998) The prevention of cancer. Drug Metab Rev 30:201–223

Ames BN, Gold LS, Willett WC (1995) The causes and prevention of cancer. Proc Natl Acad Sci U S A 92:5258–5265

Ames BN, Wakimoto P (2002) Are vitamin and mineral deficiencies a major cancer risk? Nat Rev Cancer 2:694–704

Anderson D, Phillips BJ, Yu TW, Edwards AJ, Ayesh R, Butterworth KR (1997) The effects of vitamin C supplementation on biomarkers of oxygen radical generated damage in human volunteers with "low" or "high" cholesterol levels. Environ Mol Mutagen 30:161–174

Anderson R (1991) Assessment of the roles of vitamin C, vitamin E, and beta-carotene in the modulation of oxidant stress mediated by cigarette smoke-activated phagocytes. Am J Clin Nutr 53:S358–S361

Antoniades C, Tousoulis D, Tentolouris C, Toutouza M, Marinou K, Goumas G, Tsioufis C, Toutouzas P, Stefanadis C (2003) Effects of antioxidant vitamins C and E on endothelial function and thrombosis/fibrinolysis system in smokers. Thromb Haemost 89:990–995

Block G, Dietrich M, Norkus EP, Morrow JD, Hudes M, Caan B, Packer L (2002) Factors associated with oxidative stress in human populations. Am J Epidemiol 156:274–285

Blot WJ, Li JY, Taylor PR, Guo W, Dawsey S, Wang GQ, Yang CS, Zheng SF, Gail M, Li GY (1993) Nutrition intervention trials in Linxian, China: supplementation with specific vitamin/mineral combinations, cancer incidence, and disease-specific mortality in the general population. J Natl Cancer Inst 85:1483–1492

Blumenthal RD, Lew W, Reising A, Soyne D, Osorio L, Ying Z, Goldenberg DM (2000) Anti-oxidant vitamins reduce normal tissue toxicity induced by radio-immunotherapy. Int J Cancer 86:276–280

Bode AM, Cunningham L, Rose RC (1990) Spontaneous decay of oxidized ascorbic acid (dehydro-L-ascorbic acid) evaluated by high-pressure liquid chromatography. Clin Chem 36:1807–1809

Brennan LA, Morris GM, Wasson GR, Hannigan BM, Barnett YA (2000) The effect of vitamin C or vitamin E supplementation on basal and H2O2-induced DNA damage in human lymphocytes. Br J Nutr 84:195–202

Buettner GR (1993) The pecking order of free radicals and antioxidants: lipid peroxidation, alpha-tocopherol, and ascorbate. Arch Biochem Biophys 300:535–543

Buettner GR, Schafer FQ (2004) Ascorbate as an antioxidant. In: Asard H, May JM, Smirnoff N (eds) Vitamin C: its functions and biochemistry in animals and plants. BIOS Scientific, Oxford, pp 173–188

Carr A, Frei B (2000) The role of natural antioxidants in preserving the biological activity of endothelium-derived nitric oxide. Free Radic Biol Med 28:1806–1814

Carr A, Frei B (1999a) Does vitamin C act as a pro-oxidant under physiological conditions? FASEB J 13:1007–1024

Carr AC, Frei B (1999b) Toward a new recommended dietary allowance for vitamin C based on antioxidant and health effects in humans. Am J Clin Nutr 69:1086–1107

Chambers JC, McGregor A, Jean-Marie J, Obeid OA, Kooner JS (1999) Demonstration of rapid onset vascular endothelial dysfunction after hyperhomocysteinemia: an effect reversible with vitamin C therapy. Circulation 99:1156–1160

Chazan JA, Mistilis SP (1963) The pathophysiology of scurvy. A report of seven cases. Am J Med 34:350–358

Colditz GA, Stampfer MJ, Willett WC (1987) Diet and lung cancer. A review of the epidemiologic evidence in humans. Arch Intern Med 147:157–160

Dallongeville J, Marecaux N, Fruchart JC, Amouyel P (1998) Cigarette smoking is associated with unhealthy patterns of nutrient intake: a meta-analysis. J Nutr 128:1450–1457

de la Asuncion JG, Millan A, Pla R, Bruseghini L, Esteras A, Pallardo FV, Sastre J, Vina J (1996) Mitochondrial glutathione oxidation correlates with age-associated oxidative damage to mitochondrial DNA. FASEB J 10:333–338

Del Bello B, Maellaro E, Sugherini L, Santucci A, Comporti M, Casini, AF (1994) Purification of NADPH-dependent dehydroascorbate reductase from rat liver and its identification with 3 alpha-hydroxysteroid dehydrogenase. Biochem J 304:385–390

Dietrich M, Block G, Hudes M, Morrow JD, Norkus EP, Traber MG, Cross CE, Packer L (2002) Antioxidant supplementation decreases lipid peroxidation biomarker F2-isoprostanes in plasma of smokers. Cancer Epidemiol Biomarkers Prev 11:7–13

Dietrich M, Block G, Norkus EP, Hudes M, Traber MG, Cross CE, Packer L (2001) Plasma antioxidant status in passive smokers, smokers, and nonsmokers with adjustment for dietary intake. Proceedings of the Second International Conference on Oxidative Stress and Aging, April 2001, Maui, HI

Dietrich M, Block G, Norkus EP, Hudes M, Traber MG, Cross CE, Packer L (2003) Smoking and exposure to environmental tobacco smoke decrease some plasma antioxidants and increase gamma-tocopherol in vivo after adjustment for dietary antioxidant intakes. Am J Clin Nutr 77:160–166

Doll R, Peto R, Wheatley K, Gray R, Sutherland I (1994) Mortality in relation to smoking: 40 years' observations on male British doctors. Brit Med J 309:901–911

Eichholzer M, Stahelin HB, Gey KF, Ludin E, Bernasconi F (1996) Prediction of male cancer mortality by plasma levels of interacting vitamins: 17-year follow-up of the prospective Basel study. Int J Cancer 66:145–150

Eiserich JP, van d, V, Handelman GJ, Halliwell B, Cross CE (1995) Dietary antioxidants and cigarette smoke-induced biomolecular damage: a complex interaction. Am J Clin Nutr 62:S1490–S1500

Elneihoum AM, Falke P, Hedblad B, Lindgarde F, Ohlsson K (1997) Leukocyte activation in atherosclerosis: correlation with risk factors. Atherosclerosis 131:79–84

Faruque MO, Khan MR, Rahman MM, Ahmed F (1995) Relationship between smoking and antioxidant nutrient status. Brit J Nutr 73:625–632

Frei B (1999) On the role of vitamin C and other antioxidants in atherogenesis and vascular dysfunction. Proc Soc Exp Biol Med 222:196–204

Frei B, England L, Ames BN (1989) Ascorbate is an outstanding antioxidant in human blood plasma. Proc Natl Acad Sci U S A 86:6377–6381

Frei B, Forte TM, Ames BN, Cross CE (1991) Gas phase oxidants of cigarette smoke induce lipid peroxidation and changes in lipoprotein properties in human blood plasma. Protective effects of ascorbic acid. Biochem J 277:133–138

Frei B, Stocker R, Ames BN (1988) Antioxidant defenses and lipid peroxidation in human blood plasma. Proc Natl Acad Sci U S A 85:9748–9752

Frei B, Stocker R, England L, Ames BN (1990) Ascorbate: the most effective antioxidant in human blood plasma. Adv Exp Med Biol 264:155–163

Gale CR, Martyn CN, Winter PD, Cooper C (1995) Vitamin C and risk of death from stroke and coronary heart disease in cohort of elderly people. BMJ 310:1563–1566

Genkinger JM, Platz EA, Hoffman SC, Comstock GW, Helzlsouer KJ (2004) Fruit, vegetable, and antioxidant intake and all-cause, cancer, and cardiovascular disease mortality in a community-dwelling population in Washington County, Maryland. Am J Epidemiol 160:1223–1233

Gey KF (1986) On the antioxidant hypothesis with regard to arteriosclerosis. Bibl Nutr Dieta 53–91

Gey KF, Moser UK, Jordan P, Stahelin HB, Eichholzer M, Ludin E (1993a) Increased risk of cardiovascular disease at suboptimal plasma concentrations of essential antioxidants: an epidemiological update with special attention to carotene and vitamin C. Am J Clin Nutr 57:S787–S797

Gey KF, Stahelin HB, Eichholzer M (1993b) Poor plasma status of carotene and vitamin C is associated with higher mortality from ischemic heart disease and stroke: Basel Prospective Study. Clin Investig 71:3–6

Gey KF, Stahelin HB, Puska P, Evans A (1987) Relationship of plasma level of vitamin C to mortality from ischemic heart disease. Ann N Y Acad Sci 498:110–123

Gokce N, Frei B (1996) Basic research in antioxidant inhibition of steps in atherogenesis. J Cardiovasc Risk 3:352–357

Gokce N, Keaney JF Jr, Frei B, Holbrook M, Olesiak M, Zachariah BJ, Leeuwenburgh C, Heinecke JW, Vita JA (1999) Long-term ascorbic acid administration reverses endothelial vasomotor dysfunction in patients with coronary artery disease. Circulation 99:3234–3240

Green MH, Lowe JE, Waugh AP, Aldridge KE, Cole J, Arlett CF (1994) Effect of diet and vitamin C on DNA strand breakage in freshly-isolated human white blood cells. Mutat Res 316:91–102

Greenberg ER, Baron JA, Tosteson TD, Freeman DH Jr, Beck GJ, Bond JH, Colacchio TA, Coller JA, Frankl HD, Haile RW (1994) A clinical trial of antioxidant vitamins to prevent colorectal adenoma. Polyp Prevention Study Group. N Engl J Med 331:141–147

Halliwell B (1996) Vitamin C: antioxidant or pro-oxidant in vivo? Free Radic Res 25:439–454

Hampl JS, Taylor CA, Johnston CS (2004) Vitamin C deficiency and depletion in the United States: the Third National Health and Nutrition Examination Survey, 1988 to 1994. Am J Public Health 94:870–875

Heart Protection Study Collaborative Group (2002) MRC/BHF Heart Protection Study of antioxidant vitamin supplementation in 20,536 high-risk individuals: a randomised placebo-controlled trial. Lancet 360:23–33

Heitzer T, Brockhoff C, Mayer B, Warnholtz A, Mollnau H, Henne S, Meinertz T, Munzel T (2000) Tetrahydrobiopterin improves endothelium-dependent vasodilation in chronic smokers : evidence for a dysfunctional nitric oxide synthase. Circ Res 86:E36–E41

Heitzer T, Just H, Munzel T (1996) Antioxidant vitamin C improves endothelial dysfunction in chronic smokers. Circulation 94:6–9

Helen A, Vijayammal PL (1997) Vitamin C supplementation on hepatic oxidative stress induced by cigarette smoke. J Appl Toxicol 17:289–295

Heller R, Munscher-Paulig F, Grabner R, Till U (1999) L-Ascorbic acid potentiates nitric oxide synthesis in endothelial cells. J Biol Chem 274:8254–8260

Hercberg S, Preziosi P, Galan P, Devanlay M, Keller H, Bourgeois C, Potier dC, Cherouvrier F (1994) Vitamin status of a healthy French population: dietary intakes and biochemical markers. Int J Vitam Nutr Res 64:220–232

Hirvonen T, Virtamo J, Korhonen P, Albanes D, Pietinen P (2000) Intake of flavonoids, carotenoids, vitamins C and E, and risk of stroke in male smokers. Stroke 31:2301–2306

Hodges RE, Hood J, Canham JE, Sauberlich HE, Baker EM (1971) Clinical manifestations of ascorbic acid deficiency in man. Am J Clin Nutr 24:432–443

Hornig B, Arakawa N, Kohler C, Drexler H (1998) Vitamin C improves endothelial function of conduit arteries in patients with chronic heart failure. Circulation 97:363–368

Howard DJ, Ota RB, Briggs LA, Hampton M, Pritsos CA (1998) Oxidative stress induced by environmental tobacco smoke in the workplace is mitigated by antioxidant supplementation. Cancer Epidemiol Biomarkers Prev 7:981–988

Huang A, Vita JA, Venema RC, Keaney JF Jr (2000a) Ascorbic acid enhances endothelial nitric-oxide synthase activity by increasing intracellular tetrahydrobiopterin. J Biol Chem 275:17399–17406

Huang HY, Helzlsouer KJ, Appel LJ (2000b) The effects of vitamin C and vitamin E on oxidative DNA damage: results from a randomized controlled trial. Cancer Epidemiol Biomarkers Prev 9:647–652

International Agency for Research on Cancer WHO (2005) vol. 8: Fruit and vegetables

Ito K, Akita H, Kanazawa K, Yamada S, Terashima M, Matsuda Y, Yokoyama M (1998) Comparison of effects of ascorbic acid on endothelium-dependent vasodilation in patients with chronic congestive heart failure secondary to idiopathic dilated cardiomyopathy versus patients with effort angina pectoris secondary to coronary artery disease. Am J Cardiol 82:762–767

Jackson TS, Xu A, Vita JA, Keaney JF Jr (1998) Ascorbate prevents the interaction of superoxide and nitric oxide only at very high physiological concentrations. Circ Res 83:916–922

Jacob RA, Aiello GM, Stephensen CB, Blumberg JB, Milbury PE, Wallock LM, Ames BN (2003) Moderate antioxidant supplementation has no effect on biomarkers of oxidant damage in healthy men with low fruit and vegetable intakes. J Nutr 133:740–743

Jacobson JS, Begg MD, Wang LW, Wang Q, Agarwal M, Norkus E, Singh VN, Young TL, Yang D, Santella RM (2000) Effects of a 6-month vitamin intervention on DNA damage in heavy smokers. Cancer Epidemiol Biomarkers Prev 9:1303–1311

Jarvinen R, Knekt P, Seppanen R, Reunanen A, Heliovaara M, Maatela J, Aromaa A (1994) Antioxidant vitamins in the diet: relationships with other personal characteristics in Finland. J Epidemiol Community Health 48:549–554

Johnston CS (1999) Biomarkers for establishing a tolerable upper intake level for vitamin C. Nutrition Reviews 57:71–77

Johnston CS, Luo B (1994) Comparison of the absorption and excretion of three commercially available sources of vitamin C. J Am Diet Assoc 94:779–781

Kaikkonen J, Porkkala-Sarataho E, Morrow JD, Roberts LJ, Nyyssonen K, Salonen R, Tuomainen TP, Ristonmaa U, Poulsen HE, Salonen JT (2001) Supplementation with vitamin E but not with vitamin C lowers lipid peroxidation in vivo in mildly hypercholesterolemic men. Free Radic Res 35:967–978

Kallner AB, Hartmann D, Hornig DH (1981) On the requirements of ascorbic acid in man: steady-state turnover and body pool in smokers. Am J Clin Nutr 34:1347–1355

Kalra VK, Ying Y, Deemer K, Natarajan R, Nadler JL, Coates TD (1994) Mechanism of cigarette smoke condensate induced adhesion of human monocytes to cultured endothelial cells. J Cell Physiol 160:154–162

Kaufmann PA, Gnecchi-Ruscone T, di TM, Schafers KP, Luscher TF, Camici PG (2000) Coronary heart disease in smokers: vitamin C restores coronary microcirculatory function. Circulation 102:1233–1238

Khaw KT, Bingham S, Welch A, Luben R, Wareham N, Oakes S, Day N (2001) Relation between plasma ascorbic acid and mortality in men and women in EPIC-Norfolk prospective study: a prospective population study. European Prospective Investigation into Cancer and Nutrition. Lancet 357:657–663

Kirk SF, Cade JE, Barrett JH, Conner M (1999) Diet and lifestyle characteristics associated with dietary supplement use in women. Public Health Nutr 2:69–73

Knekt P, Jarvinen R, Seppanen R, Rissanen A, Aromaa A, Heinonen OP, Albanes D, Heinonen M, Pukkala E, Teppo L (1991a) Dietary antioxidants and the risk of lung cancer. Am J Epidemiol 134:471–479

Knekt P, Jarvinen R, Seppanen R, Rissanen A, Aromaa A, Heinonen OP, Albanes D, Heinonen M, Pukkala E, Teppo L (1991b) Dietary antioxidants and the risk of lung cancer [see comments]. Am J Epidemiol 134:471–479

Knekt P, Reunanen A, Jarvinen R, Seppanen R, Heliovaara M, Aromaa A (1994) Antioxidant vitamin intake and coronary mortality in a longitudinal population study. Am J Epidemiol 139:1180–1189

Krebs-Smith SM, Cook A, Subar AF, Cleveland L, Friday J (1995) US adults' fruit and vegetable intakes, 1989 to 1991: a revised baseline for the Healthy People 2000 objective. Am J Pub Health 85:1623–1629

Kugiyama K, Motoyama T, Hirashima O, Ohgushi M, Soejima H, Misumi K, Kawano H, Miyao Y, Yoshimura M, Ogawa H, Matsumura T, Sugiyama S, Yasue H (1998) Vitamin C attenuates abnormal vasomotor reactivity in spasm coronary arteries in patients with coronary spastic angina. J Am Coll Cardiol 32:103–109

Kuipers GK, Lafleur MV (1998) Characterization of DNA damage induced by gamma-radiation-derived water radicals, using DNA repair enzymes. Int J Radiat Biol 74:511–519

Langlois M, Duprez D, Delanghe J, De BM, Clement DL (2001a) Serum vitamin C concentration is low in peripheral arterial disease and is associated with inflammation and severity of atherosclerosis. Circulation 103:1863–1868

Langlois M, Duprez D, Delanghe J, De Buyzere M, Clement DL (2001b) Serum vitamin C concentration is low in peripheral arterial disease and is associated with inflammation and severity of atherosclerosis. Circulation 103:1863–1868

Larkin FA, Basiotis PP, Riddick HA, Sykes KE, Pao EM (1990) Dietary patterns of women smokers and non-smokers. J Am Diet Assoc 90:230–237

Lee BM, Lee SK, Kim HS (1998) Inhibition of oxidative DNA damage, 8-OHdG, and carbonyl contents in smokers treated with antioxidants (vitamin E, vitamin C, beta-carotene and red ginseng). Cancer Lett 132:219–227

Leggott PJ, Robertson PB, Rothman DL, Murray PA, Jacob RA (1986) The effect of controlled ascorbic acid depletion and supplementation on periodontal health. J Periodontol 57:480–485

Lehr HA, Kress E, Menger MD, Friedl HP, Hubner C, Arfors KE, Messmer K (1993) Cigarette smoke elicits leukocyte adhesion to endothelium in hamsters: inhibition by CuZn-SOD. Free Radic Biol Med 14:573–581

Lehr HA, Weyrich AS, Saetzler RK, Jurek A, Arfors KE, Zimmerman GA, Prescott SM, McIntyre TM (1997) Vitamin C blocks inflammatory platelet-activating factor mimetics created by cigarette smoking. J Clin Invest 99:2358–2364

Levine GN, Frei B, Koulouris SN, Gerhard MD, Keaney JF Jr, Vita JA (1996a) Ascorbic Acid Reverses Endothelial Vasomotor Dysfunction in Patients With Coronary Artery Disease. Circulation 93:1107–1113

Levine M, Conry-Cantilena C, Wang Y, Welch RW, Washko PW, Dhariwal KR, Park JB, Lazarev A, Graumlich JF, King J, Cantilena LR (1996b) Vitamin C pharmacokinetics in healthy volunteers: evidence for a recommended dietary allowance. Proc Natl Acad Sci U S A 93:3704–3709

Levine M, Dhariwal KR, Welch RW, Wang Y, Park JB (1995) Determination of optimal vitamin C requirements in humans. Am J Clin Nutr 62:S1347–S1356

Levine M, Padayatty SJ, Katz A, Kwon O, Eck P, Corpe C, Lee J-H, Wang Y (2004) Dietary allowances for vitamin C: recommended dietary allowances and optimal nutrient ingestion. In: Asard H, May JM, Smirnoff N (eds) Vitamin C: its functions and biochemistry in animals and plants. BIOS Scientific, Oxford, pp 291–317

Levine M, Rumsey S, Wang Y (1997) Principles involved in formulating recommendations for vitamin C intake: a paradigm for water-soluble vitamins. Methods Enzymol 279:43–54

Loria CM, Klag MJ, Caulfield LE, Whelton PK (2000) Vitamin C status and mortality in US adults. Am J Clin Nutr 72:139–145

Lykkesfeldt J (2002) Measurement of ascorbic acid and dehydroascorbic acid in biological samples. In: Maines M, Costa LG, Hodson E, Reed JC (eds) Current protocols in toxicology. Wiley, New York, pp 7.6.1–7.6.15

Lykkesfeldt J, Bolbjerg ML, Poulsen HE (2003a) Effect of smoking on erythorbic acid pharmacokinetics. Br J Nutr 89:667–671

Lykkesfeldt J, Christen S, Wallock LM, Chang HH, Jacob RA, Ames BN (2000) Ascorbate is depleted by smoking and repleted by moderate supplementation: a study in male smokers and nonsmokers with matched dietary antioxidant intakes. Am J Clin Nutr 71:530–536

Lykkesfeldt J, Loft S, Nielsen JB, Poulsen HE (1997) Ascorbic acid and dehydroascorbic acid as biomarkers of oxidative stress caused by smoking. Am J Clin Nutr 65:959–963

Lykkesfeldt J, Prieme H, Loft S, Poulsen HE (1996) Effect of smoking cessation on plasma ascorbic acid concentration. Brit Med J 313:91

Lykkesfeldt J, Viscovich M, Poulsen HE (2004) Plasma malondialdehyde is induced by smoking: a study with balanced antioxidant profiles. Br J Nutr 92:203–206

Lykkesfeldt J, Viscovich M, Poulsen HE (2003b) Ascorbic acid recycling in human erythrocytes is induced by smoking in vivo. Free Radic Biol Med 35:1439–1447

Lynch SM, Morrow JD, Roberts LJ, Frei B (1994) Formation of non-cyclooxygenase-derived prostanoids (F2-isoprostanes) in plasma and low density lipoprotein exposed to oxidative stress in vitro. J Clin Invest 93:998–1004

Ma J, Hampl JS, Betts NM (2000) Antioxidant intakes and smoking status: data from the continuing survey of food intakes by individuals 1994–1996. Am J Clin Nutr 71:774–780

MacDonald L, Thumser AE, Sharp P (2002) Decreased expression of the vitamin C transporter SVCT1 by ascorbic acid in a human intestinal epithelial cell line. Br J Nutr 87:97–100

Macfarlane GJ, Zheng T, Marshall JR, Boffetta P, Niu S, Brasure J, Merletti F, Boyle P (1995) Alcohol, tobacco, diet and the risk of oral cancer: a pooled analysis of three case-control studies. European J Cancer B Oral Oncol 31B:181–187

Mangels AR, Block G, Frey CM, Patterson BH, Taylor PR, Norkus EP, Levander OA (1993) The bioavailability to humans of ascorbic acid from oranges, orange juice and cooked broccoli is similar to that of synthetic ascorbic acid. J Nutr 123:1054–1061

Marangon K, Herbeth B, Lecomte E, Paul-Dauphin A, Grolier P, Chancerelle Y, Artur Y, Siest G (1998a) Diet, antioxidant status, and smoking habits in French men. Am J Clin Nutr 67:231–239

Marangon K, Herbeth B, Lecomte E, Paul-Dauphin A, Grolier P, Chancerelle Y, Artur Y, Siest G (1998b) Diet, antioxidant status, and smoking habits in French men. Am J Clin Nutr 67:231–239

May JM (2000) How does ascorbic acid prevent endothelial dysfunction? Free Radic Biol Med 28:1421–1429

May JM, Mendiratta S, Hill KE, Burk RF (1997) Reduction of dehydroascorbate to ascorbate by the selenoenzyme thioredoxin reductase. J Biol Chem 272:22607–22610

May JM, Qu Z, Morrow JD (2001) Mechanisms of ascorbic acid recycling in human erythrocytes. Biochim Biophys Acta 1528:159–166

Mayland CR, Bennett MI, Allan K (2005) Vitamin C deficiency in cancer patients. Palliat Med 19:17–20

McCall MR, Frei B (1999) Can antioxidant vitamins materially reduce oxidative damage in humans? Free Radic Biol Med 26:1034–1053

McNaughton SA, Mishra GD, Paul AA, Prynne CJ, Wadsworth MEJ (2005) Supplement use is associated with health status and health-related behaviors in the 1946 British birth cohort. J Nutr 135:1782–1789

Miller ER, III, Pastor-Barriuso R, Dalal D, Riemersma RA, Appel LJ, Guallar E (2005) Meta-analysis: high-dosage vitamin E supplementation may increase all-cause mortality. Ann Intern Med 142:37–46

Moller P, Viscovich M, Lykkesfeldt J, Loft S, Jensen A, Poulsen HE (2004) Vitamin C supplementation decreases oxidative DNA damage in mononuclear blood cells of smokers. Eur J Nutr 43:267–274

Morabia A, Wynder EL (1990) Dietary habits of smokers, people who never smoked, and exsmokers. Am J Clin Nutr 52:933–937

Morrow JD, Frei B, Longmire AW, Gaziano JM, Lynch SM, Shyr Y, Strauss WE, Oates JA, Roberts LJ (1995) Increase in circulating products of lipid peroxidation (F2-isoprostanes) in smokers. Smoking as a cause of oxidative damage. N Engl J Med 332:1198–1203

Mosca L, Rubenfire M, Tarshis T, Tsai A, Pearson T (1997) Clinical predictors of oxidized low-density lipoprotein in patients with coronary artery disease. Am J Cardiol 80:825–830

Motoyama T, Kawano H, Kugiyama K, Hirashima O, Ohgushi M, Yoshimura M, Ogawa H, Yasue H (1997) Endothelium-dependent vasodilation in the brachial artery is impaired in smokers: effect of vitamin C. Am J Physiol 273:H1644–H1650

Munoz KA, Krebs-Smith SM, Ballard-Barbash R, Cleveland LE (1997) Food intakes of US children and adolescents compared with recommendations. Pediatrics 100:323–329

Munro LH, Burton G, Kelly FJ (1997) Plasma *RRR*-alpha-tocopherol concentrations are lower in smokers than in non-smokers after ingestion of a similar oral load of this antioxidant vitamin. Clin Sci (Lond) 92:87–93

Newton HM, Schorah CJ, Habibzadeh N, Morgan DB, Hullin RP (1985) The cause and correction of low blood vitamin C concentrations in the elderly. Am J Clin Nutr 42:656–659

Nyyssonen K, Porkkala E, Salonen R, Korpela H, Salonen JT (1994) Increase in oxidation resistance of atherogenic serum lipoproteins following antioxidant supplementation: a randomized double-blind placebo-controlled clinical trial. Eur J Clin Nutr 48:633–642

Nyyssonen K, Parviainen MT, Salonen R, Tuomilehto J, Salonen JT (1997) Vitamin C deficiency and risk of myocardial infarction: prospective population study of men from eastern Finland. BMJ 314:634

Oreopoulos DG, Lindeman RD, VanderJagt DJ, Tzamaloukas AH, Bhagavan HN, Garry PJ (1993) Renal excretion of ascorbic acid: effect of age and sex. J Am Coll Nutr 12:537–542

Palmer S (1985) Diet, nutrition, and cancer. Prog Food Nutr Sci 9:283–341

Panayiotidis M, Collins AR (1997) Ex vivo assessment of lymphocyte antioxidant status using the comet assay. Free Radic Res 27:533–537

Panda K, Chattopadhyay R, Chattopadhyay DJ, Chatterjee IB (2000) Vitamin C prevents cigarette smoke-induced oxidative damage in vivo. Free Radic Biol Med 29:115–124

Park JB, Levine M (1996) Purification, cloning and expression of dehydroascorbic acid-reducing activity from human neutrophils: identification as glutaredoxin. Biochem J 315:931–938

Pellegrini MP, Newby DE, Johnston NR, Maxwell S, Webb DJ (2004) Vitamin C has no effect on endothelium-dependent vasomotion and acute endogenous fibrinolysis in healthy smokers. J Cardiovasc Pharmacol 44:117–124

Pelletier O (1968) Smoking and vitamin C levels in humans. Am J Clin Nutr 21:1259–1267

Pelletier O (1970) Vitamin C status of cigarette smokers and nonsmokers. Am J Clin Nutr 23:520–524

Porkkala-Sarataho E, Salonen JT, Nyyssonen K, Kaikkonen J, Salonen R, Ristonmaa U, Diczfalusy U, Brigelius-Flohe R, Loft S, Poulsen HE (2000) Long-term effects of vitamin E, vitamin C, and combined supplementation on urinary 7-hydro-8-oxo-2'-deoxyguanosine, serum cholesterol oxidation products, and oxidation resistance of lipids in nondepleted men. Arterioscler Thromb Vasc Biol 20:2087–2093

Poulsen HE, Loft S, Prieme H, Vistisen K, Lykkesfeldt J, Nyyssonen K, Salonen JT (1998) Oxidative DNA damage in vivo: relationship to age, plasma antioxidants, drug metabolism, glutathione-S-transferase activity and urinary creatinine excretion. Free Radic Res 29:565–571

Poulsen HE, Møller P, Lykkesfeldt J, Weimann A, Loft S (2004) Ascorbic acid and DNA damage. In: Asard H, May JM, Smirnoff N (eds) Vitamin C: its functions and biochemistry in animals and plants. BIOS Scientific, Oxford, pp 189–202

Preston AM (1991) Cigarette smoking—nutritional implications. Prog Food Nutr Sci 15:183–217

Prieme H, Loft S, Nyyssonen K, Salonen JT, Poulsen HE (1997) No effect of supplementation with vitamin E, ascorbic acid, or coenzyme Q10 on oxidative DNA damage estimated by 8-oxo-7,8-dihydro-2'-deoxyguanosine excretion in smokers. Am J Clin Nutr 65:503–507

Proteggente AR, Rehman A, Halliwell B, Rice-Evans CA (2000) Potential problems of ascorbate and iron supplementation: pro-oxidant effect in vivo? Biochem Biophys Res Commun 277:535–540

Pryor WA (1997) Cigarette smoke radicals and the role of free radicals in chemical carcinogenicity. Environ Health Perspect 105:S875–S882

Pryor WA, Stone K (1993) Oxidants in cigarette smoke. Radicals, hydrogen peroxide, peroxynitrate, and peroxynitrite. Ann N Y Acad Sci 686:12–27

Raitakari OT, Adams MR, McCredie RJ, Griffiths KA, Stocker R, Celermajer DS (2000) Oral vitamin C and endothelial function in smokers: short-term improvement, but no sustained beneficial effect. J Am Coll Cardiol 35:1616–1621

Rehman A, Collis CS, Yang M, Kelly M, Diplock AT, Halliwell B, Rice-Evans C (1998) The effects of iron and vitamin C co-supplementation on oxidative damage to DNA in healthy volunteers. Biochem Biophys Res Commun 246:293–298

Reuler JB, Broudy VC, Cooney TG (1985) Adult scurvy. JAMA 253:805–807

Riemersma RA, Wood DA, Macintyre CC, Elton RA, Gey KF, Oliver MF (1991) Risk of angina pectoris and plasma concentrations of vitamins A, C, and E and carotene. Lancet 337:1–5

Ritzel G, Bruppacher R (1977) Vitamin C and tobacco. Int J Vitam Nutr Res 16:171–183

Rogers MA, Simon DG, Zucker LB, Mackessy JS, Newman-Palmer NB (1995) Indicators of poor dietary habits in a high risk population. J Am Coll Nutr 14:159–164

Sahyoun NR, Jacques PF, Russell RM (1996) Carotenoids, vitamins C and E, and mortality in an elderly population. Am J Epidemiol 144:501–511

Salonen JT, Nyyssonen K, Salonen R, Lakka HM, Kaikkonen J, Porkkala-Sarataho E, Voutilainen S, Lakka TA, Rissanen T, Leskinen L, Tuomainen TP, Valkonen VP, Ristonmaa U, Poulsen HE (2000) Antioxidant Supplementation in Atherosclerosis Prevention (ASAP) study: a randomized trial of the effect of vitamins E and C on 3-year progression of carotid atherosclerosis. J Intern Med 248:377–386

Salonen JT, Salonen R, Seppanen K, Rinta-Kiikka S, Kuukka M, Korpela, Alfthan G, Kantola M, Schalch W (1991) Effects of antioxidant supplementation on platelet function: a randomized pair-matched, placebo-controlled, double-blind trial in men with low antioxidant status. Am J Clin Nutr 53:1222–1229

Salonen RM, Nyyssonen K, Kaikkonen J, Porkkala-Sarataho E, Voutilainen S, Rissanen TH, Tuomainen TP, Valkonen VP, Ristonmaa U, Lakka HM, Vanharanta M, Salonen JT, Poulsen HE (2003) Six-year effect of combined vitamin C and E supplementation on atherosclerotic progression: the Antioxidant Supplementation in Atherosclerosis Prevention (ASAP) Study. Circulation 107:947–953

Schectman G (1993) Estimating ascorbic acid requirements for cigarette smokers. Ann N Y Acad Sci 686:335–345

Schectman G, Byrd JC, Gruchow HW (1989) The influence of smoking on vitamin C status in adults. Am J Public Health 79:158–162

Schectman G, Byrd JC, Hoffmann R (1991) Ascorbic acid requirements for smokers: analysis of a population survey. Am J Clin Nutr 53:1466–1470

Schectman G, McKinney WP, Pleuss J, Hoffman RG (1990) Dietary intake of Americans reporting adherence to a low cholesterol diet (NHANES II). Am J Public Health 80:698–703

Schindler TH, Magosaki N, Jeserich M, Olschewski M, Nitzsche E, Holubarsch C, Solzbach U, Just H (2000) Effect of ascorbic acid on endothelial dysfunction of epicardial coronary arteries in chronic smokers assessed by cold pressor testing. Cardiology 94:239–246

Schneider M, Diemer K, Engelhart K, Zankl H, Trommer WE, Biesalski HK (2001) Protective effects of vitamins C and E on the number of micronuclei in lymphocytes in smokers and their role in ascorbate free radical formation in plasma. Free Radic Res 34:209–219

Schorah CJ, Newill A, Scott DL, Morgan DB (1979) Clinical effects of vitamin C in elderly inpatients with low blood-vitamin-C levels. Lancet 1:403–405

Scott DA, Poston RN, Wilson RF, Coward PY, Palmer RM (2005) The influence of vitamin C on systemic markers of endothelial and inflammatory cell activation in smokers and non-smokers. Inflamm Res 54:138–144

Serdula MK, Byers T, Mokdad AH, Simoes E, Mendlein JM, Coates RJ (1996) The association between fruit and vegetable intake and chronic disease risk factors. Epidemiology 7:161–165

Simon JA, Hudes ES, Tice JA (2001) Relation of serum ascorbic acid to mortality among US adults. J Am Coll Nutr 20:255–263

Simon JA, Murtaugh MA, Gross MD, Loria CM, Hulley SB, Jacobs DR Jr (2004) Relation of ascorbic acid to coronary artery calcium: The Coronary Artery Risk Development in Young Adults Study. Am J Epidemiol 159:581–588

Singh RB, Ghosh S, Niaz MA, Singh R, Beegum R, Chibo H, Shoumin Z, Postiglione A (1995) Dietary intake, plasma levels of antioxidant vitamins, and oxidative stress in relation to coronary artery disease in elderly subjects. Am J Cardiol 76:1233–1238

Sinha R, Frey CM, Kammerer WG, McAdams MJ, Norkus EP, Ziegler RG (1994) Importance of supplemental vitamin C in determining serum ascorbic acid in controls from a cervical cancer case-control study: implications for epidemiological studies. Nutr Cancer 22:207–217

Smith JL, Hodges RE (1987) Serum levels of vitamin C in relation to dietary and supplemental intake of vitamin C in smokers and nonsmokers. Ann N Y Acad Sci 498:144–152

Solzbach U, Hornig B, Jeserich M, Just H (1997) Vitamin C improves endothelial dysfunction of epicardial coronary arteries in hypertensive patients. Circulation 96:1513–1519

Stein Y, Harats D, Stein O (1993) Why is smoking a major risk factor for coronary heart disease in hyperlipidemic subjects? Ann N Y Acad Sci 686:66–69

Steinberg D (1997) Low-density lipoprotein oxidation and its pathobiological significance. J Biol Chem 272:20963–20966

Taddei S, Virdis A, Ghiadoni L, Magagna A, Salvetti A (1998) Vitamin C improves endothelium-dependent vasodilation by restoring nitric oxide activity in essential hypertension. Circulation 97:2222–2229

Timimi FK, Ting HH, Haley EA, Roddy MA, Ganz P, Creager MA (1998) Vitamin C improves endothelium-dependent vasodilation in patients with insulin-dependent diabetes mellitus. J Am Coll Cardiol 31:552–557

Ting HH, Timimi FK, Boles KS, Creager SJ, Ganz P, Creager MA (1996) Vitamin C improves endothelium-dependent vasodilation in patients with non-insulin-dependent diabetes mellitus. J Clin Invest 97:22–28

Ting HH, Timimi FK, Haley EA, Roddy MA, Ganz P, Creager MA (1997) Vitamin C improves endothelium-dependent vasodilation in forearm resistance vessels of humans with hypercholesterolemia. Circulation 95:2617–2622

Traber MG, van der Vliet A, Reznick AZ, Cross CE (2000) Tobacco-related diseases. Is there a role for antioxidant micronutrient supplementation? [Review] Clin Chest Med 21:173–187

Valkonen MM, Kuusi T (2000) Vitamin C prevents the acute atherogenic effects of passive smoking. Free Radic Biol Med 28:428–436

Van Hoydonck PG, Schouten EG, Manuel YK, van CA, Hoppenbrouwers KP, Temme EH (2004) Does vitamin C supplementation influence the levels of circulating oxidized LDL, sICAM-1, sVCAM-1 and vWF-antigen in healthy male smokers? Eur J Clin Nutr 58:1587–1593

Viscovich M, Lykkesfeldt J, Poulsen HE (2004) Vitamin C pharmacokinetics of plain and slow-release formulations in smokers. Clin Nutr 23:1043–1050

Vita JA, Treasure CB, Nabel EG, McLenachan JM, Fish RD, Yeung AC, Vekshtein VI, Selwyn AP, Ganz P (1990) Coronary vasomotor response to acetylcholine relates to risk factors for coronary artery disease. Circulation 81:491–497

Vojdani A, Bazargan M, Vojdani E, Wright J (2000) New evidence for antioxidant properties of vitamin C. Cancer Detect Prev 24:508–523

Washko PW, Welch RW, Dhariwal KR, Wang Y, Levine M (1992) Ascorbic acid and dehydroascorbic acid analyses in biological samples. Anal Biochem 204:1–14

Waters DD, Alderman EL, Hsia J, Howard BV, Cobb FR, Rogers WJ, Ouyang P, Thompson P, Tardif JC, Higginson L, Bittner V, Steffes M, Gordon DJ, Proschan M, Younes N, Verter JI (2002) Effects of hormone replacement therapy and antioxidant vitamin supplements on coronary atherosclerosis in postmenopausal women: a randomized controlled trial. JAMA 288:2432–2440

Weber C, Erl W, Weber K, Weber PC (1996a) Increased adhesiveness of isolated monocytes to endothelium is prevented by vitamin C intake in smokers. Circulation 93:1488–1492

Weber P, Bendich A, Schalch W (1996b) Vitamin C and human health—a review of recent data relevant to human requirements. Int J Vitam Nutr Res 66:19–30

Weijl NI, Cleton FJ, Osanto S (1997) Free radicals and antioxidants in chemotherapy-induced toxicity. Cancer Treat Rev 23:209–240

Welch RW, Turley E, Sweetman SF, Kennedy G, Collins AR, Dunne A, Livingstone MB, McKenna PG, McKelvey-Martin VJ, Strain JJ (1999) Dietary antioxidant supplementation and DNA damage in smokers and nonsmokers. Nutr Cancer 34:167–172

Wells WW, Xu DP (1994) Dehydroascorbate reduction. J Bioenerg Biomembr 26:369–377

Wells WW, Xu DP, Washburn MP (1995) Glutathione: dehydroascorbate oxidoreductases. Methods Enzymol 252:30–38

Wells WW, Xu DP, Yang YF, Rocque PA (1990) Mammalian thioltransferase (glutaredoxin) and protein disulfide isomerase have dehydroascorbate reductase activity. J Biol Chem 265:15361–15364

White KL, Chalmers DM, Martin IG, Everett SM, Neville PM, Naylor G, Sutcliffe AE, Dixon MF, Turner PC, Schorah CJ (2002) Dietary antioxidants and DNA damage in patients on long-term acid-suppression therapy: a randomized controlled study. Br J Nutr 88:265–271

WHO Health for All Database, Copenhagen, 2000

Witt EH, Reznick AZ, Viguie CA, Starke-Reed P, Packer L (1992) Exercise, oxidative damage and effects of antioxidant manipulation. J Nutr 122:766–773

Witting PK, Stocker R (2004) Ascorbic acid in atherosclerosis. In: Asard H, May JM, Smirnoff N (eds) Vitamin C: its functions and biochemistry in animals and plants. BIOS Scientific, Oxford, pp 261–290

Wrieden WL, Hannah MK, Bolton-Smith C, Tavendale R, Morrison C, Tunstall-Pedoe H (2000) Plasma vitamin C and food choice in the third Glasgow MONICA population survey. J Epidemiol Community Health 54:355–360

Yokoyama T, Date C, Kokubo Y, Yoshiike N, Matsumura Y, Tanaka H (2000) Serum vitamin C concentration was inversely associated with subsequent 20-year incidence of stroke in a Japanese rural community: the Shibata Study. Stroke 31:2287–2294

Zeiher AM, Drexler H, Wollschlager H, Just H (1991) Modulation of coronary vasomotor tone in humans. Progressive endothelial dysfunction with different early stages of coronary atherosclerosis. Circulation 83:391–401

Zeisel SH (2004) Antioxidants suppress apoptosis. J Nutr 134:S3179–S3180

Zondervan KT, Ocke MC, Smit HA, Seidell JC (1996) Do dietary and supplementary intakes of antioxidants differ with smoking status? Int J Epidemiol 25:70–79

Chapter 10

Experimental In Vitro Exposure Methods for Studying the Effects of Inhalable Compounds

Michaela Aufderheide

Contents

10.1	Introduction		262
10.2	In Vitro Exposure Systems		262
10.2.1	Requirements for Exposure Systems		262
10.2.2	Analysis of Endpoints		263
10.2.3	Exposure		263
10.2.4	Modified Exposure Systems		264
10.2.4.1	Rolling Inserts		264
10.2.4.2	Microporous Membranes		265
10.2.4.3	Models for Epithelial Exposure		266
10.2.4.4	Delivery of Constant Gas Concentrations		268
10.2.4.5	Sidestream Tobacco Smoke Exposure		270
10.2.4.6	Filtered Mainstream Tobacco Smoke Exposure		271
10.2.4.7	Mainstream Cigarette Smoke Exposure		272
10.3	Conclusions		274
	References		274

10.1 Introduction

Analysis of the cellular reactions to complex mixtures such as ambient air, diesel exhaust, or cigarette smoke in vitro is a comprehensive approach because of the complexity of the test atmosphere. Smoke, in particular, represents a mixture of thousands of substances, including short- and long-living radicals in both the gaseous and particulate phases of the aerosol (Hoffmann and Wynder 1986). These compounds undergo chemical reactions that will change the mixture qualitatively and quantitatively in a short time after smoke generation (Pryor 1992, 1997). Thus, all toxicological investigations should be carried out under conditions that are as relevant as possible to the in vivo smoking situation.

The exposure of lung cells to such complex atmospheres will be responsible for either cell injury or cell activation associated with the overexpression of mRNA or the release of various mediators. Therefore, attention should be given to cellular reactions induced by cigarette smoke as a possible cause for the development of chronic lung disorders. Characterization of the early cellular and molecular events plays an important role in understanding the mechanisms involved in chronic lung diseases. Bronchial epithelial cells, alveolar macrophages, and alveolar epithelial cells are in close and permanent contact with inhalable compounds. They participate, at least in part, for example, in the development of inflammatory reactions, commonly described after exposure to air pollutants. The understanding of the functional and pathological disorders resulting from the inhalation of toxic gases and of complex mixtures like cigarette smoke in the respiratory tract requires investigations of the direct effect of such compounds concerning the state and activity of the cells. Here, in vitro systems offer (1) a variety of human cells including bronchial and alveolar cells as well as macrophages for use in monolayer or coculture systems; (2) the analysis of individual cell type responses to complex mixtures or fractions, allowing a better understanding of the independent contribution of this cell type to a particular response; and (3) in vitro exposure conditions that in general can be controlled and reproduced more easily (Leikauf and Driscoll 1993; Wallaert et al. 1996, 2000).

10.2 In Vitro Exposure Systems

10.2.1 Requirements for Exposure Systems

For the exposure of cultivated cells to native atmospheres, "several requirements must be met for in vitro exposure systems," as reported by Rasmussen (1984) and Ritter et al. (2004): (1) The precise control of smoke generation, (2) the age and the physicochemical properties of the smoke when brought into contact with the biological test system, (3) the test atmosphere should have as close as possible contact with the cells, and (4) the system should be designed to allow significant exposure times. Normally, the exposure of cells to ambient atmosphere results in their rapid inactivation because of drying. Therefore, methods have to be developed to maintain a humidified atmosphere or to moisten the cells to establish relevant exposure times.

10.2.2 Analysis of Endpoints

After exposure, representative endpoints should be analyzed as indicators of the toxicological effect, like reduced glutathione, which plays a key role in the cellular reactions following exposure to a wide range of reactive oxygen and nitrogen species (Comhair and Erzurum 2002) as well as to cigarette smoke (Rahman and MacNee 1999). Acute exposure to a variety of different oxidants, including cigarette smoke extracts, has been shown to induce a drastic depletion of the intracellular glutathione in vivo and in vitro (Li et al. 1994; Park et al. 1998; Rahman et al. 1995; Uejima et al. 1990). Following acute depletion, induction of glutathione biosynthesis may occur (Dickinson et al. 2003; Rahman et al. 1996) to remedy the situation.

Because of the need to test the toxic potency of complex mixtures using endpoints considered predictive, as demonstrated by in vivo studies or human evidence, a number of experimental approaches have been made to test the biological effects of such compounds in vitro. Nevertheless, most of them are limited to the testing of pure gases without particulate phase.

10.2.3 Exposure

The easiest way, without great technical effort, is to flush the cells with the test gas. Pace et al. (1961, 1969) measured the cytotoxic effects of nitrogen dioxide (NO_2) and ozone (O_3) on liver cells that were cultured in specially designed flasks (T-60 Pyrex) fitted with ground joints and tubes to permit continuous gas flow and exchange of culture medium. When the cells were covered with medium, little effect was produced by the NO_2 at concentrations below 2,400 ppm. When the medium was removed from the cells and the flasks inverted so that the gas could contact the cells more directly, then as little as 5 ppm NO_2 induced significant inhibition of cell proliferation. This effect was attributed to the physical protection of the liquid layer, as well as to the reaction of NO_2 with serum or other components of the medium. A major conclusion from these studies was that thin layers of liquid are sufficient to protect cells from NO_2, and therefore, it was recommended to use exposure systems that allow more-direct contact between the gases and the cells. These results were confirmed by experiments with O_3 (Pace et al. 1969).

Another possibility is the bubbling of a test atmosphere through a cell suspension. Voisin et al. (1974) used such a method for exposing alveolar macrophages to NO_2, whereby the gas was generated continuously by catalytic reactions with NO. Such an approach was also used in studies with O_3 (Cardile et al. 1995, Van der Zee et al. 1987). However, under these conditions, the cells are covered with culture medium, and consequently, there is no direct contact between cells and the test atmosphere.

To reduce the diffusion barrier for gas-phase toxicants by decreasing the thickness of the media overlay, various techniques have been developed to realize a more realistic and susceptible exposure condition. In this regard, in vitro systems have been described, incorporating roller bottles and rotating or rocking platforms (Baker and Tumasonis 1971; Bolton et al. 1982; Fischer and Placke, 1987; Friedman et al. 1992; Guerrero et al. 1979a,b; Madden et al. 1991; Valentine, 1985; Wenzel et al. 1979) where the culture medium is periodically placed over the apical surfaces of the cells, thus acting as a variable diffuse barrier. Additional systems that perfuse media past cells attached to membrane filters have also been mentioned (Samuelson et al. 1978; Rasmussen and Crocker 1982).

In 1969, these concepts were used to expose cells to O_3 (Pace et al. 1969) or volatile compounds (Muckter et al. 1998) in culture flasks on rocker platforms. Bombick et al. (1997) used this approach to analyze the biological activity of whole smoke, including the vapour/gas phase under periodically submerged conditions. Typical exposure times needed in such setups are in the range of several hours to a number of days (Boland et al. 2000; Don Porto Carero et al. 2001).

Culture dishes were also integrated for such strategies. Placed inside an incubation chamber on a rocker platform or a rotating holder at an angle, they could be tilted back and forth to realize an intermittent exposure to the test atmosphere without medium overlay (Rusznak et al. 1996; Wenzel et al. 1979, 1982). Guerrero et al. (1979a) used such a system for exposing human fibroblasts to O_3. Under such conditions, cells were sensitive to killing by concentrations of around 1 ppm and showed effects on alkaline phosphatase as well as some indications of genotoxic effects (Guerrero et al. 1979b).

Roller bottles with adherent growing cells on the inside offer another possibility for a periodic exposure procedure. The bottles, filled only with a minimal amount of medium to supply the cells with nutrients, rotate, thus creating a situation where the cells are without a medium layer and could be exposed to gases for a certain length of time (Bolton et al. 1982). In addition, other investigators (Madden et al. 1991) used such a technique for the treatment of rat alveolar macrophages with O_3. The system (Friedman et al. 1985) allowed direct exposure of the cells (>90%) to O_3 at any time with minimal interaction of the toxicant with the culture medium.

10.2.4 Modified Exposure Systems

10.2.4.1 Rolling Inserts

Modified exposure systems were also used to study the toxicological effects of complex mixtures composed of particulate and gaseous compounds. Morin et al. (1999) developed an in vitro system for the continuous exposure of lung tissue slices to diesel exhaust. The design of such an exposure chamber is shown in Fig. 10.1. It consists of two concentric cylinders placed over a continuous Wheaton rolling system, placed in an incubator at 37 °C. The external cylinder contained a solution of 1% copper sulfate ($CuSO_4$) solution in water to achieve adequate hygrometry (85–90%) of the atmosphere. The internal cylinder had slits at the periphery, and it is possible that the humidity from the external cylinder reach the inside of the internal cylinder where a constant and controlled flow (gas debimeters) is applied. The whole-exposure system was placed in a slight vacuum to ensure that the flow through the chamber is without physical obstruction to the progression of particulate compounds of the test atmosphere.

Freshly prepared lung slices of female Wistar rats, transferred onto a titanium grid of a Teflon rolling insert, were placed in scintillation vials with opened caps to have free access to the gaseous and particulate phase of the exhaust, or with caps bearing a Paleflex filter for free exchange of the gaseous compounds but without the penetration of particles. Short-term exposure to diesel exhaust (1 h) resulted in a significant decrease of the intracellular ATP and glutathione (GSH) levels, whereas filtered exhaust showed less marked effects. An exposure of 3 or 6 h induced an inflammatory response (tumor

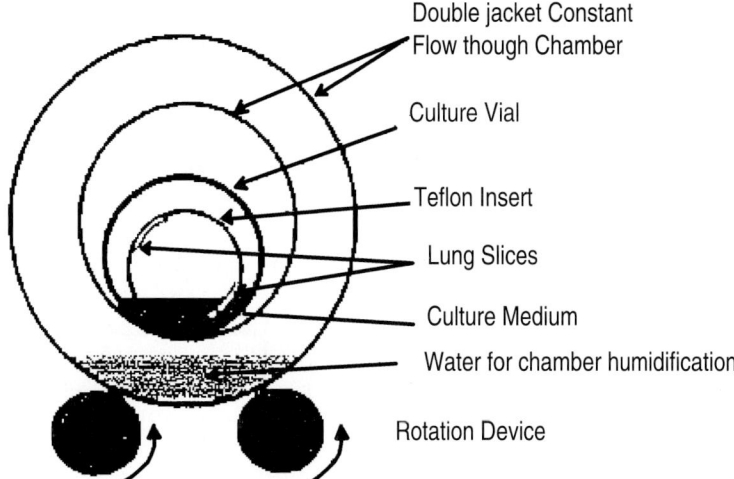

Fig. 10.1 Cross-section of the flow through exposure chambers. The two external concentric circles delimit the humidification compartment. The culture vial rotates freely on the internal wall of the chamber, and the lung slices are alternately fed by culture medium and exposed to the flow of complex atmosphere (Morin et al. 1999)

necrosis factor-α [TNF-α]) and apoptotic processes, as shown by the terminal transferase dUTP nick end-labeling (TUNEL) method and the determination of nucleosomes (Le Prieur et al. 2000). Here, under controlled conditions, a complex mixture containing particulate as well as gaseous compounds was tested, showing different activities of the whole and filtered smoke. All these systems were characterized by an undefined contact between cells, medium, and the test atmosphere, but they demonstrated the possibility to determine biological effects of inhalable test compounds such as gases and complex mixtures with regard to endpoints like cytotoxicity, inflammation, oxidative stress, and DNA damage.

10.2.4.2 Microporous Membranes

A further and more realistic strategy is to expose cells cultured on collagen gels (Jabbour et al. 1998; Zamora et al. 1986) or microporous membranes (Rasmussen 1984; Voisin et al. 1974, 1977).

In the first case, lung alveolar cells were grown on hydrated and nutrified collagen gel prepared from rat tail collagen (Zamora et al. 1986) and exposed to different NO_2 concentrations for 1 h in a modified modular exposure chamber (Fig. 10.2).

The exposure atmosphere was generated by metering 500 ppm of NO_2 in the air through a rotameter into a stream of 95% air-5% CO_2. This system supplied the desired NO_2 concentrations to the cells while maintaining environmental conditions necessary for cell survival (pH ~7.4, high relative humidity). The horizontal gas flow through the chamber was between 2.6 and 2.8 l/min.

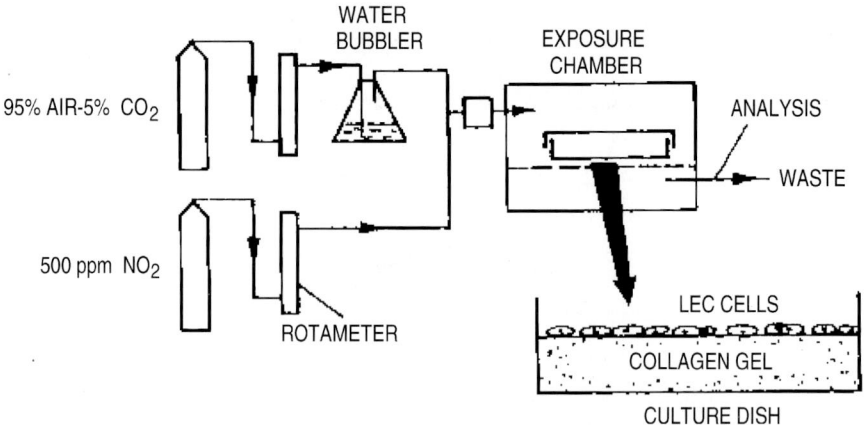

Fig. 10.2 Schematic drawing of the cell exposure system (Zamora et al. 1986)

The introduction of microporous membranes for biphasic cultures offered a new way to make progress in the field of inhalation toxicology by using in vitro methods. In this strategy, called air–liquid exposure, the cells are fed and humidified from the basal side and exposed from the apical side. This method provides the best and closest contact between the test atmosphere and the cells, compared with the in vivo situation.

Voisin and coworkers (1975, 1977a, b) described a method where macrophages were layered on a polysulfone membrane of 0.2-µm porosity, which was placed on a plastic ring in a culture dish, filled with medium (Fig. 10.3).

In such a way, the cells can be exposed and nutrified. Gas exposure was conducted in an exposure chamber for various time durations to various gas concentrations in a continuous flow of 2 l/min. Control cells were exposed in the same manner to purified air with 5% CO_2. Immediately after gas exposure, cell injury was determined by measuring the ATP content and lactate dehydrogenase (LDH) release. The biological effects of gas exposure could also be estimated by the release of various bioactive mediators or cytokines into the medium.

10.2.4.3 Models for Epithelial Exposure

Another in vitro system (Adler et al. 1987; Whitcutt et al. 1988) was developed for maintaining guinea pig respiratory epithelial cells between the air and liquid phases. The cells, which were plated onto a collagen gel substratum, formed on the top of a nitrocellulose membrane and were fed from below through the membrane and collagen gel, whereas the upper surface was not exposed to medium, but to an air interface, as it occurs in vivo. The system is ideally suited for studies on airway epithelial function, such as secretory responses to irritants and mediators of inflammation, studies involving cell differentiation and gene expression, as well as exposure studies to study the effects of pollutants.

This cultivation method at the air–liquid interface was favored for the development of exposure strategies to analyze the biological effects of inhalable substances, especially

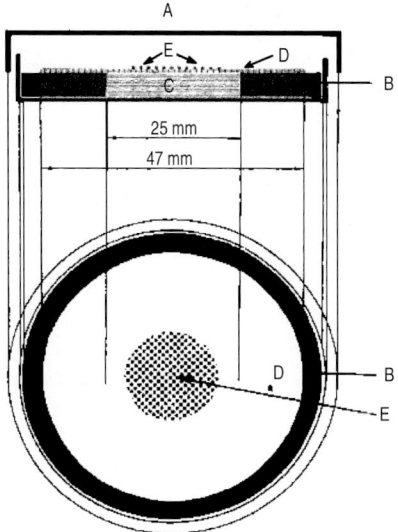

Fig. 10.3 a Petri dish. **b** Plastic ring. **c** Medium reservoir. **d** Microporous membrane. **e** Zone for the cultivation of the macrophages (Voisin et al. 1977)

on cells from the respiratory tract in order to simulate the in vivo situation. In general, mainly gases were analyzed for their adverse effects on alveolar macrophages, bronchial, and alveolar epithelial cells by using static or dynamic exposure conditions. However, each of these experimental approaches is complex, because of the biological and technical efforts that have to be made to create a reproducible exposure method for the determination of dose-dependent effects.

By using a biphasic culture system in aerobiosis, Aerts et al. (1992) demonstrated the roles of antioxidant enzymes and of GHS in providing protection against hyperoxia in alveolar type II cells of the guinea pig. In all studies, cell cultures were maintained at 37 °C in humidified airtight incubation chambers, which were flushed with gas mixture (containing 50 or 95% O_2, 5% CO_2, and balanced purified N_2) and then closed. Control cells were exposed to purified air under the same conditions. The chambers were then sealed and incubated for 2 days at 37 °C. Afterwards, cells were harvested for ATP cell content and biochemical analyses. Exposure of type II cells did not induce significant changes in the cell protein content, superoxide dismutase (SOD), catalase, GHS peroxidase (GPx), or GSH content when compared with control cells under normoxia. With ATP content expressed as a cell injury index (CII), type II cell injury was found to increase with increasing O_2 concentrations. Cell injury effects of hyperoxia did not correlate with the endogenous antioxidant enzyme activities (SOD, manganese [MN]-SOD, catalase), whereas a significant correlation between the CII and total GSH content of the cells was estimated. This correlation was largely because of the close relationship between CII and reduced GSH. Hyperoxic-induced cell injury was clearly associated with significantly lower intracellular GSH levels when compared with control cells under normoxia.

10.2.4.4 Delivery of Constant Gas Concentrations

With in vitro systems, a major problem is the proper design of the exposure system to deliver constant and reproducible concentrations of a test gas, especially when using a highly reactive chemical like O_3. Another challenge is to mimic in vivo conditions where the luminal surfaces of respiratory epithelial cells are exposed almost directly to the inspired air, except for a mucus or surfactant layer of variable thickness. Exposure of cell cultures through a stationary liquid layer is undesirable for the following reasons: (1) relatively insoluble gases such as O_3 have little effect except at very high concentrations (Pace et al. 1969, Hager et al. 1981), and (2) the mechanism of action may be different if an oxidant first reacts with the components of a liquid layer rather than reacting directly with the cell or its surface layer (Wenzel and Morgan 1982). To solve this problem, Whitcutt and coworkers (1988) developed a biphasic cell culture system where the cells are maintained between air and the liquid medium to realize a direct exposure of the apical surface of the epithelial cells, e.g., to O_3.

Based on this culture device, Tarkington et al. (1994) designed a new in vitro exposure system for the direct exposure of cultured airway epithelial cells and of tracheal explants in several replicate vessels to O_3, and simultaneously allowing cells to be exposed to an experimental atmosphere without O_3 as a control. This system was designed to generate and monitor consistent, reproducible levels of O_3 over a broad range of concentrations in a humidified atmosphere. Application of earlier versions of the exposure device to tracheal explants has been described by Nikula et al. (1988, 1990). A schematic diagram of the in vitro system is shown in Fig. 10.4.

One vessel for O_3 exposure and one control vessel were used, placed in an incubator. Lines pass through a port in the incubator and convey the gas stream to the exposure and control vessels (Fig. 10.5).

The gas streams are humidified by bubbling through bottles containing sterile distilled water. The humidified gases are then conveyed to jars, serving as exposure and control vessels that have a surface area of 75 cm², an appropriate volume to contain five culture vials (Fig. 10.6).

Inside each vessel, the gases enter at the top through a jet orientated in such a way that the atmosphere is injected tangentially to the wall and swirls across the tops of the culture vials. This promotes mixing and even exposure among each of the five vials. Exhaust from each vessel is taken from the bottom in the center. Here, for the first time, a system was described using a directed gas stream to the cells, whereas in other systems, the gas was guided horizontally above the cells. After exposing human tracheobronchial epithelial cells and rat tracheal epithelium to 0.1–1.0 ppm of O_3, cell viability was measured also dependent on the medium layer above the cells. As shown in Fig. 10.7, without any fluid on the top surface of the epithelial cells, O_3 caused substantial cell damage (cell viability 20%) in comparison with cultures exposed to filtered air (85%). When culture medium was added, viability increased, thus demonstrating the importance of direct exposure in order to assess the toxicity of O_3 in vitro. Furthermore, a good correlation between the duration of exposure and the loss of cell viability could be found. In summary, such an exposure method offers the possibility to study functional and morphological effects of gaseous compounds under controlled conditions also in human cell systems.

For the exposure of cells of the respiratory tract to reactive gases, exposure at the air–liquid interface was favored, based on the experience gained so far. Different experimental setups were described in the following years, based on a biphasic culture system.

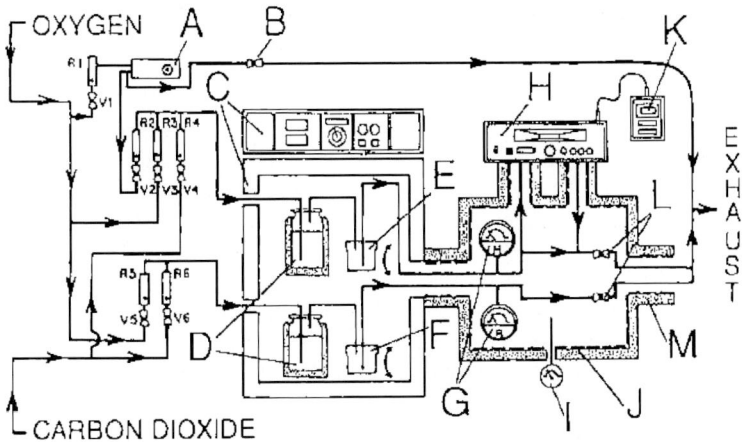

Fig. 10.4 Schematic diagram of in vitro exposure system. **a** Ozonizer. **b** Ozone bypass valve. **c** Incubator. **d** Humidification bottles. **e** Exposure vessel. **f** Control vessel. **g** Pressure gauges. **h** Ozone analyzer. **i** Thermometer. **j** Heating tape. **k** Thermometer. **l** Thermal insulation (Tarkington et al. 1994)

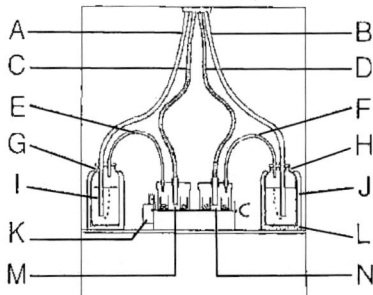

Fig. 10.5 Ozone exposure system: view within incubator. **a** Inlet exposure atmosphere. **b** Inlet control atmosphere. **c** Exhaust exposure atmosphere. **d** Exhaust control atmosphere. **e** Humidified exposure atmosphere. **f** Humidified control atmosphere. **g** Humidifier bottle, exposure. **h** Humidifier bottle, control. **i** Distilled water. **j** Heating mat. **k** Motorized rocker. **l** Thermal insulation. **m** Exposure vessel. **n** Control vessel (Tarkington et al. 1994)

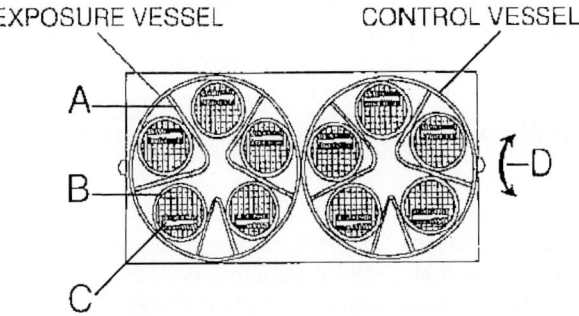

Fig. 10.6 Rocking platform supporting exposure and control vessels. (Tarkington et al. 1994)

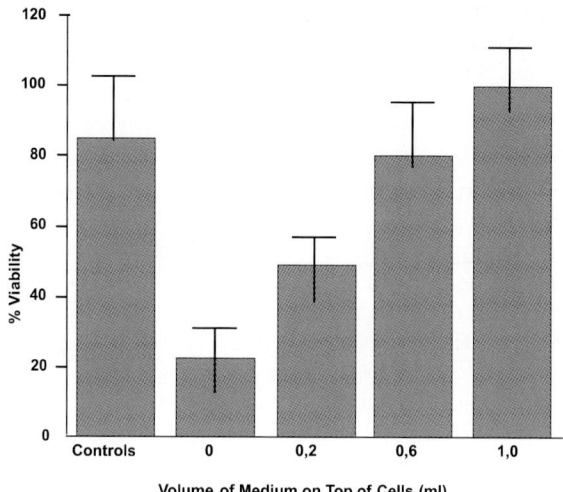

Fig. 10.7 Effects of culture surface fluid volume on ozone toxicity. The human cell line S6 was maintained biphasically. Cultures were exposed to 1 ppm ozone or to filtered air for 2 h. Before ozone exposure, various volumes of cell culture medium, as shown in the figure, were added. (Tarkington et al. 1994)

Janic et al. (2003) studied the effects of O_3 and other gaseous agents in THP-1 cells (monocyte/macrophage lineage) also under dynamic exposure conditions, i.e., a continuous flow of the test atmosphere. The system used for in vitro exposure (Umstead et al. 2002) also delivered precisely controlled flow rates of gases to the exposure vessel, with precise O_3 concentrations and appropriate humidification. To avoid any interaction of O_3 with the components in the media, all the exposures were done using Hanks Balanced Salt Solution (HBSS). To facilitate direct contact of the test gas with cells and accurate O_3 doses, no HBSS remained on the top during exposures; cells were moistened from below with 1.6 ml HBSS. THP-1 cells exposed to different O_3 concentrations ranging from 0.1 to 0.5 ppm for 1 h were analyzed for cell viability and apoptosis either immediately after exposure or at later time points. The studies demonstrated the absence of apoptosis and a small decrease in cell viability after O_3 exposure. In addition, THP-1 cell expression of cell surface proteins (CD14 and CD11b) appeared to be unaltered. However, the response to a stimulus (i.e., lipopolysaccharide [LPS]) following gas exposure, resulted in a decrease in TNF-α levels, compared with filtered air/LPS-exposed cells.

10.2.4.5 Sidestream Tobacco Smoke Exposure

Encouraged by the positive results gained under the exposure conditions at the air–liquid interface, this experimental approach was also used to study the biological effects of complex mixtures. Sun et al. (1995) studied the effects of sidestream tobacco smoke (STS) as a surrogate for environmental tobacco smoke (ETS) under biphasic culture conditions. BEAS-2B cells (a human bronchial epithelial line immortalized by viral transformation), cultured in the biphasic Millicell-CM system, were exposed in an exposure system described by Teague et al. (1994). The cells were placed in a 37 °C incubator (lid off) with apical exposure to a defined atmosphere (filtered air and 5% CO_2 saturated with water vapor) and the addition of STS generated from an ADL/II smoking system. The machine delivers a standard puff of 35 ml in 2 s at 30-s intervals on 1KR4F cigarettes. The proliferating cells were exposed to 1 mg/m³ RSP (total respirable suspended particles) STS for 0, 2, 4, or 6 h, and then their viability and functional status were evaluated by measuring DNA synthesis, the mitochondrial metabolic activity, and cell counting. The results clearly demonstrated that STS is cytotoxic to BEAS-2B cells; it inhibited the metabolism as well as the proliferative ability of the cells. The extent of cell injury was directly related to the concentration of STS to which the cells were exposed. Furthermore, exposed cells were analyzed for their protein synthesis pattern. In general, the exposure inhibited total cellular protein synthesis; however, there were several proteins whose synthesis was upregulated after smoke exposure. Among them, a 45-kDa protein was most significantly induced. Expression of classical heat shock proteins with molecular masses around 70 kDa was not increased in these cells. In addition, the exposure of BEAS-2B cells to mainstream smoke resulted in an increased synthesis of the 45-kDa protein, whereas the exposure to cigarette smoke condensate (CSC) showed no induction in protein synthesis. These results suggest that the particular chemical components responsible for this reaction probably exist in the gas phase of tobacco products or are chemically quite labile.

Especially when dealing with complex atmospheres, the biological activity of the particulate and gas phase has to be taken into consideration to characterize the toxicologic activity of such test compounds.

10.2.4.6 Filtered Mainstream Tobacco Smoke Exposure

For studying in particular the effects of the gas phase and the biological mechanisms of its action, Piperi and coworkers (2003) exposed mouse lung epithelial cells (LA-4 and NCI-H157 cells) to filtered cigarette smoke in a plastic chamber, containing the 96-well or 6-well plate cultures. The medium was replaced with serum-free medium before exposure and, after exposure, the cells were washed with phosphate-buffered saline (PBS), and complete medium was added. The dose ranged between one and nine puffs, generated according to International Organization for Standardization (ISO) rules. The cytotoxicity of the gas phase was found to be dose dependent. Exposure to low doses (one to three puffs) had minimal effects on cell proliferation (WST-1) and viability (LDH leakage), whereas higher doses were associated with a significant increase in cell mortality. These observations were evident even 2 and 8 h postexposure, thus pointing to significant effects of the gas phase that do not immediately cause loss of viability, but lead to progressive loss of metabolic activity.

The mechanisms of cell death were found to be both apoptotic and necrotic, depending on the concentrations used. Because of the high amount of oxidants and free radicals, the gas phase mediated its effects primarily by depleting cellular GSH or by modifying protein cysteine residues. Cells that have been exposed to the gas phase showed a rapid but dose-dependent depletion of GSH as measured immediately, 2 and 4 h after exposure. Dose dependency was identical to that observed in cell proliferation and viability assays, suggesting that gas-phase cigarette smoke exerts its effects via oxidative damage. In parallel, increased nitrotyrosine immunoreactivity and phosphorylation of p44/42 mitogen-activated protein kinase (MAPK) proteins were observed. Interestingly, activation of MAPK appeared to coincide with the depletion of cellular GSH, which suggests that the effects of the gas phase may be the results of redox changes of critical protein cysteine residues secondary to GSH depletion or to direct oxidation of protein thiol residues that may occur with, or subsequently to, the loss of GSH.

By using the same experimental setup, the gas phase of cigarette smoke deprived of its volatile constituents (VOCs) was used to study the role of the nonorganic compounds on the cytotoxicity of mouse lung epithelial cells (Pouli et al. 2003). The exposure of cells to this gas fraction showed no toxic effects, and cell viability was found to be equivalent to control cultures, indicating that the removal of the VOCs almost eliminated the cytotoxic potency of the gas phase.

10.2.4.7 Mainstream Cigarette Smoke Exposure

Taking into consideration the importance of the particulate and gas phase of cigarette smoke with regard to their qualitative and quantitative contribution to the biological effects, it would be desirable to analyze these compounds in biphasic systems where the cells are in direct contact with the test atmosphere.

In a specially designed exposure device, CULTEX® (Fig. 10.8), human cells of the respiratory tract (bronchial epithelial cell line, HFBE21; A549 cells) were exposed at the air–liquid interface (Ritter et al. 2003, 2004) to mainstream cigarette smoke as well as to its gas–vapor phase. To test the native atmosphere, exposures were done without heating, humidification, or addition of CO_2. This strategy has already been successfully used for the in vitro testing of native gaseous compounds (Ritter et al. 2001), complex mixtures like sidestream cigarette smoke (Aufderheide et al. 2001), and automobile exhaust (Knebel et al. 2002).

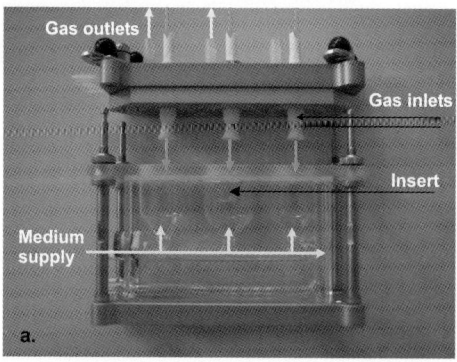
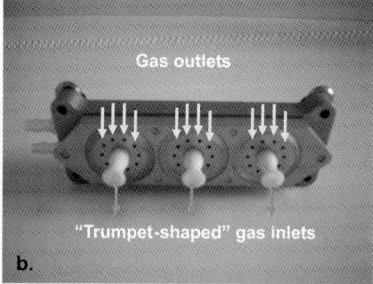

Fig. 10.8: CULTEX® exposure module. **a** The basic part of the exposure module housing the Transwell inserts in three vessels connected via a glass tube system for medium supply. The inner space of the module is insulated against the Transwell vessels to be filled with water at a defined temperature. **b** Exposure top with specially designed trumpet-shaped gas inlets for homogenous distribution of the test atmosphere above the cells and outlets placed in a circle around the inlets

Cells were seeded on Transwell membranes and placed in the basic part of the exposure unit (Fig. 10.8a) housing three Transwell inserts and exposed to the atmosphere without humidification or other modifications. The vessels for the inserts are insulated against the inner space of the module, which can be floated in warm water (37 °C). The vessels are filled with medium, thus providing the humidification and supply of the cells with nutrients. The exposure top of the module (Fig. 10.8b) has three specially designed inlet tubes that guarantee homogenous distribution of the test atmosphere above the cells. In contrast to systems described so far, the smoke is guided vertically, directly to the cells in a continuous flow. The smoke is sucked by negative pressure through the system, exiting the exposure chamber via several outlets. This exposure technique results in an effective and direct contact. By using the CULTEX® system, A549 cells, which are described to share several fundamental characteristics with human lung alveolar type II cells (Lieber et al. 1976; Mendelson and Boggaram, 1991; Nardone and Andrews 1979; Smith 1977; Smith et al. 1982; Young and Mendelson, 1997) and competence of xenobiotic metabolism (Hukkanen et al. 2000; Iwanari et al. 2002; Urani et al. 1998), were exposed to mainstream smoke and the gas phase of three cigarettes, two of comparable tar content (Ritter et al. 2004). Fresh cigarette smoke, generated according to ISO norms by the smoking robot VC10 (Vitrocell, Germany) was sucked at different dilutions (1.67 to 17.67) above the cells for 32 min. To characterize the biological effect of smoke, protein content and intracellular reduced GSH were analyzed directly after exposure. Cellular protein revealed no statistically relevant changes in comparison with control populations exposed to synthetic air throughout all tested cigarettes, dilutions, and exposures to whole and filtered smoke. Under these nontoxic conditions, all cigarettes induced a significant dose-dependent depletion of reduced GHS, which has been shown to be of high relevance with respect to human lung cells and cigarette smoke.

In addition, exposure to whole smoke throughout depleted the GSH more effectively than did exposure to filtered smoke (Fig. 10.9). Based on a detailed analysis of one of the concentrations, the quantitative effects of whole smoke and the gas phase were statisti-

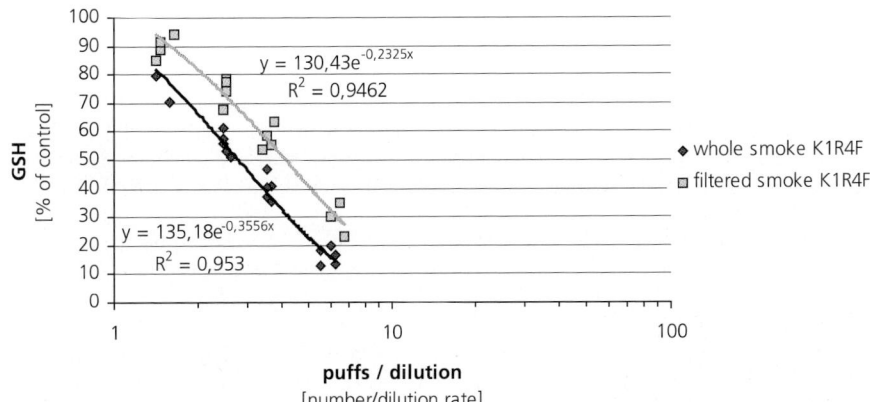

Fig. 10.9 Dose–response curves from exposures of A549 cells to fresh filtered or whole smoke from K1R4F. Intracellular glutathione contents were plotted as a percentage of control values against exposure dose calculated as the ratio of number of smoked cigarette puffs and dilution rate used. Each *dot* represents the result of a single exposure experiment. For determination of effective glutathione (GSH) dose for 50% of the cells ($ED_{50\text{-}GSH}$) values, an exponential regression (K1R4F) was applied (Ritter et al. 2004)

cally significantly distinguishable for the different cigarettes. In conclusion, these studies have shown that the experimental approach allows the investigation of complex mixtures composed of particulate matter and gaseous compounds. By using such a system with a directed flow of the test atmosphere to the cells on the basis of a biphasic cell culture, basic mechanisms of cigarette smoke can be evaluated, e.g., with human lung cells.

10.3 Conclusions

In summary, new developments in the cultivation of isolated cells and optimized exposure methods using direct exposure principles at the air–liquid interface open up new research fields for the analysis of complex mixtures like cigarette smoke. The complexity of such an aerosol, including short- and long-lived radicals in both the gaseous and particulate phase can now be described by analyzing biological effects after exposure to native, unmodified test atmospheres.

References

Aerts C, Wallaert B, Voisin C (1992) In vitro hyperoxia on alveolar type II pneumocytes: inhibition of glutathione synthesis increases hyperoxic cell injury. Exp Lung Res 18: 845–861
Adler KB, Schwarz JE, Whitcutt MJ, Wu R (1987) A new chamber system for maintaining differentiated guinea pig respiratory epithelial cells between air and liquid phases. Biotech 5:462–465
Aufderheide M, Mohr U (1999) CULTEX—a new system and technique for the cultivation and exposure of cells at the air/liquid interface. Exp Toxic Pathol 51:489–490
Aufderheide M, Mohr U (2000) CULTEX—an alternative technique for the cultivation and exposure of cells of the respiratory tract to airborne pollutants at the air/liquid interface. Exp Toxic Pathol 52:265–270
Aufderheide M, Ritter D, Knebel JW, Scherer G (2001) A method for in vitro analysis of the biological activity of complex mixtures such as sidestream cigarette smoke. Exp Toxic Pathol 53141–152
Baker FD, Tumasonis CF (1971) Modified roller drum apparatus for analysing effects of pollutant gases on tissue culture systems. Atmos Environ 5891–893
Boland S, Bonvallot V, Fournier T, Baeza-Squiban A, Aubier M, Marano F (2000) Mechanisms of GM-CSF increase by diesel exhaust particles in human airway epithelial cells. Am J Physiol 278: L25–L32
Bolton DC, Tarkington BK, Zee YC, Osebold JW (1982) An in vitro system for studying the effects of ozone on mammalian cell cultures and viruses. Environ Res 27:466–475
Bombick DW, Bombick BR, Ayres PH, Putnam K, Avalos J, Borgerding MF, Doolittle DJ (1997) Evaluation of the genotoxic and cytotoxic potential of mainstream whole smoke and smoke condensate from a cigarette containing a novel carbon filter. Fundam Appl Toxicol 39:11–17
Cardile V, Jiang X, Russo A, Casella F, Renis M, Bindoni M (1995) Effects of ozone on some biological activities of cells in vitro. Cell Biol Toxicol 11:11–21
Comhair SA, Erzurum SC (2002) Antioxidant responses to oxidant-mediated lung diseases. Am J Physiol 283:L246–L255
Dickinson DA, Moellering DR, Iles KE, Patel RP, Levonen AL, Wigley A, Darley-Usmar VM, Forman H (2003) Cytoprotection against oxidative stress and the regulation of glutathione synthesis. Biol Chem 384:527–537

Don Porto Carero A, Hoet PH, Verschaeve L, Schoeters G, Nemery B (2001) Genotoxic effects of carbon black particles, diesel exhaust particles, and urban air particulates and their extracts on a human alveolar epithelial cell line (A549) and a human monocytic cell line (THP-1). Environ Mol Mutagen 37:155–163

Fischer GL, Placke ME (1987) In vitro models of lung toxicity. Toxicology 47:71–93

Friedman M, Madden MC, Saunders DS, Gammon K, White GC II, Kwock L (1985) Ozone inhibits prostacyclin synthesis in pulmonary epithelium. Prostaglandins 30:1069–1085

Friedman M, Madden MC, Samet JM, Koren HS (1992) Effects of ozone exposure on lipid metabolism in human alveolar macrophages. Environ Health Perspect. 97:95–101

Guerrero RR, Rounds DE, Booher J, Olson RS, Hackney JD (1979a) Ozone sensitivity in aging WI-38 cells based on acid phosphatase content. Arch Environ Health 34:407–412

Guerrero RR, Rounds DE, Booher J, Olson RS, Hackney JD (1979b) Mutagenic effects of ozone on human cells exposed in vivo and in vitro based on sister chromatid exchange analysis. Environ Res 18:336–346

Hagar WL, Sweet WE, Sweet F (1981) An in vitro system for assessing lung cell response to ozone. J Air Pollut Control Assoc 31:993–995

Hoffmann D, Wynder EL (1986) Chemical constituents and bioactivity of tobacco smoke. IARC Sci Pub 74:145–165

Hukkanen J, Lassila A, Paivarinta K, Valanne S, Sarpo S, Hakkola J, Pelkonen O, Raunio H (2000) Induction and regulation of xenobiotic-metabolizing cytochrome P450s in the human A549 lung adenocarcinoma cell line. Am J Respir Cell Mol Biol 22:360–366

Iwanari M, Nakajima M, Kizu R, Hayakawa K, Yokoi T (2002) Induction of CYP1A1, CYP1A2, and CYP1B1 mRNAs by nitropolycyclic aromatic hydrocarbons in various human tissue-derived cells: chemical-, cytochrome P450 isoform-, and cell-specific differences. Arch Toxicol 76:287–298

Janic B, Umstead TM, Phelps DS, Floros J (2003) An in vitro model system for the study of the effects of ozone and other gaseous agents on phagocytic cells. J Immunol Methods 272:125–134

Leikauf G, Driscoll K (1993) Cellular approaches in respiratory tract toxicology. In Gardner DE et al. (eds) Toxicology of the lung, 2nd ed. Raven, New York, pp 335–370

Lieber M, Smith B, Szakal A, Nelson-Rees W, Todaro G (1976) A continuous tumor-cell line from a human lung carcinoma with properties of type II alveolar epithelial cells. Int J Cancer 17:62–70

Le Prieur E, Vaz E, Bion A, Dionnet F, Morinn J-P (2000) Toxicity of diesel engine exhaust in an in vitro model of lung slices in biphasic organotypic culture: induction of a proinflammatory and apoptotic response. Arch Toxicol 74:460–466

Li XY, Donaldson K, Rahman I, MacNee W (1994) An investigation of the role of glutathione in increased epithelial permeability induced by cigarette smoke in vivo and in vitro. Am J Respir Crit Care Med 149:1518–1525

Madden MC, Eling TE, Dailey LA, Friedman M (1991) The effect of ozone exposure on rat alveolar macrophage arachidonic acid metabolism. Exp Lung Res 17:47–63

Mendelson CR, Boggaram V (1991) Hormonal control of the surfactant system in fetal lung. Annu Rev Physiol 53:415–440

Morin J-P, Fouquet F, Monteil C, Le Prieur E, Dionnet F (1999) Development of a new in vitro system for continuous in vitro exposure of lung tissue to complex atmospheres: Application to diesel exhaust toxicology. Cell Biol Toxicol 15:143–152

Muckter H, Zwing M, Bader S, Marx T, Doklea E, Liebl B, Fichtl B, Georgieff M (1998) A novel apparatus for the exposure of cultured cells to volatile agents. J Pharmacol Toxicol Methods 40:63–69

Nardone LL, Andrews SB (1979) Cell line A549 as a model of type II pneumocytes. Phospholipid biosynthesis from native and organometallic precursors. Biochim Biophys Acta 573:276–295

Nikula KJ, Wilson DW, Dungworth DL, Plopper CG (1988) In vitro evidence of cellular adaptation to ozone toxicity in the rat trachea. Toxicol Appl Pharmacol 93:394–402

Nikula KJ, Wilson DW (1990) Response of rat tracheal epithelium to ozone and oxygen exposure in vitro. Fund Appl Toxicol 15:121–131

Pace DM, Landolt PA, Aftonomos BT (1969) Effects of ozone on cells in vitro. Arch Environ Health 18:165–170

Pace DM, Thompson JR, Aftonomos BT (1961) The effects of NO_2 and salts of NO_2 upon established cell lines. Can J Biochem Physiol 39:1247–1255

Park EM, Park YM, Gwak YS (1998) Oxidative damage in tissues of rats exposed to cigarette smoke. Free Radical Biol Med 25:79–86

Piperi C, Pouli AE, Katerelos NA, Hatzinikolaou DG, Stavridou A, Psallidopoulus AC (2003) Study of the mechanisms of cigarette smoke gas phase cytotoxicity. Anticancer Res 23:2185–2190

Pouli AE, Hatzinikolaou DG, Piperi C, Stavridou A, Psallidopoulos MC, Stavrides (2003) The cytotoxic effects of volatile organic compounds of the gas phase of cigarette smoke on lung epithelial cells. Free Radical Biol Med 34:345–355

Pryor WA (1992) Biological effects of cigarette smoke, wood smoke, and the smoke from plastics: the use of electron spin resonance. Free Radical Biol Med 13:659–676

Pryor WA (1997) Cigarette smoke radicals and the role of free radicals in chemical carcinogenicity. Environ Health Perspect 105:S875–S882

Rahman I, Li XY, Donaldson K, Harrison DJ, MacNee W (1995) Glutathione homeostasis in alveolar epithelial cells in vitro and lung in vivo under oxidative stress. Am J Physiol 269(3 Pt 1): L285–L292

Rahman I, Smith CA, Lawson MF, Harrison DJ, MacNee W (1996) Induction of gamma-glutamylcysteine synthetase by cigarette smoke is associated with AP-1 in human alveolar epithelial cells. FEBS Lett 396:21–25

Rahman I, MacNee W (1999) Lung glutathione and oxidative stress: implications in cigarette smoke-induced airway disease. Am J Physiol 277(6 Pt 1):L1067–L1088

Rasmussen RE, Crocker TT (1982) Lung cells grown on cellulose membrane filters as an in vitro model of the respiratory epithelium. In: Tice RR, Costa DL, Schaich KM (eds) Genotoxic effects of airborne agents. Plenum, New York, pp 105–120

Rasmussen RE (1984) In vitro system for exposure of lung cells to NO_2 and O_3. J Toxicol Environ Health 13:397–411

Ritter D, Knebel JW, Aufderheide M (2003) Exposure of human lung cells to inhalable substances: a novel test strategy involving clean air exposure periods using whole diluted cigarette mainstream smoke. Inhalation Toxicol 15:67–84

Ritter D, Knebel JW, Aufderheide M (2004) Comparative assessment of toxicities of mainstream smoke from commercial cigarettes. Inhal Toxicol 16:691–700

Rusznak C, Devalia JL, Sapsford RJ, Davies RJ (1996) Ozone-induced mediator release from human bronchial epithelial cells in vitro and the influence of nedocromil sodium. Eur Respir J 9:2298–2305

Samuelson GS, Rasmussen RE, Nair BK, Crocker TT (1978) Novel culture and exposure system for measurement of effects of airborne pollutants on mammalian cells. Environ Sci Technol 12:426–430

Smith BT (1977) Cell line A549: a model system for the study of alveolar type II cell function. Am Rev Respir Dis 115:285–293

Smith FB, Kikkawa Y, Diglio CA, Dalen RC (1982) Increased saturated phospholipid in cultured cells grown with linoleic acid. In Vitro 18:331–338

Sun W, Wu R, Last JA (1995) Effects of exposure to environmental tobacco smoke on a human tracheobronchial epithelial cell line. Toxicol 100:163–174

Tarkington BK, Wu R, Sun W-M, Nikula KJ, Wilson DW, Last JA (1994) In vitro exposure of tracheobronchial epithelial cells and of tracheal explants to ozone. Toxicol 88:51–68

Teague SV, Pinkerton KE, Goldsmith M, Gebremichael A, Chang S, Jenkins RA, Moneylun JH (1994) A sidestream cigarette smoke generation and exposure system for environmental tobacco smoke studies. Inhal Toxicol 6:79–93

Umstead TM, Wang G, Phelps DS, Floros J, Tarkington BK (2002) In vitro exposure of proteins to ozone. Toxicol Mech Methods 12:1–16

Uejima Y, Fukuchi Y, Nagase T, Matsuse T, Yamaoka M, Tabata R, Orimo H (1990) Influence of inhaled tobacco smoke on the senescence accelerated mouse (SAM). Eur Respir J 3:1029–1036

Urani C, Doldi M, Crippa S, Camatini M (1998) Human-derived cell lines to study xenobiotic metabolism. Chemosphere 37(14–15):2785–2795

Valentine R (1985) An in vitro system for exposure of lung cells to gases: effects of ozone on rat macrophages. J Toxicol Environ Health 16:115–126

Van der Zee J, Tijssen Christianse K, Dubbelman TM, Van Steveninck J (1987) The influence of ozone on human red blood cells. Comparison with other mechanisms of oxidative stress. Biochim Biophys Acta 924:111–118

Voisin C, Aerts C, Houdret JL, Tonnel AB (1974) Effect of NO_2 on alveolar macrophages. In: Voisin C (ed) Réactions bronchopulmonaires aux pollutants atmosphes [in French]. INSERM, Paris, pp 273–288

Voisin C, Aerts C, Jakubsczak E, Houdret JL, Tonnel AB (1977a) Effets du bioxyde d'azote sur les macrophages alvéolaires en survie en phase gazeuse: un nouveau modèle expérimental pour l'étude in vitro de la cytotoxicité des gaz nocifs [in French]. Bull Eur Physiopath Respir 13:137–144

Voisin C, Aerts C, Jakubsczak E, Tonnel AB (1977b) La culture cellulaire en phase gazeuse. Un nouveau modèle expérimental d'étude in vitro des activités des macrophages [in French]. Bull Eur Physiopath Respir 13:69–82

Voisin C, Aerts C, Tonnel AB (1975) Mise en survie en phase gazeuse et reconstitution in vitro du microenvironnement naturel des macrophages alvéolaires [in French]. Pathol Biol 23:453–459

Wallaert B, Coursier JM, Gosset Ph, Saison JY, Tonnel AB (1998) Effects of urban air solution on cytokines secretion by alveolar macrophages in vitro. Eur Resp J 12:260S

Wallaert B, Fahy O, Tsicopoulos A, Gosset Ph, Saison JY, Tonnel AB (2000) Experimental systems for mechanistic studies of toxicant induced lung inflammation. Toxicol Letters 112–113:157–163

Wallaert B, Gosset Ph, Boitelle A, Tonnel AB (1996) In vitro assessment of environmental toxicology using alveolar cells as a target. Cell Biol Toxicol 12:251–256

Wenzel DG, Wrobel WJ, Kotek JJ, Morgan DL (1979) An ozone-generating system and chamber for testing injury to cultured cells. Arch Environ Health 34:454–460

Wenzel DG, Morgan DL (1982) Role of in vitro factors in ozone toxicity for cultured rat lung fibroblasts. Drug Chem Toxicol 5:201–217

Whitcutt MJ, Adler KB, Wu R (1988) A biphasic chamber system for maintaining polarity of differentiation of cultured respiratory tract epithelial cells. In vitro Cell Develop Biol 24:420–428

Young PP, Mendelson CR (1997) A GT box element is essential for basal and cyclic adenosine 3′,5′-monophosphate regulation of the human surfactant protein A2 gene in alveolar type II cells: evidence for the binding of lung nuclear factors distinct from Sp1. Mol Endocrinol 11:1082–1093

Zamora PO, Gregory RE, Li AP, Brooks AL (1986) An in vitro model for the exposure of lung alveolar epithelial cells to toxic gases. J Environ Pathol Toxicol Oncol 7:159–168

Chapter 11

Oxidative Stress in Laboratory Animals Exposed to Cigarette Smoke, with Special Reference to Chronic Obstructive Pulmonary Disease

Chris Coggins

Contents

11.1	Introduction	280
11.2	Cigarette Smoke	280
11.3	Smoking Machines	281
11.4	Markers of Oxidative Stress in Smoke-Exposed Animals	282
11.5	COPD	283
11.5.1	Epidemiology of COPD	283
11.5.2	Basic Pathways Mediating Cigarette-Smoke-Induced COPD	284
11.5.3	Animal Models of COPD	285
11.6	Future Models	286
	References	286

11.1 Introduction

The historical concept of oxygen as a major air pollutant has already been well documented (Halliwell and Gutteridge 1999), putting into balance the fact that virtually all life on Earth needs oxygen, with the fact that oxygen is biologically very reactive. The two are in balance because of the evolutionary development of antioxidant-defense mechanisms. Organisms that have antioxidant defense mechanisms can use oxygen for the production of energy, mainly in the cellular mitochondria.

Oxidative stress comes about when organisms are exposed to excessive amounts of oxygen, as higher atmospheric concentrations, higher partial pressures in such activities as diving, disease and/or malnutrition, and in the case of higher species such as vertebrates, by alterations in the oxygen transport system. The lung is uniquely susceptible to oxidative stress, as several cell types are continuously exposed to oxygen at atmospheric concentrations, unlike virtually all other cells in the body. The major components of ambient air that contribute to oxidative damage in the lungs include cigarette smoke, exhaust from internal combustion engines (fueled by both diesel and gasoline), and gases such as ozone and nitrogen dioxide.

Antioxidant protective mechanisms in the lungs include the presence of surfactant (from serous and goblet cells), which in turn contains such compounds as reduced glutathione (GSH), α-tocopherol, and ascorbic acid (MacNee and Rahman 2004). The deeper, nonciliated parts of the lung contain free protective cells such as alveolar macrophages, neutrophils, and lymphocytes. Many of the antioxidant protective mechanisms can be upregulated in the presence of oxidative stress; pulmonary disease results when the normal balance between oxidants and antioxidants is lost. Many pulmonary diseases thought to result from such imbalances are hypothesized to do so through inflammatory processes (Reuben et al. 2004). This is especially thought to be the case for smoking-induced diseases, such as pulmonary neoplasia, cardiovascular disease, and chronic obstructive pulmonary disease (COPD).

11.2 Cigarette Smoke

The chemistry of smoke from reference cigarettes has been described in a number of publications (Hoffman and Hoffman 1997; Hoffmann et al. 2001; Rodgman and Green 2003; Roemer 2004; Stabbert 2003), including those that have concentrated in particular on radicals and the role radicals may play in disease (Pryor 1997; Pryor et al. 1998). An integral part of this chemistry is the complicated sequence of processes that occur during the combustion of tobacco. The conditions in the burning cone are highly reducing (temperatures up to 950 °C), as oxygen is consumed by carbonized tobacco to produce heat, carbon monoxide, carbon dioxide, and water (Baker 1999).

Immediately behind the combustion zone is a pyrolysis/distillation zone. Temperatures here are between 200° and 600 °C, still with low concentrations of oxygen (Baker 1999). Aerosol formation occurs as chemicals pass from the burning cone, through the unburned tobacco and (usually) through the cigarette filter.

The smoke that emerges from the cigarette filter is termed mainstream smoke. It is available to smokers, and to machines that mimic human smoking for analytical purposes or for dilution and subsequent distribution to experimental animals. This mainstream smoke is arbitrarily divided into a particulate phase, which does not pass through a Cambridge pad, and a vapor or gas phase, which does. Additional complications include added ingredients (Baker et al. 2004), selective absorption (e.g., phenols by the cellulose acetate fibers used in most cigarette filters), and the use of ventilation holes and additional materials (e.g., activated charcoal) in the filter (Hoffman et al. 2001).

Both particulate and gas phases of cigarette smoke have been reported to contain large numbers (e.g., 10^{15-16}) of so-called free radicals (Pryor et al. 1998), low-molecular-weight compounds, often carbon- or oxygen-centered radicals. The carbon-centered radicals can react with oxygen to produce other reactive oxygen species (ROS).

Although the concentrations of oxygen are reduced in the burning cone of the cigarette, it is unlikely that this would translate into reduced concentrations in the smoke inhaled by smokers. This is because the puffs taken from the cigarette (puffs usually with volumes of 20–100 ml) are diluted substantially with air at the point of inhalation into the respiratory tract (Bernstein 2004).

Nonsmokers may be exposed to a different kind of smoke, termed environmental tobacco smoke, or ETS (Baker and Proctor 1990). This is the aged and diluted mixture of exhaled smoke from the smoker, with smoke emitted from the burning tip of the cigarette between puffs (the latter being termed sidestream smoke). No filtration is involved in the formation of ETS; because of the dilution that takes place, ETS concentrations are very much smaller than are those of the mainstream smoke taken in by smokers (Jenkins et al. 2000). The free radicals mentioned above for mainstream smoke have also been reported to be present in large numbers in sidestream smoke (Pryor 1997); concentrations in ETS are likely to be very much lower.

11.3 Smoking Machines

A number of designs have been published for smoking machines to expose experimental animals (largely rodents) nose-only to diluted mainstream smoke. The designs have attempted to balance a short path length from the cigarette to the animal, with the ability to expose large numbers of animals. Long path lengths may prevent any short-lived components of the smoke from reaching the experimental animals. A typical range would be short path length, small number of animals (Guerin et al. 1979), medium path length, and medium-large number of animals (Baumgartner and Coggins 1980), and long path length, large number of animals (Henry et al. 1985). Designs involving whole-body exposures (Chen et al. 1992) would appear to have very long path lengths, along with other disadvantages. Long-term inhalation studies with a variety of different animal species have not resulted in useful animal models for human smoking-related disease (Coggins 2002).

Machines for exposing animals to surrogates of ETS (surrogates are required because of the logistical constraint in producing smoke exhaled by smokers) have in general used appropriate aging periods (Ayres et al. 1994; Haussmann et al. 1998a; Teague et al. 1994). In general, responses noted in animals exposed to ETS surrogates have been restricted to localized hyperplasia in the nasal passages (Coggins et al. 1993; Haussmann et al. 1998b; Stinn et al. 2005). By contrast, an inhalation study with mice exposed nose-only to sidestream smoke showed systemic inflammatory responses and accentuated systemic lipid peroxidation (Zhang et al. 2003). This same group had earlier shown that antioxidant supplementation in healthy, old mice prevented inflammatory responses induced by exposure to sidestream smoke (Zhang et al. 2001). Unfortunately, neither of these two studies made measurements of the amounts of smoke presented—they were almost certainly extremely high.

Although there are reports of measurements of radicals in mainstream smoke (Pryor 1997), there do not appear to any such measurements reported in mainstream smoke presented to experimental animals in smoking machines, or in similar studies using ETS surrogates as the test material.

11.4 Markers of Oxidative Stress in Smoke-Exposed Animals

The National Institute of Environmental Health Sciences (NIEHS) has "taken the lead in initiating the first comparative study for determining which of the available biomarkers of oxidative stress are most specific, sensitive, and selective," using animals treated with carbon tetrachloride (Kadiiska et al. 2000). The original list of biomarkers was α-tocopherol, coenzyme Q, ascorbic acid and uric acid, GHS, and total oxidant capacity (Kadiiska et al. 2000). Very recently, an update was published (Kadiiska et al. 2005), giving a series of analytes for the oxidation products of lipids, proteins, and DNA in different body fluids. For oxidation products in lipids, the following assays are suggested: lipid hydroperoxide, malondialdehyde (MDA), thiobarbituric acid reactive substances (TBARS), and 8-iso-$PGF_{2\alpha}$ (free and esterified) (Kadiiska et al. 2005). For oxidation products of proteins, the list is protein carbonyls, methionine sulfoxidation, and tyrosine products. Finally, for oxidation products of DNA, the list is the Comet assay, leukocyte MDA–DNA adducts, and urinary 8-hydroxy-2'-deoxyguanosine (8-OHdG) (Kadiiska et al. 2005). A variety of different assays is given for different body fluids (Kadiiska et al. 2005).

Very few of the NIEHS list (Kadiiska et al. 2005) have been measured in smoke-exposed animals. The subject of markers of oxidative stress in animals exposed to smoke was included as part of a recent review (van der Vaart et al. 2004), a review which also included studies in humans and which also assessed the effects of smoke on inflammation. A supplemental online report (van der Vaart et al. 2004) lists the various studies examined in the review and lists the various parameters that have been examined.

A total of six studies were included in the review (van der Vaart et al. 2004). The following parameters were reported: 8-OHdG, a DNA oxidation product (Evans et al. 2004) in both lung tissues and bronchoalveolar lavage fluid (BALF), GSH in lung homogenate, BALF and in blood, ascorbic acid in lung homogenate and in BALF, and cysteine in blood and lung tissue (van der Vaart et al. 2004).

Other studies have concentrated on the 8-OHdG endpoint. In a study using whole-body exposures of rats to sidestream smoke, no effect was noted on 8-OHdG concentrations in lung tissue (Arif et al. 2001). This is in contrast to work with both mainstream smoke (Aoshiba et al. 2003a) and ETS (Izzotti et al. 1999), where increased concentrations were noted.

There are some studies that reported an impact of smoke exposure on GSH concentrations. Thus mainstream smoke increased total GSH in BALF (March et al. 2002), with no effect of concurrent treatment with ozone. Work has shown that it is the particulate phase of the smoke that is responsible for the oxidative damage, and that it can be blocked by vitamin C (Panda et al. 2001). Various antioxidants have also been effective (D'Agostini 2001; De Flora 2003; Izzotti 2001; Sadowska 2005).

A study with only an indirect assessment of oxidative stress examined the effects after smoke exposure of an instilled catalytic antioxidant, manganese (III) *meso*-tetrakis(*N*,*N*'-diethyl-1,3-imidazolium-2-yl) porphyrin (Smith et al. 2002). The catalyst was given by intratracheal instillation to groups of rats exposed to filtered air or cigarette smoke, for up to 8 weeks (6 h/day, 3days/week). Smoke exposures were well characterized and were at conventional concentrations. The experimental treatment significantly reduced the number of cells recovered in BALF, specifically macrophages, neutrophils, and lymphocytes. The authors concluded that the catalysts decreased the adverse effects of smoke exposure. Metalloporphyrins are known to have multiple antioxidant properties, including scavenging superoxide, hydrogen peroxide, peroxynitrite, and lipid peroxyl radicals (Smith et al. 2002).

11.5 COPD

COPD is a disease state characterized by airflow limitation that is not fully reversible. The airflow limitation is usually progressive and is associated with an abnormal inflammatory response of the lungs to noxious particles and gases (Pauweis et al. 2001). The "abnormal" or chronic inflammation leads to a narrowing of the small airways (bronchiolitis) and to alveolar wall destruction (Hogg 2002; Snider 2003). The chronic inflammation is characterized by increased numbers of alveolar macrophages, neutrophils, and cytotoxic T lymphocytes (Barnes and Cosio 2004), and the release of multiple inflammatory mediators (lipids, chemokines, cytokines, growth factors) (Barnes 2003, 2004; Rennard 1998). The abnormal inflammatory response may be the key to susceptibility (Agusti et al. 2003). Although many types of inflammatory cells and mediators have been identified in COPD patients, their role in the progression of the disease remains largely unknown (Barnes 2003).

The chronic obstructive bronchitis with mucus hypersecretion may contribute to, but is not necessarily associated with, airflow limitation (Barnes 2003; Cosio-Piqueras and Cosio 2001). *Emphysema* is defined as a condition of the lung characterized by abnormal permanent enlargement of airspaces distal to the terminal bronchiole, accompanied by destruction of the lung parenchyma with or without obvious fibrosis and loss of lung elasticity (Cosio-Piqueras and Cosio 2001; Snider 1992a, b, 2003). Subjects with COPD do not often show emphysema without bronchitis and small airway disease (March et al. 2000).

11.5.1 Epidemiology of COPD

COPD is considered a major health concern, with an overall prevalence in adults estimated at between 4 and 10% in countries where it has been rigorously measured (Halbert et al. 2003). A recent estimate for the incidence of COPD in the United States was given as 16 million people (Mahadeva and Shapiro 2002). The major risk factors for COPD are considered to be cigarette smoking, use of biomass fuels, and air pollution

(Halbert et al. 2003); the population-attributable incidence for cigarette smoking and COPD is about 80–90% (Halbert et al. 2003).

Epidemiological studies have shown that it is mainly susceptible smokers that develop COPD (Siafakas and Tzortzaki 2002).

11.5.2 Basic Pathways Mediating Cigarette-Smoke-Induced COPD

Cigarette smoke exposure has been shown to cause severe oxidative stress in the lung (Aoshiba 2003; MacNee and Rahman 2001, 2004). The oxidants present in cigarette smoke, together with abundant infiltration and activation status of inflammatory cells in the smoker's lung, releasing even more oxygen-based free radicals, may be involved in a proteolytic/antiproteolytic imbalance, leading to tissue destruction (Churg et al. 2003; Seagrave 2000; Seagrave et al. 2004). The incidence of such an imbalance in human populations was the subject of a recent review (deSerres 2003).

A recent study characterized the inflammatory and mucus hypersecretory changes in the lungs of smoke-exposed rats, examining both the role of cytokine-induced neutrophil attractants (CINCs) and a possible mediator of the hypersecretion (Stevenson et al. 2005). The results showed that generation of a neutrophilic/mucus hypersecretory lung phenotype could be produced by just two exposures to smoke, 15 h apart (no details were given on smoke composition). There was a time-dependent increase in the number of CINCs in lung tissue and in lavage fluid over the 24-h period following exposure to smoke. These temporal changes in CINCs mirrored increases in neutrophil infiltration, indicative of a likely role in neutrophil influx, in turn thought to correlate well with matrix destruction (Churg and Wright 2005). The smoke-induced neutrophil infiltration could be inhibited in a dose-related manner (Stevenson et al. 2005).

Recent work has indicated that cigarette smoke is the main etiologic factor, through a mechanism that may involve enhanced proinflammatory gene transcription (Marwick et al. 2004). Other work has indicated that the oxidative stress produced by exposure to cigarette smoke (MacNee and Rahman 2001; Moodie et al. 2004) is a highly relevant factor. The responsiveness of the nuclear factor erythroid 2-related factor 2 (Nrf2) pathway may act as a major determinant of the susceptibility to tobacco-smoke-induced airway disease, by upregulating antioxidant defenses and by decreasing inflammation and alveolar cell apoptosis (Rangasamy et al. 2004).

Oxidative stress has been shown to directly inactivate antiproteinases such as α1-antitrypsin (α1-AT) and secretory leukoprotease inhibitor (SLPI) (Betsuyaku et al. 2002; Cavarra et al. 2001b; Hill et al. 2000), as well as activating matrix metalloproteinases (MMPs) (Belvisi 2003; Selman 2003). Moreover, oxidative stress induces the transcription of many proinflammatory genes controlled by transcription factors such as nuclear factor-κB (NF-κB) (Di Stefano 2002; Moodie et al. 2004). Oxidative stress is also thought to be involved in the accumulation of macrophages in the alveolar interstitial spaces, independent of other proinflammatory stimuli (Kirkham et al. 2003). This latter group has hypothesized that the oxidative stress promotes the macrophage accumulation through the production of reactive carbonyls (particularly acrolein) (Kirkham et al. 2003).

11.5.3 Animal Models of COPD

A number of animal models have been reported that exhibit at least one of the features of the complicated pathology of COPD, such as chronic bronchitis (Nikula and Green 2000) and emphysema (Mahadeva and Shapiro 2002; March et al. 2000; Taraseviciene-Stewart 2004; Wright and Churg 2002). In these models, airspace enlargement has been demonstrated after chronic exposure to mainstream smoke, and also in shorter exposures to high concentrations of smoke. Ideally, such models need to represent the various patterns of alveolar wall destruction that have been reported in humans, as well as host factors that parallel the etiology of the pathological condition. Animal models with genetic predisposition (e.g., an inherent α1-AT deficiency or increased sensitivity to oxidative stress) to develop emphysema are probably the most relevant in mimicking the susceptible human population (deSerres 2003; Kodavanti et al. 1998, 2001). The application of genetic engineering strategies in mice offers a great potential to dissect the pathogenetic pathways of emphysema (Kodavanti 2001; Mahadeva et al. 2002). A few examples of susceptible and genetically engineered models are described below.

Promising susceptible animal models have been described that develop emphysema following whole body exposure to mainstream smoke (Caverra et al. 2001b; Takubo et al. 2002). C57Bl/6J mice, which have a mild deficiency in their antielastase screen, and DBA/2 mice, which are sensitive to oxidants, developed emphysema following 6 months of exposure to cigarette smoke, whereas the mouse strain with normal antielastase screen and nonsensitivity to oxidants (ICR-mouse) did not (Cavarra et al. 2001a). It appears that there are considerable strain differences in the extent of emphysema produced in smoke-exposed mice (Churg et al. 2004; Guerassimov et al. 2004; Obot et al. 2004; Shapiro et al. 2004; Valenca et al. 2004). The situation is complicated by large differences in the degree of detail in characterizing the smoke exposures used to produce emphysema.

The pallid mouse (C57Bl/6J, pa$^{+/+}$), with a severe α1-AT deficiency (DeSanti et al. 1995; Martorana et al. 1993), developed panlobular emphysema after only 4 months of whole-body exposure to cigarette smoke (Cavarra et al. 2001a; Takubo et al. 2002). The pallid mice exhibited features similar to the human situation, including a T-lymphocytic inflammatory response and increased lung compliance (after 6 months of exposure).

The development of spontaneous emphysema has been studied in various transgenic mouse models (Mahadeva and Shapiro 2002). Most of these models have contributed to the knowledge of certain aspects of the development of emphysema, but unfortunately, they have not been challenged by exogenous noxious agents.

Recently, a transgenic mouse model was established that expresses low levels of human α1-AT (Churg et al. 2003), as part of an effort to produce a treatment for cigarette smoke-induced emphysema. The transgenic mice were tolerant to exogenously applied human α1-AT. Mice were exposed to mainstream smoke for up to 6 months; some of them received human α1-AT repeatedly. The latter treatment abolished smoke-induced elevations of neutrophil counts in lavage fluide, as well as the elastin and collagen breakdown products desmosine and hydroxyproline, respectively. Treatment also provided some protection against airspace size. It was concluded that α1-AT therapy reduced the inflammation and partially protects the animals against emphysema.

A murine model deficient for macrophage elastase (MME$^{-/-}$) has been used to shown to be protected against development of mainstream smoke-induced emphysema (Hautamaki et al. 1997). The authors concluded that macrophage elastase is probably sufficient for the development of emphysema that results from chronic inhalation of mainstream smoke. The role of the macrophage elastase in the smoke-induced inflammation and tissue destruction has been corroborated by elegant studies carried out by Ofulue and coworkers (1998).

Recent work has suggested that a further consideration should be taken when examining the role of inflammation and excessive proteolysis in the pulmonary tissue destruction (Aoshiba et al. 2003b). This work provided evidence that alveolar epithelial apoptosis causes emphysema in C57Bl/6J mice. The authors used a novel protein transfection agent (Chariot) to introduce active caspase-3 into bronchial epithelial cells in vivo. These findings indicate that inflammation, proteolysis, oxidative stress, apoptosis, or cell hemostasis in general are interrelated mechanisms contributing to cigarette smoke-induced emphysema (Tuder et al. 2003).

11.6 Future Models

In many of the studies described relatively minor attention was made to the abnormal inflammatory process mentioned earlier (Siafakas and Tzortzaki 2002; Rangasamy 2004). Future models should provide a tool to understand the exact role of inflammation on the etiology and progression of the disease (Adcock et al. 2005; Reuben et al. 2004; Sadowska et al. 2005).

A prototypic chain of events might be as follows: cigarette smoke exposure → oxidative stress → proinflammatory mediators → inflammation → COPD. Support for this hypothesis is given from a recent paper that showed adverse effects of oxygen supplementation in COPD patients (Carpagnano et al. 2004), in conjunction with increased oxidative stress and with airway inflammation.

Novel designs for cigarette designs, and the potential use of antioxidants and other agents (Adcock et al. 2005; Xu et al. 2004), may be able to break this chain for those people unable to quit smoking.

References

Adcock IM, Cosio B, Tsaoprouni L, Barnes PJ, Ito K (2005) Redox regulation of histone deacetylases and glucocorticoid-mediated inhibition of the inflammatory response. Antioxid Redox Signal 7:144–152

Agusti A, MacNee W, Donaldson K, Cosio MG (2003) Hypothesis: does COPD have an autoimmune component? Thorax 58:832–834

Aoshiba K, Koinuma M, Yokohori N, Nagai A (2003a) Immunohistochemical evaluation of oxidative stress in murine lungs after cigarette smoke exposure. Inhal Toxicol 15:1029–1038

Aoshiba K, Yokohori N, Nagai A (2003b) Alveolar wall apoptosis causes lung destruction and emphysematous changes. Am J Respir Cell Mol Biol 28:555–562

Arif JM, Vadhanam MV, DeGroot AJL, VanZeeland AA, Gairola CG, Gupta RC (2001) Effect of cigarette smoke exposure on the modulation of 8-oxo-2′-deoxyguanosine in rat lungs as analyzed by 32P postlabeling and HPLC-ECD. Int J Oncol 19:763–766

Ayres PH, Mosberg AT, Coggins CRE (1994) Design, construction and operation of an inhalation system for exposing laboratory animals to environmental tobacco smoke. Am Ind Hyg Assoc J 55:806–810

Baker RR (1999) Smoke chemistry. In: Davis DL, Nielsen MT (eds) Tobacco: production, chemistry, and technology. Blackwell, Oxford, pp 398–439

Baker RR, Proctor CJ (1990) The origins and properties of environmental tobacco smoke. Environ Int 16:231245

Baker RR, Massey ED, Smith G (2004) An overview of the effects of tobacco ingredients on smoke chemistry and toxicity. Food Chem Toxicol 42:S53–S83

Barnes PJ (2003) New concepts in chronic obstructive pulmonary disease. Ann Rev Med Selected Topics Clin Sci 54:113–129

Barnes PJ (2004) Mediators of chronic obstructive pulmonary disease. Pharmacol Rev 56:515–548

Barnes PJ, Cosio MG (2004) Characterization of T lymphocytes in chronic obstructive pulmonary disease. PLoS Med 1:25–27

Baumgartner H, Coggins CRE (1980) Description of a continuous-smoking inhalation machine for exposing small animals to tobacco smoke. Beitr Tabakforsch Int 10:169–174

Belvisi MG, Bottomley KM (2003) The role of matrix metalloproteinases (MMPs) in the pathophysiology of chronic obstructive pulmonary disease (COPD): a therapeutic role for inhibitors of MMPs? Inflamm Res 52:95–100

Bernstein DM (2004) A review of the influence of particle size, puff volume, and inhalation pattern on the deposition of cigarette smoke particles in the respiratory tract. Inhal Toxicol 16:675–689

Betsuyaku T, Takeyabu K, Tanino M, Nishimura M (2002) Role of secretory leukocyte protease inhibitor in the development of subclinical emphysema. Eur Respir J 19:1051–1057

Carpagnano GE, Kharitonov SA, Foschino-Barbaro MP, Resta O, Gramiccioni E, Barnes PJ (2004) Supplementary oxygen in healthy subjects and those with COPD increases oxidative stress and airway inflammation. Thorax 59:1016–1019

Cavarra E, Bartelesi B, Lucatelli M, Fineschi S, Lunghi B, Gambelli F, Ortiz LA, Martorana PA, Lungarella G (2001a) Effects of cigarette smoke in mice with different levels of alpha-1 proteinase inhibitor and sensitivity to oxidants. Am J Respir Crit Care Med 164:886–890

Cavarra E, Lucatelli M, Gambelli F, Bartelesi B, Fineschi S, Szarka A, Giannerini F, Martorana PA, Lungarella G (2001b) Human SLPI inactivation after cigarette smoke exposure in a new in vivo model of pulmonary oxidative stress. Am J Physiol 281:L412–L417

Chen BT, Bechtold WE, Mauderly JL (1992) Description and evaluation of a cigarette smoke generation system for inhalation studies. J Aerosol Med 5:19–30

Churg A, Wright CW (2005) Proteases and emphysema. Curr Opin Pulm Med 11:153–159

Churg A, Wang RD, Xie CS, Wright JL (2003) Alpha-1-antitrypsin ameliorates cigarette smoke-induced emphysema in the mouse. Am J Respir Crit Care Med 168:199–207

Churg A, Wang RD, Tai H, Wang X, Xie CS, Wright JL (2004) Tumor necrosis factor-alpha drives 70% of cigarette smoke-induced emphysema in the mouse. Am J Respir Crit Care Med 170:492–498

Coggins CRE (2002) A minireview of chronic animal inhalation studies with mainstream cigarette smoke. Inhal Toxicol 14:991–1002

Coggins CRE, Ayres PH, Mosberg AT, Sagartz JW, Hayes AW (1993) Subchronic inhalation study in rats, using aged and diluted sidestream smoke from a reference cigarette. Inhal Toxicol 5:77–96

Cosio-Piqueras MG, Cosio MG (2001) Disease of the airways in chronic obstructive pulmonary disease. Eur Respir J 18:S41–S49

D'Agostini F, Balansky RM, Izzotti A, Lubet RA, Kelloff GJ, DeFlora S (2001) Modulation of apoptosis by cigarette smoke and cancer chemopreventive agents in the respiratory tract of rats. Carcinogenesis 22:375–380

De Flora S, D'Agostini F, Balansky R, Camoirano A, Bennicelli C, Bagnasco M, Cartiglia C, Tampa E, Longobardi MG, Lubet RA, Izzotti A (2003) Modulation of cigarette smoke-related endpoints in mutagenesis and carcinogenesis. Mutat Res 523:237–252

DeSanti MM, Martorana PA, Cavarra E (1995) Pallid mice with genetic emphysema. Neutrophil elastase burden and elastin loss occur without alteration in the bronchoalveolar lavage cell population. Lab Invest 73:40–47

deSerres FTJ (2003) Alpha-1 antitrypsin deficiency is not a rare disease but a disease that is rarely diagnosed. Environ Health Perspect 111:161851–161854

Di Stefano A, Caramori G, Oates T, Capelli A, Lusuardi M, Gnemmi I, Ioli F, Chung KF, Donner CF, Barnes PJ, Adcock IM (2002) Increased expression of nuclear factor-κB in bronchial biopsies from smokers and patients with COPD. Eur Respir J 20:556–563

Evans MD, Dizdaroglu M, Cooke MS (2004) Oxidative DNA damage and disease: induction, repair and significance. Mutat Res 567:1–61

Guerassimov A, Hoshino Y, Takubo Y, Turcotte A, Yamamoto M, Ghezzo H, Triantafillopoulos A, Whittaker K, Hoidal JR, Cosio MG (2004) The development of emphysema in cigarette smoke-exposed mice is strain dependent. Am J Respir Crit Care Med 170:974–980

Guerin MR, Stokely JR, Higgins CE, Moneyhun JH, Holmberg RW (1979) Inhalation bioassay chemistry—Walton horizontal smoking machine for inhalation exposure of rodents to cigarette smoke. J Nat Cancer Inst 63:441–448

Halbert RJ, Isonaka S, George D, Iqbal A (2003) Interpreting COPD prevalence estimates: What is the true burden of disease? Chest 123:1684–1692

Halliwell B, Gutteridge JMC (1999) Free radicals in biology and medicine, 3rd ed. Oxford University Press, Oxford

Haussmann H-J, Anskeit E, Becker D, Kuhl P, Stinn W, Teredesai A, Voncken P, Walk R-A (1998a) Comparison of fresh and room-aged cigarette sidestream smoke in a subchronic inhalation study on rats. Toxicol Sci 41:100–116

Haussmann H-J, Gerstenberg B, Gocke W, Kuhl P, Schepers G, Stabbert R, Stinn W, Teredesai A, Tewes F, Anskeit E, Terpstra P (1998b) 12-Month inhalation study on room-aged cigarette sidestream smoke in rats. Inhal Toxicol 10:663–697

Hautamaki RD, Kobayashi DK, Senior RM, Shapiro SD (1997) Requirement for macrophage elastase for cigarette smoke-induced emphysema in mice. Science 277:2002–2004

Henry CJ, Dansie DR, Kanagalingam KK, Kouri RE, Gayle T, Guerin M, Holmberg R, Florant L, Greenspan J (1985) Chronic inhalation studies in mice. 1. Facilities and equipment for "nose-only" exposure to cigarette smoke. Beitr Tabakforsch Int 13:37–53

Hill AT, Bayley DL, Campbell EJ, Hill SL, Stockley RA (2000) Airways inflammation in chronic bronchitis: the effects of smoking and alpha1-antitrypsin deficiency. Eur Respir J 15:886–890

Hoffmann D, Hoffmann I (1997) The changing cigarette, 1950–1995. J Toxicol Environ Health 50:307–364

Hoffmann D, Hoffmann I, El-Bayoumy K (2001) The less harmful cigarette: a controversial issue. A tribute to Ernst L. Wynder. Chem Res Toxicol 14:768–790

Hogg JC, Senior RM (2002) Chronic obstructive pulmonary disease center dot 2: pathology and biochemistry of emphysema. Thorax 57:830–834

Izzotti A, Bagnasco M, D'Agostini F, Cartiglia C, Lubet RA, Kelloff GJ, De Flora S (1999) Formation and persistence of nucleotide alterations in rats exposed whole-body to environmental cigarette smoke. Carcinogenesis 20:1499–1505

Izzotti A, Balansky RM, D'Agostini F, Bennicelli C, Myers SR, Grubbs CJ, Lubet RA, Kelloff GJ, DeFlora S (2001) Modulation of biomarkers by chemopreventive agents in smoke-exposed rats. Cancer Res 61:2472–2479

Jenkins RA, Guerin MR, Tomkins BA (2000) Eisenberg M (ed) The chemistry of environmental tobacco smoke: composition and measurement, 2nd edn. Lewis, Boca Raton

Kadiiska MB, Gladen BC, Baird DD, Dikalova AE, Sohal RS, Hatch GA, Jones DP, Mason RP, Barrett JC (2000) Biomarkers of oxidative stress study: are plasma antioxidants markers of CCl4 poisoning? Free Radic Biol Med 28:838–845

Kadiiska MB, Gladen BC, Baird DD, Germolec D, Graham LB, Parker CE, Nyska A, Wachsman JT, Ames BN, Basu S, Brot N, Fitzgerald GA, Floyd RA, George M, Heinecke JW, Hatch GE, Hensley K, Lawson JA, Marnett LJ, Morrow JD, Murray DM, Plastaras J, Roberts LJ, Rokach J, Shigenaga MK, Sohal RS, Sun J, Tice RR, Van Thiel DH, Wellner D, Walter PB, Tomer KB, Mason RP, Barrett JC (2005) Biomarkers of oxidative stress study II. Are oxidation products of lipids, proteins, and DNA markers of CCl_4 poisoning? Free Radic Biol Med 38:698–710

Kirkham PA, Spooner G, Ffoulkes-Jones C, Calvez R (2005) Cigarette smoke triggers macrophage adhesion and activation: role of lipid peroxidation products and scavenger receptor. Free Radic Biol Med 35:697–710

Kodavanti UP, Costa DL (2005) Rodent models of susceptibility: what is their place in inhalation toxicology? Respir Physiol 128:57–70

Kodavanti UP, Costa DL, Bromberg PA (1998) Rodent models of cardiopulmonary disease: their potential applicability in studies of air pollutant susceptibility. Environ Health Perspect 106:111–130

MacNee W, Rahman I (2001) Is oxidative stress central to the pathogenesis of chronic obstructive pulmonary disease? Trends Mol Med 7:55–62

MacNee W, Rahman I (2004) Oxidative stress in chronic obstructive pulmonary disease. In: Vallyathan V, Castranova V, Shi X (eds) Oxygen/nitrogen radicals: lung injury and disease. Marcel Dekker, New York, pp 317–360

Mahadeva R, Shapiro SD (2002) Chronic obstructive pulmonary disease center dot 3: experimental animal models of pulmonary emphysema. Thorax 57:908–914

March TH, Green FHY, Hahn FF, Nikula KJ (2000) Animal models of emphysema and their relevance to studies of particle-induced disease. Inhal Toxicol 12:155–187

March TH, Barr EB, Finch GL, Nikula KJ, Seagrave JC (2002) Effects of concurrent ozone exposure on the pathogenesis of cigarette smoke-exposed emphysema in B6C3F1 mice. Inhal Toxicol 14:1187–1213

Martorana PA, Brand T, Gardi C, vanEven P, deSanti MM, Calzoni P, Marcolongo P, Lungarella G (1993) The pallid mouse: a model of genetic $alpha_1$-antitrypsin deficiency. Lab Invest 68:233–241

Marwick JA, Kirkham PA, Stevenson CS, Danahay H, Giddings J, Butler K, Donaldson K, MacNee W, Rahman I (2004) Cigarette smoke alters chromatin remodeling and induces proinflammatory genes in rat lungs. Am J Respir Cell Mol Biol 31:633–642

Moodie FM, Marwick JA, Anderson CS, Szulakowski P, Biswas SK, Bauter MR, Kilty I, Rahman I (2004) Oxidative stress and cigarette smoke alter chromatin remodeling but differentially regulate NF-κB activation and proinflammatory cytokine release in alveolar epithelial cells. FASEB J 18:1897–1899

Nikula KJ, Green FHY (2000) Animal models of chronic bronchitis and their relevance to studies of particle-induced disease. Inhal Toxicol 12:123–153

Obot CJ, Lee KM, Fuciarelli AF, Renne RA, McKinney WJ (2004) Characterization of mainstream cigarette smoke (MS)-induced biomarker responses in ICR and C57BL/6 mice. Inhal Toxicol 16:701719

Ofulue AF, Ko M, Abboud RT (1998) Time course of neutrophil and macrophage elastinolytic activities in cigarette smoke-induced emphysema. Am J Physiol 19:L1134–L1144

Panda K, Chattopadhyay R, Chattopadhyay D, Chatterjee IB (2001) Cigarette smoke-induced protein oxidation and proteolysis is exclusively caused by its tar phase: prevention by vitamin C. Toxicol Lett 123:21–32

Pauweis RA, Buist AS, Calverley PM (2001) Global strategy for the diagnosis, management, and prevention of chronic obstructive pulmonary disease. NHLBI/WHO Global Initiative for Chronic Obstructive Lung Disease (GOLD) workshop summary. Am J Respir Crit Care Med 163:1256–1276

Pryor WA (1997) Cigarette smoke radicals and the role of free radicals in chemical carcinogenicity. Environ Health Perspect 105:S875–S882

Pryor WA, Stone K, Zang LY, Bermudez E (1998) Fractionation of aqueous cigarette tar extracts: fractions that contain the tar radical cause DNA damage. Chem Res Toxicol 11:441–448

Rangasamy T, Cho CY, Thimmulappa RK, Zhen L, Srisuma SS, Kensler TW, Yamamoto M, Petrache I, Tuder RM, Biswal S (2004) Genetic ablation of Nrf2 enhances susceptibility to cigarette smoke-induced emphysema in mice. J Clin Invest 114:1248–1259

Rennard SI (1998) COPD: Overview of definitions, epidemiology, and factors influencing its development. Chest113:S235–S241

Reuben JS, Guo R-F, Ward PA (2004) Mediators of lung inflammation. Role of reactive oxygen and nitrogen species. In: Vallyathan V, Castranova V, Shi X (eds) Oxygen/nitrogen radicals: lung injury and disease. Marcel Dekker, New York, pp 91–110

Rodgman A, Green CR (2003) Toxic chemicals in cigarette mainstream smoke—hazard and hoopla. Beit Tabakforsch Int 20:481–545

Roemer E, Stabbert R, Rustemeier K, Veltel DJ, Meisgen TJ, Reininghaus W, Carchman RA, Gaworski CL, Podraza KF (2004) Chemical composition, cytotoxicity and mutagenicity of smoke from US commercial and reference cigarettes smoked under two sets of machine smoking conditions. Toxicol 195:31–52

Sadowska AM, van Overveld FJ, Gorecka D, Zdral A, Filewska M, Demkow UA, Luyten C, Saenen E, Zielinski J, De Backer WA (2005) The interrelationship between markers of inflammation and oxidative stress in chronic obstructive pulmonary disease: modulation by inhaled steroids and antioxidant. Respir Med 99:241–249

Seagrave J (2000) Oxidative mechanisms in tobacco smoke-induced emphysema. J Toxicol Environ Health 61:69–78

Seagrave J, Barr EB, March TH, Nikula KJ (2004) Effects of cigarette smoke exposure and cessation on inflammatory cells and matrix metalloproteinase activity in mice. Exp Lung Res 30:1–15

Selman M, Cisneros-Lira J, Gaxiola M, Ramirez R, Kudlacz EM, Mitchell PG, Pardo A (2003) Matrix metalloproteinases inhibition attenuates tobacco smoke-induced emphysema in guinea pigs. Chest 123:1633–1641

Shapiro SD, DeMeo DL, Silverman EK (2004) Smoke and mirrors: mouse models as a reflection of human chronic obstructive pulmonary disease. Am J Respir Crit Care Med 170:929–931

Siafakas NM, Tzortzaki EG (2002) Few smokers develop COPD. Why? Respir Med 96:615–624

Smith KR, Uyeminami DL, Kodavanti UP, Crapo JD, Chang LY, Pinkerton KE (2002) Inhibition of tobacco smoke-induced lung inflammation by a catalytic antioxidant. Free Radic Biol Med 33:1106–1114

Snider GL (1992a) Emphysema: the first two centuries—and beyond. A historical overview, with suggestions for future research: part 1. Am Rev Respir Dis 146:1334–1344

Snider GL (1992b) Emphysema: the first two centuries—and beyond. A historical overview, with suggestions for future research: part 2. Am Rev Respir Dis 146:1615–1622

Snider GL (2003) Nosology for our day—its application to chronic obstructive pulmonary disease. Am J Respir Crit Care Med 167:678–683

Stabbert R, Voncken P, Rustemeier K, Haussmann H-J, Roemer E, Schaffernicht H, Patskan G (2003) Toxicological evaluation of an electrically heated cigarette. Part 2. Chemical composition of mainstream smoke. J Appl Toxicol 23:329–339

Stevenson CS, Coote K, Webster R, Johnston A, Atherton HC, Nicholls A, Giddings J, Sugar R, Jackson A, Press NJ, Brown Z, Butler K, Danahay H (2005) Characterization of cigarette smoke-induced inflammatory and mucus hypersecretory changes in rat lung and the role of CXCR2 ligands in mediating this effect. Am J Physiol 88:L514–L522

Stinn W, Teredesai A, Anskeit E, Rustemeier K, Schepers G, Schnell P, Haussmann H-J, Carchman RA, Coggins CRE, Reininghaus W (2005) Chronic nose-only inhalation study in rats, comparing room-aged sidestream smoke and diesel engine exhaust. Inhal Toxicol 17:549–576

Takubo Y, Guerassimov A, Ghezzo H, Triantafillopoulos A, Bates JHT, Hoidal JR, Cosio MG (2002) α_1-Antitrypsin determines the pattern of emphysema and function in tobacco smoke-exposed mice parallels with human disease. Am J Respir Crit Care Med 166:1596–1603

Taraseviciene-Stewart L, Scerbavicius R, Choe K-H, Moore M, Sullivan A, Nicolls MR, Fontenot AP, Tuder RM, Voelkel NF (2004) An animal model of autoimmune emphysema. Am J Respir Crit Care Med 171:734–742

Teague SV, Pinkerton KE, Goldsmith M, Gebremichael A, Chang S, Jenkins RA (1994) Sidestream cigarette smoke generation and exposure system for environmental tobacco smoke studies. Inhal Toxicol 6:79–93

Tuder RM, Petrache I, Elias JA, Voelkel NF, Henson PM (2003) Apoptosis and emphysema—the missing link. Am J Respir Cell Mol Biol 28:551–554

Valenca S, Da Hora K, Castro P, Moraes VG, Carvalho L, Porto LC (2004) Emphysema and metalloelastase expresion in mouse lung induced by cigarette smoke. Toxicol Pathol 32:351–356

van der Vaart H, Postma DS, Timens W, Ten Hacken NHT (2004) Acute effects of cigarette smoke on inflammation and oxidative stress: a review. Thorax 59:713–721

Wright JL, Churg A (2002) Animal models of cigarette smoke-induced COPD. Chest 122: S301–S306

Xu L, Cai BQ, Zhu YJ (2004) Pathogenesis of cigarette smoke-induced chronic obstructive pulmonary disease and therapeutic effects of glucocorticoids and N-acetylcysteine in rats. Chin Med J 117:1611–1619

Zhang J, Jiang S, Watson RR (2001) Antioxidant supplementation prevents oxidation and inflammation responses induced by sidestream cigarette smoke in old mice. Environ Health Perspect 109:1007–1009

Zhang J, Liu YL, Shi JQ, Larson DF, Watson RR (2002) Side-stream cigarette smoke induces dose-response in systemic inflammatory cytokine production and oxidative stress. Exp Biol Med 227:823–829

Chapter 12

Pulmonary Effects of Cigarette Smoke in Humans

Nick H.T. ten Hacken and Dirkje S. Postma

Contents

12.1	Diseases Associated or Caused by Tobacco Smoke	294
12.2	Composition and Inhalation Patterns	295
12.3	Healthy Smokers	296
12.3.1	Epidemiology and Clinical Presentation	296
12.3.2	The First Steps of Inflammation	299
12.3.3	Oxidative Stress	300
12.3.4	Inflammation and Pathological Changes	301
12.3.4.1	Changes in Sputum and BAL Fluid	301
12.3.4.2	Mucosal Changes in the Airways	302
12.3.5	Smoking Cessation	304
12.4	Chronic Bronchitis	304
12.4.1	Epidemiology and Clinical Presentation	304
12.4.2.	Inflammation and Pathological Changes	305
12.4.3	Smoking Cessation	306
12.4.4	Antioxidative Therapy	306
12.5	COPD	307
12.5.1	Epidemiology and Clinical Presentation	307
12.5.2	Inflammation and Pathological Changes	308
12.5.3	Oxidative Stress	309
12.5.4	Smoking Cessation	311
12.5.3	Antioxidative Treatment	312
12.6	Asthma	314
12.6.1	Smoking and Induction of Asthma	314
12.6.2	Smoking and Clinical Severity of Asthma	315
12.6.3	Smoking and Inflammation	317

Contents

12.6.4	Smoking Cessation		317
12.7	Lung Cancer		318
12.7.1	Epidemiology		318
12.7.2	Mutagens, Carcinogens, and Molecular Changes in the Lung		320
12.7.3	Lung Cancer and COPD		321
12.7.4	Chemoprevention		321
12.8	Smoking-Related Interstitial Lung Diseases		322
12.9	Summary		323
	References		323

12.1 Diseases Associated or Caused by Tobacco Smoke

Tobacco use is the leading cause of preventable death in the world today. At present, it is estimated that tobacco kills over 3 million people per year. Based on current trends, the death toll will rise to 10 million deaths per year by the 2020s or 2030s, with 70% of those deaths occurring in developing countries. According to estimates of the World Health Organization, there are approximately 1.1 thousand million smokers in the world, about one third of the global population aged 15 years and over. Globally, approximately 47% of men and 12% of women smoke. In developing countries, available data suggest that 48% of men smoke as do 7% of women, whereas in developed countries, 42% of men and 24% of women smoke. Smoking is an established or probable cause of death from cancers of the oral cavity, larynx, lung, esophagus, bladder, pancreas, renal pelvis, stomach, and cervix. It is also a cause of heart disease, stroke, peripheral vascular disease, chronic obstructive lung diseases (COPD) and other respiratory diseases, and low-birth-weight babies. Finally, smoking is associated with peptic ulcer disease, infertility, unsuccessful pregnancies, and increased infant mortality.

Obviously, the first target to be hit by tobacco smoke is the respiratory tract. This chapter addresses the various abnormalities and diseases that may develop in the lung because of cigarette smoking. Cigarette smoke contains a very high amount of free radicals and carcinogens, which may injure the human lung via various mechanisms. If a smoker is lucky, the lungs remain "healthy." Nevertheless, healthy smokers frequently experience respiratory symptoms and demonstrate signs of underlying inflammation. About 50% of the smokers develop chronic respiratory symptoms belonging to chronic bronchitis, whereas about 15–20% develop full-blown chronic obstructive pulmonary disease, i.e., with airflow limitation. It is generally accepted that asthma is induced by inhalation of allergens in susceptible individuals; however, exposure to cigarette smoke at childhood or adulthood is also associated with a higher prevalence of asthma and asthma-like symptoms. Cigarette smoking is also the single most important risk factor for development of lung cancer; unfortunately, the risk decreases only modestly after smoking cessation. Finally, four smoking-related interstitial lung diseases have been described, prevalence rates being relatively rare as compared with other smoking-induced lung diseases. Therefore, this chapter summarizes the present knowledge of the pulmonary effects of cigarette smoking in humans. Discussed are (1) cigarette smoke, (2) healthy smokers, (3) chronic bronchitis, (4) COPD, (5) asthma, (6) lung cancer, and (7) smoking-related interstitial lung diseases.

When possible, these topics are discussed in the context of cigarette smoking (current/past) and exposure to oxidative stress. In addition, the effect of smoking cessation and of antioxidant therapies is summarized.

12.2 Composition and Inhalation Patterns

Mainstream cigarette smoke is a complex mixture of more than 4,700 chemicals including many potent free radicals and carcinogens (Langen et al. 2003; Pryor and Stone 1993). The less stable gas phase contains 10^{15} free radicals per puff, whereas the more stable tar phase contains 10^{17} radicals per gram. Sidestream cigarette smoke contains more than 10^{15} reactive organic compounds per puff including carbon monoxide, ammonia, N-nitrosamines, benzopyrene, ethane, pentane, acrolein, nicotine, isoprene, and acetaldehyde formaldehyde. Studies (Bernstein 2004) with smoking machines (mostly 35-ml puffs, 2-s duration) have shown that particle size of cigarette smoke varies between 0.18 and 0.34 µm. Particle size of cigarette smoke does not differ between the different cigarette types, whether filtered or not filtered, ventilated or not ventilated (Bernstein 2004). In contrast, particle concentration of cigarette smoke is significantly reduced using filters, showing efficiencies between 22 and 94%. Most subjects inhale smoke in two phases (Higenbottam et al. 1980b). The first phase is the mouth phase when smoke is drawn into the mouth. After a pause, the inhalation phase starts when smoke is drawn into the lung. The smoking pattern varies importantly between individuals. The mean (range) number of puffs per cigarette is 11 (8–16), interval between puffs, 28 (18–64) s; duration per cigarette, 351 (232–414) s; duration per puff, 1.9 (1.6–2.4) s; volume per puff, 42.5 (21–66) ml; peak flow of inhalation, 35.5 (28–40) ml/s; and volume of inhalation, 560 (413–918) ml (US Department of Health and Human Services 1988). It has been shown that puff volume determines mainly the concentration of plasma nicotine and expired carbon monoxide; the volume and duration of inhalation does not affect these parameters (Zacny et al. 1987). Smokers who switch to low-tar cigarettes may compensate their relative nicotine lack by increasing puff volume and frequency, inhalation volume, and number of cigarettes per day. Unfortunately, little is known about the effect of breathing pattern on the deposition of cigarette smoke in the human lung. Using a mathematical model, a particle size range of 0.1–0.4 µm is predicted to result in a near-zero bronchial deposition (Nazir et al. 2002) and in a 15–25% total lung deposition fraction. This mathematical model approximates the real-life figures of the particle deposition study of Altshuler et al. (1957), who showed a 26–41% total lung deposition, using particles ranging in size from 0.14–3.2 µm. After being deposited, the free radicals in cigarette smoke may injure the human lungs via various mechanisms: depletion of antioxidants, initiation of redox-cycling reactions, direct damage to lipids-nucleic acids-proteins, enhancement of respiratory burst in macrophages and neutrophils, inactivation of protease inhibitors, inhibition of steroid receptor function, activation of nuclear transcription factors such as nuclear factor (NF)-κB and activated protein (AP)-1, and epigenetic modulation of gene expression.

12.3 Healthy Smokers

12.3.1 Epidemiology and Clinical Presentation

Healthy smokers generally more often experience respiratory symptoms, like cough, phlegm and wheeze, than do nonsmokers (Bjornsson et al. 1994; Brown et al. 1991b; Enright et al. 1994; Jansen et al. 1999; Lundback et al. 1991; Rijcken et al. 1987b; Sherman et al. 1992; Sherrill et al. 1993; Viegi et al. 1988; Vollmer et al. 1989). The prevalence of these symptoms in smokers increases with the number of cigarettes smoked per day (Brown et al. 1991b; Higenbottam et al. 1980a; Jansen et al. 1999; Lindstrom et al. 2001; Silverman et al. 2000) and/or the number of pack years (Enright et al. 1994; Silverman et al. 2000; Viegi et al. 1988). Low-tar cigarettes as compared with normal (high) tar cigarettes have been associated with a lower risk for cough and mucus hypersecretion (Higenbottam et al. 1980a; Schenker et al. 1982), although this is not confirmed in all studies (Rimpela and Teperi 1989; Withey et al. 1992a, b). The prevalence of dyspnea in healthy smokers varies between 2 and 42%, and is higher in those who smoke more than 25 cigarettes per day (Rijcken et al. 1987b; Silverman et al. 2000). Healthy smokers without respiratory symptoms have a higher risk to develop these symptoms later in life than have nonsmokers (Jansen et al. 1999; Krzyzanowski and Lebowitz 1992; Xu et al. 1997). Healthy smokers also have a higher risk for acute upper and lower respiratory infections than have nonsmokers (US Department of Health and Human Services 2004). This has been demonstrated for influenza-like illnesses (Finklea et al. 1969, 1971; Kark and Lebiush 1981; Kark et al. 1982), Legionella (Straus et al. 1996), tuberculosis (Alcaide et al. 1996; Alderson et al. 1985; Buskin et al. 1994; Liu et al. 1998), and community-acquired pneumonia (Almirall et al. 1999a, b; Ferrari et al. 2000; Nuorti et al. 2000; von Hertzen et al. 1998a, b). When current smokers are classified according to the number of cigarettes smoked per day, positive exposure–response relationships have been demonstrated in some but not all studies for influenza (Finklea et al. 1969), tuberculosis (Alcaide et al. 1996; Alderson et al. 1985; Liu et al. 1998), and community-acquired pneumonia (Almirall et al. 1999b; Nuorti et al. 2000). Lower tar content of cigarettes was associated with a lower risk for pneumonia and influenza in one study (Petitti and Friedman 1985)

Above observations are compatible with the finding that cigarette smoking decreases the local cellular defense mechanisms in the human lung. Phytohemagglutinin/concanavalin A-stimulated production by lung lymphocytes was lower in smokers than nonsmokers, and reversed 6 weeks after smoking cessation (Daniele et al. 1977). Lipopolysaccharide (LPS)-stimulated interleukin (IL)-1 production by alveolar macrophages was lower in smokers than in nonsmokers (Yamaguchi et al. 1989). Concentration of IL-1 receptor antagonists in bronchoalveolar lavage (BAL) fluid was significantly lower in chronic smokers than in nonsmokers (Mikuniya et al. 1999). In the same study, LPS stimulated IL-6 production, and IL-1 receptor antagonist concentration was lower in chronic smokers than in nonsmokers (Mikuniya et al. 1999). The spontaneous release of tumor necrosis factor (TNF)-α, IL-1β, IL-8, and macrophage inflammatory protein (MIP)-1α by human alveolar macrophages from smokers is significantly lower than from nonsmokers (Dandrea et al. 1997). Recently, Laan et al. (2004) demonstrated that cigarette smoke suppressed the LPS-stimulated granulocyte-macrophage colony-stimulating factor (GM-CSF) and IL-8 production of human bronchial epithelial cells (Beas-2B) via suppression of AP-1 activation. The higher risk for pulmonary infections in smokers as demonstrated in epidemiological studies could thus be because of changes in cellular function, but also because of other mechanisms like (1) dysregulation of the cytokine network by proinflammatory cytokines (Capelli et al. 1999; Chalmers et al. 2001; Keatings et al. 1996; Linden et al. 1993; Morrison et al. 1998a; Sun et al. 1998); (2) lower nitric oxide (NO) production (Balint et al. 2001; Delen et al. 2000; Montuschi et al. 2001; Persson et al. 1994; Rutgers et al. 1999; Schilling et al. 1994); (3) inhibition of local immunoglobulin (Ig)A function because of decreased expression of epithelial secretory component (Rusznak et al. 2001); (4) skewing of the immune response to a T-helper (Th)-2 phenotype (Burrows et al. 1981; Byron et al. 1994); (5) impaired mucociliary clearance (Janoff et al. 1987); (6) metaplastic changes of the airway epithelium (Sherman 1992); and (7) increased bacterial adherence on mucosal surfaces (Piatti et al. 1997). Indeed, bacterial colonization of the bronchial tree occurs more frequently in healthy smokers than in nonsmokers (Qvarfordt et al. 2000; Soler et al. 1999).

Active smoking during childhood and adolescence has been investigated in a limited number of studies and consistently demonstrated that lung function growth is slower, prematurely ceases, and begins to decline earlier (US Department of Health and Human Services 2004). In particular, adolescent girls seem to be more vulnerable, as smoking five or more cigarettes per day slowed the increase in forced expiratory volume in 1 second (FEV_1) by 31 ml/year versus 9 ml/year in boys (Gold et al. 1996). Healthy adult smokers have a faster decline in FEV_1 than have nonsmokers (Burchfiel et al. 1995), ranging from –2 to –85 ml/year in smokers versus 0 to –56 ml/year in nonsmokers (Beaty et al. 1984; Bosse et al. 1981; Camilli et al. 1987; Krzyzanowski et al. 1986, 1990; Lange et al. 1989; Pelkonen et al. 2001; Samet and Lange 1996; Sherman et al. 1992; Tager et al. 1988; Tashkin et al. 1984; Taylor et al. 1985b; Townsend et al. 1991; Xu et al. 1992, 1994). This accelerated decline in FEV_1 in healthy adult smokers is related to age, actual cigarette consumption per day, and duration of smoking (Burchfiel et al. 1995; Lange et al. 1989; Xu et al. 1992, 1994), but not clearly to the number of pack years (Buist et al. 1979; Lange et al. 1989; Tashkin et al. 1984; Taylor et al. 1985b; Townsend et al. 1991; Xu et al. 1994). Healthy smokers who are young or who smoke less than 15 cigarettes per day have a similar decline in FEV_1 than have nonsmokers (Lange et al. 1989). Decline in FEV_1 is associated with the presence of respiratory symptoms and bronchial hyperresponsiveness (Bosse et al. 1981; Camilli et al. 1987; Krzyzanowski et al. 1990; Rijcken et al. 1987a, b; Sherrill et al. 1991, 1993). In healthy smokers, the prevalence of airway hyperresponsiveness to methacholine or histamine has found to be higher (Burney et al. 1987; Cerveri et al. 1989; Gerrard et al. 1980; Paoletti et al. 1995; Rijcken et al. 1987b; Sunyer et al. 1997; Taylor et al. 1985b), similar (Brown et al. 1977; Kennedy et al. 1984; Lim et al. 1988; Paoletti et al. 1995; Rijcken et al. 1987b; Sunyer et al. 1997; Xu et al. 1997), and lower (Cockcroft et al. 1983) than in nonsmokers.

Hogg et al. (1968) demonstrated that the increased airway resistance in healthy smokers is because of changes in the peripheral airways. Using the single-breath N_2 washout test, Cosio and coworkers (1978) demonstrated that unevenness of ventilation is associated with structural changes in the small airways of healthy smokers with normal spirometry. In line with this, Verbanck et al. (2004) used the more sophisticated multiple-breath N_2 washout test, and demonstrated in smokers with more than 10 pack years that the earliest manifestations of small airway alterations because of smoking were located around the acinair airway entrance (Fig. 12.1). This is completely in line with the data from Lee et al. (2000), who demonstrated on thin section expiratory computer tomography (CT) scans increased air trapping in asymptomatic individuals with a smoking history of more than 10 pack years (Fig. 12.2). In addition, Berger et al. (2003) demonstrated that increased air trapping on thin-section CT scans was associated with reduced diameters of the small airways because of inflammation in apparently healthy smokers. Importantly, cigarette smokers have already signs of air trapping and hyperinflation regardless of the presence of functional characteristics of emphysema (Kubo et al. 1999).

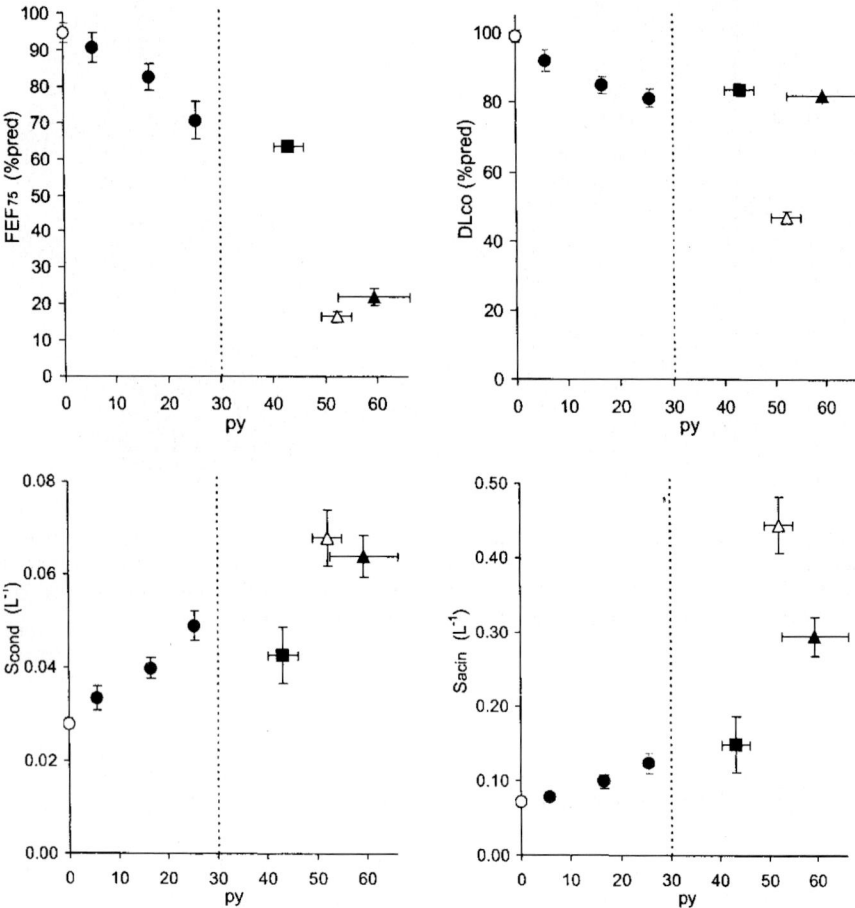

Fig. 12.1 Lung function and ventilation distribution as a function of smoking history for forced expiratory flow between 25 and 75% forced vital capacity (FVC) (FEF_{75}), carbon monoxide diffusing capacity (DL_{CO}), index of acinair conductive ventilation heterogeneity (S_{cond}), and index of acinair ventilation heterogeneity (S_{acin}). *Right* of the *vertical dashed lines* are data representing smokers with a 30-or-more-pack years smoking history classified into three categories: 25 healthy subjects with forced expiratory volume in 1 second (FEV_1)/FVC ≥70% (*solid square*), 26 chronic obstructive lung disease (COPD) subjects with FEV_1/FVC <70%, D_{LCO} ≥60% predicted (*solid triangle*), and 27 COPD subjects with FEV_1/FVC <70%, D_{LCO} <60% predicted and high-resolution computed tomography (CT)-confirmed emphysema (*open triangle*). *Left* of the *vertical dashed line* are data representing 63 never smokers (*open circle*), 27 healthy smokers with <10-pack years smoking history (*solid circle*), 35 healthy smokers with ≥10 and <20 pack years (*solid circle*), and 29 healthy smokers with ≥20 and <30 pack years (*solid circle*). After 10 pack years, healthy smokers demonstrated significantly higher S_{acin} values than the nonsmoking controls ($p<0.05$). After >30 pack years smoking, the COPD patients without emphysema demonstrated higher S_{acin} values than did the healthy smokers ($p<0.05$), and the COPD patients with emphysema demonstrated higher values than did the ones without emphysema ($p<0.05$). (Reproduced with permission from Verbanck et al. 2004)

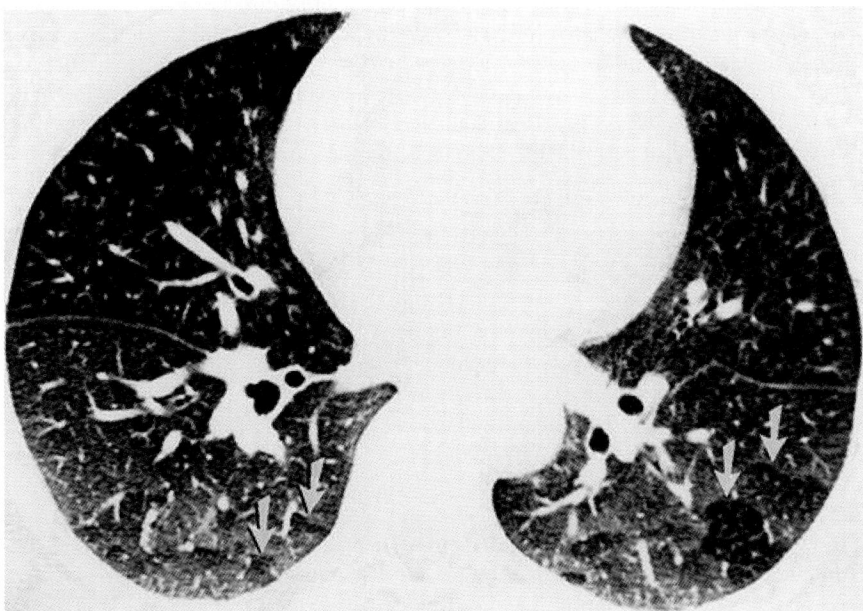

Fig. 12.2 Expiratory transverse, thin-section computer tomography (CT) scan in a 51-year-old man with normal pulmonary function test and without any history of pulmonary disease or symptoms. In contrast to an inspiratory scan at the same level (not shown), this expiratory scan demonstrates air trapping (*arrows*) with a mosaic pattern. (Reproduced with permission from Lee et al. 2000)

12.3.2 The First Steps of Inflammation

Directly after cigarette smoking, increased numbers of neutrophils in BAL fluid have been reported in chronic smokers (Morrison et al. 1998b). The first step in the recruitment of neutrophils toward the airspaces is the sequestration of these cells in the microcirculation of the lung (Macnee and Selby 1993; Macnee et al. 1989), which might be because of decreased deformability and thus stiffening of circulating neutrophils. In vitro and ex vivo experiments have demonstrated such stiffening after exposure to cigarette smoke (Drost et al. 1992, 1993), an effect that was abolished by glutathione (Drost et al. 1992). Once sequestered, cigarette smoke may enhance neutrophil adhesion to the endothelium by upregulating neutrophilic and endothelial adhesion molecules (Patiar et al. 2002). Afterward, the sequestered neutrophils may be attracted by chemotactic components in cigarette smoke, or by chemotactic components (IL-8, leukotriene B_4 [LTB_4]) released from inflammatory and resident cells in lung tissue. NO in cigarette smoke may induce local vasodilatation and plasma exudation, and enhance in this way diapedesis of sequestered neutrophils. Cigarette smoke may activate neutrophils and enhance the formation of reactive oxygen intermediates and release of proteases. Indeed, 1 h after smoking a cigarette, elastase activity was found to be increased in BAL fluid

(Janoff et al. 1983). Consequently, the epithelial integrity may become compromised, leading to a disturbed air space epithelial barrier and allowing in this way the entrance of noxious agents and inflammatory cells. Epithelial permeability has shown to increase immediately after acute exposure to cigarette smoke, compared with nonsmokers and chronic cigarette smokers (Morrison et al. 1999). However, Gil et al. (1995) showed no difference in epithelial permeability between acute and chronic smokers.

12.3.3 Oxidative Stress

Cigarette smoke is a major exogenous source of oxidants containing, e.g., hydroxyl radicals, NO, and hydrogen peroxide. In the lung, these radicals may initiate a number of redox-cycling reactions and give rise to newly formed free radicals. Furthermore, cigarette smoke promotes the recruitment and activation of neutrophils and macrophages, which may act as endogenous sources of free radicals, like superoxide anion and hydrogen peroxide. The only direct method to measure excessive free radical production is electron spin resonance. Using this technique, Otha et al. demonstrated in the lungs of smokers darkly pigmented areas of high electron spin resonance containing heme iron, nonheme iron, and carbon-centered radicals (Fahn et al. 1998; Ohta et al. 1985). Indirect measures of oxidative stress (by determining antioxidant status, tissue damage, or physiological effects) provide overwhelming evidence that cigarette smoking induces oxidative stress inside the human lung (Macnee 2001b; Rahman and Macnee 1996; Repine et al. 1997). Interpretation of these studies has to be done carefully, taking into account conditions of acute, acute on chronic, and chronic cigarette smoke exposure. The following summary includes indirect measures in the lung, BAL fluid, or exhaled air.

One study investigated markers of oxidative stress in BAL fluid from healthy smokers abstaining from smoking for 12 h (chronic smoking) and 1 h after smoking two cigarettes (acute smoking) (Morrison et al. 1999). The superoxide release from PMA-stimulated and unstimulated BAL fluid leukocytes was increased both after acute and chronic smoking. Other studies have also demonstrated increased amounts of superoxide anion in alveolar macrophages of chronic smokers (Hoidal et al. 1981; Nakashima et al. 1987; Schaberg et al. 1992a).

After acute cigarette smoking, the Trolox-equivalent antioxidant capacity (TEAC) in serum was lower, and in BAL fluid higher, than values in chronic smoking (Morrison et al. 1999). In line, after acute cigarette smoking, lower-than-normal serum glutathione levels have been demonstrated, suggesting temporary depletion. In contrast, glutathione in epithelial lining fluid is increased in chronic smokers as compared with nonsmokers (Cantin et al. 1987; Morrison et al. 1999; Rahman et al. 2000), suggesting a compensatory upregulation of the glutathione system. This is associated with an increased expression of γ-glutamylcysteine synthetase mRNA in the lungs (Rahman et al. 2000). In contrast, Harju et al. (2002) found decreased protein γ-glutamylcysteine synthetase immunoreactivity in the lungs of smokers. An explanation for this discrepancy is not available.

Hydrogen peroxide in exhaled breath condensate of healthy smokers increased about 25% 30 min after smoking only one cigarette (Guatura et al. 2000). The same study showed that current smokers had similar hydrogen peroxide concentrations as nonsmokers at baseline. Contradictory results were reported about exhaled NO immediately after cigarette smoking. No differences were observed at 15 (Kharitonov et al. 1995), 30

(Balint et al. 2001), and 90 min (Balint et al. 2001) after smoking. One study reported an increase in NO at 1 and 10 min after smoking a single cigarette (Chambers et al. 1998), whereas another study reported a decrease after 5 min (Kharitonov et al. 1995). Breath condensate levels of nitrate increased 30 min after cigarette smoking, but nitrite and nitrotyrosine levels in this study did not change (Balint et al. 2001). Exhaled NO in *chronic* smokers is consistently lower than in nonsmokers (Balint et al. 2001; Delen et al. 2000; Montuschi et al. 2001; Persson et al. 1994; Rutgers et al. 1999; Schilling et al. 1994). Recently, Comhair et al. (2000) showed that cigarette smoke did not upregulate inducible NO synthase (*iNOS*) mRNA expression in human epithelial cells and alveolar macrophages. Maestrelli (2001) demonstrated that heme oxygenase (HO)-1 is induced in the alveolar spaces of smokers, probably leading to increased carbon monoxide in exhaled air. Indeed, carbon monoxide in exhaled breath condensate of healthy smokers is higher than in healthy nonsmokers (Carpagnano et al. 2003)

8-Isoprostane concentrations in exhaled breath condensate of healthy smokers increased about 50% 15 min after inhaling cigarette smoke (Montuschi et al. 2000). In the same study, it was shown that current smokers had about 2.2-fold higher 8-isoprostane concentrations than had nonsmokers. In addition, ethane (Paredi et al. 2000a) and pentane (Euler et al. 1996) concentrations in exhaled breath condensate were increased. Higher levels of carcinogen–DNA adducts have been demonstrated in lung tissue of smokers, which have been associated with increased iron burden in the lower respiratory tract (Phillips et al. 1988; Thompson et al. 1991).

12.3.4 Inflammation and Pathological Changes

It is generally accepted that long-term cigarette smoking elicits an inflammatory reaction involving the entire tracheobronchial tree.

12.3.4.1 Changes in Sputum and BAL Fluid

More inflammatory cells have been demonstrated in sputum and BAL fluid of healthy smokers, suggesting more inflammation both in the central and peripheral airways (Balzano et al. 1999; Chalmers et al. 2001; Costabel et al. 1986, 1992; Dippolito et al. 2001; Keatings et al. 1996; Koyama et al. 1991; Kuschner et al. 1996; Linden et al. 1993; Morrison et al. 1998a; Schaberg et al. 1992b; Sun et al. 1998). In addition, macrophages in BAL fluid of healthy smokers seemed to be activated, because they express more CD11, CD18, and have increased chemotactic activity (Holt 1987; Schaberg et al. 1992b). When analyzing subsets of lymphocytes in BAL fluid from healthy smokers, the percentage of $CD4^+$ cells was lower, whereas the percentage of $CD8^+$ cells was higher, resulting in a lower CD4/CD8 ratio in healthy smokers than in nonsmokers (Costabel et al. 1986, 1992). Proinflammatory cytokines like TNF-α, IL-6, and chemokines like monocyte-chemoattractactic protein-1 and IL-8 were elevated in sputum supernatant or BAL fluid of healthy smokers (Capelli et al. 1999; Chalmers et al. 2001; Keatings et al. 1996; Linden et al. 1993; Morrison et al. 1998a; Sun et al. 1998). One study demonstrated that healthy smokers have higher IL-6 and LTB_4 concentrations in exhaled breath condensate than have nonsmoking controls (Carpagnano et al. 2003). In addition, IL-6 correlated positively with the number of cigarettes smoked per day and negatively with FEV_1 %predicted.

12.3.4.2 Mucosal Changes in the Airways

In the submucosa of central airways, the density of neutrophils, eosinophils, CD3, CD4, and CD8 immunopositive cells was similar between healthy smokers and nonsmokers. Only the number of macrophages in the epithelium and the number of CD8 immunopositive cells near the pulmonary arteries in the peripheral airways were higher in healthy smokers (Fournier et al. 1989; Lams et al. 2000; Saetta et al. 1999, 2000; Wallace et al. 1992). Pathological changes because of smoking have been reported mostly in older subjects; however, already at a young age smoking leads to changes. Niewoehner et al. (1974) demonstrated an inflammatory cell infiltrate consisting of mononuclear cells and clusters of pigmented macrophages in the wall of the respiratory bronchioles from young smokers (aged 25 years) who suddenly died outside the hospital setting. These lesions were present in the absence of noteworthy tissue destruction and fibrosis, suggesting that such changes are largely reversible. Alternatively, it will take longstanding smoking before such changes occur. Cigarette smokers older than 40 years showed increased goblet cell metaplasia and smooth muscle hypertrophy in the small airways, and inflammation in the walls of bronchioles and respiratory bronchioles (Cosio et al. 1980). A pathological score on the degree of inflammatory cell infiltrate, squamous cell metaplasia of the airway epithelium and airway fibrosis in the small airways was associated with unevenness of ventilation in smokers, although they showed normal spirometry (Cosio et al. 1980). In the central airways, no differences in pathological changes between young healthy smokers and nonsmokers were reported (Sobonya and Kleinerman 1972). However, at an older age, the central airways showed higher numbers of goblet cells and inflammatory cells (Wright et al. 1988), smooth muscle hypertrophy, and a lower number of alveolar attachments (Cosio et al. 1980; Saetta et al. 1985). Thus, smoking-induced changes seem to start in the peripheral airways and to involve the larger airways later in life. Most likely, in the large airways, the mucus layer is protective to a certain extent. These findings are in line with the observed radiological changes that were present without overt lung function changes in healthy smokers, as described above.

A higher occurrence of basal cell hyperplasia, stratification, goblet cell hyperplasia, basement membrane thickening, and increased nucleus/cytoplasma (NC) ratio was found in bronchial biopsies of 31 healthy smokers (age 37 years, 25 pack years) than in 53 nonsmokers (Fligiel et al. 1997). In addition, a higher occurrence of DNA ploidy and higher immunohistochemical expression of epidermal growth factor (EGF) receptor have been demonstrated in the bronchial epithelium of smokers (Barsky et al. 1998), suggesting that smokers are at increased risk for the subsequent development of lung cancer. Recently, O'Donnell et al. (2004) demonstrated in bronchial biopsies from long-term current smokers a higher expression of EGF receptor (including ErbB3) and MU-C5AC expression (Fig. 12.3) than in nonsmokers. The group of current smokers in this study consisted of healthy smokers, chronic bronchitis (Global Initiative for Chronic Obstructive Lung Disease [GOLD] stage 0) and COPD (GOLD stage I and II) patients, but demonstrated no differences between subgroups in this respect. Current smoking

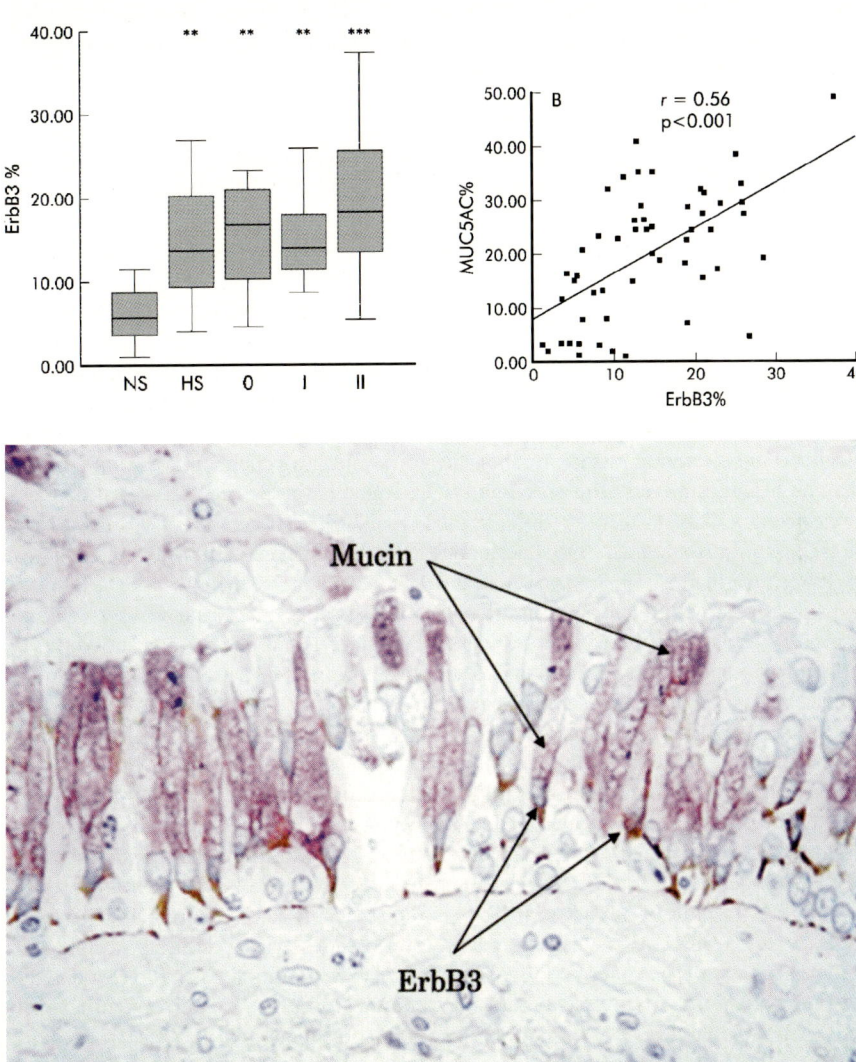

Fig. 12.3 *Left panel* demonstrates the ErbB3 receptor expression in bronchial epithelium of nonsmokers vs current smokers without or with chronic obstructive pulmonary disease (COPD). The *box* and *whisker plots* show median, range and interquartile ranges of the percentages of the epithelial area staining with the antibody. The percentage area expressing ErbB3 was significantly increased in all smoker groups, compared with nonsmokers. *NS* Nonsmokers ($n=10$), *HS* healthy smokers ($n=11$), *0* stage 0 COPD ($n=17$), *I* stage I COPD ($n=9$), *II* stage II COPD ($n=14$). *$p<0.05$ vs NS, **$p<0.01$ vs NS, ***$p<0.001$ vs NS. *Right panel* is a *scatter plot* showing the correlation between MUC5AC and ErbB3 expression in bronchial epithelium in all subjects (smokers and nonsmokers). *Lower panel* demonstrates colocalization of ErbB3 and mucin in goblet cells in a bronchial biopsy specimen from a smoker with COPD. The *photomicrograph* shows epithelial cells with intracellular mucin stained *pink* with periodic acid-Schiff (PAS) and membrane–bound ErbB3 stained *brown* with 3,3-diaminobenzidine (DAB). Magnification ×40. (Reproduced with permission from O'Donnell et al. 2004)

(number of cigarettes per day) correlated weakly but significantly with ErbB3 expression ($r=0.37$, $p<0.05$). Neutrophil numbers in sputum, epithelium, and submucosa were not associated with MUC5AC and EGF receptor expression. Interestingly, MUC5AC expression was significantly associated with ErbB3 expression, suggesting that cigarette smoking promotes epithelial goblet cell hyperplasia via activation of ErbB3 receptors. This study did not find a higher expression of ErbB2, although ErbB2 expression has been associated with malignant transformations (Selvaggi et al. 2002), whereas premalignant changes have been demonstrated in healthy smokers (Fligiel et al. 1997). Unfortunately, this study did not include ex-smokers, thus we are not informed about the possible reversibility of these changes.

12.3.5 Smoking Cessation

Healthy subjects who quit smoking show lower prevalence of cough, phlegm, and wheeze than do healthy smokers. The prevalence in ex-smokers was 5–21%, 5–30%, and 1–19% respectively, and in smokers 10–40%, 10–40%, and 7–32% (Bjornsson et al. 1994; Brown et al. 1991b; Enright et al. 1994; Lundback et al. 1991; Rijcken et al. 1987b; Sherman et al. 1992; Sherrill et al. 1993; Sparrow et al. 1987; Viegi et al. 1988). Most of these symptoms decreased within 1–2 months after smoking cessation (Barbee et al. 1991; Buczko et al. 1984; Buist et al. 1976; Comstock et al. 1970; Israel et al. 1988; Krzyzanowski et al. 1993; Lange et al. 1990b; Peterson et al. 1968; Tashkin et al. 1984; Wilhelmsen 1967). The prevalence of cough and wheeze in healthy smokers decreased to the level of nonsmokers, whereas the prevalence of phlegm remained slightly higher (Comstock et al. 1970; Tashkin et al. 1984). Not only did symptoms decrease on smoking cessation, but they were also less likely to develop if healthy smokers quit smoking than when they continued to smoke (Krzyzanowski et al. 1993; Lange et al. 1990b). The effect of smoking cessation on dyspnea in healthy smokers is controversial. Three studies showed no difference in the prevalence of dyspnea after smoking cessation (Israel et al. 1988; Krzyzanowski et al. 1993; Tashkin et al. 1984). In these studies, dyspnea was defined as the feeling of "shortness of breath" or "having to stop for a breath while walking up a slight hill" or "walking with other people of the same age on level ground." Also, the incidence of dyspnea was similar in those who quit and continued smoking: 17 and 16%, respectively (Krzyzanowski et al. 1993). In contrast, another study suggested that 5 years smoking cessation led to an increase in dyspnea when hurrying on the level or walking up a slight hill (41–52%) (Comstock et al. 1970).

12.4 Chronic Bronchitis

12.4.1 Epidemiology and Clinical Presentation

Chronic bronchitis has been clinically defined by the American Thoracic Society (1995) as "the production of sputum on most days for at least 3 months in at least 2 consecutive years when another cause of chronic cough has been excluded." Chronic bronchitis has been classified into simple bronchitis, chronic or recurrent mucopurulent bronchitis, and obstructive bronchitis. Recently, GOLD emphasized that chronic cough and sputum production may precede the development of airflow limitation. Consequently, subjects with chronic cough and sputum production, but with still normal spirometry, were classified as being "at risk" of COPD (GOLD stage 0). Chronic smoking in almost every person leads to the universally called smokers cough (and phlegm); however, awareness of these symptoms varies enormously between persons. In smoking patients with chronic bronchitis the prevalence of wheeze, a respiratory symptom not included in the definition of chronic bronchitis, is significantly higher (39%) than in healthy nonsmokers (12%) (Ekberg-Jansson et al. 2001). In contrast, smokers with chronic bronchitis hardly experience dyspnea (Ekberg-Jansson et al. 2001). There are insufficient data as to whether smoking constitutes an independent risk factor for acute respiratory infections in chronic bronchitis (US Department of Health and Human Services 2004).

Epidemiological studies on the prevalence of chronic nonobstructive bronchitis may have problems in recognizing this condition because of the use of self-administrated questionnaires, without the use of spirometry to rule out COPD. Considering the methodological differences between studies, the prevalence of chronic bronchitis in general population studies varies between 0.7 and 14% (Cerveri et al. 2001; Cetinkaya et al. 2000; Collins 1997; Dutu and Paun 1998; Huchon et al. 2002; Liard et al. 1980; Lundback et al. 1993; Menezes et al. 1994; von Hertzen et al. 2000), which strongly depends on smoking habits. Recently, the European Community Respiratory Health Survey reported on the prevalence of chronic bronchitis and smoking habits in 18,966 young adults across 16 European countries (Cerveri et al. 2001). The median (range) prevalence of chronic bronchitis was 2.6% (0.7–9.7%) and of current smoking, 40% (20–57%). Current smoking was the major risk factor for chronic bronchitis, especially in males. In males the odds ratio was 3.51 (confidence interval [CI] = 2.21–5.32) in 1–14 pack-years smokers, which increased to 17.32 (9.97–30.11) in ≥45 pack-years smokers. Comparable odds ratios for current smoking were demonstrated in 1,053 subjects, aged ≥40 years, living in a southern area of Brazil (Menezes et al. 1994). Interestingly, smokers using filter cigarettes showed the lowest risk. In a study of 10,359 subjects (2,801 current smokers), aged 40–59 years and living in Scotland, daily cigarette consumption and number of pack years smoked was the most important risk factor for chronic bronchitis symptoms (Brown et al. 1991a). This study demonstrated that cigarette tar content was a small but significant risk factor for chronic bronchitis in females only.

12.4.2 Inflammation and Pathological Changes

Hyperplasia of goblet cells together with an increase in glands size and increased numbers of inflammatory cells have been reported in the central and peripheral airways (Mullen et al. 1985; Spurzem et al. 1991). In addition, the percentage of abnormal bronchial cilia is increased (Trevisani et al. 1992). Inhalation of cigarette smoke may paralyze the cilia and stimulate irritant receptors in the bronchial wall. This may give rise to an increased mucus production, unfortunately without being cleared effectively. A nonspecific inflammation has been demonstrated in chronic bronchitis with higher numbers of macrophages, neutrophils, eosinophils, and mast cells in BAL fluid as compared with healthy smokers and nonsmokers. In addition, the number of CD8 immunopositive lymphocytes was increased (Sun et al. 1998). In bronchial biopsies, a higher protein expression of IL-4 positive cells has been demonstrated in the submucosal airways from chronic bronchitis patients as compared with normal healthy controls (Mueller et al.

1996). In line with this, Zhu et al. (2001) demonstrated in a semiquantitative way strong IL-4 and IL-5 mRNA expression in the submucosal glands and in the subepithelium of smokers with chronic bronchitis. Recently, a higher IL-4 and IL-13 submucosal immunoreactivity was demonstrated in a quantitative way in smoking chronic bronchitis patients as compared with smoking healthy controls (Miotto et al. 2003). The most abundant sources of these Th-2 type cytokines were CD4- and CD8-immunopositive lymphocytes. Immunoreactivity of the Th-1 type cytokine interferon-γ did not differ between chronic bronchitis patients and healthy smokers in this study. In particular, IL-13 might play a supportive role in the mucus hypersecretion of chronic bronchitis patients, e.g., via the activation of the EGF receptor cascade as discussed above.

12.4.3 Smoking Cessation

Longitudinal data about the effects of smoking cessation in patients with chronic bronchitis are scarce. Friedman and Siegelaub (1980) showed in almost all persons with chronic bronchitis who quit smoking that chronic cough had disappeared 1.5 years later. Decline in FEV_1 in smokers with chronic bronchitis who quit smoking decreased, compared with those who continued smoking (Comstock et al. 1970). Mullen and coworkers (1987) compared the large and small airways of current and ex-smokers. In the central airways, goblet cell hyperplasia was lower in ex-smokers than in current smokers. In contrast, inflammation near the glands was higher in ex-smokers as compared with current smokers (Mullen et al. 1987). In the peripheral airways, goblet cell hyperplasia was similar in ex- and current smokers. Again, inflammation in ex-smokers was higher than in current smokers. In contrast, macrophages in the airway lumen were lower in ex-smokers than in current smokers with chronic bronchitis (Mullen et al. 1987). Taken together, the above studies suggest that smoking cessation decreases respiratory symptoms and the underlying mucus producing elements in the central airways. However, the apparent increases in airway inflammation in the walls of the central and peripheral airways are hard to explain.

12.4.4 Antioxidative Therapy

Only one study did investigate the effect of antioxidant therapy in patients with non-obstructive chronic bronchitis. This open study in 1,392 patients in general practice did show that *N*-acetylcysteine (600 mg per day) after 2 months treatment effectively changed the viscosity and character of sputum, with resultant ease of expectoration and cough severity. There was a notable improvement in associated abnormal physical signs such as the presence of rhonchi, crepitations, and symptoms including dyspnea at rest (Tattersall et al. 1983). Three meta-analyses have been published on the clinical efficacy of *N*-acetylcysteine in chronic bronchitis patients (Grandjean et al. 2000; Poole and Black 2001; Stey et al. 2000). Because they included also obstructive chronic bronchitis patients, they are presented in the following section.

12.5 COPD

12.5.1 Epidemiology and Clinical Presentation

COPD is defined by the GOLD standard as "a disease state characterized by airflow limitation that is not fully reversible. The airflow limitation is usually both progressive and associated with an abnormal inflammatory response of the lungs to noxious particles or gases" (www.goldcopd.com). The major environmental factors are tobacco smoke, occupational dusts and chemicals, and indoor/outdoor pollution. The risk to develop chronic airflow limitation because of tobacco smoke increases with increasing pack years, and after >10 pack years, 15–20% of all smokers have developed full-blown COPD. This means that the inflammatory response to tobacco smoke is probably different between susceptible and nonsusceptible individuals; however, at this time we have no clue about the underlying genetic factors that modify an individual's risk. A large national survey conducted in the United States between 1988 and 1994 demonstrated that airflow limitation (FEV_1/forced vital capacity [FVC] <70%) in white males was present in 14.2% of the current smokers, 6.9% of ex-smokers, and 3.3% of never smokers (National Center for Health Statistics 1995). Among white females, the prevalence was 13.6, 6.8, and 3.1% respectively. Prevalence of physician-diagnosed COPD in the United Kingdom between 1990 and 1997 demonstrated that men reached a plateau of 1.6% in the mid 1990s, while the women rose continuously from 0.8 to 1.36% (Soriano et al. 2000). A formal analysis on past smoking behavior was not performed in this study, but the trends (comparable to lung cancer) may fit with changed smoking habits in the past. Worldwide the prevalence of COPD in 1990 was estimated to be 0.9% in all men, and 0.7% in all women (Murray and Lopez 1996). Across countries, the prevalence varies between 0.3 and 3%, and strongly relates to tobacco consumption.

Progressive airflow limitation is one of the hallmarks of COPD. Smoking COPD patients have a decline in FEV_1 of more than 60 ml/year and sometimes even more than 100 ml/year (Campbell et al. 1985; Postma and Sluiter 1989). This decline is strongly related to current and the number of pack years smoking (Postma et al. 1986; Scanlon et al. 2000). Decline in FEV_1 is not related to use of filter-tipped cigarettes (containing on average 23 mg tar) or unfiltered cigarettes (containing on average 35 mg tar) (Lange et al. 1992). Increased airway hyperresponsiveness frequently occurs both in smoking and nonsmoking patients with COPD (Tashkin et al. 1992; Yan et al. 1985). A large prospective cohort study in mild-to-moderately severe COPD patients demonstrated that 67% had increased airway hyperresponsiveness to methacholine, being partially dependent on FEV_1 (Tashkin et al. 1992). The severity of airway hyperresponsiveness was not related to current or past smoking in males, but there was a positive association between increased airway hyperresponsiveness and the number of pack years in females. In smoking patients with severe COPD, the small airways showed increased numbers of leukocytes, which correlated with reduced expiratory flow, lung hyperinflation, carbon monoxide diffusion impairment, and radiological emphysema (Turato et al. 2002). Verbanck et al. (2004), using the multiple breath N_2 washout test, demonstrated that COPD patients with a smoking history of more than 30 pack years have a disproportional larger unevenness of ventilation originating from the small airways (S_{cond}), irrespective of the presence of emphysema (Fig. 12.1).

Chronic cough and phlegm are frequently reported symptoms in COPD. Therefore, in the past the American Thoracic Society based its definition of COPD partly on the presence of at least 3 months' cough and phlegm during at least 2 consecutive years. In the new mondial GOLD standard (www.goldcopd.com), the presence of these symptoms is not obligatory any more. One population-based study reported cough and phlegm in 84% of the patients with mild disease, and 68% of the patients with severe disease (von Hertzen et al. 2000). Dyspnea is more prevalent in patients with severe COPD (80%) than in patients with mild (33%) or moderate (53%) COPD (von Hertzen et al. 2000). COPD is associated with a greater risk of acute respiratory infections (Monto and Ross 1977, 1978). The effects of current smoking on this risk are strongest in men with chronic bronchitis symptoms and show a positive exposure–response relationship. Many studies have demonstrated a higher prevalence of potentially pathogenic bacteria isolated from sputa of patients with an exacerbation. The impact of current smoking on this prevalence, however, is not formally investigated. One study demonstrated similar prevalence of positive cultures for gram-negative bacilli in former and current smokers (23 vs 32%), whereas another study demonstrated an increased risk of current smoking for quantitative sputum cultures yielding *Haemophilus influenza* (odds ratio = 8.16, CI = 1.9–43). The prevalence of positive serology for respiratory viral infections was higher in COPD patients than in healthy individuals (74 vs 48%) (Omenaas et al. 1996). Finally, a population-based study demonstrated that cigarette smoking was a strong independent risk factor for invasive pneumococcal infection in COPD patients (Nuorti et al. 2000).

12.5.2 Inflammation and Pathological Changes

Inflammatory and pathological changes in smokers with established COPD have received much attention in the last two decades as summarized in a number of excellent reviews (Cosio and Guerassimov 1999; Hogg 2001; Jeffery 1991, 1998, 2001; Saetta et al. 2001). Briefly, the peripheral airways show inflammatory wall infiltration, fibrosis, smooth muscle hypertrophy, goblet cell metaplasia, and luminal occlusion because of mucus plugging. Central airway walls show increased infiltration with macrophages and T lymphocytes (especially $CD8^+$ cells), whereas the airway lumen contains a neutrophilic inflammation. In sputum, the anti-inflammatory cytokine IL-10 is decreased, whereas the proinflammatory cytokines IL-8 and TNF-α are increased. The adhesion molecules E-selectin and intercellular adhesion molecule (ICAM)-1 were upregulated on the bronchial epithelium and on submucosal vessels, suggesting a role in the recruitment of neutrophils. The lung parenchyma also shows inflammation, especially $CD8^+$ T lymphocytes. Even the pulmonary arteries are involved in the inflammatory process in established COPD, showing endothelial dysfunction, intimal thickening, medial thickening, and adventitial inflammation (especially with $CD8^+$ cells). Some patient may show signs of emphysema, which is defined anatomically as a permanent destructive enlargement of airspaces distal to the terminal bronchioles, without fibrosis. COPD patients can develop centriacinar emphysema (mainly in upper lobes) or panacinar emphysema (mainly in lower lobes). Centriacinar emphysema is the most common form in smokers. The destruction is associated with the presence of an inflammatory process in the alveolar walls, consisting predominantly of $CD8^+$ T cells and correlating with reduced airflow limitation (Saetta et al. 1999). Apparently, cytotoxic $CD8^+$ T cells infiltrate the complete lung and seem to play a causal role in the development of COPD (Saetta et al. 2001).

An imbalance between proteases and antiproteases because of cigarette smoking has been postulated as one important factor in its etiology of emphysema. Among the various proteases and antiproteases that have been proposed to affect the extracellular matrix, there is now increasing evidence that matrix metalloproteinases (MMPs) and their inhibitors (tissue inhibitors of MMP [TIMPs]) play an important role. Patients with emphysema have increased MMP-9 expression and production by alveolar macrophages (Finlay et al. 1997a) and have elevated levels in BAL fluid (Finlay et al. 1997b). Furthermore, increased MMP-2, MMP-9, and TIMP-1 levels have been demonstrated in sputum of COPD patients (Beeh et al. 2003; Cataldo et al. 2000; Vignola et al. 1998). One study showed that FEV_1 %predicted correlated negatively with MMP-9 expression in lung tissue protein extracts from subjects undergoing lung surgery because of (suspected) malignancy (Kang et al. 2003). Moreover, FEV_1 %predicted correlated negatively with the MMP-9/TIMP-1 molar ratio. In contrast, a sputum study demonstrated that FEV_1 %predicted correlated positively with this ratio (Vignola et al. 1998). These cross-sectional studies cannot elucidate whether there is a causal relationship between smoking and development of COPD. Supportive evidence stems from the observation that alveolar macrophages from healthy cigarette smokers produce more MMP-9 and TIMP-1 than healthy nonsmokers (Lim et al. 2000). In addition, MMP-9 expression and the MMP-9/TIMP-1 ratio in lung tissue from subjects with and without airway obstruction correlate positively with the amount of past and current cigarette smoking (Kang et al. 2003). At this time, it is not clear how cigarette smoking exactly induces the functional imbalance between proteases and antiproteases. Interestingly, many oxidants present in smoke itself, or those generated by inflammatory cells may inactivate proteinase inhibitors and stimulate the release and activation of proteases (Seagrave 2000).

Comparable to nonobstructive chronic bronchitis, increased numbers of neutrophils together with goblet cell hyperplasia have been demonstrated in the bronchial epithelium of smokers with COPD (Jeffery 1991; Saetta et al. 2000). In addition, neutrophils are increased in the bronchial glands of these subjects and may support mucus hypersecretion via the release of neutrophil elastase (Saetta et al. 1997). However, increased $CD8^+$ cells, mast cells, and macrophages have also been demonstrated in the airway epithelium. Similar to smoking healthy controls and smoking chronic bronchitis patients, higher MUC5AC and EGF receptor (ErbB1 and ErbB3) expression have been demonstrated in the epithelium of smoking COPD patients (GOLD stages II–III) as compared with nonsmoking healthy controls (Fig. 12.3) (O'Donnell et al. 2004). Neutrophil numbers in sputum from COPD stage III patients were also higher in this study, and they correlated negatively with FEV_1 levels, but not with the expression of mucins and ErbB receptors. Obviously, more studies are needed to understand better the exact role of smoking-induced airway inflammation and mucus hypersecretion in COPD. Apparently, the EGF receptor cascade does not play a role in the development of airway obstruction.

12.5.3 Oxidative Stress

Several reviews have summarized the studies on the presence and consequences of oxidative stress in the lungs of smokers with COPD (Dekhuijzen 2004; Macnee 2000, 2001a; Macnee and Rahman 1996, 1999; Repine et al. 1997). Evidence for local oxidative stress has been found in sputum, BAL fluid, exhaled air, and exhaled breath condensates of patients with COPD.

Hydrogen peroxide production seems to be elevated in COPD patients. Measured in exhaled breath hydrogen peroxide is higher in patients with stable COPD as compared with healthy controls (Dekhuijzen et al. 1996; Nowak et al. 1999), and even more so during exacerbations (Dekhuijzen et al. 1996). Current smokers have shown similarly increased hydrogen peroxide levels as ex-smokers or never smokers with COPD (Nowak et al. 1998, 1999). In addition, no correlation was found between hydrogen peroxide and daily cigarette consumption or cumulative cigarette consumption in current smokers or ex-smokers with COPD (Nowak et al. 1998). One study showed that smoking patients with COPD (GOLD stage >0) had significantly higher hydrogen peroxide levels in exhaled breath condensate than in smoking patients with chronic bronchitis (GOLD stage 0) (Kostikas et al. 2003). Moreover, hydrogen peroxide levels correlated significantly with FEV_1 ($r = -0.83$, $p<0.0001$), Medical Research Council (MRC) dyspnea score ($r = 0.68$, $p<0.0001$), and percentage of neutrophils in induced sputum ($r = 0.83$, $p<0.0001$) in the COPD group (Kostikas et al. 2003). Apparently, the level of hydrogen peroxide is determined by endogenous hydrogen peroxide production and not by cigarette smoking.

Exhaled NO has been reported to be elevated (Corradi et al. 1999; Maziak et al. 1998) and to be normal (Ichinose et al. 2000; Rutgers et al. 1998, 1999) in stable COPD patients. Despite normal exhaled NO levels, Ichinose et al. (2000) demonstrated higher numbers of iNOS-positive and nitrotyrosine-positive cells in induced sputum in nonsmoking COPD patients than in healthy controls. In addition, there was a negative correlation between the number of nitrotyrosine-immunopositive cells and the degree of airway obstruction ($r = -68$, $p<0.05$). Kanazawa et al. demonstrated that nitrite and nitrate levels in induced sputum were significantly higher in patients with stable COPD than in normal healthy controls. Peroxynitrite inhibitory activity in induced sputum was significantly lower in patients with COPD than in normal controls. In addition, there was a negative correlation between peroxynitrite inhibitory activity and FEV_1 %predicted ($r=0.539$, $p=0.004$) and the percentage of neutrophils ($r = -0.754$, $p<0.001$). In contrast, Corradi et al. (2003a) demonstrated in exhaled breath condensate of COPD patients that the amount of nitrate is not higher than in condensate of nonsmoking controls. In the study of Rutgers et al. (1999), exhaled NO was also not increased, but it correlated positively with percentage sputum eosinophils ($r=0.65$, $p=0.009$), suggesting that patients with less stable COPD have more airway inflammation as reflected by exhaled NO. Carbon monoxide also has shown to be elevated in exhaled breath of COPD patients (Choi and Alam 1996).

Lipid peroxidation because of oxidative stress can be demonstrated in various ways in COPD. Increased immunostaining expression for adducts of the lipid peroxidation product 4-hydroxy-2-nonenal (4-HNE) have been demonstrated in the bronchi and alveoli of smokers with and without COPD (Rahman et al. 2002). Levels of 4-HNE adducts in alveolar and airway epithelium correlated negatively with FEV_1 in this study, suggesting a role for 4-HNE in the development of irreversible airway obstruction in COPD. Aldehydes (malondialdehyde, hexanal, heptanal) were higher in exhaled breath condensate of COPD patients than of nonsmoking controls; however, only malondialdehyde was higher than in condensate of smoking controls (Corradi et al. 2003b). Thiobarbituric acid-reactive substances (TBARs) in exhaled breath condensate have shown to be higher in smokers and ex-smokers with stable COPD than in healthy subjects who had never smoked (Nowak et al. 1999), without significant correlation with actual or cumulative cigarette consumption. TBARs plasma levels increased significantly in patients with COPD exacerbations as compared with healthy nonsmokers (Rahman et al. 1997). Exhaled ethane in stable COPD patients was higher than in healthy controls, and correlated with FEV_1 ($r = -0.67$, $p<0.05$) (Paredi et al. 2000b). 8-Isoprostanes because of peroxidation of arachidonic acid can be measured in exhaled breath and urine. Patients with stable COPD demonstrated higher exhaled breath condensate levels than healthy controls (Kostikas et al. 2003; Montuschi et al. 2000); whereas ex-smokers had similar levels as current smokers (Montuschi et al. 2000). One study demonstrated increased 8-isoprostane levels in exhaled breath condensate during exacerbation, a decrease 2 weeks after treatment, and normalization after 2 months (Biernacki et al. 2003). In urine, F_2-isoprostanes were elevated in patients with stable COPD (Pratico et al. 1998); levels further increased during exacerbations (Pratico et al. 1998). This elevation in urine was independent of age, sex, COPD duration, or smoking history.

We conclude in line with a number of reviews that there is overwhelming evidence that the lungs of COPD patients suffer from oxidative stress. Interestingly, the level of oxidative stress in ex-smokers seems to be similar as in current smokers, suggesting that an endogenous source is responsible for persistence of oxidative tress. This is in line with the observation that there is ongoing inflammation after smoking cessation.

12.5.4 Smoking Cessation

The Lung Healthy Study is a large prospective cohort study on smoking cessation in 5,887 mild-to-moderate COPD patients. One year after successful quitting the proportion of subjects that reported at the start of the study respiratory symptoms (cough, phlegm, wheeze, or dyspnea) reduced to approximately 20%, and this was maintained in the next 4 years of follow-up. Moreover, smoking cessation was associated with a lower risk to develop new respiratory symptoms: about 5% in sustained quitters versus 25% in continuous smokers (Kanner et al. 1999; Pride 2001). A cross-sectional population study suggested that dyspnea improves in mild-to-moderate COPD patients who were ex-smokers, but persists in severe COPD patients who quitted smoking (von Hertzen et al. 2000). A large population study with a mean follow-up of 14 years demonstrated that the risk of hospital admission because of COPD was approximately 40% lower in those who quitted smoking (Godtfredsen et al. 2002). In line, the Lung Health Study demonstrated that smoking cessation reduced the frequency of self-reported lower respiratory illnesses resulting in physician visits (Kanner et al. 2001).

Cross-sectional studies show that increased airway hyperresponsiveness to histamine and methacholine is not different between smokers and ex-smokers with COPD (Oosterhoff et al. 1993; Postma et al. 1988). In contrast, increased airway hyperresponsiveness to adenosine 5'-monophosphate is present in many smoking individuals with COPD, whereas it is less severe or absent in ex-smoking COPD patients (Pesci et al. 1994). A longitudinal study in 16 patients with mild-to-moderate COPD showed that both airway hyperresponsiveness to methacholine and adenosine 5'-monophosphate improved significantly after 1 year smoking cessation, though with 1.6 doubling doses with methacholine and 2.1 with AMP (Willemse et al. 2004b). The Lung Health Study showed that both persistent smokers and sustained quitters over a 5-year period had more severe airway hyperresponsiveness to methacholine than at baseline (Wise et al. 2003). However, airway hyperresponsiveness in quitters was over 3-fold less severe than in sustained smokers and closely associated with decline in FEV_1. Sustained quitters had a less rapid decline in FEV_1 over 5 years than persistent smokers: –34 ml/year and –63 ml/year, respectively (Anthonisen et al. 1994, 1997; Murray et al. 1998; Scanlon et al. 2000). During the first year after smoking cessation, FEV_1 improved by 57 ml in quitters, whereas it fell with –32 ml in persistent smokers (Anthonisen et al. 1994). After 11 years' follow-up, the decline in FEV_1 in quitters was –30 ml/year for men and –22 ml/year for women, values for persistent smokers being –66 and –54 ml/year, respectively (Fig. 12.4) (Anthonisen et al. 2002). Heavy smokers showed larger declines in FEV_1 than light smokers, and these heavy smokers had greater improvements after smoking cessation than light smokers (Scanlon et al. 2000). If symptoms, hyperresponsiveness, and decline in FEV_1 all improve after smoking cessation, one would expect that local inflammation improves also. Unfortunately, the few available sputum studies do not confirm this (Willemse et al. 2004a). Similar levels of IL-6, IL-8, myeloperoxidase, and eosinophil cation protein were demonstrated in sputum from ex- and current smokers (Bhowmik et al. 1998; Yamamoto et al. 1997). A longitudinal study even demonstrated an increase in the percentage of neutrophils and IL-8 levels after smoking cessation, suggesting deterioration of airway inflammation (Willemse et al. 2004b). The few available histological studies provide contradictory results. In the peripheral airway walls, squamous metaplasia, inflammatory cell density, fibrosis, and muscle hypertrophy are similar in ex- and current smokers with mild COPD (Wright et al. 1983). In contrast, goblet cell hypertrophy tended to be lower in ex-smokers (Wright et al. 1983), which may explain improvement in cough and sputum production with smoking cessation. In the central airways, Pesci et al. (1994) showed that ex-smokers tended to have lower numbers of mast cells in the epithelium and lamina propria than current smokers with mild-to-moderately severe COPD. As adenosine 5'-monophosphate triggers mast cells to release the bronchoconstrictive agent histamine, this finding might explain why hyperresponsiveness to AMP decreases after smoking cessation (Willemse et al. 2004b). De Boer et al. (2000) found no differences in expression of IL-8, monocyte chemotactic protein (MCP)-1 and its receptor, CCR2, in the central airways from current and ex-smokers with moderate-to-severe COPD (de Boer et al. 2000). In line, Turato et al. (1995) found no differences in expression of a number of inflammatory cells, cytokines, and adhesion molecules. However, Lapperre et al. (2003) found a higher number of submucosal $CD3^+$ and $CD4^+$ T cells in central airway biopsies from ex-smokers than from current smokers with COPD. The latter study is in line with earlier described sputum findings (Willemse et al. 2004b), suggesting that central airway inflammation increases immediately after smoking cessation. Together, these data suggest that some components of airway inflammation improve, whereas most components persist or even deteriorate after smoking cessation. However, this might reflect a beneficial healing process more than a detrimental effect.

12.5.3 Antioxidative Treatment

N-Acetylcysteine is the only commercially available antioxidative agent that can be prescribed in patients with COPD. The presently available experimental and clinical data on the antioxidative effects of *N*-acetylcysteine in COPD have recently been reviewed (Dekhuijzen 2004).

In a randomized 1-year study after 9 and 12 months treatment with *N*-acetylcysteine (600 mg/day), exhaled hydrogen peroxide was 2.3-fold less than with placebo treatment (Kasielski and Nowak 2001). In this study, no significant effects of *N*-acetylcysteine administration were noted on exhaled levels of TBARs or on serum levels of TBARs and lipid peroxides. After administration of a higher dose of 1,200 mg *N*-acetylcysteine per day, the concentrations of hydrogen peroxide in exhaled breath condensate reduced within a 1-month treatment (De Benedetto et al. 2000).

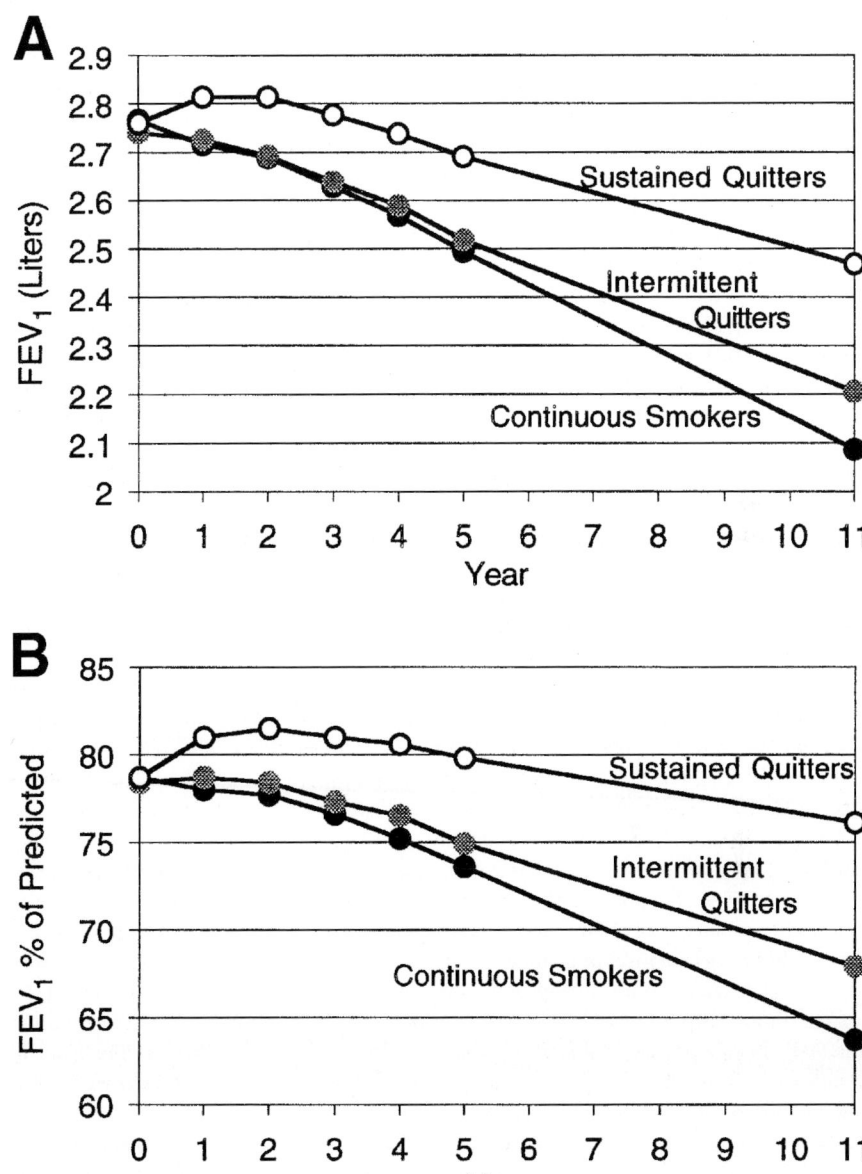

Fig. 12.4 Loss of lung function over the years of the Lung Health Study among 722 sustained quitters (*white circles*), 2,369 continuing smokers (*black circles*), and 1,054 intermittent smokers (*gray circles*). Average values of post bronchodilator forced expiratory volume in 1 second (FEV_1) are shown expressed in absolute terms in **a**, and as a percentage of predicted normal value in **b**. (Reproduced with permission from Anthonisen et al. 2002)

Only a few randomized controlled studies are presently available on the effects of N-acetylcysteine on clinical outcome variables in COPD patients. In a small ($n=2\times25$) placebo-controlled study N-acetylcysteine did not improve recovery of FEV_1, oxygen saturation, or length of hospital stay in COPD patients admitted to the hospital because of an exacerbation (Black et al. 2004). However, the risk of rehospitalization within 1 year after hospitalization was reduced by approximately 30% if COPD patients (>55 years) used prophylactic N-acetylcysteine (Gerrits et al. 2003). In addition, in this post hoc analysis the relative risk significantly decreased with increasing average daily dose of N-acetylcysteine. In a systematic review, 286 of 466 (61.4%) chronic bronchitis patients who received N-acetylcysteine reported improvements of respiratory symptoms versus 160 of 462 (34.6%) patients who received placebo. Of 723 actively treated patients, 351 (48.5%) did not have an exacerbation, versus 229 of 733 (31.2%) placebo-treated patients (Stey et al. 2000). The percentage of patients (per randomized controlled trial) who were smokers or ex-smokers ranged from 72 to 100%. These findings are in line with two previous meta-analyses (Grandjean et al. 2000; Poole and Black 2001), but interpretation is difficult, as many studies included both obstructive and nonobstructive patients. We have to await the definite results of a large prospective placebo-controlled study that included only COPD patients (BRONCUS trial: Bronchitis Randomized on NAC Cost-Utility Study) (Decramer et al. 2001). This 3-year study included 523 COPD patients with moderate-to-severe disease, 46% being current smokers and 54% ex-smokers. This study will also provide data about the possible effect of N-acetylcysteine administration on decline of lung function in COPD.

12.6 Asthma

12.6.1 Smoking and Induction of Asthma

Epidemiological studies suggest that both active (mainstream) and passive (sidestream) exposure to tobacco smoke may contribute to induction of asthma at childhood as well as adulthood. In utero exposure to maternal smoking was associated with a higher incidence and an earlier onset of asthma (Agabiti et al. 1999; Weitzman et al. 1990). Smoking 20 cigarettes or more during pregnancy was associated with an odds ratio of 2.1 for childhood asthma at age 0–5 years, as compared with nonsmoking (Weitzman et al. 1990). Postnatal maternal smoking was positively associated with the prevalence of childhood asthma at age 7–13 years (Soyseth et al. 1995). A large review article including 37 studies concluded that there is compelling evidence that parental smoking induces asthma at childhood (odds ratio = 1.75–2.25) (Cook and Strachan 1999). Hu et al. (1997) demonstrated in young adults a dose–response relationship with the number of cigarettes smoked and the number of parents who smoked. At older ages, passive smoking seemed to increase the risk of asthma only slightly (Coultas 1998; Greer et al. 1993; Leuenberger et al. 1994; Wang et al. 1999).

There are contradictory results about the role of active (mainstream) smoking. Rasmussen et al. (2000) demonstrated in a longitudinal study of 271 asymptomatic adolescents an independent contribution of smoking to the development of respiratory symptoms (odds ratio = 2.1). In cross-sectional studies the risk of asthma was either increased (Arif et al. 2003; Backer et al. 2002; Flodin et al. 1995; Kim et al. 2002; Kiviloog et al. 1974; Piipari et al. 2004) or similar (Hjern et al. 2001; Lebowitz 1977; Pilotto et al. 1999;

Senthilselvan et al. 1993; Walraven et al. 2001) compared with never smokers. Contradictory results were also reported in longitudinal studies, demonstrating an increased (Plaschke et al. 2000; Toren and Hermansson 1999); equal (Vesterinen et al. 1988); or decreased risk (Troisi et al. 1995) in current smokers. Piipari et al. (2004) investigated in a prospective case control study the associations between new adult asthma ($n=521$) and smoking habits. The risk to develop asthma was slightly but significantly higher among current smokers (odds ratio = 1.33) and among ex-smokers (odds ratio = 1.49), compared with never smokers. Among current smokers, the risk increased up to 14 cigarettes per day, but was normal in heavy smokers. A similar trend was detected for cumulative lifetime smoking. Females in this study were at higher risk than males, both in current (odds ratio = 2.43) and ex-smokers (odds ratio = 2.38). In a large review, the Surgeon General's report concluded recently that available studies provide inconsistent findings on the causal relationship between active smoking and the induction of asthma (US Department of Health and Human Services 2004). Inconsistent findings may be caused by not fully controlling for known risk factors for asthma in childhood and adolescence studies, and by different definitions of asthma, different study designs, recall bias, and healthy smoker bias in adult-onset studies (US Department of Health and Human Services 2004).

12.6.2 Smoking and Clinical Severity of Asthma

Cigarette smoking has without doubt far-fetching detrimental effects on the outcome of asthma. In a cross-sectional study of 225 asthmatics, aged 20–54 years, actual smoking was strongly associated with bothersome asthma symptoms that affect daily life activities (Althuis et al. 1999). In a large European epidemiological study (the EGEA Study), active current smoking was associated with asthma severity (Siroux et al. 2000). Cigarette smoking in asthma was associated with increased wheeze (Althuis et al. 1999; Siroux et al. 2000); increased sputum production (Lange et al. 1990b); acute bronchoconstriction (Higenbottam et al. 1980c; Jensen et al. 2000); greater need for rescue medication (Gallefoss and Bakke 2003); unresponsiveness to steroids (Chalmers et al. 2002; Chaudhuri et al. 2003; Kerstjens et al. 1993; Pedersen et al. 1996; Thomson and Spears 2005); accelerated decline in lung function (Almind et al. 1992; Apostol et al. 2002; James et al. 2005; Lange et al. 1998); signs of hyperinflation and emphysema (Lynch et al. 1993; Mitsunobu et al. 2004); greater risk for invasive pneumococcal pneumonia (Nuorti et al. 2000); higher number of hospital admissions (Prescott et al. 1997; Sippel et al. 1999); and higher number of life-threatening asthma attacks (LeSon and Gershwin 1996; Mitchell et al. 2002; Ryan et al. 1991). The Surgeon General concluded that there is sufficient evidence to infer a causal relationship between active smoking and poor asthma control (US Department of Health and Human Services 2004).

There are several reports suggesting that cigarette smoking decreases the responsiveness to inhaled glucocorticosteroids in asthma (Thomson and Spears 2005). Kerstjens et al. (1993) showed that smokers on treatment with inhaled beclomethasone (800 µg/day) had a 383-ml smaller improvement in FEV_1 after 3 months' treatment than nonsmokers did. Pedersen et al. (1996) showed that smoking asthmatics did not improve on treatment with high doses of budesonide (1,600 µg/day) with respect to FEV_1, PC_{20} histamine, serum eosinophil cation protein (ECP), and eosinophil protein X (EPX), bronchodilator use, whereas nonsmoking asthmatics did improve significantly. In line with this,

Chalmers et al. (2002) showed that smoking asthmatics did not improve on treatment with fluticasone propionate (1,000 μg/day) with respect to morning PEF, FEV_1, PC_{20} methacholine, and sputum eosinophilia, in contrast to nonsmoking asthmatics. The detrimental effects of smoking on hyperresponsiveness can not solely be explained by decreased deposition of inhaled corticosteroids in these studies, as smoking has also shown to affect hyperresponsiveness after oral corticosteroid administration (Fig. 12.5) (Chaudhuri et al. 2003). The effect of smoking on corticosteroid responsiveness seems

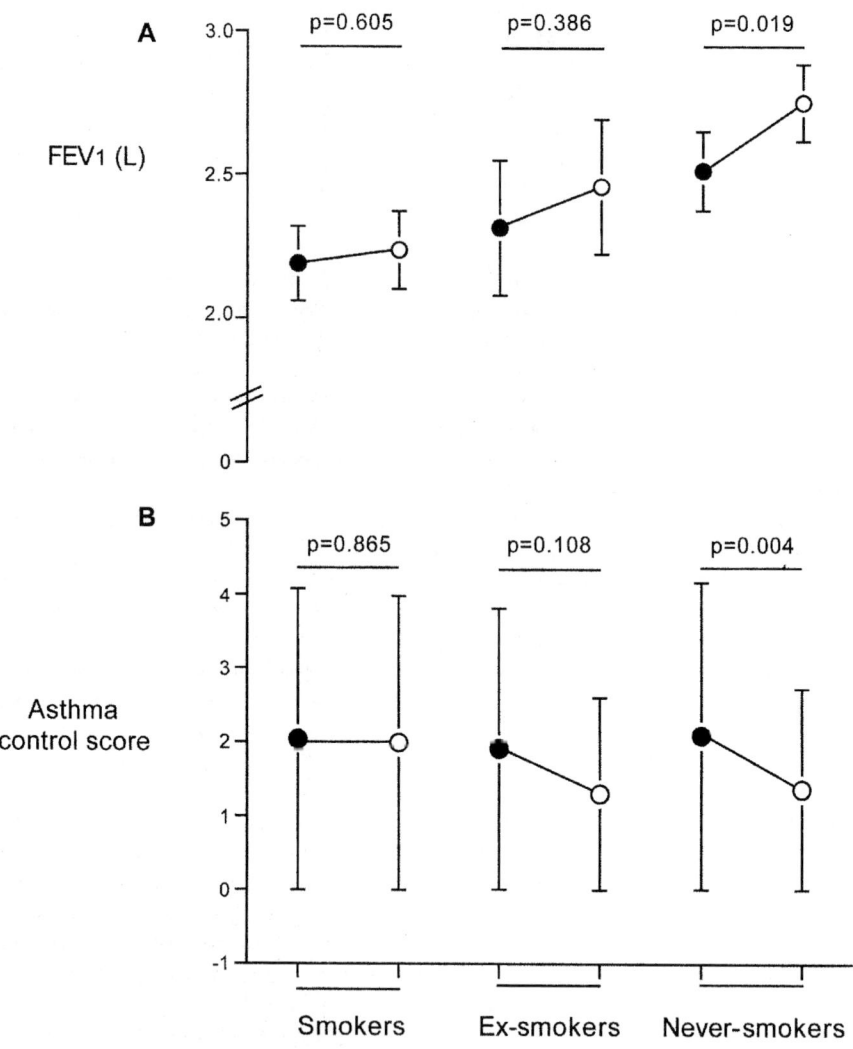

Fig. 12.5 Mean difference (95% confidence interval) after placebo (*solid circle*) and after prednisolone, 40 mg/day for 2 weeks, in smokers with asthma, ex-smokers with asthma, and never smokers with asthma for **a** change in forced volume in one second (FEV_1), and **b** asthma control score. A reduction in the asthma control score implies an improvement. (Reproduced with permission from Chaudhuri et al. 2003)

partially reversible, as ex-smokers in contrast to current smokers show improved morning PEF values after oral corticosteroid treatment (Chaudhuri et al. 2003). The underlying mechanisms of smoking-induced steroid unresponsiveness in asthma are not clear. Possible mechanisms are changed corticosteroid pharmacokinetics, interaction with corticosteroid and β-2 adrenergic receptors, increased airway neutrophil and $CD8^+$ lymphocyte numbers, reduced airway eosinophil numbers, changed cytokine and mediator levels, overexpression of glucocorticoid receptor-β, reduced expression of glucocorticoid receptor-α, overexpression of proinflammatory transcription factors, and reduced histone deacetylase activity (Thomson et al. 2004).

12.6.3 Smoking and Inflammation

Limited data in humans are available with respect to effects of cigarette smoking on airways inflammation and systemic inflammation in asthmatics. Chalmers et al. (2001) demonstrated that asthmatic smokers had higher sputum cell counts, neutrophil numbers, and IL-8 concentrations than did asthmatic nonsmokers. Furthermore, a lower lung function (FEV_1 %predicted) was present in smoking asthmatics, which was related to higher levels of sputum IL-8 and percent neutrophils, whereas higher levels of sputum IL-8 were related to higher numbers of pack years smoking and higher percentages sputum neutrophils. In peripheral blood, the leucocytes from asthmatic smokers produced higher LTB_4 levels than from nonasthmatic smokers (Mitsunobu et al. 2004). In contrast, circulating MPO concentrations in peripheral blood of asthmatic smokers were similar to those of asthmatic nonsmokers (Pedersen et al. 1996).

Sputum eosinophils and ECP levels in the study of Chalmers et al. were lower in asthmatics smokers than in asthmatic nonsmokers. This is in line with the results of studies on circulating blood cells (Halonen et al. 1982; Jensen et al. 1998; Taylor et al. 1985a). Together, these findings suggest that cigarette smoking may alter the balance of Th-1/Th-2 cytokine production; however, we can only speculate about the underlying mechanisms. A reduction in eosinophil numbers may be because of exogenous Nitric Oxide in cigarette smoke, which may increase apoptosis of activated eosinophils (Zhang et al. 2003). On the other hand, a reduced endogenous NO production was demonstrated in mild steroid-naïve asthmatic smokers as compared with asthmatic nonsmokers (Verleden et al. 1999). Interestingly, Melgert et al. (2004) demonstrated in ovalbumine-sensitized mice that short-term exposure to cigarette smoke significantly reduced airway obstruction 24 h after ovalbumine challenge, accompanied by reduced eosinophil numbers in lung lavage fluid and lung tissue. This might have been because of carbon monoxide in cigarette smoke.

Taken together, cigarette smoking seems to both increase and decrease aspects of airway inflammation. Obviously, histological studies are needed to assess whether the airways of smoking asthmatics predominantly show airway pathology characteristic for asthma or COPD, or a combination of these two diseases.

12.6.4 Smoking Cessation

Little data are available about the impact of smoking cessation in asthma. One small cross-sectional study reported less cough and sputum production in ex-smokers, compared with current smokers (Higenbottam et al. 1980c). However, another study not designed for this purpose reported similar asthma-symptom scores in current smokers and ex-smokers (Chaudhuri et al. 2003). In a small longitudinal study, 14 asthmatic patients managed to stop for 24 h, and 7 for 1 week. Twenty-four hours after smoking cessation, airway obstruction improved significantly; after 7 days, there was a further improvement (Fennerty et al. 1987). Seven days after smoking cessation, bronchial responsiveness to histamine improved, and four of the seven subjects recorded an improvement in symptoms. In another longitudinal study, blood samples were collected in 160 asthmatics who quit smoking, and in 30 continuing smokers (Jensen et al. 1998). In particular, the asthmatic subjects with decreased lung function and heavy smoking showed significant increases in blood eosinophil counts after smoking cessation. Gotfretson et al. (2001) demonstrated in a large epidemiological cohort study that ex-smokers had a higher incidence of self-reported asthma than did never smokers (Godtfredsen et al. 2001). The risk to develop self-reported asthma in ex-smokers, compared with never smokers was also increased in two small clinical studies (Hillerdahl and Rylander 1984; Troisi et al. 1995).

12.7 Lung Cancer

12.7.1 Epidemiology

Lung cancer is one of the leading causes of death from neoplastic disease in most developed countries. About 87% of all lung cancer cases are caused by cigarette smoking (American Cancer Society 2001). Diseases such as lung cancer were rare before the widespread use of tobacco; however, after the 1940s, lung cancer was increasing at alarming rates (Auerbach et al. 1957; Cornfield et al. 1959). In the United States, the incidence of lung cancer peaked in 1990 and since has fallen (Cole and Rodu 1996). In Europe, the incidence of lung cancer in men in Denmark, Finland, Germany, Italy, The Netherlands, Switzerland, and the United Kingdom decreased since the 1980s; however, the age-adjusted rate for men in other European countries increased at least until the 1990s. In women, the peak in incidence had not been reached in the 1990s (Janssen-Heijnen and Coebergh 2003). A meta-analysis including 48 studies published between 1970 and 1999 provided additional evidence for a causal relationship between smoking and all histological subtypes of lung cancer (Khuder 2001). The association was stronger with squamous cell carcinoma and small cell carcinoma than was the association with large cell cancer and adenocarcinoma. Combined odd ratios for heavy smoking (>30 cig/day) ranged from 4.1 (CI = 3.16–5.31) for adenocarcinoma to 18.3 (CI = 9.26–36.4) for small cell lung cancer (Khuder 2001).

The ratio of adenocarcinoma and squamous cell carcinoma in the United States was about 1:18 in the 1950s, whereas it was 1:1.2–1.4 in the 1990s. This shift to a higher proportion of adenocarcinoma has also been demonstrated in Europe (Janssen-Heijnen and Coebergh 2003) and other parts of the world (Janssen-Heijnen and Coebergh 2001). The shift to low-tar filter cigarettes during the 1960s and 1970s is the most likely cause (Wynder and Muscat 1995). Ironically, low-tar cigarette smokers may compensate for their low-nicotine delivery by inhaling deeper, in this way exposing the peripheral parts of the lung to increased amounts of carcinogens. In addition, a more intense smoking pattern may increase the generation of N-nitrosamines in smoke 3-fold (Wynder and Muscat

1995). An increase in the nitrate content of cigarette tobacco blends may be another explanation for the observed shift in subtypes (Wynder and Muscat 1995). Because there is an overwhelming body of evidence linking cigarette smoking to lung cancer, smoking cessation might be the most effective way to decrease risk of lung cancer. Indeed, smoking cessation reduces the risk to develop lung cancer; however, 15 years after smoking cessation the risk is still higher as compared with never smokers (Halpern et al. 1993). The relative benefits of smoking cessation in this respect appear to be larger for persons with shorter smoking histories (Halpern et al. 1993; Sobue et al. 1993). This is also reflected by the mortality rates of 34,439 male British doctors who have been followed for 50 years (Doll et al. 2004). Continuous smokers born between 1900 and 1930 died, on average, 10 years younger than lifelong nonsmokers (Fig. 12.6). Smoking cessation at age 60, 50, 40, or 30 years gained respectively about 6, 9, 9, or 10 years of life expectancy. Excess mortality associated with cigarette smoking involved vascular, respiratory, and neoplastic diseases; 1,052 of them died because of lung cancer. Age-standardized lung cancer mortality rates (per 100 men per year) of current cigarette smokers depended on the number of cigarettes smoked per day; mortality rates of light (<15/day), moderate (15–24/day), and heavy (>24/day) smokers being 1.31, 2.33, and 4.17 respectively. Lung cancer mortality rates of lifelong nonsmokers, current smokers, and former smokers were 0.17, 0.68, and 2.49, respectively. Those who stopped at age 55–64 were at lower risk to die of lung cancer than continuous smokers, but still were at higher risk than lifelong nonsmokers. Stopping at earlier ages protected even more, but until about age 40 there was still some excess risk to develop lung cancer at older ages. Evidently, smoking cessation at an early age is the most effective way to decrease lung cancer risk; however, many smokers are not able to quit smoking, and those who successfully quit still have a higher risk of lung cancer.

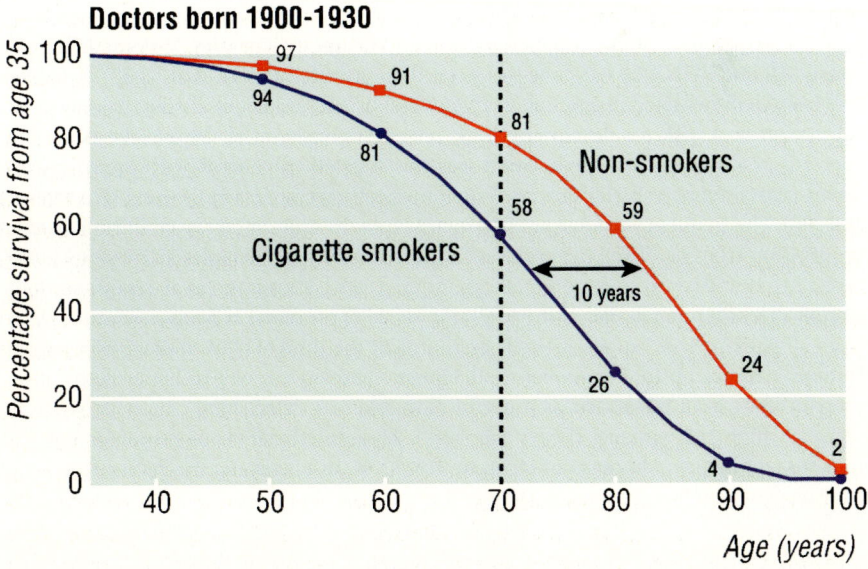

Fig. 12.6 Survival from age 35 for continuing cigarette smokers and life-long nonsmokers among UK male doctors born between 1900 and 1930, with percentage alive at each decade of age. (Reproduced with permission from Doll et al. 2004)

12.7.2 Mutagens, Carcinogens, and Molecular Changes in the Lung

Cigarette smoking results in the exposure to more than 60 established mutagens and carcinogens (Hoffmann and Hoffmann 1997). The strongest carcinogens are polycyclic aromatic hydrocarbons (PAHs) and N-nitrosamines. Metabolic detoxification of these agents may lead to excretion; however, sometimes reactive intermediates are formed, which may result in the formation of covalently bound DNA products (DNA adducts). PAHs are formed from the incomplete pyrolysis of tobacco leaves, and many types are present as a complex mixture in tobacco smoke (Lodovici et al. 1998; Seto et al. 1993). Parent PAHs and PAH-related DNA adducts have been demonstrated in the human lung (Lodovici et al. 1998; Seto et al. 1993). N-Nitrosamines are formed at higher burning temperatures of the cigarette, e.g., in case smokers inhale faster to compensate for low nicotine contents. N-Nitrosamines undergo metabolic activation by cytochrome P450s in the lung and may form three different classes of DNA adducts (Hecht 1999a). They include methylation of different nucleotides (Hecht 1999a), oxidative DNA damage (Hecht 1999a), and bulky DNA adducts (Hecht 1999b). N-Nitrosamines adducts have also been demonstrated in human lung tissue. Once DNA adducts are present in the lung cellular DNA repair processes may remove adducts and return the DNA to its normal structure. However, some adducts may escape repair and cause persistent miscoding. Such mutations can activate oncogens (like *RAS*), or inactivate tumor suppressor genes (like *p53*), leading to self-sufficiency in growth signals, insensitivity to antigrowth signals, evasion of apoptosis, tissue invasion and metastasis, sustained angiogenesis, and limitless replicative potential (Hanahan and Weinberg 2000).

Theoretically, cigarette smoking may cause lung cancer also through hypermethylation of promoter regions of tumor suppressor genes. In bronchial brush samples from ex-smokers, hypermethylation of the promoter region of multiple genes including *GSTP1*, *p16* (*INK4a*) tumor suppressor gene, and O^6-methylguanine DNA methyltransferase (*MGMT*) DNA repair gene has been demonstrated (Soria et al. 2002). This has also been demonstrated in sputum and bronchial brush samples of current smokers and subjects at high risk for developing lung cancer (Belinsky et al. 2002). The degree of aberrant *p16* and *MGMT* methylation was investigated in patients with premalignant lesions, carcinoma in situ lesions, and squamous cell carcinomas of the lung (Herman et al. 1996). The frequency of aberrant p16 methylation in sputum increased during disease progression from basal cell hyperplasia (17%), to squamous metaplasia (24%), to carcinoma in situ (50%), to squamous cell carcinoma (80%). Palmisano et al. (2000) demonstrated aberrant methylation of the *p16* (and *MGMT*) promoter regions in sputum DNA from all patients with squamous cell carcinoma at the time of clinical diagnosis, and in sputum samples up to 3 years before diagnosis. Assessment of p16 hypermethylation therefore has been advocated as a useful biomarker to detect lung cancer in an early phase in high-risk patients (heavy smokers). Hypermethylation of promoter regions in a susceptible gene because of cigarette smoke is an epigenetic mechanism demonstrating gene–environmental interaction.

12.7.3 Lung Cancer and COPD

Airway obstruction because of COPD has been associated with increased risk of lung cancer, independent of smoking history. This has been demonstrated both in cross-sectional (Kishi et al. 2002; Tockman et al. 1987) and longitudinal studies (Lange et al. 1990c; Mannino et al. 2003a; Nomura et al. 1991; Skillrud et al. 1986), and one study demonstrated it specifically in COPD patients with a more rapid decline of FEV_1 (Islam and Schottenfeld 1994). Both in current and past smokers the relative risk of lung cancer, when adjusted for age and pack years smoked, ranged from 2 to 6, depending on the degree of airflow obstruction (Lange et al. 1990a; Mannino et al. 2003b; Nomura et al. 1991; Tockman et al. 1987). An explanation for the higher risk of lung cancer in COPD patients might be the decreased mucociliary clearance and pooling of inhaled carcinogens in the central airways. Important in this respect is that Nomura (1991) found only an association between COPD and lung cancer for centrally located lung tumors. Another explanation might be a common etiological factor such as the inability of the lung to dispose free radicals and oxidants in cigarette smoke, leading to oxidative stress. Recently, Papi et al. (2004) demonstrated in patients with resectable non–small cell carcinoma lung cancer (NSCLC) that COPD increased the risk for the squamous cell histological subtype by more than four times. In accordance with previous studies, they also demonstrated that chronic bronchitis (without airflow obstruction) increased the risk for the adenocarcinoma subtype by more than four times. The authors speculated that the latter might be because of a more peripheral distribution of tobacco smoke, causing activation of cell signaling pathways (e.g., via the EGF receptor) and inducing increased mucus, producing elements together with adenocarcinoma differentiation of preneoplastic lesions of the bronchial/bronchiolar epithelium.

12.7.4 Chemoprevention

Chemoprevention has been advocated as an alternative for smoking cessation. *Chemoprevention* is defined as the use of agents to prevent, inhibit, or reverse the process of carcinogenesis (Bertram et al. 1987). Two major categories of compounds have been investigated. The first group consists of naturally occurring dietary micronutrients and their synthetic analogues. The second group is composed of synthetic agents like non-steroidal anti-inflammatory drugs (NSAIDs) and difluoromethyl ornithine. Such agents have been tested in three settings: primary prevention (in healthy subjects being at high risk because of smoking), secondary prevention (in subjects with premalignant lesions), and tertiary prevention (in previously treated lung cancer patients). No randomized trials, in human, in any setting, have shown evidence for efficacy of any agents tested, including α-tocopherol, β-carotene, selenium, retinyl palmitate, isotretinoin, and *N*-acetylcysteine (Cohen and Khuri 2004; Goodman 2002; Hecht 2002; Kelley and McCrory 2003; Lippman and Spitz 2001). Many of these agents might act as scavengers for cigarette smoke-induced free radicals. For example, *N*-acetylcysteine, 600 mg/day, as a potent glutathione donor, and retinyl palmitate were investigated in a randomized controlled trial of 2,592 patients who previously had been treated for head/neck (60%) or lung cancer (40%) (van Zandwijk et al. 2000). Of these patients, 93.5% had smoked, and 25% were still smoking. After a median follow-up of 49 months, no beneficial effect of retinyl palmitate and/or *N*-acetylcysteine on second primary cancer incidence could be demonstrated. Although the results of the above-described studies all are negative, there still is hope for a future role of chemoprevention in lung cancer. A better understanding of human uptake of tobacco carcinogens and of individual differences in the metabolic activation and detoxification of carcinogens may help to effectively tailor chemoprevention, using promising new agents that are still in a preclinical phase (Hecht 2002).

12.8 Smoking-Related Interstitial Lung Diseases

Four interstitial lung disorders have been linked to cigarette smoking; the clinical, radiological, and histopathological features have been summarized in a concise review recently (Ryu et al. 2001).

Desquamative interstitial pneumonia is characterized by the presence of increased numbers of pigmented macrophages evenly dispersed within the alveolar spaces (Katzenstein and Myers 1998). Honeycombing is minimal, and the overall architecture is maintained in most cases. Ninety percent of the patients smoke or have smoked; however, there is also an association with systemic disorders or infections, as well as exposures to environmental agents and drugs. Untreated, about two thirds of patients show clinical worsening. Patients treated with smoking cessation and steroids generally have a good prognosis and may recover completely.

Respiratory bronchiolitis-associated interstitial lung disease is characterized by the presence of pigmented macrophages and mild interstitial inflammatory changes centering around respiratory bronchioles and neighboring alveoli. This clinicopathological entity is seen almost exclusively in current and former cigarette smokers (Myers et al. 1987) and extends the normally occurring respiratory bronchiolitis because of smoking. Patients with respiratory bronchiolitis-associated interstitial lung disease have a good prognosis and show complete recovery, especially with smoking cessation.

Pulmonary Langerhans cell histiocytosis is characterized by nodular sclerosing lesions containing Langerhans cells, accompanied by mixed cellular infiltrates (Travis et al. 1993). The isolated pulmonary form of Langerhans cell histiocytosis in adults occurs almost exclusively in cigarette smokers. In addition, in young healthy individuals, the accumulation of Langerhans cells on the epithelial surface of the respiratory tract is strongly associated with cigarette smoking (Casolaro et al. 1988). Radiological improvement and even complete resolution after smoking cessation has been described in two case reports (Mogulkoc et al. 1999; Von Essen et al. 1990).

Idiopathic pulmonary fibrosis or cryptogenic fibrosing alveolitis is defined as a specific form of chronic fibrosing interstitial pneumonia limited to the lung and associated with the histological appearance of usual interstitial pneumonia on surgical lung biopsy. The morphological findings range from a normal appearance in early cases to diffuse honeycombing in the later stages. The prevalence of current or former cigarette smoking varies between 41 and 83%. Baumgartner et al. (1997) found a history of smoking to be associated with a lightly increased risk to develop idiopathic pulmonary fibrosis (odds ratio = 1.6). Unfortunately, smoking cessation does not affect the poor prognosis. Although *N*-acetylcysteine administration intravenously or orally has led to increased glutathione levels in BAL fluid and epithelial lining fluid of idiopathic pulmonary fibrosis (IPF) patients (Meyer et al. 1994, 1995), its clinical efficacy has not been demonstrated in long-term studies.

We conclude that cigarette smoking has been implicated in the development of the four interstitial lung diseases described above. Nevertheless, the exact role of cigarette smoking still needs to be defined; the relatively low prevalence of interstitial lung disease makes epidemiologic studies difficult (Flaherty and Martinez 2004).

12.9 Summary

Many studies have shown the detrimental role of smoking on development and progression of pulmonary diseases such as chronic bronchitis, COPD, asthma, lung cancer, and some interstitial lung diseases. The role of oxidative stress is in this respect variable, clearly established in COPD, and either less explicitly present or not reported because lack of studies in the other diseases.

References

(1995) Standards for the diagnosis and care of patients with chronic obstructive pulmonary disease. American Thoracic Society. Am J Respir Crit Care Med 152:S77–S121

(2000) American Thoracic Society. Idiopathic pulmonary fibrosis: diagnosis and treatment. International consensus statement. American Thoracic Society (ATS), and the European Respiratory Society (ERS). Am J Respir Crit Care Med 161:646–664

Agabiti N et al. (1999) The impact of parental smoking on asthma and wheezing. SIDRIA Collaborative Group. Studi Italiani sui Disturbi Respiratori nell'Infanzia e l'Ambiente. Epidemiology 10:692–698

Alcaide J et al. (1996) Cigarette smoking as a risk factor for tuberculosis in young adults: a case-control study. Tuber Lung Dis 77:112–116

Alderson MR et al. (1985) Risks of lung cancer, chronic bronchitis, ischaemic heart disease, and stroke in relation to type of cigarette smoked. J Epidemiol Community Health 39:286–293

Almind M et al. (1992) A seven-year follow-up study of 343 adults with bronchial asthma. Dan Med Bull 39:561–565

Almirall J et al. (1999a) Risk factors for community-acquired pneumonia in adults: a population-based case-control study. Eur Respir J 13:349–355

Almirall J et al. (1999b) Proportion of community-acquired pneumonia cases attributable to tobacco smoking. Chest 116:375–379

Althuis MD et al. (1999) Cigarette smoking and asthma symptom severity among adult asthmatics. J Asthma 36:257–264

Altshuler B et al. (1957) Aerosol deposition in the human respiratory tract. I. Experimental procedures and total deposition. AMA Arch Ind Health 15:293–303

American Cancer Society (2001) Cancer facts and figures 2001. In: American Cancer Society (ed) Cancer facts and figures 2001. American Cancer Society, Atlanta, pp 29–32

Anthonisen NR (1997) Epidemiology and the Lung Health Study. Eur Respir Rev 7:202–205

Anthonisen NR et al. (1994) Effects of smoking intervention and the use of an inhaled anticholinergic bronchodilator on the rate of decline of FEV1. The Lung Health Study. JAMA 272:1497–1505

Anthonisen NR et al. (2002) Smoking and lung function of lung health study participants after 11 years. Am J Respir Crit Care Med 166:675–679

Apostol GG et al. (2002) Early life factors contribute to the decrease in lung function between ages 18 and 40: the Coronary Artery Risk Development in Young Adults study. Am J Respir Crit Care Med 166:166–172

Arif AA et al. (2003) Prevalence and risk factors of asthma and wheezing among US adults: an analysis of the NHANES III data. Eur Respir J 21:827–833

Auerbach O et al. (1957) Changes in the bronchial epithelium in relation to smoking and cancer of the lung; a report of progress. N Engl J Med 256:97–104

Backer V et al. (2002) Factors associated with asthma in young Danish adults. Ann Allergy Asthma Immunol 89:148–154

Balint B et al. (2001) Increased nitric oxide metabolites in exhaled breath condensate after exposure to tobacco smoke. Thorax 56:456–461

Balzano G et al. (1999) Eosinophilic inflammation in stable chronic obstructive pulmonary disease. Relationship with neutrophils and airway function. Am J Respir Crit Care Med 160:1486–1492

Barbee RA et al. (1991) A longitudinal study of respiratory symptoms in a community population sample. Correlations with smoking, allergen skin-test reactivity, and serum IgE [see comments]. Chest 99:20–26

Barsky SH et al. (1998) Histopathologic and molecular alterations in bronchial epithelium in habitual smokers of marijuana, cocaine, and/or tobacco. J Natl Cancer Inst 90:1198–1205

Baumgartner KB et al. (1997) Cigarette smoking: a risk factor for idiopathic pulmonary fibrosis. Am J Respir Crit Care Med 155:242–248

Beaty TH et al. (1984) Risk factors associated with longitudinal change in pulmonary function. Am Rev Respir Dis 129:660–667

Beeh KM et al. (2003) Sputum matrix metalloproteinase-9, tissue inhibitor of metalloprotinease-1, and their molar ratio in patients with chronic obstructive pulmonary disease, idiopathic pulmonary fibrosis and healthy subjects. Respir Med 97:634–639

Belinsky SA et al. (2002) Aberrant promoter methylation in bronchial epithelium and sputum from current and former smokers. Cancer Res. 62:2370–2377

Berger P et al. (2003) Structure and function of small airways in smokers: relationship between air trapping at CT and airway inflammation. Radiology 228:85–94

Bernstein D (2004) A review of the influence of particle size, puff volume, and inhalation pattern on the deposition of cigarette smoke particles in the respiratory tract. Inhal Toxicol 16:675–689

Bertram JS et al. (1987) Rationale and strategies for chemoprevention of cancer in humans. Cancer Res. 47:3012–3031

Bhowmik A et al. (1998) Comparison of spontaneous and induced sputum for investigation of airway inflammation in chronic obstructive pulmonary disease. Thorax 53:953–956

Biernacki WA et al. (2003) Increased leukotriene B4 and 8-isoprostane in exhaled breath condensate of patients with exacerbations of COPD. Thorax 58:294–298

Bjornsson E et al. (1994) Symptoms related to asthma and chronic bronchitis in three areas of Sweden. Eur Respir J 7:2146–2153

Black PN et al. (2004) Randomised, controlled trial of N-acetylcysteine for treatment of acute exacerbations of chronic obstructive pulmonary disease [ISRCTN21676344]. BMC Pulm Med 4:13

Bosse R et al. (1981) Longitudinal effect of age and smoking cessation on pulmonary function. Am Rev Respir Dis 123:378–381

Brown CA et al. (1991a) Cigarette tar content and symptoms of chronic bronchitis: results of the Scottish Heart Health Study. J Epidemiol Community Health 45:287–290

Brown CA et al. (1991b) The impact of quitting smoking on symptoms of chronic bronchitis: results of the Scottish Heart Health Study. Thorax 46:112–116

Brown NE et al. (1977) Airway responses to inhaled histamine in asymptomatic smokers and non-smokers. J Appl Physiol 42:508–513

Buczko GB et al. (1984) Effects of cigarette smoking and short-term smoking cessation on airway responsiveness to inhaled methacholine. Am Rev Respir Dis 129:12–14

Buist AS et al. (1976) The effect of smoking cessation and modification on lung function. Am Rev Respir Dis 114:115–122

Buist AS et al. (1979) The effect of smoking cessation on pulmonary function: a 30-month follow-up of two smoking cessation clinics. Am Rev Respir Dis 120:953–957

Burchfiel CM et al. (1995) Effects of smoking and smoking cessation on longitudinal decline in pulmonary function. Am J Respir Crit Care Med 151:1778–1785

Burney PG et al. (1987) Descriptive epidemiology of bronchial reactivity in an adult population: results from a community study. Thorax 42:38–44

Burrows B et al. (1981) The relationship of serum immunoglobulin E to cigarette smoking. Am Rev Respir Dis 124:523–525

Buskin SE et al. (1994) Tuberculosis risk factors in adults in King County, Washington, 1988 through 1990. Am J Public Health 84:1750–1756

Byron KA et al. (1994) IL-4 production is increased in cigarette smokers. Clin Exp Immunol. 95:333–336

Camilli AE et al. (1987) Longitudinal changes in forced expiratory volume in one second in adults. Effects of smoking and smoking cessation. Am Rev Respir Dis 135:794–799

Campbell AH et al. (1985) Factors affecting the decline of ventilatory function in chronic bronchitis. Thorax 40:741–748

Cantin AM et al. (1987) Normal alveolar epithelial lining fluid contains high levels of glutathione. J Appl Physiol 63:152–157

Capelli A et al. (1999) Increased MCP-1 and MIP-1beta in bronchoalveolar lavage fluid of chronic bronchitics. Eur Respir J 14:160–165

Carpagnano GE et al. (2003) Increased inflammatory markers in the exhaled breath condensate of cigarette smokers. Eur Respir J 21:589–593

Casolaro MA et al. (1988) Accumulation of Langerhans' cells on the epithelial surface of the lower respiratory tract in normal subjects in association with cigarette smoking. Am Rev Respir Dis 137:406–411

Cataldo D et al. (2000) MMP-2- and MMP-9-linked gelatinolytic activity in the sputum from patients with asthma and chronic obstructive pulmonary disease. Int Arch Allergy Immunol 123:259–267

Cerveri I et al. (2001) Variations in the prevalence across countries of chronic bronchitis and smoking habits in young adults. Eur Respir J 18:85–92

Cerveri I et al. (1989) Smoking habit and bronchial reactivity in normal subjects. A population-based study. Am Rev Respir Dis. 140:191–196

Cetinkaya F et al. (2000) Prevalence of chronic bronchitis and associated risk factors in a rural area of Kayseri, Central Anatolia, Turkey. Monaldi Arch Chest Dis 55:189–193

Chalmers GW et al. (2001) Smoking and airway inflammation in patients with mild asthma. Chest 120:1917–1922

Chalmers GW et al. (2002) Influence of cigarette smoking on inhaled corticosteroid treatment in mild asthma. Thorax 57:226–230

Chambers DC et al. (1998) Acute inhalation of cigarette smoke increases lower respiratory tract nitric oxide concentrations. Thorax 53:677–679

Chaudhuri R et al. (2003) Cigarette smoking impairs the therapeutic response to oral corticosteroids in chronic asthma. Am J Respir Crit Care Med 168:1308–1311

Choi AM, Alam J (1996) Heme oxygenase-1: function, regulation, and implication of a novel stress-inducible protein in oxidant-induced lung injury. Am J Respir Cell Mol Biol 15:9–19

Cockcroft DW et al. (1983) Bronchial response to inhaled histamine in asymptomatic young smokers. Eur J Respir Dis 64:207–211

Cohen V, Khuri FR (2004) Chemoprevention of lung cancer. Curr Opin Pulm Med 10:279–283

Cole P, Rodu B (1996) Declining cancer mortality in the United States. Cancer 78:2045–2048

Collins JG (1997) Prevalence of selected chronic conditions: United States, 1990–1992. Vital Health Stat.10:1–89

Comhair SA et al. (2000) Differential induction of extracellular glutathione peroxidase and nitric oxide synthase 2 in airways of healthy individuals exposed to 100% O_2 or cigarette smoke. Am J Respir Cell Mol Biol 23:350–354

Comstock GW et al. (1970) Cigarette smoking and changes in respiratory findings. Arch Environ Health 21:50–57

Cook DG, Strachan DP (1999) Health effects of passive smoking-10: summary of effects of parental smoking on the respiratory health of children and implications for research. Thorax 54:357–366

Cornfield J et al. (1959) Smoking and lung cancer: recent evidence and a discussion of some questions. J Natl Cancer Inst 22:173–203

Corradi M et al. (1999) Increased exhaled nitric oxide in patients with stable chronic obstructive pulmonary disease [see comments]. Thorax 54:572–575

Corradi M et al. (2003a) Nitrate in exhaled breath condensate of patients with different airway diseases. Nitric Oxide 8:26–30

Corradi M et al. (2003b) Aldehydes in exhaled breath condensate of patients with chronic obstructive pulmonary disease. Am J Respir Crit Care Med 167:1380–1386

Cosio M et al. (1978) The relations between structural changes in small airways and pulmonary-function tests. N Engl J Med 298:1277–1281

Cosio MG, Guerassimov A (1999) Chronic obstructive pulmonary disease. Inflammation of small airways and lung parenchyma. Am J Respir Crit Care Med 160:S21–S25

Cosio MG et al. (1980) Morphologic and morphometric effects of prolonged cigarette smoking on the small airways. Am Rev Respir Dis 122:265–221

Costabel U et al. (1986) Alterations in immunoregulatory T-cell subsets in cigarette smokers. A phenotypic analysis of bronchoalveolar and blood lymphocytes. Chest 90:39–44

Costabel U et al. (1992) Local immune components in chronic obstructive pulmonary disease. Respiration 59:S17–S19

Coultas DB (1998) Health effects of passive smoking. 8. Passive smoking and risk of adult asthma and COPD: an update. Thorax 53:381–387

Dandrea T et al. (1997) Differential inhibition of inflammatory cytokine release from cultured alveolar macrophages from smokers and non-smokers by NO_2. Hum Exp Toxicol 16:577–588

Daniele RP et al. (1977) Lymphocyte studies in asymptomatic cigarette smokers. A comparison between lung and peripheral blood. Am Rev Respir Dis 116:997–1005

De Benedetto F et al. (2000) Long-term treatment with N-acetylcysteine (NAC) decreases hydrogen peroxide level in the exhaled air of patients with moderate COPD. Am J Respir Crit Care Med 163:A725–A725

de Boer WI et al. (2000) Monocyte chemoattractant protein 1, interleukin 8, and chronic airways inflammation in COPD. J Pathol 190:619–626

Decramer M et al. (2001) The Bronchitis Randomized on NAC Cost-Utility Study (BRONCUS): hypothesis and design. BRONCUS-Trial Committee. Eur Respir J 17:329–336

Dekhuijzen PN (2004) Antioxidant properties of N-acetylcysteine: their relevance in relation to chronic obstructive pulmonary disease. Eur Respir J 23:629–636

Dekhuijzen PN et al. (1996) Increased exhalation of hydrogen peroxide in patients with stable and unstable chronic obstructive pulmonary disease. Am J Respir Crit Care Med 154:813–816

Delen FM et al. (2000) Increased exhaled nitric oxide in chronic bronchitis: comparison with asthma and COPD. Chest 117:695–701

Dippolito R et al. (2001) Eosinophils in induced sputum from asymptomatic smokers with normal lung function. Respir Med 95:969–974

Doll R et al. (2004) Mortality in relation to smoking: 50 years' observations on male British doctors. BMJ 328:1519–1533

Drost EM et al. (1992) Changes in neutrophil deformability following in vitro smoke exposure: mechanism and protection. Am J Respir Cell Mol Biol 6:287–295

Drost EM et al. (1993) Decreased leukocyte deformability after acute cigarette smoking in humans. Am Rev Respir Dis 148:1277–1283

Dutu S, Paun G (1998) [The prevalence of respiratory symptoms, bronchial asthma and chronic bronchitis (simple and obstructive) in a representative sample of the adult rural population]. Pneumoftiziologia 47:151–160

Ekberg-Jansson A et al. (2001) Respiratory symptoms relate to physiological changes and inflammatory markers reflecting central but not peripheral airways. A study in 60-year-old "healthy" smokers and never-smokers. Respir Med 95:40–47

Enright PL et al. (1994) Prevalence and correlates of respiratory symptoms and disease in the elderly. Cardiovascular Health Study. Chest 106:827–834

Euler DE et al. (1996) Effect of cigarette smoking on pentane excretion in alveolar breath. Clin Chem 42:303–308

Fahn HJ et al. (1998) Smoking-associated mitochondrial DNA mutations and lipid peroxidation in human lung tissues. Am J Respir Cell Mol Biol 19:901–909

Fennerty AG et al. (1987) The effect of cigarette withdrawal on asthmatics who smoke. Eur J Respir Dis 71:395–399

Ferrari M et al. (2000) Seroprevalence of *Chlamydia pneumoniae* antibodies in a young adult population sample living in Verona. European Community Respiratory Health Survey (ECRHS) Verona. Infection 28:38–41

Finklea JF et al. (1969) Cigarette smoking and epidemic influenza. Am J Epidemiol 90:390–399

Finklea JF et al. (1971) Cigarette smoking and hemagglutination inhibition response to influenza after natural disease and immunization. Am Rev Respir Dis 104:368–376

Finlay GA et al. (1997a) Matrix metalloproteinase expression and production by alveolar macrophages in emphysema [see comments]. Am J Respir Crit Care Med 156:240–247

Finlay GA et al. (1997b) Elevated levels of matrix metalloproteinases in bronchoalveolar lavage fluid of emphysematous patients [see comments]. Thorax 52:502–506

Flaherty KR, Martinez FJ (2004) Cigarette smoking in interstitial lung disease: concepts for the internist. Med Clin North Am 88:1643–1653, xiii

Fligiel SE et al. (1997) Tracheobronchial histopathology in habitual smokers of cocaine, marijuana, and/or tobacco. Chest 112:319–326

Flodin U et al. (1995) An epidemiologic study of bronchial asthma and smoking. Epidemiology 6:503–505

Fournier M et al. (1989) Intraepithelial T-lymphocyte subsets in the airways of normal subjects and of patients with chronic bronchitis. Am Rev Respir Dis 140:737–742

Friedman GD, Siegelaub AB (1980) Changes after quitting cigarette smoking. Circulation 61:716–723

Gallefoss F, Bakke PS (2003) Does smoking affect the outcome of patient education and self-management in asthmatics? Patient Educ Couns 49:91–97

Gerrard JW et al. (1980) Increased nonspecific bronchial reactivity in cigarette smokers with normal lung function. Am Rev Respir Dis 122:577–581

Gerrits CM et al. (2003) N-acetylcysteine reduces the risk of re-hospitalisation among patients with chronic obstructive pulmonary disease. Eur Respir J 21:795–798

Gil E et al. (1995) Acute and chronic effects of marijuana smoking on pulmonary alveolar permeability. Life Sci 56:2193–2199

Godtfredsen NS et al. (2001) Changes in smoking habits and risk of asthma: a longitudinal population based study. Eur Respir J 18:549–554

Godtfredsen NS et al. (2002) Risk of hospital admission for COPD following smoking cessation and reduction: a Danish population study. Thorax 57:967–972

Gold DR et al. (1996) Effects of cigarette smoking on lung function in adolescent boys and girls. N Engl J Med 335:931–937

Goodman GE (2002) Lung cancer. 1: Prevention of lung cancer. Thorax 57:994–999

Grandjean EM et al. (2000) Efficacy of oral long-term N-acetylcysteine in chronic bronchopulmonary disease: a meta-analysis of published double-blind, placebo-controlled clinical trials. Clin Ther 22:209–221

Greer JR et al. (1993) Asthma related to occupational and ambient air pollutants in nonsmokers. J Occup Med 35:909–915

Guatura SB et al. (2000) Increased exhalation of hydrogen peroxide in healthy subjects following cigarette consumption. Sao Paulo Med J 118:93–98

Halonen M et al. (1982) An epidemiologic study of interrelationships of total serum immunoglobulin E, allergy skin-test reactivity, and eosinophilia. J Allergy Clin Immunol 69:221–228

Halpern MT et al. (1993) Patterns of absolute risk of lung cancer mortality in former smokers. J Natl Cancer Inst 85:457–464

Hanahan D, Weinberg RA (2000) The hallmarks of cancer. Cell 100:57–70

Harju T et al. (2002) Diminished immunoreactivity of gamma-glutamylcysteine synthetase in the airways of smokers' lung. Am J Respir Crit Care Med 166:754–759

Hecht SS (1999a) DNA adduct formation from tobacco-specific N-nitrosamines. Mutat Res 424:127–142

Hecht SS (1999b) Tobacco smoke carcinogens and lung cancer. J Natl Cancer Inst 91:1194–1210

Hecht SS (2002) Cigarette smoking and lung cancer: chemical mechanisms and approaches to prevention. Lancet Oncol 3:461–469

Herman JG et al. (1996) Methylation-specific PCR: a novel PCR assay for methylation status of CpG islands. Proc Natl Acad Sci U S A 93:9821–9826

Higenbottam T et al. (1980a) Lung function and symptoms of cigarette smokers related to tar yield and number of cigarettes smoked. Lancet 1:409–411

Higenbottam T et al. (1980b) Cigarette smoke inhalation and the acute airway response. Thorax 35:246–254

Higenbottam TW et al. (1980c) Cigarette smoking in asthma. Br J Dis Chest 74:279–284

Hillerdahl G, Rylander R (1984) Asthma and cessation of smoking. Clin Allergy 14:45–47

Hjern A et al. (2001) Does tobacco smoke prevent atopic disorders? A study of two generations of Swedish residents. Clin Exp Allergy 31:908–914

Hoffmann D, Hoffmann I (1997) The changing cigarette, 1950–1995. J Toxicol Environ Health 50:307–364

Hogg JC (2001) Chronic obstructive pulmonary disease: an overview of pathology and pathogenesis. Novartis Found Symp 234:4–19

Hogg JC et al. (1968) Site and nature of airway obstruction in chronic obstructive lung disease. N Engl J Med 278:1355–1360

Hoidal JR et al. (1981) Altered oxidative metabolic responses in vitro of alveolar macrophages from asymptomatic cigarette smokers. Am Rev Respir Dis 123:85–89

Holt PG (1987) Immune and inflammatory function in cigarette smokers. Thorax 42:241–249

Hu FB et al. (1997) An epidemiological study of asthma prevalence and related factors among young adults. J Asthma 34:67–76

Huchon GJ et al. (2002) Chronic bronchitis among French adults: high prevalence and underdiagnosis. Eur Respir J 20:806–812

Ichinose M et al. (2000) Increase in reactive nitrogen species production in chronic obstructive pulmonary disease airways. Am J Respir Crit Care Med 162:701–706

Islam SS, Schottenfeld D (1994) Declining FEV1 and chronic productive cough in cigarette smokers: a 25-year prospective study of lung cancer incidence in Tecumseh, Michigan. Cancer Epidemiol Biomarkers Prev 3:289–298

Israel RH et al. (1988) Bronchial provocation tests before and after cessation of smoking. Respiration 54:247–254

James AL et al. (2005) Decline in lung function in the busselton health study: the effects of asthma and cigarette smoking. Am J Respir Crit Care Med 171:109–114

Janoff A et al. (1983) Levels of elastase activity in bronchoalveolar lavage fluids of healthy smokers and nonsmokers. Am Rev Respir Dis 127:540–544

Janoff A et al. (1987) NHLBI workshop summary. Effects of tobacco smoke components on cellular and biochemical processes in the lung. Am Rev Respir Dis 136:1058–1064

Jansen DF et al. (1999) Smoking and airway hyperresponsiveness especially in the presence of blood eosinophilia increase the risk to develop respiratory symptoms: a 25-year follow-up study in the general adult population. Am J Respir Crit Care Med 160:259–264

Janssen-Heijnen ML, Coebergh JW (2001) Trends in incidence and prognosis of the histological subtypes of lung cancer in North America, Australia, New Zealand and Europe. Lung Cancer 31:123–137

Janssen-Heijnen ML, Coebergh JW (2003) The changing epidemiology of lung cancer in Europe. Lung Cancer 41:245–258

Jeffery PK (1991) Morphology of the airway wall in asthma and in chronic obstructive pulmonary disease. Am Rev Respir Dis 143:1152–1158

Jeffery PK (1998) Structural and inflammatory changes in COPD: a comparison with asthma. Thorax 53:129–136

Jeffery PK (2001) Remodeling in asthma and chronic obstructive lung disease. Am J Respir Crit Care Med 164:S28–S38

Jensen EJ et al. (2000) Bronchial reactivity to cigarette smoke; relation to lung function, respiratory symptoms, serum-immunoglobulin E and blood eosinophil and leukocyte counts. Respir Med 94:119–127

Jensen EJ et al. (1998) Blood eosinophil and monocyte counts are related to smoking and lung function. Respir Med 92:63–69

Kang MJ et al. (2003) Lung matrix metalloproteinase-9 correlates with cigarette smoking and obstruction of airflow. J Korean Med Sci 18:821–827

Kanner RE et al. (2001) Lower respiratory illnesses promote FEV_1 decline in current smokers but not ex-smokers with mild chronic obstructive pulmonary disease. Results from the Lung Health Study. Am J Respir Crit Care Med 164:358–364

Kanner RE et al. (1999) Effects of randomized assignment to a smoking cessation intervention and changes in smoking habits on respiratory symptoms in smokers with early chronic obstructive pulmonary disease: the Lung Health Study. Am J Med 106:410–416

Kark JD, Lebiush M (1981) Smoking and epidemic influenza-like illness in female military recruits: a brief survey. Am J Public Health 71:530–532

Kark JD et al. (1982) Cigarette smoking as a risk factor for epidemic a (h1n1) influenza in young men. N Engl J Med 307:1042–1046

Kasielski M, Nowak D (2001) Long-term administration of N-acetylcysteine decreases hydrogen peroxide exhalation in subjects with chronic obstructive pulmonary disease. Respir Med 95:448–456

Katzenstein AL, Myers JL (1998) Idiopathic pulmonary fibrosis: clinical relevance of pathologic classification. Am J Respir Crit Care Med 157:1301–1315

Keatings VM et al. (1996) Differences in interleukin-8 and tumor necrosis factor-alpha in induced sputum from patients with chronic obstructive pulmonary disease or asthma. Am J Respir Crit Care Med 153:530–534

Kelley MJ, McCrory DC (2003) Prevention of lung cancer: summary of published evidence. Chest 123:S50–S59

Kennedy SM et al. (1984) Increased airway mucosal permeability of smokers. Relationship to airway reactivity. Am Rev Respir Dis 129:143–148

Kerstjens HA et al. (1993) Airways hyperresponsiveness, bronchodilator response, allergy and smoking predict improvement in FEV1 during long-term inhaled corticosteroid treatment. Dutch CNSLD Study Group. Eur Respir J 6:868–876

Kharitonov SA et al. (1995) Acute and chronic effects of cigarette smoking on exhaled nitric oxide. Am J Respir Crit Care Med 152:609–612

Khuder SA (2001) Effect of cigarette smoking on major histological types of lung cancer: a meta-analysis. Lung Cancer 31:139–148

Kim YK et al. (2002) High prevalence of current asthma and active smoking effect among the elderly. Clin Exp Allergy 32:1706–1712

Kishi K et al. (2002) The correlation of emphysema or airway obstruction with the risk of lung cancer: a matched case-controlled study. Eur Respir J 19:1093–1098

Kiviloog J et al. (1974) The prevalence of bronchial asthma and chronic bronchitis in smokers and non-smokers in a representative local Swedish population. Scand J Respir Dis 55:262–276

Kostikas K et al. (2003) Oxidative stress in expired breath condensate of patients with COPD. Chest 124:1373–1380

Koyama S et al. (1991) Bronchoalveolar lavage fluid obtained from smokers exhibits increased monocyte chemokinetic activity. J Appl Physiol 70:1208–1214

Krzyzanowski M, Lebowitz MD (1992) Changes in chronic respiratory symptoms in two populations of adults studied longitudinally over 13 years. Eur Respir J 5:12–20

Krzyzanowski M et al. (1986) Factors associated with the change in ventilatory function and the development of chronic obstructive pulmonary disease in a 13-year follow-up of the Cracow Study. Risk of chronic obstructive pulmonary disease. Am Rev Respir Dis 134:1011–1019

Krzyzanowski M et al. (1990) Relationships between pulmonary function and changes in chronic respiratory symptoms. Comparison of Tucson and Cracow longitudinal studies. Chest 98:62–70

Krzyzanowski M et al. (1993) Smoking cessation and changes in respiratory symptoms in two populations followed for 13 years. Int J Epidemiol 22:666–673

Kubo K et al. (1999) Expiratory and inspiratory chest computed tomography and pulmonary function tests in cigarette smokers. Eur Respir J 13:252–256

Kuschner WG et al. (1996) Dose-dependent cigarette smoking-related inflammatory responses in healthy adults. Eur Respir J 9:1989–1994

Laan M et al. (2004) Cigarette smoke inhibits lipopolysaccharide-induced production of inflammatory cytokines by suppressing the activation of activator protein-1 in bronchial epithelial cells. J Immunol 173:4164–4170

Lams BE et al. (2000) Subepithelial immunopathology of the large airways in smokers with and without chronic obstructive pulmonary disease. Eur Respir J 15:512–516

Lange P et al. (1989) Effects of smoking and changes in smoking habits on the decline of FEV1. Eur Respir J 2:811–816

Lange P et al. (1990a) Decline of the lung function related to the type of tobacco smoked and inhalation. Thorax 45:22–26

Lange P et al. (1990b) Phlegm production in plain cigarette smokers who changed to filter cigarettes or quit smoking. J Intern Med 228:115–120

Lange P et al. (1990c) Ventilatory function and chronic mucus hypersecretion as predictors of death from lung cancer. Am Rev Respir Dis 141:613–617

Lange P et al. (1992) Relationship of the type of tobacco and inhalation pattern to pulmonary and total mortality. Eur Respir J 5:1111–1117

Lange P et al. (1998) A 15-year follow-up study of ventilatory function in adults with asthma. N Engl J Med 339:1194–1200

Langen RC et al. (2003) ROS in the local and systemic pathogenesis of COPD. Free Radic Biol Med 35:226–235

Lapperre S et al. (2003) Bronchial T lymphocyte infiltrate is associated with smoking status in patients with COPD. Eur Respir J 22:S549

Lebowitz MD (1977) Smoking habits and changes in smoking habits as they relate to chronic conditions and respiratory symptoms. Am J Epidemiol 105:534–543

Lee KW et al. (2000) Correlation of aging and smoking with air trapping at thin-section CT of the lung in asymptomatic subjects. Radiology 214:831–836

LeSon S, Gershwin ME (1996) Risk factors for asthmatic patients requiring intubation. III. Observations in young adults. J Asthma 33:27–35
Leuenberger P et al. (1994) Passive smoking exposure in adults and chronic respiratory symptoms (SAPALDIA Study). Swiss Study on Air Pollution and Lung Diseases in Adults, SAPALDIA Team. Am J Respir Crit Care Med 150:1222–1228
Liard R et al. (1980) Smoking and chronic respiratory symptoms: prevalence in male and female smokers. Am J Public Health 70:271–273
Lim S et al. (2000) Balance of matrix metalloprotease-9 and tissue inhibitor of metalloprotease-1 from alveolar macrophages in cigarette smokers. Regulation by interleukin-10. Am J Respir Crit Care Med 162:1355–1360
Lim TK et al. (1988) Changes in bronchial responsiveness to inhaled histamine over four years in middle aged male smokers and ex-smokers. Thorax 43:599–604
Linden M et al. (1993) Airway inflammation in smokers with nonobstructive and obstructive chronic bronchitis. Am Rev Respir Dis 148:1226–1232
Lindstrom M et al. (2001) Smoking, respiratory symptoms, and diseases: a comparative study between northern Sweden and northern Finland: report from the FinEsS study. Chest 119:852–861
Lippman SM, Spitz MR (2001) Lung cancer chemoprevention: an integrated approach. J Clin Oncol 19:S74–S82
Liu BQ et al. (1998) Emerging tobacco hazards in China: 1. Retrospective proportional mortality study of one million deaths. BMJ 317:1411–1422
Lodovici M et al. (1998) Benzo[a]pyrene diol-epoxide DNA adducts and levels of polycyclic aromatic hydrocarbons in autoptic samples from human lungs. Chem Biol Interact 116:199–212
Lundback B et al. (1991) Obstructive lung disease in northern Sweden: respiratory symptoms assessed in a postal survey. Eur Respir J 4:257–266
Lundback B et al. (1993) An interview study to estimate prevalence of asthma and chronic bronchitis. The obstructive lung disease in northern Sweden study. Eur J Epidemiol 9:123–133
Lynch DA et al. (1993) Uncomplicated asthma in adults: comparison of CT appearance of the lungs in asthmatic and healthy subjects. Radiology 188:829–833
Macnee W (2000) Oxidants/antioxidants and COPD. Chest 117:S303–S317
Macnee W (2001a) Oxidants/antioxidants and chronic obstructive pulmonary disease: pathogenesis to therapy. Novartis Found Symp 234:169–185
Macnee W (2001b) Oxidative stress and lung inflammation in airways disease. Eur J Pharmacol 429:195–207
Macnee W, Rahman I (1999) Oxidants and antioxidants as therapeutic targets in chronic obstructive pulmonary disease. Am J Respir Crit Care Med 160:58–SS6
Macnee W, Selby C (1993) New perspectives on basic mechanisms in lung disease. 2. Neutrophil traffic in the lungs: role of haemodynamics, cell adhesion, and deformability. Thorax 48:79–88
Macnee W et al. (1989) The effect of cigarette smoking on neutrophil kinetics in human lungs [see comments]. N Engl J Med 321:924–928
Maestrelli P et al. (2001) Increased expression of heme oxygenase (HO)-1 in alveolar spaces and HO-2 in alveolar walls of smokers. Am J Respir Crit Care Med 164:1508–1513
Mannino DM et al. (2003a) Low lung function and incident lung cancer in the United States: data from the First National Health and Nutrition Examination Survey follow-up. Arch Intern Med 163:1475–1480
Mannino DM et al. (2003b) Obstructive and restrictive lung disease and markers of inflammation: data from the Third National Health and Nutrition Examination. Am J Med 114:758–762
Maziak W et al. (1998) Exhaled nitric oxide in chronic obstructive pulmonary disease. Am J Respir Crit Care Med 157:998–1002
Melgert BN et al. (2004) Short-term smoke exposure attenuates ovalbumin-induced airway inflammation in allergic mice. AmJ Respir Cell Mol Biol 30:880–885

Menezes AM et al. (1994) Prevalence and risk factors for chronic bronchitis in Pelotas, RS, Brazil: a population-based study. Thorax 49:1217–1221

Meyer A et al. (1995) Intravenous N-acetylcysteine and lung glutathione of patients with pulmonary fibrosis and normals. Am J Respir Crit Care Med 152:1055–1060

Meyer A et al. (1994) The effect of oral N-acetylcysteine on lung glutathione levels in idiopathic pulmonary fibrosis. Eur Respir J 7:431–436

Mikuniya T et al. (1999) Proinflammatory or regulatory cytokines released from BALF macrophages of healthy smokers. Respiration 66:419–426

Miotto D et al. (2003) Interleukin-13 and -4 expression in the central airways of smokers with chronic bronchitis. Eur Respir J 22:602–608

Mitchell I et al. (2002) Near-fatal asthma: a population-based study of risk factors. Chest 121:1407–1413

Mitsunobu F et al. (2004) Influence of long-term cigarette smoking on immunoglobulin E-mediated allergy, pulmonary function, and high-resolution computed tomography lung densitometry in elderly patients with asthma. Clin Exp Allergy 34:59–64

Mogulkoc N et al. (1999) Pulmonary Langerhans' cell histiocytosis: radiologic resolution following smoking cessation. Chest 115:1452–1455

Monto AS, Ross H (1977) Acute respiratory illness in the community: effect of family composition, smoking, and chronic symptoms. Br J Prev Soc Med 31:101–108

Monto AS, Ross HW (1978) The Tecumseh study of respiratory illness. X. Relation of acute infections to smoking, lung function and chronic symptoms. Am J Epidemiol 107:57–64

Montuschi P et al. (2000) Exhaled 8-isoprostane as an in vivo biomarker of lung oxidative stress in patients with COPD and healthy smokers. Am J Respir Crit Care Med 162:1175–1177

Montuschi P et al. (2001) Exhaled carbon monoxide and nitric oxide in COPD. Chest 120:496–501

Morrison D et al. (1998a) Neutrophil chemokines in bronchoalveolar lavage fluid and leukocyte-conditioned medium from nonsmokers and smokers. Eur Respir J 12:1067–1072

Morrison D et al. (1998b) Neutrophil chemokines in bronchoalveolar lavage fluid and leukocyte-conditioned medium from nonsmokers and smokers. Eur Respir J 12:1067–1072

Morrison D et al. (1999) Epithelial permeability, inflammation, and oxidant stress in the air spaces of smokers. Am J Respir Crit Care Med 159:473–479

Mueller R et al. (1996) Different cytokine patterns in bronchial biopsies in asthma and chronic bronchitis. Respir Med 90:79–85

Mullen JB et al. (1985) Reassessment of inflammation of airways in chronic bronchitis. Br Med J (Clin Res Ed) 291:1235–1239

Mullen JB et al. (1987) Structure of central airways in current smokers and ex-smokers with and without mucus hypersecretion: relationship to lung function. Thorax 42:843–848

Murray CJ, Lopez AD (1996) Evidence based health policy—lessons from the Global Burden of Disease Study. Science 274:740–743

Murray RP et al. (1998) Effects of multiple attempts to quit smoking and relapses to smoking on pulmonary function. Lung Health Study Research Group. J Clin Epidemiol 51:1317–1326

Myers JL et al. (1987) Respiratory bronchiolitis causing interstitial lung disease. A clinicopathologic study of six cases. Am Rev Respir Dis 135:880–884

Nakashima H et al. (1987) Receptor-mediated O_2-release by alveolar macrophages and peripheral blood monocytes from smokers and nonsmokers. Priming and triggering effects of monomeric IgG, concanavalin A, N-formyl-methionyl-leucyl-phenylalanine, phorbol myristate acetate, and cytochalasin D. Am Rev Respir Dis 136:310–315

National Center for Health Statistics (1995) Current estimates from the National Health Interview Survey, United States

Nazir J et al. (2002) Artificial neural network prediction of aerosol deposition in human lungs. Pharm Res 19:1130–1136

Niewoehner DE et al. (1974) Pathologic changes in the peripheral airways of young cigarette smokers. N Engl J Med 291:755–758
Nomura A et al. (1991) Prospective study of pulmonary function and lung cancer. Am Rev Respir Dis 144:307–311
Nowak D et al. (1999) Increased content of thiobarbituric acid-reactive substances and hydrogen peroxide in the expired breath condensate of patients with stable chronic obstructive pulmonary disease: no significant effect of cigarette smoking. Respir Med 93:389–396
Nowak D et al. (1998) Cigarette smoking does not increase hydrogen peroxide levels in expired breath condensate of patients with stable COPD. Monaldi Arch Chest Dis 53:268–273
Nuorti JP et al. (2000) Cigarette smoking and invasive pneumococcal disease. Active Bacterial Core Surveillance Team. N Engl J Med 342:681–689
O'Donnell RA et al. (2004) Expression of ErbB receptors and mucins in the airways of long term current smokers. Thorax 59:1032–1040
Ohta Y et al. (1985) An electron spin resonance study of free radicals in black dust deposited in human lungs. Arch Environ Health 40:279–282
Omenaas E et al. (1996) Serum respiratory virus antibodies: predictor of reduced one-second forced expiratory volume (FEV1) in Norwegian adults. Int J Epidemiol 25:134–141
Oosterhoff Y et al. (1993) Airway responsiveness to adenosine 5'-monophosphate in chronic obstructive pulmonary disease is determined by smoking. Am Rev Respir Dis 147:553–558
Palmisano WA et al. (2000) Predicting lung cancer by detecting aberrant promoter methylation in sputum. Cancer Res 60:5954–5958
Paoletti P et al. (1995) Distribution of bronchial responsiveness in a general population: effect of sex, age, smoking, and level of pulmonary function. Am J Respir Crit Care Med 151:1770–1777
Papi A et al. (2004) COPD increases the risk of squamous histological subtype in smokers who develop non-small cell lung carcinoma. Thorax 59:679–681
Paredi P et al. (2000a) Exhaled ethane, a marker of lipid peroxidation, is elevated in chronic obstructive pulmonary disease. Am J Respir Crit Care Med 162:369–373
Paredi P et al. (2000b) Exhaled ethane, a marker of lipid peroxidation, is elevated in chronic obstructive pulmonary disease. Am J Respir Crit Care Med 162:369–373
Patiar S et al. (2002) Smoking causes a dose-dependent increase in granulocyte-bound L-selectin. Thromb Res 106:1–6
Pedersen B et al. (1996) Eosinophil and neutrophil activity in asthma in a one-year trial with inhaled budesonide. The impact of smoking. Am J Respir Crit Care Med 153:1519–1529
Pelkonen M et al. (2001) Smoking cessation, decline in pulmonary function and total mortality: a 30-year follow up study among the Finnish cohorts of the Seven Countries Study. Thorax 56:703–707
Persson MG et al. (1994) Single-breath nitric oxide measurements in asthmatic patients and smokers. Lancet 343:146–147
Pesci A et al. (1994) Mast cells in the airway lumen and bronchial mucosa of patients with chronic bronchitis. Am J Respir Crit Care Med 149:1311–1316
Peterson DI et al. (1968) Smoking and pulmonary function. Arch Environ Health 16:215–218
Petitti DB, Friedman GD (1985) Respiratory morbidity in smokers of low- and high-yield cigarettes. Prev Med 14:217–225
Phillips DH et al. (1988) Correlation of DNA adduct levels in human lung with cigarette smoking. Nature 336:790–792
Piatti G et al. (1997) Bacterial adherence in smokers and non-smokers. Pharmacol Res 36:481–484
Piipari R et al. (2004) Smoking and asthma in adults. Eur Respir J 24:734–739
Pilotto LS et al. (1999) Industry, air quality, cigarette smoke and rates of respiratory illness in Port Adelaide. Aust N Z J Public Health 23:657–660
Plaschke PP et al. (2000) Onset and remission of allergic rhinitis and asthma and the relationship with atopic sensitization and smoking. Am J Respir Crit Care Med 162:920–924

Poole PJ, Black PN (2001) Oral mucolytic drugs for exacerbations of chronic obstructive pulmonary disease: systematic review. BMJ 322:1271–1274

Postma DS, Sluiter HJ (1989) Prognosis of chronic obstructive pulmonary disease: the Dutch experience. Am Rev Respir Dis 140:S100–S105

Postma DS et al. (1986) Independent influence of reversibility of air-flow obstruction and nonspecific hyperreactivity on the long-term course of lung function in chronic air-flow obstruction. Am Rev Respir Dis 134:276–280

Postma DS et al. (1988) Association between nonspecific bronchial hyperreactivity and superoxide anion production by polymorphonuclear leukocytes in chronic air-flow obstruction. Am Rev Respir Dis 137:57–61

Pratico D et al. (1998) Chronic obstructive pulmonary disease is associated with an increase in urinary levels of isoprostane F_2alpha-III, an index of oxidant stress. Am J Respir Crit Care Med 158:1709–1714

Prescott E et al. (1997) Effect of gender on hospital admissions for asthma and prevalence of self-reported asthma: a prospective study based on a sample of the general population. Copenhagen City Heart Study Group. Thorax 52:287–289

Pride NB (2001) Smoking cessation: effects on symptoms, spirometry and future trends in COPD. Thorax 56:SII7–SII10

Pryor WA, Stone K (1993) Oxidants in cigarette smoke. Radicals, hydrogen peroxide, peroxynitrate, and peroxynitrite. Ann N Y Acad Sci 686:12–27

Qvarfordt I et al. (2000) Lower airway bacterial colonization in asymptomatic smokers and smokers with chronic bronchitis and recurrent exacerbations. Respir Med 94:881–887

Rahman I, Macnee W (1996) Oxidant/antioxidant imbalance in smokers and chronic obstructive pulmonary disease [editorial]. Thorax 51:348–350

Rahman I et al. (1997) Attenuation of oxidant/antioxidant imbalance during treatment of exacerbations of chronic obstructive pulmonary disease. Thorax 52:565–568

Rahman I et al. (2000) Localization of gamma-glutamylcysteine synthetase messenger rna expression in lungs of smokers and patients with chronic obstructive pulmonary disease. Free Radic Biol Med 28:920–925

Rahman I et al. (2002) 4-Hydroxy-2-nonenal, a specific lipid peroxidation product, is elevated in lungs of patients with chronic obstructive pulmonary disease. Am J Respir Crit Care Med 166:490–495

Rasmussen F et al. (2000) Impact of airway lability, atopy, and tobacco smoking on the development of asthma-like symptoms in asymptomatic teenagers. Chest 117:1330–1335

Repine JE et al. (1997) Oxidative stress in chronic obstructive pulmonary disease. Oxidative Stress Study Group. Am J Respir Crit Care Med 156:341–357

Rijcken B et al. (1987a) The association of airways responsiveness to respiratory symptom prevalence and to pulmonary function in a random population sample. Bull Eur Physiopathol Respir 23:391–394

Rijcken B et al. (1987b) The relationship of nonspecific bronchial responsiveness to respiratory symptoms in a random population sample. Am Rev Respir Dis 136:62–68

Rimpela A, Teperi J (1989) Respiratory symptoms and low tar cigarette smoking—a longitudinal study on young people. Scand J Soc Med 17:151–156

Rusznak C et al. (2001) Cigarette smoke decreases the expression of secretory component in human bronchial epithelial cells, in vitro. Acta Microbiol Immunol Hung 48:81–94

Rutgers SR et al. (1998) Nitric oxide measured with single-breath and tidal-breathing methods in asthma and COPD. Eur Respir J 12:816–819

Rutgers SR et al. (1999) Markers of nitric oxide metabolism in sputum and exhaled air are not increased in chronic obstructive pulmonary disease [see comments]. Thorax 54:576–580

Ryan G et al. (1991) Risk factors for death in patients admitted to hospital with asthma: a follow-up study. Aust N Z J Med 21:681–685

Ryu JH et al. (2001) Smoking-related interstitial lung diseases: a concise review. Eur Respir J 17:122–132
Saetta M et al. (1985) Loss of alveolar attachments in smokers. A morphometric correlate of lung function impairment. Am Rev Respir Dis 132:894–900
Saetta M et al. (1999) CD8+ve cells in the lungs of smokers with chronic obstructive pulmonary disease. Am J Respir Crit Care Med 160:711–717
Saetta M et al. (2000) Goblet cell hyperplasia and epithelial inflammation in peripheral airways of smokers with both symptoms of chronic bronchitis and chronic airflow limitation. Am J Respir Crit Care Med 161:1016–1021
Saetta M et al. (1997) Inflammatory cells in the bronchial glands of smokers with chronic bronchitis. Am J Respir Crit Care Med 156:1633–1639
Saetta M et al. (2001) Cellular and structural bases of chronic obstructive pulmonary disease. Am J Respir Crit Care Med 163:1304–1309
Samet JM, Lange P (1996) Longitudinal studies of active and passive smoking. Am J Respir Crit Care Med 154:S257–S265
Scanlon PD et al. (2000) Smoking cessation and lung function in mild-to-moderate chronic obstructive pulmonary disease. The Lung Health Study. Am J Respir Crit Care Med 161:381–390
Schaberg T et al. (1992a) Superoxide anion release induced by platelet-activating factor is increased in human alveolar macrophages from smokers. Eur Respir J 5:387–393
Schaberg T et al. (1992b) Increased number of alveolar macrophages expressing adhesion molecules of the leukocyte adhesion molecule family in smoking subjects. Association with cell-binding ability and superoxide anion production [see comments]. Am Rev Respir Dis 146:1287–1293
Schenker MB et al. (1982) Effect of cigarette tar content and smoking habits on respiratory symptoms in women. Am Rev Respir Dis 125:684–690
Schilling J et al. (1994) Reduced endogenous nitric oxide in the exhaled air of smokers and hypertensives. Eur Respir J 7:467–471
Seagrave J (2000) Oxidative mechanisms in tobacco smoke-induced emphysema. J Toxicol Environ Health A 61:69–78
Selvaggi G et al. (2002) HER-2/neu overexpression in patients with radically resected nonsmall cell lung carcinoma. Impact on long-term survival. Cancer 94:2669–2674
Senthilselvan A et al. (1993) Predictors of asthma and wheezing in adults. Grain farming, sex, and smoking. Am Rev Respir Dis 148:667–670
Seto H et al. (1993) Determination of polycyclic aromatic hydrocarbons in the lung. Arch Environ Contam Toxicol 24:498–503
Sherman CB (1992) The health consequences of cigarette smoking. Pulmonary diseases. Med Clin North Am 76:355–375
Sherman CB et al. (1992) Longitudinal lung function decline in subjects with respiratory symptoms. Am Rev Respir Dis 146:855–859
Sherrill DL et al. (1991) Smoking and symptom effects on the curves of lung function growth and decline. Am Rev Respir Dis 144:17–22
Sherrill DL et al. (1993) Longitudinal methods for describing the relationship between pulmonary function, respiratory symptoms and smoking in elderly subjects: the Tucson Study [see comments]. Eur Respir J 6:342–348
Silverman EK et al. (2000) Gender-related differences in severe, early-onset chronic obstructive pulmonary disease. Am J Respir Crit Care Med 162:2152–2158
Sippel JM et al. (1999) Associations of smoking with hospital-based care and quality of life in patients with obstructive airway disease. Chest 115:691–696
Siroux V et al. (2000) Relationships of active smoking to asthma and asthma severity in the EGEA study. Epidemiological study on the Genetics and Environment of Asthma. Eur Respir J 15:470–477
Skillrud DM et al. (1986) Higher risk of lung cancer in chronic obstructive pulmonary disease. A prospective, matched, controlled study. Ann Intern Med 105:503–507

Sobonya RE, Kleinerman J (1972) Morphometric studies of bronchi in young smokers. Am Rev Respir Dis 105:768–775

Sobue T et al. (1993) Lung cancer incidence rate for male ex-smokers according to age at cessation of smoking. Jpn J Cancer Res 84:601–607

Soler N et al. (1999) Airway inflammation and bronchial microbial patterns in patients with stable chronic obstructive pulmonary disease. Eur Respir J 14:1015–1022

Soria JC et al. (2002) Aberrant promoter methylation of multiple genes in bronchial brush samples from former cigarette smokers. Cancer Res. 62:351–355

Soriano JB et al. (2000) Recent trends in physician diagnosed COPD in women and men in the UK. Thorax 55:789–794

Soyseth V et al. (1995) Postnatal maternal smoking increases the prevalence of asthma but not of bronchial hyperresponsiveness or atopy in their children. Chest 107:389–394

Sparrow D et al. (1987) The relationship of nonspecific bronchial responsiveness to the occurrence of respiratory symptoms and decreased levels of pulmonary function. The Normative Aging Study. Am Rev Respir Dis 135:1255–1260

Spurzem JR et al. (1991) Chronic inflammation is associated with an increased proportion of goblet cells recovered by bronchial lavage. Chest 100:389–393

Stey C et al. (2000) The effect of oral N-acetylcysteine in chronic bronchitis: a quantitative systematic review. Eur Respir J 16:253–262

Straus WL et al. (1996) Risk factors for domestic acquisition of legionnaires disease. Ohio legionnaires Disease Group. Arch Intern Med 156:1685–1692

Sun G et al. (1998) Cellular and molecular characteristics of inflammation in chronic bronchitis. Eur J Clin Invest 28:364–372

Sunyer J et al. (1997) Smoking and bronchial responsiveness in nonatopic and atopic young adults. Spanish Group of the European Study of Asthma. Thorax 52:235–238

Tager IB et al. (1988) The natural history of forced expiratory volumes. Effect of cigarette smoking and respiratory symptoms. Am Rev Respir Dis 138:837–849

Tashkin DP et al. (1992) The lung health study: airway responsiveness to inhaled methacholine in smokers with mild to moderate airflow limitation. The Lung Health Study Research Group. Am Rev Respir Dis 145:301–310

Tashkin DP et al. (1984) The UCLA population studies of chronic obstructive respiratory disease. VIII. Effects of smoking cessation on lung function: a prospective study of a free-living population. Am Rev Respir Dis 130:707–715

Tattersall AB et al. (1983) Acetylcysteine (Fabrol) in chronic bronchitis—a study in general practice. J Int Med Res 11:279–284

Taylor RG et al. (1985a) Smoking, allergy, and the differential white blood cell count. Thorax 40:17–22

Taylor RG et al. (1985b) Bronchial reactivity to inhaled histamine and annual rate of decline in FEV_1 in male smokers and ex-smokers. Thorax 40:9–16

Thompson AB et al. (1991) Lower respiratory tract iron burden is increased in association with cigarette smoking. J Lab Clin Med 117:493–499

Thomson NC, Spears M (2005) The influence of smoking on the treatment response in patients with asthma. Curr Opin Allergy Clin Immunol 5:57–63

Thomson NC et al. (2004) Asthma and cigarette smoking. Eur Respir J 24:822–833

Tockman MS et al. (1987) Airways obstruction and the risk for lung cancer. Ann Intern Med 106:512–518

Toren K, Hermansson BA (1999) Incidence rate of adult-onset asthma in relation to age, sex, atopy and smoking: a Swedish population-based study of 15813 adults. Int J Tuberc Lung Dis 3:192–197

Townsend MC et al. (1991) Pulmonary function in relation to cigarette smoking and smoking cessation. MRFIT Research Group. Prev Med 20:621–637

Travis WD et al. (1993) Pulmonary Langerhans cell granulomatosis (histiocytosis X). A clinicopathologic study of 48 cases. Am J Surg Pathol 17:971–986
Trevisani L et al. (1992) Structural characterization of the bronchial epithelium of subjects with chronic bronchitis and in asymptomatic smokers. Respiration 59:136–144
Troisi RJ et al. (1995) Cigarette smoking and incidence of chronic bronchitis and asthma in women. Chest 108:1557–1561
Turato G et al. (1995) Effect of smoking cessation on airway inflammation in chronic bronchitis. Am J Respir Crit Care Med 152:1262–1267
Turato G et al. (2002) Airway inflammation in severe chronic obstructive pulmonary disease: relationship with lung function and radiologic emphysema. Am J Respir Crit Care Med 166:105–110
US Department of Health and Human Services (1988) US Department of Health and Human Services, Rockville, pp 156–157
US Department of Health and human Services (2004) The health consequences of smoking: a report of the Surgeon General. In: Department of Health and Human Services, National Center for Chronic Disease Prevention and Health Promotion, Office on Smoking and Health (eds) The health consequences of smoking; a report of the Surgeon General. Atlanta, pp 421–524
van Zandwijk N et al. (2000) EUROSCAN, a randomized trial of vitamin A and N-acetylcysteine in patients with head and neck cancer or lung cancer. For the European Organization for Research and Treatment of Cancer Head and Neck and Lung Cancer Cooperative Groups. J Natl Cancer Inst 92:977–986
Verbanck S et al. (2004) Noninvasive assessment of airway alterations in smokers: the small airways revisited. Am J Respir Crit Care Med 170:414–419
Verleden GM et al. (1999) The effect of cigarette smoking on exhaled nitric oxide in mild steroid-naive asthmatics. Chest 116:59–64
Vesterinen E et al. (1988) Prospective study of asthma in relation to smoking habits among 14,729 adults. Thorax 43:534–539
Viegi G et al. (1988) Prevalence of respiratory symptoms in an unpolluted area of northern Italy. Eur Respir J 1:311–318
Vignola AM et al. (1998) Sputum metalloproteinase-9/tissue inhibitor of metalloproteinase-1 ratio correlates with airflow obstruction in asthma and chronic bronchitis. Am J Respir Crit Care Med 158:1945–1950
Vollmer WM et al. (1989) Respiratory symptoms, lung function, and mortality in a screening center cohort. Am J Epidemiol 129:1157–1169
Von Essen S et al. (1990) Complete resolution of roentgenographic changes in a patient with pulmonary histiocytosis X. Chest 98:765–767
von Hertzen L et al. (1998a) Humoral immune response to *Chlamydia pneumoniae* in twin discordant for smoking. J Intern Med 244:227–234
von Hertzen L et al. (1998b) Immune responses to *Chlamydia pneumoniae* in twins in relation to gender and smoking. J Med Microbiol 47:441–446
von Hertzen L et al. (2000a) Airway obstruction in relation to symptoms in chronic respiratory disease—a nationally representative population study. Respir Med 94:356–363
Wallace WA et al. (1992) Intra-alveolar macrophage numbers in current smokers and non-smokers: a morphometric study of tissue sections. Thorax 47:437–440
Walraven GE et al. (2001) Asthma, smoking and chronic cough in rural and urban adult communities in The Gambia. Clin Exp Allergy 31:1679–1685
Wang TN et al. (1999) Association between indoor and outdoor air pollution and adolescent asthma from 1995 to 1996 in Taiwan. Environ Res 81:239–247
Weitzman M et al. (1990) Maternal smoking and childhood asthma. Pediatrics 85:505–511
Wilhelmsen L (1967) Effects on bronchopulmonary symptoms, ventilation, and lung mechanics of abstinence from tobacco smoking. Scand J Respir Dis 48:407–414

Willemse BW et al. (2004a) The impact of smoking cessation on respiratory symptoms, lung function, airway hyperresponsiveness and inflammation. Eur Respir J 23:464–476

Willemse BW et al. (2004b) Smoking cessation improves both direct and indirect airway hyperresponsiveness in COPD. Eur Respir J 24:391–396

Wise RA et al. (2003) The Effect of smoking intervention and an inhaled bronchodilator on airways reactivity in COPD: the Lung Health Study. Chest 124:449–458

Withey CH et al. (1992a) Respiratory effects of lowering tar and nicotine levels of cigarettes smoked by young male middle tar smokers. I. Design of a randomised controlled trial. J Epidemiol Community Health 46:274–280

Withey CH et al. (1992b) Respiratory effects of lowering tar and nicotine levels of cigarettes smoked by young male middle tar smokers. II. Results of a randomised controlled trial. J Epidemiol Community Health 46:281–285

Wright JL et al. (1988) Airway inflammation and peribronchiolar attachments in the lungs of nonsmokers, current and ex-smokers. Lung 166:277–286

Wright JL et al. (1983) Morphology of peripheral airways in current smokers and ex-smokers. Am Rev Respir Dis 127:474–477

Wynder EL, Muscat JE (1995) The changing epidemiology of smoking and lung cancer histology. Environ Health Perspect 103:S143–S148

Xu X et al. (1992) Effects of cigarette smoking on rate of loss of pulmonary function in adults: a longitudinal assessment. Am Rev Respir Dis 146:1345–1348

Xu X et al. (1997) Airways responsiveness and development and remission of chronic respiratory symptoms in adults. Lancet 350:1431–1434

Xu X et al. (1994) Smoking, changes in smoking habits, and rate of decline in FEV1: new insight into gender differences. Eur Respir J 7:1056–1061

Yamaguchi E et al. (1989) Interleukin 1 production by alveolar macrophages is decreased in smokers. Am Rev Respir Dis 140:397–402

Yamamoto C et al. (1997) Airway inflammation in COPD assessed by sputum levels of interleukin-8. Chest 112:505–510

Yan K et al. (1985) Prevalence and nature of bronchial hyperresponsiveness in subjects with chronic obstructive pulmonary disease. Am Rev Respir Dis 132:25–29

Zacny JP et al. (1987) Human cigarette smoking: effects of puff and inhalation parameters on smoke exposure. J Pharmacol Exp Ther 240:554–564

Zhang X et al. (2003) Regulation of eosinophil apoptosis by nitric oxide: Role of c-Jun-N-terminal kinase and signal transducer and activator of transcription 5. J Allergy Clin Immunol 112:93–101

Zhu J et al. (2001) Interleukin-4 and interleukin-5 gene expression and inflammation in the mucus-secreting glands and subepithelial tissue of smokers with chronic bronchitis. Lack of relationship with CD8$^+$ cells. Am J Respir Crit Care Med 164:2220–2228

Chapter 13

Smoking and Oxidative Stress: Vascular Damage

Thomas Münzel, Felix Post, and Ascan Warnholtz

Contents

13.1	Introduction	340
13.2	Active and Passive Smoking and the Epidemiology of Cardiovascular Disease	340
13.3	Endothelium and Vascular Tone	341
13.4	ROS and Endothelial Dysfunction	341
13.4.1	Endothelial Dysfunction and Cardiovascular Risk Factors	342
13.4.2	Endothelial Dysfunction and Prognosis	342
13.5	Constituents of Cigarette Smoke and Oxidative Stress	343
13.6	Smoking and Oxidative Stress Parameters	343
13.7	Active Smoking and Endothelial Dysfunction	344
13.8	Passive Smoking and Endothelial Dysfunction	345
13.9	Evidence for Direct Toxic Effects of Smoke-Derived Free Radicals	345
13.10	Smoking-Related Activation of Superoxide-Producing Enzymes	346
13.10.1	eNOS	346
13.10.2	NAD(P)H Oxidase	350
13.10.3	Xanthine Oxidase	350
13.11	Smoking and Inflammation	351
13.12	Smoking and Lipid Profile	351
13.13	Smoking and Thrombosis	352
13.14	Effects of Smoking on Antioxidant Levels	352
13.15	Cessation of Smoking and Oxidative Stress	352
13.16	Treatment of Smoking-Induced Endothelial Dysfunction	353

Contents

13.16.1	Vitamin C	353
13.16.2	Vitamin E	353
13.16.3	Folic Acid and Tetrahydrobiopterin	354
13.16.4	Angiotensin-Converting Enzyme Inhibitor	354
13.16.5	Statins	355
13.16.6	Nebivolol	355
13.17	Summary	355
13.18	Conclusions	356
	References	357

13.1 Introduction

Chronic smoking is one of the important risk factors for the development of atherosclerosis. Although the precise mechanisms underlying smoking-induced atherosclerosis remain unclear, it became evident that oxidants delivered by the tar and by the gas phase become deposited in the lung but are also delivered directly to the plasma and the vasculature, thereby activating superoxide producing enzymes within the vascular wall (Heitzer et al. 2000). In addition, there is a marked activation of neutrophils, monocytes, platelets and T cells, all of which will significantly enhance the damage to the vasculature. Endothelial dysfunction, which has been demonstrated to be present in active but also passive smokers, is markedly improved by the antioxidant vitamin C, pointing to a crucial role of reactive oxygen species (ROS) in mediating this phenomenon (Heitzer et al. 1996). Because oxidative stress has been shown to be associated with an increased cardiovascular event rate including death, myocardial infarction, stroke and coronary revascularization procedures, the therapeutic strategy should include treatment forms, which effectively reduce ROS-induced damage to the vascular wall (Heitzer et al. 2001). This chapter reviews experimental and clinical studies addressing the mechanisms underlying smoking-induced vascular damage, with a special focus on oxidative stress.

13.2 Active and Passive Smoking and the Epidemiology of Cardiovascular Disease

Smoking has been shown to cause about 140,000 deaths per year from cardiovascular disease in the United States (for detailed review, see Burns 2003). Smoking as a cardiovascular risk factor exponentially enhances the detrimental effects of other risk factor such as diabetes, hypertension, and hypercholesterolemia. Importantly, in other countries than the United States, where the blood pressure is less well controlled, numbers concerning the cardiovascular risk in smokers may be substantially higher. It has been shown that smoking increases the risk of cardiovascular events during surgery performed for noncardiac reasons, and it also increases ischemic episodes after coronary bypass surgery. In addition, smoking increases the risk of reocclusion after myocardial infarction. Nonsmokers exposed to environmental smoke are at 25–30% increased risk for cardiovascular morbidity and mortality, and over 35,000 deaths per year have been attributed to ischemic heart disease caused by second-hand smoke (Law and Wald 2003).

Endothelial dysfunction represents one of the early stages of atherosclerosis. In the next paragraphs, we focus on the mechanisms by which the endothelium regulates vascular tone and which mechanisms lead to increased oxidative stress within vascular tissue, thereby leading to endothelial dysfunction.

13.3 Endothelium and Vascular Tone

The endothelium, a single-layered continuous cell sheet lining the luminal vessel wall separates the intravascular (blood) from the interstitial compartment and the vascular smooth muscle. Based on cell count (6×10^{13}), mass (1.5 kg), and surface area (1,000 m^2) the endothelium is an autonomous organ. Though for long time regarded as a passive barrier for blood cells and macrosolutes, this view completely changed with the discovery of endothelial autacoids like prostacyclin (PGI$_2$) (Moncada et al. 1978) and nitric oxide, NO· (Palmer et al. 1987), as well as with the discovery of integrins and other surface signals (Stupack and Cheresh 2004). It is now evident that the endothelium is not only at the crossbridges of communication between blood and tissue cells, but actively controls this process and the function of surrounding cells by a plethora of signaling routes. One of the prominent communication lines is established by the so-called L-arginine-NO·-cyclic GMP pathway (Busse and Fleming 1998). This signaling cascade starts with endothelial NO· synthase (eNOS, NOSIII), which generates NO· and L-citrulline from L-arginine and O$_2$ in response to receptor-dependent agonists (bradykinin, acetylcholine, ATP) and physicochemical stimuli (shear, stretch) (Fleming and Busse 2003). Reducing equivalents are provided by NADPH, and electrons are passed via a flavin chain to the catalytic center, the enzyme's heme iron. The first step of the normal NOS reaction is a classical monooxygenation, which consumes 1 mol of NADPH and O$_2$. Molecular oxygen bound to the iron is activated and split to accomplish a hydroxylation of the substrate, the guanidino-nitrogen of L-arginine, forming N^G-hydroxy-L-arginine. The second step is an atypical monooxygenation, which consumes 1 mol O$_2$ and 0.5 mol NADPH. It is a three-electron oxidation of N^G-hydroxy-L-arginine to afford the final products NO· and L-citrulline. In order to guarantee this reaction path, the enzyme has to be homodimeric and the cofactor tetrahydrobiopterin must be present. For details, the reader is referred to excellent reviews on this topic (Alderton et al. 2001; Ghosh and Salerno 2003).

13.4 ROS and Endothelial Dysfunction

The endothelium-derived relaxing factor, previously identified as nitric oxide (NO·) (Palmer et al. 1987) or a closely related compound (Myers et al. 1990), has potent antiatherosclerotic properties. NO· released from endothelial cells works in concert with prostacyclin to inhibit platelet aggregation (Radomski et al. 1987), it inhibits the attachment of neutrophils to endothelial cells and the expression of adhesion molecules. NO· in high concentrations inhibits the proliferation of smooth muscle cells (Garg and Hassid 1989). Therefore, under all conditions, where an absolute or relative NO· deficit is encountered, the process of atherosclerosis is being initiated or accelerated. The half-life of NO· and therefore its biological activity is decisively determined by oxygen-derived free radicals such as superoxide (Gryglewski et al 1986). Superoxide rapidly reacts with NO· to form the highly reactive intermediate peroxynitrite (ONOO⁻) (Beckman 1996). The rapid bimolecular reaction between NO· and superoxide yielding peroxynitrite (rate constant: $5–10 \times 10^9 \ M^{-1}s^{-1}$) is about three to four times faster than the dismutation of superoxide by the superoxide dismutase. Therefore, peroxynitrite formation represents a major potential pathway of NO· reactivity pending on the rates of tissue superoxide production. Peroxynitrite in high concentrations is cytotoxic and may cause oxidative damage to proteins, lipids, and DNA (Beckman 1996). Recent studies also indicate that peroxynitrite may have deleterious effects on activity and function of the prostacyclin synthase (Zou and Ullrich 1996) and the endothelial NOS (Zou et al. 2002). Other ROS such as the dismutation product of superoxide, hydrogen peroxide, and the hypochlorous acid released by activated neutrophils, are not free radicals, but have a powerful oxidizing capacity, which will further contribute to oxidative stress within vascular tissue. In addition, myeloperoxidase (MPO) secreted by neutrophils has been demonstrated to be a potent producer of HOCl and to have NO· consuming activity (Baldus et al. 2001, 2002, 2003).

13.4.1 Endothelial Dysfunction and Cardiovascular Risk Factors

It is well known that in the presence of cardiovascular risk factors endothelial dysfunction is frequently encountered. This has been shown for chronic smokers (Heitzer et al. 1996), patients with increased low-density lipoprotein (LDL) levels (Vita et al. 1990), patients with type I diabetes (Johnstone et al. 1993) and type 2 diabetes (Nitenberg et al. 1993), for hypertensive patients (Treasure et al. 1993), and for patients with metabolic syndrome (Deedwania 2003). There are several potential abnormalities that could account for reductions in endothelium-dependent vascular relaxation including changes in the activity and/or expression of the endothelial NOS, decreased sensitivity of vascular smooth muscle cells to NO·, or increased degradation of NO· via its interaction with ROS such as superoxide. The NO·-degradation concept is the most attractive one because in the presence of cardiovascular risk factors endothelial dysfunction is established and even more importantly, it is markedly improved by the acute administration of the antioxidant vitamin C (Duffy et al. 2001; Heitzer et al. 1996; Levine et al. 1996; Ting et al. 1996). Superoxide and/or peroxynitrite have/has also been shown to act further downstream by oxidative inactivation of soluble guanylyl cyclase (sGC) as well as activation of cGMP/cGMP-dependent protein kinase (cGK-I) (for review see Munzel et al. 2003).

13.4.2 Endothelial Dysfunction and Prognosis

Recent studies have demonstrated that endothelial dysfunction of the coronary as well as peripheral arteries has prognostic implications. This has been shown for patients with coronary artery disease (Heitzer et al. 2001; Schachinger et al. 2000), arterial hypertension (Perticone et al. 2001), peripheral vascular disease (Gokce et al. 2002, 2003), and chronic congestive heart failure (Fischer et al. 2005). Importantly, Heitzer et al. (2001) have shown that the degree of oxidative stress within vascular tissue assessed by acute vitamin C challenges is an independent predictor of future vascular events such as death because of myocardial infarction, stroke, and coronary revascularization.

13.5 Constituents of Cigarette Smoke and Oxidative Stress

In general, cigarette smoke can be divided into two phases (Ambrose and Barua 2004). The tar or particulate phase is defined as material that is trapped when the smoke stream is passed through the Cambridge glass-fiber filter that retains 99.9% of all particulate material with a size >0.1μm. The gas phase is therefore the material that passes the filter. The tar phase of cigarette smoke contains 10^{17} radicals per gram, and the gas phase contains >10^{15} free radicals per puff (Smith and Fischer 2001). The radicals associated with the tar phase are long lived (hours to months), whereas the radicals associated with the gas phase have a shorter life span (seconds) (Ambrose and Barua 2004).

Cigarette smoke that is drawn through the tobacco into an active smoker's mouth is known as mainstream smoke. Sidestream smoke is the smoke emitted from the burning end of a cigarette. Mainstream smoke is composed of 8% tar and 92% gaseous phase (Ambrose and Barua 2004). Environmental tobacco smoke results from the combination of sidestream smoke (85%) from smokers and a small fraction of exhaled mainstream smoke (15%) from smokers. Sidestream smoke contains a relatively higher concentration of the toxic gaseous component than mainstream cigarette smoke.

Of all the known constituents, nicotine is the addictive substance of cigarette smoke (Powell 1998).

13.6 Smoking and Oxidative Stress Parameters

The radicals in the gas and tar phase will not only produce oxidative stress when deposited in the lung, but will also cause oxidative damage to the vasculature remote from the lung. There are several possibilities to quantify smoking induced oxidative stress. Spin trapping as well as chemiluminescence techniques have been used (Munzel et al. 2002). In addition, fingerprinting methods that largely detect oxidatively modified biomolecules, such as lipid peroxides, have been used to detect oxidative stress in living organisms. Markers for lipid peroxidation include malondialdehyde and the gold standard for detection of oxidative stress such as isoprostanes (Meagher and Fitzgerald 2000). Isoprostane levels in blood and urine can be increased in a dose-dependent fashion, and they decrease immediately during quitting of smoking, although complete normalization of isoprostane levels may require almost 1 year (Morrow et al. 1995). Markers of protein oxidation include assays for nitrotyrosine, which can be used as a footprint for increased peroxynitrite formation (Beckman 1996).

Measurements of antioxidant capacity can also be performed. The total peroxyl trapping antioxidant parameter is the most popular one to detect if there is a depletion of antioxidants because of increased oxidative stress (Ghiselli et al. 1995).

13.7 Active Smoking and Endothelial Dysfunction

Endothelial dysfunction represents the first detectable manifestation of atherosclerotic disease. Direct evidence that smoking could result in endothelial injury was provided by morphological observations on the umbilical arteries from smoking mothers. Animals exposed to cigarette smoke have been shown to have marked morphological alterations that were accompanied by reductions in prostacyclin production (Pittilo et al. 1982). Later, endothelial dysfunction has been demonstrated for large coronary arteries in response to intracoronary acetylcholine and flow dependent dilation (Nitenberg et al. 1993; Zeiher et al. 1995) and peripheral conductance (Celermajer et al. 1993) and resistance vessels (Heitzer et al. 1996). Importantly, in patients with angiographically normal coronary arteries, intracoronary infusion of acetylcholine has been shown to cause potent coronary artery constriction, compatible with severe endothelial dysfunction (Nitenberg et al. 1993). Previously, we could demonstrate that risk factors such as smoking or hypercholesterolemia reduced endothelium-dependent vasodilation to a similar degree. When both risk factors were present, however, endothelium dependent dilation was strikingly reduced (Fig. 13.1a; Heitzer et al. 1996). α-Receptor blockade was not able to improve endothelium-dependent vasodilation, indicating that increased sympathetic tone did not contribute to this phenomenon (Heitzer et al. 1996). In contrast, acute treatment with vitamin C was able to improve endothelial function in peripheral conductance (Raitakari et al. 2000) and resistance vessels (Fig. 13.1b; Heitzer et al. 1996)

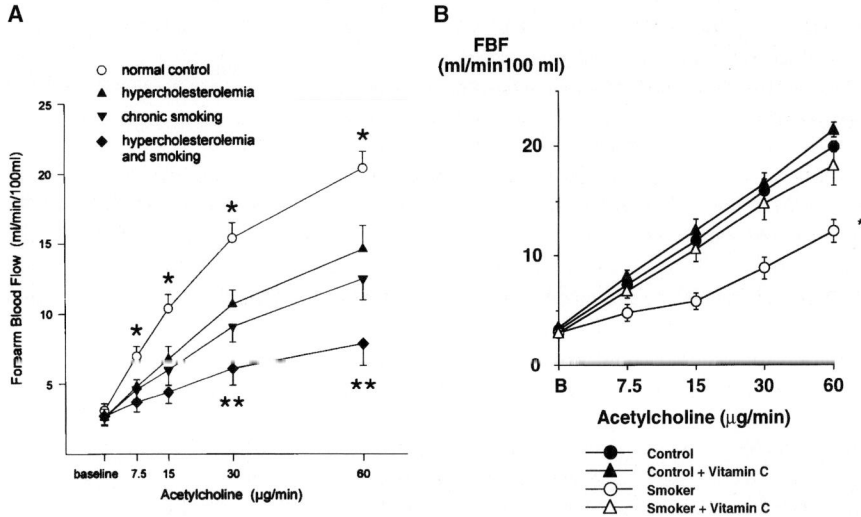

Fig. 13.1 The figure summarizes the effects of cardiovascular risk factors on endothelial function as assessed by forearm plethysmography and the effects of vitamin C on endothelial dysfunction in chronic smokers. **a** Increased low-density lipoprotein (LDL) (mean LDL 236±10 mg/dl) as well as a history of chronic smoking (mean 46±3 pack years) caused a significant degree of endothelial dysfunction on its own. When patients had both hypercholesterolemia as well as a history of chronic smoking, the endothelial function was drastically impaired. **b** Intra-arterial infusion of vitamin C almost completely normalized endothelial dysfunction in chronic smokers, pointing to a crucial role of reactive oxygen species in mediating this phenomenon

as well as in the coronary artery (Schindler et al. 2000), suggesting that increased concentrations of ROS mediate this phenomenon to a large part. Using the technique of flow-dependent dilation of the brachial artery, Neunteufl et al. (2002) recently demonstrated that nicotine also contributes to endothelial dysfunction in chronic smokers, but to a lesser extent than smoking a cigarette of the same nicotine yield.

There has been a debate as to whether endothelial dysfunction occurs solely in response to chronic or also in response to acute smoking. Papamichael et al. (2004) showed that endothelial dysfunction was established in response to acute smoking in the brachial artery. The authors also provided insight into the mechanisms underlying this phenomenon, because red wine's antioxidants were able to correct endothelial dysfunction (Papamichael et al. 2004), indicating that, as observed in chronic smokers, ROS markedly contribute to acute smoking-induced vascular damage as well.

13.8 Passive Smoking and Endothelial Dysfunction

Passive smoking has been demonstrated to be associated with a strikingly reduced coronary flow velocity reserve in young adults (Otsuka et al. 2001). In this study, the authors speculated that endothelial dysfunction mainly accounts for this phenomenon (Otsuka et al. 2001). Indeed, abnormal endothelium-dependent vasodilation in response to passive smoking has been demonstrated in several investigations studying endothelial function in the coronary and forearm circulation (Celermajer et al. 1996; Sumida et al. 1998). Importantly, in some of these studies, there was no significant difference in the response seen in passive versus active smokers, even though cotinine levels in the passive were well below those attained in active smokers (Celermajer et al. 1996). Similar to studies with active smokers, increased oxidative stress as indicated by reduced total antioxidative capacity and increased peroxide levels has been established (Kosecik et al. 2005). Interestingly, chronic treatment with L-arginine slows down atherosclerosis and improves endothelial dysfunction in animals exposed to secondhand smoke, suggesting that a dysfunction in eNOS contributes to this phenomenon (Hutchison et al. 1997).

Despite clear evidence that active and passive smoking have negative effects on vascular function, it remains to be established, however, whether constituents of the cigarette smoke have direct toxic effects to the vasculature and/or whether these components may activate vascular superoxide producing enzymes that may further increase the free radical burden to the vasculature in a positive feedback fashion.

13.9 Evidence for Direct Toxic Effects of Smoke-Derived Free Radicals

The mechanisms underlying smoking related vascular dysfunction are unclear. Cigarette smoke contains more than 4,000 known components, and few components have been characterized in isolation.

Carbon monoxide (CO) represents one of these components, but the precise role in mediating vascular disease remains unclear. Carboxyhemoglobin levels average about 5%, but may reach levels of 10% in heavy smokers. CO exposure increases the number and complexity of arrhythmias in patients with coronary artery disease (CAD) (Sheps et al. 1990) and also impairs left ventricular function during exercise (Sheps et al. 1990).

Polycyclic aromatic hydrocarbons (PAHs) are found in the tar fraction and have been shown to accelerate atherosclerosis in experimental animal models. Weekly injections of PAHs increase atherosclerotic plaque development in the aortas in cockerels (Penn and Snyder 1988). Likewise, inhalation of butadiene, a vapor component of cigarette smoke, increases atherosclerotic plaques in the same animal model (Penn et al. 1996), whereas the tar fraction does not.

Nicotine is so far the most studied component. It is a sympathomimetic compound that releases catecholamines both locally from neurons and systemically from the adrenal cortex. When given acutely, nicotine accounts for smoking induced-increases in heart rate, blood pressure, and cardiac output, but the precise contribution to the atherosclerotic process remains unclear. The dose of nicotine absorbed from each cigarette is about 1–2 mg. Nicotine exposure has been shown to decrease, not to change or to increase NO· bioavailability. In addition, it increases the rate of copper-induced LDL oxidation in vitro (Gouaze et al. 1998), and high concentrations of nicotine have been shown to accelerate atherogenesis in mice (Heeschen et al. 2001). Nicotine also activates dendritic cells, facilitating their ability to mediate T-cell activation and cytokine release, which also may be relevant to atherogenesis (Aicher et al. 2003). Although nicotine replacement therapy may facilitate reduced exposure to carcinogens in cigarette smoke, the long-term cardiovascular consequences of such a strategy remain to be elucidated.

13.10 Smoking-Related Activation of Superoxide-Producing Enzymes

13.10.1 eNOS

In most situations where endothelial dysfunction because of increased oxidative stress is encountered, the expression of the eNOS has been shown to be paradoxically increased rather than decreased (Guzik et al. 2002; Hink et al. 2001, Laursen et al. 2001; Vaziri et al. 1998). This has also been demonstrated in human umbilical vein endothelial cells (HUVECs) exposed to serum from chronic smokers (Barua et al. 2001, 2003). The mechanisms underlying increased expression of eNOS are likely to be secondary to increased endothelial levels of hydrogen peroxide, which has been shown to increase the expression at the transcriptional and translational level (Drummond et al. 2000). In addition in cultured HUVECs, the increase in eNOS expression in response to serum from chronic smokers was prevented by catalase, which metabolizes hydrogen peroxide to water and oxygen (Barua et al. 2003). The demonstration of endothelial dysfunction in the presence of increased expression of eNOS indicates that the capacity of the enzyme to produce NO· may be limited. Very intriguing are observations that the eNOS itself can be a superoxide source, thereby causing endothelial dysfunction. It has become clear from studies with the purified enzyme that eNOS may become "uncoupled," e.g., in the absence of the NOS substrate L-arginine or the cofactor tetrahydrobiopterin (BH_4). In such uncoupled state, electrons normally flowing from the reductase domain of one subunit to the oxygenase domain of the other subunit are diverted to molecular oxygen rather than to L-arginine (Vasquez-Vivar et al. 1998; Xia and Zweier 1997), resulting in the production of superoxide rather than NO· (Fig. 13.2). For proper function of NOS,

BH₄ seems to be essential in several ways. BH₄ stabilizes the NOS dimer, facilitates its formation, and protects NOS against proteolysis (Panda et al. 2002; Stuehr et al. 2004). It also increases the affinity of NOS for L-arginine, and affects the spin state of the heme iron, the heme redox potential, and the oxygen binding. Most importantly, however, BH₄ plays a decisive role for oxygen activation and the time-critical delivery of one electron and proton to the Fe^{II}–O_2 intermediate, which converts to an iron-oxo species and releases H_2O in the catalytic cycle of NOS (Mansuy et al. 2004). BH₄ provides the second electron in the first monooxygenation reaction, which hydroxylates L-arginine to N-hydroxy-arginine. Rapid kinetics analysis by freeze-quench electron paramagnetic resonance (EPR) revealed the transient formation of a $BH_4^{+\cdot}$ cation radical during this reaction, which rapidly splits off a proton to form a $BH_3\cdot$ radical. The $BH_3\cdot$ radical is reduced by one electron and proton delivered by the reductase domain to BH₄, which participates in a second oxygen activation step, leading to the final products NO· and L-citrulline. In the absence of BH₄, the Fe^{II}–O_2-intermediate decays to form superoxide and Fe^{III}. Dihydrobiopterin (BH₂) and other derivatives such as sepiapterin can bind to NOS, but cannot support NO· formation (for review, see Mansuy et al. 2004). Therefore,

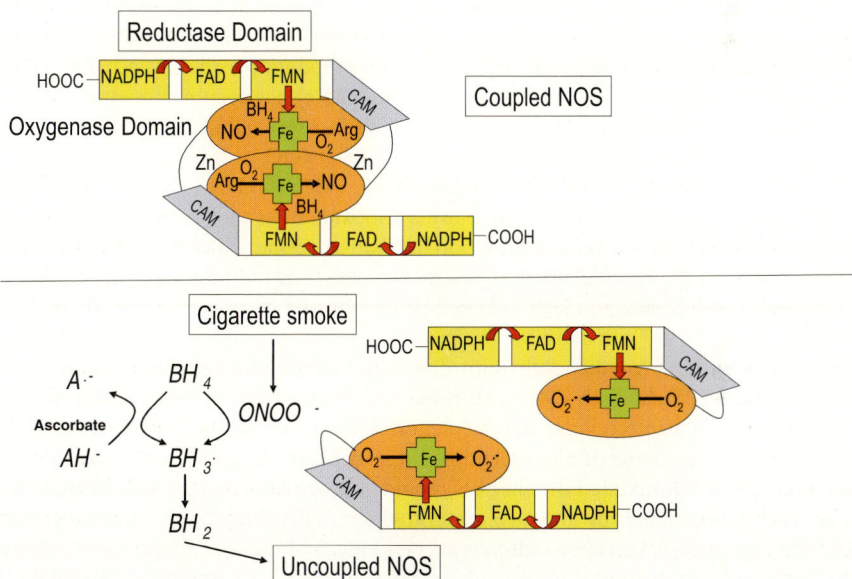

Fig. 13.2 Scheme depicting the mechanisms underlying endothelial nitric oxide (NO) synthase (eNOS) uncoupling in chronic smokers. Under normal conditions, the electron flow starts from NADPH to flavins FAD and FMN of the reductase domain, which delivers the electrons to the iron of the heme (*oxygenase domain*) and to the trihydrobiopterin radical ($BH_3\cdot$) generated as an intermediate in the catalytic cycle. Tetrahydrobiopterin (BH_4) seems to be essential to donate an electron and proton to versatile intermediates in the reaction cycle of L-arginine/O_2 to L-citrulline/NO·. Thus, when BH₄ is present in sufficiently high concentrations, eNOS exists as a dimer and couples its heme and O_2 reduction to NO· synthesis. In the absence of BH₄, e.g., because of peroxynitrite-induced oxidation of BH₄ to the $BH_3\cdot$ radical in the setting of chronic smoking, the "uncoupling reaction" is initiated, which means that significant $O_2^{-\cdot}$ production by eNOS may occur by the heme-catalyzed O_2 reduction. Acute treatment with vitamin C may improve endothelial dysfunction by reducing the $BH_3\cdot$ radical to BH₄ rather than by directly scavenging superoxide anions

limited availability of BH$_4$ for NOS will inevitably result in increased superoxide formation at the expense of NO· formation, i.e., it will uncouple NOS.

What are the mechanisms leading to BH$_4$ depletion? In vitro studies proposed that native LDL (Pritchard et al. 1995) and, even more pronounced, oxidized LDL (Vergnani et al. 2000), are able to stimulate endothelial superoxide production, and that this phenomenon is inhibited by the NOS inhibitor L-NAME, pointing to a specific role of eNOS in superoxide production. Hypercholesterolemia has also been shown to increase vascular formation of superoxide via activation of the NAD(P)H oxidase (Warnholtz et al. 1999) and/or xanthine oxidase (Ohara et al. 1993). Superoxide derived from both enzyme sources may lead to increased formation of peroxynitrite (Laursen et al. 2001; White et al. 1994). Peroxynitrite in turn rapidly oxidizes the active NOS cofactor BH$_4$ to inactive molecules such as BH$_2$ (Laursen et al. 2001; Milstien and Katusic 1999). Accordingly, treatment of HUVECs exposed to serum from smokers with BH$_4$ ex vivo markedly increased eNOS activity and NO· production, pointing to a recoupling of eNOS (Barua et al. 2003)

Recently, we were able to demonstrate that eNOS uncoupling may represent an important mechanism contributing to endothelial dysfunction in chronic smokers in vivo (Heitzer et al. 2000). As mentioned before, cigarette smoke contains free radicals such as NO· and O$_2^-$·, which may react with each other to form the strong prooxidant ONOO$^-$. Moreover, autooxidation of polyhydroxyaromatic compounds such as catechol and 1,4-hydroquinone present in cigarette tar (particulate phase) has been demonstrated to induce superoxide production in lung tissue, which in turn could react with NO· from the gas phase of cigarette smoke to form ONOO$^-$. ONOO$^-$ has been associated with increased oxidative reactions (Yoshie and Ohshima 1997) and DNA damage (Radi et al. 1991), and it may cause a reduction of plasma antioxidants as well. Nitration of tyrosine residues of proteins leads to the production of 3-nitrotyrosine, which may be considered as a marker of ONOO$^-$-dependent oxidative damage (Szabo et al. 1996). Interestingly, in plasma from chronic smokers, increased nitrotyrosine levels have been established (Petruzzelli et al. 1997). In addition, in vitro studies with saphenous veins from chronic smokers showed improved endothelium-dependent relaxation after preincubation with BH$_4$ (Pieper and Siebeneich 1997). All these observations would imply that BH$_4$ oxidation rather than intracellular BH$_4$ depletion may induce eNOS dysfunction, which in turn may be a source of altered endothelium-dependent vasorelaxation in chronic smokers. We therefore tested whether BH$_4$ could improve basal and stimulated NOS· activity in chronic smokers by measuring endothelium-dependent vasomotion using forearm plethysmography, an approach to reflect endothelial function of forearm resistance vessels. We also compared the antioxidant effects of the pteridine tetrahydroneopterin (NH$_4$) with BH$_4$ effects in vitro and in vivo to determine whether BH$_4$ induced improvements in forearm blood flow in chronic smokers are secondary to its effects as a cofactor on a dysfunctional eNOS or because of its nonspecific antioxidant effects. The results demonstrated that in chronic smokers, administration of the endothelial eNOS cofactor BH$_4$ improves both basal and stimulated NO·-mediated vasodilation (Fig. 13.3). Importantly, the improvement was observed in response to BH$_4$ and not to NH$_4$, indicating that a recoupling of eNOS and not a nonspecific antioxidant property of these reduced pteridines was responsible for this phenomenon (Fig. 13.4).

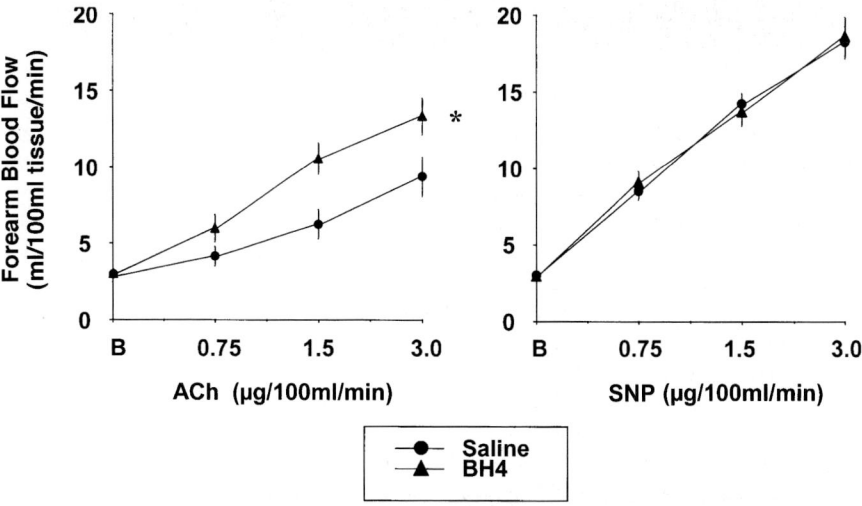

Fig. 13.3 Effects of the nitric oxide synthase (eNOS) cofactor tetrahydrobiopterin (BH_4) on endothelial dysfunction of chronic smokers. Intra-arterial infusion markedly enhanced acetylcholine-induced forearm blood flow, in chronic smokers while having no effect in healthy control subjects, indicating that eNOS uncoupling, e.g., because of BH_4 deficiency, may significantly contribute to endothelial dysfunction in chronic smokers

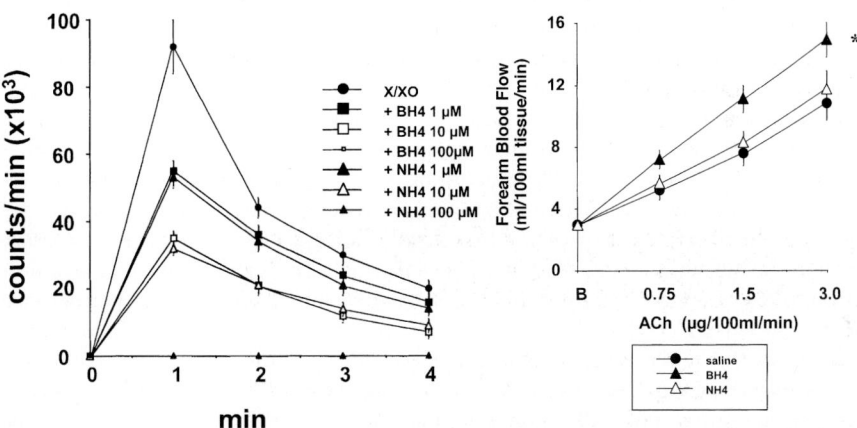

Fig. 13.4 (*left*) Effects of tetrahydrobiopterin and tetrahydroneopterin on the lucigenin-enhanced chemiluminescence signal in response to the xanthine/xanthine oxidase reaction in the presence and absence of tetrahydrobiopterin (BH_4) and tetrahydroneopterin (NH_4). Both reduced pteridines decreased the chemiluminescence signal to a similar degree with equimolar concentrations, but BH_4 only was able to improve the acetylcholine (*ACh*) dose–response relationship (*right*), suggesting that recoupling of eNOS rather than nonspecific antioxidant properties of reduced pteridines accounts for these beneficial effects

13.10.2 NAD(P)H Oxidase

NAD(P)H-oxidase is a superoxide producing enzyme, which was first characterized in neutrophils (Bastian and Hibbs 1994). We know that a similar enzyme exists also in endothelial and smooth muscle cells as well as in the adventitia. The activity of the enzyme in endothelial as well as smooth muscle cells is increased on stimulation with angiotensin II (Griendling et al. 2000). The stimulatory effects of angiotensin II on the activity of this enzyme would suggest that in the presence of an activated renin angiotensin system (local or circulating), vascular dysfunction because of increased vascular superoxide production is likely to be expected. Experimental hypercholesterolemia has been shown to be associated with an activation of the NAD(P)H-oxidase (Warnholtz et al. 1999). There is a close association with endothelial dysfunction and clinical risk factors, and the activity of this enzyme in human saphenous veins in patients with coronary artery disease (Guzik et al. 2000). At present, no data exist demonstrating that constituents of cigarette smoke are able to increase the activity and/or the expression of the vascular, nonphagocytic NADPH oxidase. With respect to inflammatory cells, acute smoking increases the oxidative burst reflecting NADPH oxidase activity, a phenomenon that is completely corrected by a 3-week abstinence from smoking (Sorensen et al. 2004).

13.10.3 Xanthine Oxidase

Xanthine oxido-reductase catalyzes the sequential hydroxylation of hypoxanthine to yield xanthine and uric acid. The enzyme can exist in two forms that differ primarily in their oxidizing substrate specificity. The dehydrogenase form preferentially utilizes NAD^+ as an electron acceptor but is also able to donate electrons to molecular oxygen. By proteolytic breakdown as well as thiol oxidation, xanthine dehydrogenase from mammalian sources can be converted to the oxidase (XO) form that readily donates electrons to molecular oxygen, thereby producing superoxide and hydrogen peroxide, but does not reduce NAD^+. Oxypurinol, an inhibitor of xanthine oxidoreductase, has been shown to reduce superoxide production and to improve endothelium-dependent vascular relaxations to acetylcholine in vessels from hyperlipidemic animals (Ohara et al. 1993). In vitro, incubation of cultured pulmonary endothelial cells with tobacco smoke condensate (TSC) significantly upregulated XO activity after 24 h of exposure. Further TSC treatment upregulated the XO mRNA expression and the *XO* promoter activity. Actinomycin was able to block the upregulation, suggesting that TSC upregulates XO activity at the transcriptional level (Kayyali et al. 2003). In agreement with these in vitro findings, treatment of smokers with the xanthine oxidase inhibitor oxypurinol was able to improve endothelial dysfunction at the conductance or resistance vessel level markedly (Guthikonda et al. 2003, 2004), providing indirect evidence for a role of XO in mediating at least in part this phenomenon.

13.11 Smoking and Inflammation

Chronic smoking leads to a strong inflammatory response, e.g., marked increases in leukocyte count as well as increases in C-reactive protein (CRP), interleukin-6, and tumor necrosis factor-α have been observed (Jensen et al. 1998; Tracy et al. 1997; Tuut and Hense 2001). In addition, increased levels of circulating soluble vascular cell adhesion molecule 1 (VCAM-1), intercellular adhesion molecule 1 (ICAM-1), and E-selectin, and simultaneously, decreased levels of NO· have been demonstrated in chronic smokers (Mazzone et al. 2001). Exposure of HUVECs to cigarette smoke condensate (CSC) markedly increased adherence of monocytes to the endothelium (Kalra et al. 1994) as a consequence of increased expression of adhesion molecules and also increased transmigration of monocytes to the subendothelial space (Shen et al. 1996). Monocytes isolated from smokers have increased expression of the integrin CD11b/CD18, which further augments the adhesiveness of monocytes to HUVECs in culture (Weber et al. 1996). In addition, exposing human monocytes and HUVECs to smoker serum markedly increases the expression of ICAM-1 (Adams et al. 1997), a phenomenon which is reversed by L-arginine but not by vitamin C treatment.

Nicotine may also contribute to the inflammatory process by acting as a chemotactic agent for neutrophil migration (Totti et al. 1984). Nicotine also causes leukocyte rolling and adhesion within the microcirculation as a parameter for enhanced leukocyte-endothelium interaction (Yong et al. 1997).

13.12 Smoking and Lipid Profile

There are several reports demonstrating that the oxidation of LDL may trigger many proatherogenic properties in vivo. In general, smokers have higher total cholesterol, triglycerides, and LDL levels, and high-density lipoprotein (HDL) levels are lower (Craig et al. 1989). Hypercholesterolemia per se is itself associated with increased oxidative stress as indicated by increased isoprostane levels (Davi et al. 1997), that are drastically increased by chronic smoking as well (Morrow 2005). Interestingly, the triglyceride/HDL abnormalities have been recently related to insulin resistance, all of which may represent a link between cigarette smoking and cardiovascular disease (Reaven and Tsao 2003). Smoking also increases oxidative modification of LDL in animal models (Yamaguchi et al. 2001) and in humans (Heitzer et al. 1996). We have shown that lipid peroxidation and antibody titers to oxLDL are markedly increased in smokers (Heitzer et al. 1996). It is also reported that exposure of LDL to CSC caused a modification of LDL, which was then rapidly taken up by macrophages to form foam cells in culture (Yokode et al. 1988). Exposure of human plasma to the gas phase of cigarette smoke caused oxidative modification of LDL (Frei et al. 1991). Further, HUVECs isolated from smokers caused significantly stronger oxidative modification of LDL than HUVECs from nonsmokers (Pech-Amsellem et al. 1996). Cigarette smoke also increases the plasma activity of paraoxonase, an enzyme that protects against LDL oxidation. In addition, injection of CSC accelerated atherosclerosis in a hyperlipidemic rabbit model, which was at least in part mediated through oxidative modification of LDL (Yamaguchi et al. 2000). Importantly, the susceptibility of LDL to oxidation decreases immediately in subjects in response to smoking cessation.

13.13 Smoking and Thrombosis

Platelet activation and subsequent focal myocardial ischemia has been implicated in sudden cardiac death, which is disproportionally increased in chronic smokers (Castelli et al. 1981). Platelet turnover is accelerated in chronic smokers and urinary thromboxane excretion—a marker of platelet activation—is increased in smokers (Nowak et al. 1987). Interestingly, this phenomenon is prevented by switching to nicotine replacement therapy. Importantly, platelets also contain eNOS, which, may become uncoupled thereby contributing to vascular dysfunction by producing large amounts of superoxide. Indeed, platelets from smokers produce less NO· (Ichiki et al. 1996), a phenomenon, which is partly corrected by L-arginine (Ichiki et al. 1996), and by vitamin C (Takajo et al. 2001). Recent data also indicate effects of smoking on thrombohemostatic factors such as tissue factor and tissue factor pathway inhibitor (TFPI-1) and on fibrinolytic factors such as NO·, tissue plasminogen activator (t-PA), and plasminogen activator inhibitor 1 (PAI-1) (Barua et al. 2002). Incubation of cultured endothelial cells (HUVECs) with serum from chronic smokers was associated with a marked decrease in the t-PA/PAI-1 ratio, and the TFPI-1 levels were lower in smokers. Basal as well as stimulated NO· were also reduced (Barua et al. 2002).

13.14 Effects of Smoking on Antioxidant Levels

Numerous studies have demonstrated decreased plasma levels of vitamins in smokers as compared with nonsmokers. In particular, vitamin C levels in smokers decrease markedly in response to not only chronic, but also to acute smoking. This remains significant when plasma levels were corrected for the decreased vitamin intake of smokers (Ma et al. 2000)

13.15 Cessation of Smoking and Oxidative Stress

As mentioned above, chronic smoking is associated with increased platelet aggregation and production of isoprostanes, lipid peroxides reflecting oxidative stress. Cessation of smoking for about 2 weeks markedly ameliorates enhanced platelet aggregability and also normalizes excretion of isoprostanes. In addition, the redox balance within platelets was restored by increasing the reduced form of reduced glutathione (GSH) and by decreasing the oxidized form of GHS (GSSG) (Morita et al. 2005).

13.16 Treatment of Smoking-Induced Endothelial Dysfunction

13.16.1 Vitamin C

In 1996, we were able to demonstrate that endothelial dysfunction of the forearm (Heitzer et al. 1996) and the coronary artery (Schindler et al. 2000) in chronic smokers is markedly improved by acute intra-arterial or intravenous administration of vitamin C. Similar has been observed in response to acute treatment with 2 g of vitamin C when taken orally (Raitakari et al. 2000). These findings clearly indicate that oxidative stress is a major player in causing endothelial dysfunction. The question is whether these beneficial effects are sustained during chronic therapy. This topic was addressed in a study by Raitakari et al (2000). The authors tested endothelial function in chronic smokers (10 pack years) in response to acute vitamin C treatment (2g orally) and in response to 8 weeks treatment with 1 g/day. Although vitamin C had a quite marked effect when given acutely on endothelial dysfunction, these beneficial effects disappeared completely during the long-term treatment period despite markedly increased plasma vitamin C levels (Raitakari et al. 2000). Based on the low rate constant for reaction of vitamin C and superoxide, this observation suggests that the vitamin C dose given was likely too low in order to scavenge superoxide within the endothelial cell. At higher doses, however, side effects and even prooxidant effects may come into play questioning this kind of treatment.

13.16.2 Vitamin E

A wealth of previous experimental and epidemiological data suggested that excess LDL oxidation was, in part, responsible for the development of atherosclerosis. Since vitamin E inhibits LDL oxidation ex vivo, it seemed logical that one strategy to reduce oxidative stress would include the administration of antioxidants, such as vitamin E. There is considerable risk with such an approach if the antioxidant is not active against all relevant oxidants. Although vitamin E effectively scavenges lipid peroxyl radicals, it has little activity against other oxidants such as superoxide, peroxynitrite, and hypochlorous acid that have also been implicated in atherosclerosis. Another risk with an antioxidant strategy relates to putative cellular compartments or microdomains in the vascular wall that do not contain appreciable amounts of the antioxidant. The sum total of these effects would be continued oxidation even in the presence of the antioxidant. Experimental evidence from both animals and patients suggests that lipid peroxidation does proceed in the vascular wall even in the presence of vitamin E (Upston et al. 1999). Attempts to increase the effectiveness of vitamin E with higher doses have generally met with worsening atherosclerosis and vascular function (Keaney et al. 1994), perhaps because of the well-described prooxidant activity of vitamin E (Bowry et al. 1992). Thus, a single-agent antioxidant strategy may not completely reduce vascular oxidative stress and may leave other important processes, such as smooth muscle proliferation and impaired vascular function untouched. Treatment of chronic smokers (23 pack years) with vitamin E (600 IU/day) for 4 weeks has been shown to improve acute and chronic endothelial dysfunction (flow-mediated vasodilation [FMD]) in chronic smokers. In another study, Heitzer et al. (1999) have shown that chronic smokers with increased oxLDL levels only had benefit with respect to endothelial dysfunction from a long-term vitamin E therapy (544 IU/day, 4 months' treatment period). Despite these beneficial effects in this small trial, recent results from a meta-analysis as well as data from the HOPE-TOO Trial (Lonn et al. 2005) indicate that long-term treatment with vitamin E might endanger people. Chronic use in a concentration of 400 IE/day markedly increased mortality and also the incidence of left heart failure as well as hospitalization because of heart failure, suggesting that treatment with vitamin E should be avoided.

13.16.3 Folic Acid and Tetrahydrobiopterin

Interesting is the observation that treatment with folic acid is able to improve endothelial dysfunction in chronic smokers (Doshi et al. 2001; Mangoni et al. 2002). As mentioned above, one of the important superoxide producing enzymes is an uncoupled eNOS because of an intracellular BH_4 deficiency. Recent work from Ton Rabelink's group clearly indicated that folic acid improves endothelial dysfunction by preventing this uncoupling phenomenon (Verhaar et al. 2002). Mechanisms discussed are a chemical stabilization of BH_4, preventing it from being degraded, antioxidant effects of folic acid itself, or a direct effect on eNOS (Verhaar et al. 2002). These findings clearly indicate the therapeutic potential of folic acid in treating smoking-induced vascular dysfunction. Another option is treatment with the NOS cofactor BH_4 itself. As pointed out before, acute treatment with intra-arterially applied BH_4 markedly improved endothelial dysfunction in the forearm of chronic smokers in response to acetylcholine and serotonin (Heitzer et al. 2000). Recent studies indicate that oral treatment with sapropterin hydrochloride, an active analogue of BH_4, markedly improved vascular NO· bioactivity, further pointing to an uncoupled NOS in chronic smokers (Ueda et al. 2000).

13.16.4 Angiotensin-Converting Enzyme Inhibitor

Angiotensin-converting enzyme (ACE) inhibitors have been shown to improve vascular function because of stimulatory effects on vascular NO· production as a consequence of the inhibition of the kinase II, which is responsible for the breakdown of bradykinin. Bradykinin in turn stimulates the release of NO·, the endothelium-derived hyperpolarizing factor as well as prostacyclin, all of which will contribute to an improvement of endothelial dysfunction (Griendling and Ushio-Fukai 2000). In addition, ACE inhibitors reduce oxidative stress within vascular tissue by blocking the ACE enzyme, which will lead to a marked reduction in circulating angiotensin II levels. Angiotensin II in turn has been shown to have potent stimulatory effects on vascular superoxide production, proliferation of cells but also on the inflammatory status of the vasculature. Butler et al. (2001) have shown that the ACE inhibitor lisinopril in a concentration of 20 mg for 8 weeks markedly improved forearm blood flow responses on intra-arterially administered acetylcholine, whereas the endothelium-independent responses to sodium nitroprusside remained unchanged. In addition, the vasoconstrictor responses to the NOS inhibitor L-NMMA were enhanced in response to lisinopril treatment. These findings clearly indicate that treatment with an ACE inhibitor is able to improve endothelial dysfunction in chronic smokers because of enhanced basal as well as stimulated NO· production.

13.16.5 Statins

Statins have been shown to have important pleiotropic effects, which include an up-regulation of vascular eNOS (Laufs et al. 1998) and therefore NO· production, and also a decrease in vascular superoxide in particular because of an inhibition of the activity and expression of important superoxide producing enzymes (Wassmann et al. 2002). Recently, Beckman et al. (2004) demonstrated that treatment of chronic smokers with atorvastatin markedly improved endothelial function, independent of changes in LDL. Endothelium-dependent FMD improved from 8.0 to 10.5%. Because the degree of endothelial function has been shown to have prognostic importance, these findings implicate that statin treatment should be initiated when endothelial dysfunction is encountered in chronic smokers.

13.16.6 Nebivolol

Nebivolol is a third-class β-receptor blocking agent with vasodilating properties, which are largely mediated by releasing NO· from the endothelium. Nebivolol also has potent antioxidant (Troost et al. 2000) properties, which may favorably influence endothelial function in animal models (Mollnau et al. 2003) and in patients with cardiovascular risk factors (Tzemos et al. 2001). Importantly, nebivolol markedly inhibits formation of reactive species in inflammatory cells such as neutrophils and macrophages (Mollnau et al. 2003), which have been shown to produce larger amounts of ROS in chronic smokers. Recently Vyssoulis et al. (2004) demonstrated that treatment of chronic smokers with nebivolol, but not treatment with celiprolol or carvedilol, was able to reduce fibrinogen, PAI-1, and homocysteine. The authors conclude that the smoking status should be an important determinant of antihypertensive treatment choice.

13.17 Summary

Smoking-induced vascular damage is likely to be secondary to the generation of ROS. There is a growing body of evidence that cigarette smoke causes damage via direct delivery of ROS, but also indirectly via delivery of ROS formed by superoxide producing enzymes within the vascular wall, all of which contribute to the acceleration of the atherosclerotic process. Oxidative stress within the blood and within vascular tissue triggers abnormalities with respect to lipid metabolism and the coagulation cascade, which will further contribute to endothelial dysfunction and vascular damage in a positive feedback fashion (Fig. 13.5). The results of treatment of smokers with classical antioxidants such as vitamin C and vitamin E are very disappointing, which may be related to the slow rate constant between the compounds and ROS and the prooxidant effects observed in response to chronic treatment. In contrast, substances that are able to stimulate NO·

production and that simultaneously have inhibitory effects on vascular superoxide production such as statins, ACE inhibitors, or angiotensin I receptor blockers may represent compounds, which will be suited to reduce the consequences of chronic smoking to the vascular wall.

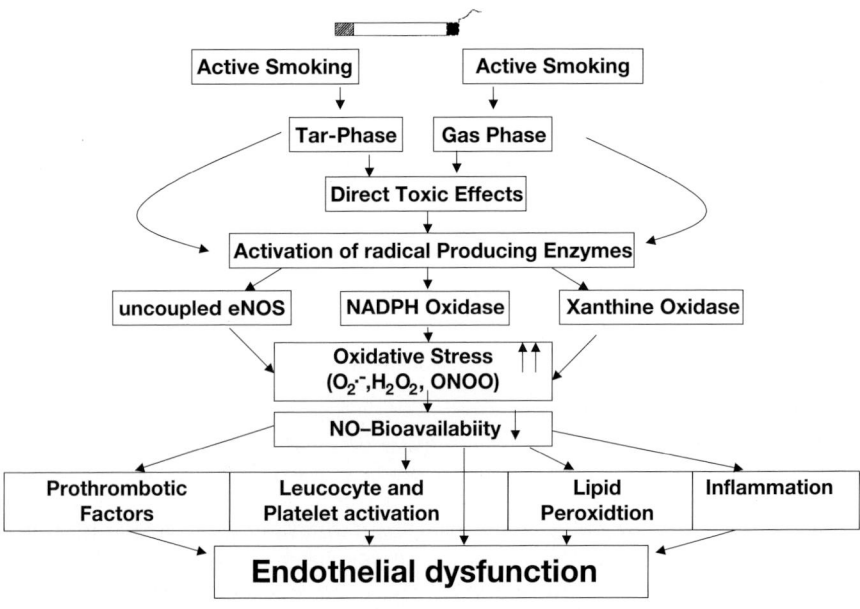

Fig. 13.5 Mechanisms causing endothelial dysfunction in active and passive smokers. Active and passive smoking has toxic effects via contact of lung tissue with the tar and gas phase of the cigarette smoke, respectively. The toxic effects of cigarette smoke may be further enhanced via activation of superoxide-producing enzymes within vascular tissue and therefore remote from the lung such as the NADPH oxidase, xanthine oxidase, and by uncoupling nitric oxide (*NO*) synthase (eNOS). Increased oxidative stress reduces vascular NO· bioavailability, which in turn triggers events that cause endothelial activation/dysfunction by platelet and thrombocyte activation, lipid peroxidation, inflammation, and by creating a prothrombotic environment

13.18 Conclusions

Epidemiological studies indicate that chronic smoking is associated with a marked incidence of cardiovascular morbidity and mortality. Experimental as well as clinical studies have demonstrated that not only active, but also passive exposure to cigarette smoke promotes the phenomenon of endothelial dysfunction. Acute administration of antioxidants markedly improves endothelial dysfunction, pointing to an involvement of reactive oxygen species in mediating this phenomenon. The principal source of free radicals is the cigarette smoke and secondary oxygen-derived free radicals produced from enzymes located within the vessel wall. Cigarette smoke has also strong proinflammatory and procoagulatory effects, all of which contribute to vascular dysfunction as well. Results from small studies suggest that substances that are able to restore eNOS function such as folic acid, and tetrahydrobiopterin as well as established substances such as ACE inhibitors and statins markedly improve smoking-induced endothelial dysfunction. However, despite potentially effective pharmacological treatment options, cessation of smoking remains the most recommended and most cost-effective treatment of smoking induced oxidative stress and endothelial dysfunction.

References

Adams MR, Jessup W, Celermajer DS (1997) Cigarette smoking is associated with increased human monocyte adhesion to endothelial cells: reversibility with oral L-arginine but not vitamin C. J Am Coll Cardiol 29:491–497

Aicher A, Heeschen C, Mohaupt M, Cooke JP, Zeiher AM, Dimmeler S (2003) Nicotine strongly activates dendritic cell-mediated adaptive immunity: potential role for progression of atherosclerotic lesions. Circulation 107:604–611

Alderton WK, Cooper CE, Knowles RG (2001) Nitric oxide synthases: structure, function and inhibition. Biochem J 357:593–615

Ambrose JA, Barua RS (2004) The pathophysiology of cigarette smoking and cardiovascular disease: an update. J Am Coll Cardiol 43:1731–1737

Baldus S, Eiserich JP, Brennan ML, Jackson RM, Alexander CB, Freeman BA (2002) Spatial mapping of pulmonary and vascular nitrotyrosine reveals the pivotal role of myeloperoxidase as a catalyst for tyrosine nitration in inflammatory diseases. Free Radic Biol Med 33:1010

Baldus S, Eiserich JP, Mani A, Castro L, Figueroa M, Chumley P, Ma W, Tousson A, White CR, Bullard DC et al (2001) Endothelial transcytosis of myeloperoxidase confers specificity to vascular ECM proteins as targets of tyrosine nitration. J Clin Invest 108:1759–1770

Baldus S, Heeschen C, Meinertz T, Zeiher AM, Eiserich JP, Munzel T, Simoons ML, Hamm CW (2003) Myeloperoxidase serum levels predict risk in patients with acute coronary syndromes. Circulation 108:1440–1445

Baldus S, Heitzer T, Eiserich JP, Lau D, Mollnau H, Ortak M, Petri S, Goldmann B, Duchstein HJ, Berger J et al (2004) Myeloperoxidase enhances nitric oxide catabolism during myocardial ischemia and reperfusion. Free Radic Biol Med 37:902–911

Barua RS, Ambrose JA, Eales-Reynolds LJ, Devoe MC, Zervas JG, Saha DC (2001) Dysfunctional endothelial nitric oxide biosynthesis in healthy smokers with impaired endothelium-dependent vasodilatation. Circulation 104:1905–1910

Barua RS, Ambrose JA, Saha DC, Eales-Reynolds LJ (2002) Smoking is associated with altered endothelial-derived fibrinolytic and antithrombotic factors: an in vitro demonstration. Circulation 106:905–908

Barua RS, Ambrose JA, Srivastava S, Devoe MC, Eales-Reynolds LJ (2003) Reactive oxygen species are involved in smoking-induced dysfunction of nitric oxide biosynthesis and upregulation of endothelial nitric oxide synthase: an in vitro demonstration in human coronary artery endothelial cells. Circulation 107:2342–2347

Bastian NR, Hibbs JB Jr (1994) Assembly and regulation of NADPH oxidase and nitric oxide synthase. Curr Opin Immunol 6:131–139

Beckman JA, Liao JK, Hurley S, Garrett LA, Chui D, Mitra D, Creager MA (2004) Atorvastatin restores endothelial function in normocholesterolemic smokers independent of changes in low-density lipoprotein. Circ Res 95:217–223

Beckman JS (1996) Oxidative damage and tyrosine nitration from peroxynitrite. Chem Res Toxicol 9:836–844

Bowry VW, Ingold KU, Stocker R (1992) Vitamin E in human low-density lipoprotein. When and how this antioxidant becomes a pro-oxidant. Biochem J 288(Pt 2):341–344

Burns DM (2003) Epidemiology of smoking-induced cardiovascular disease. Prog Cardiovasc Dis 46:11–29

Busse R, Fleming I (1998) Regulation of NO synthesis in endothelial cells. Kidney Blood Press Res 21:264–266

Butler R, Morris AD, Struthers AD (2001) Lisinopril improves endothelial function in chronic cigarette smokers. Clin Sci (Lond) 101:53–58

Castelli WP, Garrison RJ, Dawber TR, McNamara PM, Feinleib M, Kannel WB (1981) The filter cigarette and coronary heart disease: the Framingham study. Lancet 2:109–113

Celermajer DS, Adams MR, Clarkson P, Robinson J, Mccredie R, Donald A, Deanfield JE (1996) Passive smoking and impaired endothelium-dependent arterial dilatation in healthy young adults. N Engl J Med 334:150–154

Celermajer DS, Sorensen KE, Georgakopoulos D, Bull C, Thomas O, Robinson J, Deanfield JE (1993) Cigarette smoking is associated with dose-related and potentially reversible impairment of endothelium-dependent dilation in healthy young adults. Circulation 88:2149–2155

Craig WY, Palomaki GE, Haddow JE (1989) Cigarette smoking and serum lipid and lipoprotein concentrations: an analysis of published data. BMJ 298:784–788

Davi G, Alessandrini P, Mezzetti A, Minotti G, Bucciarelli T, Costantini F, Cipollone F, Bon GB, Ciabattoni G, Patrono C (1997) In vivo formation of 8-epi-prostaglandin F_2 alpha is increased in hypercholesterolemia. Arterioscler Thromb Vasc Biol 17:3230–3235

Deedwania PC (2003) Mechanisms of endothelial dysfunction in the metabolic syndrome. Curr Diab Rep 3:289–292

Doshi SN, Mcdowell IF, Moat SJ, Lang D, Newcombe RG, Kredan MB, Lewis MJ, Goodfellow J (2001) Folate improves endothelial function in coronary artery disease: an effect mediated by reduction of intracellular superoxide? Arterioscler Thromb Vasc Biol 21:1196–1202

Drummond GR, Cai H, Davis ME, Ramasamy S, Harrison DG (2000) Transcriptional and post-transcriptional regulation of endothelial nitric oxide synthase expression by hydrogen peroxide. Circ Res 86:347–354

Duffy SJ, Gokce N, Holbrook M, Hunter LM, Biegelsen ES, Huang A, Keaney JF Jr, Vita JA (2001) Effect of ascorbic acid treatment on conduit vessel endothelial dysfunction in patients with hypertension. Am J Physiol 280:H528–H534

Fischer D, Rossa S, Landmesser U, Spiekermann S, Engberding N, Hornig B, Drexler H (2005) Endothelial dysfunction in patients with chronic heart failure is independently associated with increased incidence of hospitalization, cardiac transplantation, or death. Eur Heart J 26:65–69

Fleming I, Busse R (2003) Molecular mechanisms involved in the regulation of the endothelial nitric oxide synthase. Am J Physiol 284:R1–R12

Frei B, Forte TM, Ames BN, Cross CE (1991) Gas phase oxidants of cigarette smoke induce lipid peroxidation and changes in lipoprotein properties in human blood plasma. Protective effects of ascorbic acid. Biochem J 277(Pt 1):133–138

Garg UC, Hassid A (1989) Nitric oxide-generating vasodilators and 8-bromo-cyclic guanosine monophosphate inhibit mitogenesis and proliferation of cultured rat vascular smooth muscle cells. J Clin Invest 83:1774–1777

Ghiselli A, Serafini M, Maiani G, Azzini E, Ferro-Luzzi A (1995) A fluorescence-based method for measuring total plasma antioxidant capability. Free Radic Biol Med 18:29–36

Ghosh DK, Salerno JC (2003) Nitric oxide synthases: domain structure and alignment in enzyme function and control. Front Biosci 8:d193–209

Gokce N, Keaney JF Jr, Hunter LM, Watkins MT, Menzoian JO, Vita JA (2002) Risk stratification for postoperative cardiovascular events via noninvasive assessment of endothelial function: a prospective study. Circulation 105:1567–1572

Gokce N, Keaney JF Jr, Hunter LM, Watkins MT, Nedeljkovic ZS, Menzoian JO, Vita JA (2003) Predictive value of noninvasively determined endothelial dysfunction for long-term cardiovascular events in patients with peripheral vascular disease. J Am Coll Cardiol 41:1769–1775

Gouaze V, Dousset N, Dousset JC, Valdiguie P (1998) Effect of nicotine and cotinine on the susceptibility to in vitro oxidation of LDL in healthy non smokers and smokers. Clin Chim Acta 277:25–37

Griendling KK, Sorescu D, Ushio-Fukai M (2000) NAD(P)H oxidase: role in cardiovascular biology and disease. Circ Res 86:494–501

Griendling KK, Ushio-Fukai M (2000) Reactive oxygen species as mediators of angiotensin II signaling. Regul Pept 91:21–27

Gryglewski RJ, Moncada S, Palmer RM (1986) Bioassay of prostacyclin and endothelium-derived relaxing factor (EDRF) from porcine aortic endothelial cells. Br J Pharmacol 87:685–694

Guthikonda S, Sinkey C, Barenz T, Haynes WG (2003) Xanthine oxidase inhibition reverses endothelial dysfunction in heavy smokers. Circulation 107:416–421

Guthikonda S, Woods K, Sinkey CA, Haynes WG (2004) Role of xanthine oxidase in conduit artery endothelial dysfunction in cigarette smokers. Am J Cardiol 93:664–668

Guzik TJ, Mussa S, Gastaldi D, Sadowski J, Ratnatunga C, Pillai R, Channon KM (2002) Mechanisms of increased vascular superoxide production in human diabetes mellitus: role of NAD(P)H oxidase and endothelial nitric oxide synthase. Circulation 105:1656–1662

Guzik TJ, West NE, Black E, McDonald D, Ratnatunga C, Pillai R, Channon KM (2000) Vascular superoxide production by NAD(P)H oxidase: association with endothelial dysfunction and clinical risk factors. Circ Res 86:E85–90

Heeschen C, Jang JJ, Weis M, Pathak A, Kaji S, Hu RS, Tsao PS, Johnson FL, Cooke JP (2001) Nicotine stimulates angiogenesis and promotes tumor growth and atherosclerosis. Nat Med 7:833–839

Heitzer T, Brockhoff C, Mayer B, Warnholtz A, Mollnau H, Henne S, Meinertz T, Munzel T (2000) Tetrahydrobiopterin improves endothelium-dependent vasodilation in chronic smokers: evidence for a dysfunctional nitric oxide synthase. Circ Res 86:E36–E41

Heitzer T, Just H, Munzel T (1996) Antioxidant vitamin C improves endothelial dysfunction in chronic smokers. Circulation 94:6–9

Heitzer T, Schlinzig T, Krohn K, Meinertz T, Munzel T (2001) Endothelial dysfunction, oxidative stress, and risk of cardiovascular events in patients with coronary artery disease. Circulation 104:2673–2678

Heitzer T, Yla-Herttuala S, Luoma J, Kurz S, Munzel T, Just H, Olschewski M, Drexler H (1996) Cigarette smoking potentiates endothelial dysfunction of forearm resistance vessels in patients with hypercholesterolemia. Role of oxidized LDL. Circulation 93:1346–1353

Heitzer T, Yla-Herttuala S, Wild E, Luoma J, Drexler H (1999) Effect of vitamin E on endothelial vasodilator function in patients with hypercholesterolemia, chronic smoking or both. J Am Coll Cardiol 33:499–505

Hink U, Li H, Mollnau H, Oelze M, Matheis E, Hartmann M, Skatchkov M, Thaiss F, Stahl RA, Warnholtz A et al (2001) Mechanisms underlying endothelial dysfunction in diabetes mellitus. Circ Res 88:E14–E22

Hutchison SJ, Reitz MS, Sudhir K, Sievers RE, Zhu BQ, Sun YP, Chou TM, Deedwania PC, Chatterjee K, Glantz SA et al (1997) Chronic dietary L-arginine prevents endothelial dysfunction secondary to environmental tobacco smoke in normocholesterolemic rabbits. Hypertension 29:1186–1191

Ichiki K, Ikeda H, Haramaki N, Ueno T, Imaizumi T (1996) Long-term smoking impairs platelet-derived nitric oxide release. Circulation 94:3109–3114

Jensen EJ, Pedersen B, Frederiksen R, Dahl R (1998) Prospective study on the effect of smoking and nicotine substitution on leucocyte blood counts and relation between blood leucocytes and lung function. Thorax 53:784–789

Johnstone MT, Creager SJ, Scales KM, Cusco JA, Lee BK, Creager MA (1993) Impaired endothelium-dependent vasodilation in patients with insulin-dependent diabetes mellitus. Circulation 88:2510–2516

Kalra VK, Ying Y, Deemer K, Natarajan R, Nadler JL, Coates TD (1994) Mechanism of cigarette smoke condensate induced adhesion of human monocytes to cultured endothelial cells. J Cell Physiol 160:154–162

Kayyali US, Budhiraja R, Pennella CM, Cooray S, Lanzillo JJ, Chalkley R, Hassoun PM (2003) Upregulation of xanthine oxidase by tobacco smoke condensate in pulmonary endothelial cells. Toxicol Appl Pharmacol 188:59–68

Keaney JF Jr, Gaziano JM, Xu A, Frei B, Curran-Celentano J, Shwaery GT, Loscalzo J, Vita JA (1994) Low-dose alpha-tocopherol improves and high-dose alpha-tocopherol worsens endothelial vasodilator function in cholesterol-fed rabbits. J Clin Invest 93:844–851

Kosecik M, Erel O, Sevinc E, Selek S (2005) Increased oxidative stress in children exposed to passive smoking. Int J Cardiol 100:61–64

Laufs U, La Fata V, Plutzky J, Liao JK (1998) Upregulation of endothelial nitric oxide synthase by HMG CoA reductase inhibitors. Circulation 97:1129–1135

Laursen JB, Somers M, Kurz S, McCann L, Warnholtz A, Freeman BA, Tarpey M, Fukai T, Harrison DG (2001) Endothelial regulation of vasomotion in apoE-deficient mice: implications for interactions between peroxynitrite and tetrahydrobiopterin. Circulation 103:1282–1288

Law MR, Wald NJ (2003) Environmental tobacco smoke and ischemic heart disease. Prog Cardiovasc Dis 46:31–38

Levine GN, Frei B, Koulouris SN, Gerhard MD, Keaney JF Jr, Vita JA (1996) Ascorbic acid reverses endothelial vasomotor dysfunction in patients with coronary artery disease. Circulation 93:1107–1113

Lonn E, Bosch J, Yusuf S, Sheridan P, Pogue J, Arnold JM, Ross C, Arnold A, Sleight P, Probstfield J et al (2005) Effects of long-term vitamin E supplementation on cardiovascular events and cancer: a randomized controlled trial. JAMA 293:1338–1347

Ma J, Hampl JS, Betts NM (2000) Antioxidant intakes and smoking status: data from the continuing survey of food intakes by individuals 1994–1996. Am J Clin Nutr 71:774–780

Mangoni AA, Sherwood RA, Swift CG, Jackson SH (2002) Folic acid enhances endothelial function and reduces blood pressure in smokers: a randomized controlled trial. J Intern Med 252:497–503

Mansuy D, Mathieu D, Battioni P, Boucher J-L (2004) Reactions between iron porphyrins and tetrahydropterins. J Porphyrins Phthalocyanines 8:265–278

Mazzone A, Cusa C, Mazzucchelli I, Vezzoli M, Ottini E, Ghio S, Tossini G, Pacifici R, Zuccaro P (2001) Cigarette smoking and hypertension influence nitric oxide release and plasma levels of adhesion molecules. Clin Chem Lab Med 39:822–826

Meagher EA, Fitzgerald GA (2000) Indices of lipid peroxidation in vivo: strengths and limitations. Free Radic Biol Med 28:1745–1750

Milstien S, Katusic Z (1999) Oxidation of tetrahydrobiopterin by peroxynitrite: implications for vascular endothelial function. Biochem Biophys Res Commun 263:681–684

Mollnau H, Schulz E, Daiber A, Baldus S, Oelze M, August M, Wendt M, Walter U, Geiger C, Agrawal R et al (2003) Nebivolol prevents vascular NOS III uncoupling in experimental hyperlipidemia and inhibits NADPH oxidase activity in inflammatory cells. Arterioscler Thromb Vasc Biol 23:615–621

Moncada S, Korbut R, Bunting S, Vane JR (1978) Prostacyclin is a circulating hormone. Nature 273:767–768

Morita H, Ikeda H, Haramaki N, Eguchi H, Imaizumi T (2005) Only two-week smoking cessation improves platelet aggregability and intraplatelet redox imbalance of long-term smokers. J Am Coll Cardiol 45:589–594

Morrow JD (2005) Quantification of isoprostanes as indices of oxidant stress and the risk of atherosclerosis in humans. Arterioscler Thromb Vasc Biol 25:279–286

Morrow JD, Frei B, Longmire AW, Gaziano JM, Lynch SM, Shyr Y, Strauss WE, Oates JA, Roberts LJ II (1995) Increase in circulating products of lipid peroxidation (F_2-isoprostanes) in smokers. Smoking as a cause of oxidative damage. N Engl J Med 332:1198–1203

Munzel T, Afanas'ev IB, Kleschyov AL, Harrison DG (2002) Detection of superoxide in vascular tissue. Arterioscler Thromb Vasc Biol 22:1761–1768

Munzel T, Feil R, Mulsch A, Lohmann SM, Hofmann F, Walter U (2003) Physiology and pathophysiology of vascular signaling controlled by guanosine 3',5'-cyclic monophosphate-dependent protein kinase. Circulation 108:2172–2183

Myers PR, Minor RL Jr, Guerra R Jr, Bates JN, Harrison DG (1990) Vasorelaxant properties of the endothelium-derived relaxing factor more closely resemble S-nitrosocysteine than nitric oxide. Nature 345:161163

Neunteufl T, Heher S, Kostner K, Mitulovic G, Lehr S, Khoschsorur G, Schmid RW, Maurer G, Stefenelli T (2002) Contribution of nicotine to acute endothelial dysfunction in long-term smokers. J Am Coll Cardiol 39:251–256

Nitenberg A, Antony I, Foult JM (1993) Acetylcholine-induced coronary vasoconstriction in young, heavy smokers with normal coronary arteriographic findings. Am J Med 95:71–77

Nitenberg A, Valensi P, Sachs R, Dali M, Aptecar E, Attali JR (1993) Impairment of coronary vascular reserve and ACh-induced coronary vasodilation in diabetic patients with angiographically normal coronary arteries and normal left ventricular systolic function. Diabetes 42:1017–1025

Nowak J, Murray JJ, Oates JA, Fitzgerald GA (1987) Biochemical evidence of a chronic abnormality in platelet and vascular function in healthy individuals who smoke cigarettes. Circulation 76:6–14

Ohara Y, Peterson TE, Harrison DG (1993) Hypercholesterolemia increases endothelial superoxide anion production. J Clin Invest 91:2546–2551

Otsuka R, Watanabe H, Hirata K, Tokai K, Muro T, Yoshiyama M, Takeuchi K, Yoshikawa J (2001) Acute effects of passive smoking on the coronary circulation in healthy young adults. JAMA 286:436–441

Palmer RM, Ferrige AG, Moncada S (1987) Nitric oxide release accounts for the biological activity of endothelium-derived relaxing factor. Nature 327:524–526

Panda K, Rosenfeld RJ, Ghosh S, Meade AL, Getzoff ED, Stuehr DJ (2002) Distinct dimer interaction and regulation in nitric-oxide synthase types I, II, and III. J Biol Chem 277:31020–31030

Papamichael C, Karatzis E, Karatzi K, Aznaouridis K, Papaioannou T, Protogerou A, Stamatelopoulos K, Zampelas A, Lekakis J, Mavrikakis M (2004) Red wine's antioxidants counteract acute endothelial dysfunction caused by cigarette smoking in healthy nonsmokers. Am Heart J 147: E5

Pech-Amsellem MA, Myara I, Storogenko M, Demuth K, Proust A, Moatti N (1996) Enhanced modifications of low-density lipoproteins (LDL) by endothelial cells from smokers: a possible mechanism of smoking-related atherosclerosis. Cardiovasc Res 31:975–983

Penn A, Keller K, Snyder C, Nadas A, Chen LC (1996) The tar fraction of cigarette smoke does not promote arteriosclerotic plaque development. Environ Health Perspect 104:1108–1113

Penn A, Snyder C (1988) Arteriosclerotic plaque development is "promoted" by polynuclear aromatic hydrocarbons. Carcinogenesis 9:2185–2189

Perticone F, Ceravolo R, Pujia A, Ventura G, Iacopino S, Scozzafava A, Ferraro A, Chello M, Mastroroberto P, Verdecchia P et al (2001) Prognostic significance of endothelial dysfunction in hypertensive patients. Circulation 104:191–196

Petruzzelli S, Puntoni R, Mimotti P, Pulera N, Baliva F, Fornai E, Giuntini C (1997) Plasma 3-nitrotyrosine in cigarette smokers. Am J Respir Crit Care Med 156:1902–1907

Pieper GM, Siebeneich W (1997) Diabetes-induced endothelial dysfunction is prevented by long-term treatment with the modified iron chelator, hydroxyethyl starch conjugated-deferoxamine. J Cardiovasc Pharmacol 30:734–738

Pittilo RM, Mackie IJ, Rowles PM, Machin SJ, Woolf N (1982) Effects of cigarette smoking on the ultrastructure of rat thoracic aorta and its ability to produce prostacyclin. Thromb Haemost 48:173–176

Powell JT (1998) Vascular damage from smoking: disease mechanisms at the arterial wall. Vasc Med 3:21–28

Pritchard KA Jr, Groszek L, Smalley DM, Sessa WC, Wu M, Villalon P, Wolin MS, Stemerman MB (1995) Native low-density lipoprotein increases endothelial cell nitric oxide synthase generation of superoxide anion. Circ Res 77:510–518

Radi R, Beckman JS, Bush KM, Freeman BA (1991) Peroxynitrite oxidation of sulfhydryls. The cytotoxic potential of superoxide and nitric oxide. J Biol Chem 266:4244–4250

Radomski MW, Palmer RM, Moncada S (1987) Comparative pharmacology of endothelium-derived relaxing factor, nitric oxide and prostacyclin in platelets. Br J Pharmacol 92:181–187

Raitakari OT, Adams MR, Mccredie RJ, Griffiths KA, Stocker R, Celermajer DS (2000) Oral vitamin C and endothelial function in smokers: short-term improvement, but no sustained beneficial effect. J Am Coll Cardiol 35:1616–1621

Reaven G, Tsao PS (2003) Insulin resistance and compensatory hyperinsulinemia: the key player between cigarette smoking and cardiovascular disease? J Am Coll Cardiol 41:1044–1047

Schachinger V, Britten MB, Zeiher AM (2000) Prognostic impact of coronary vasodilator dysfunction on adverse long-term outcome of coronary heart disease. Circulation 101:1899–1906

Schindler TH, Magosaki N, Jeserich M, Olschewski M, Nitzsche E, Holubarsch C, Solzbach U, Just H (2000) Effect of ascorbic acid on endothelial dysfunction of epicardial coronary arteries in chronic smokers assessed by cold pressor testing. Cardiology 94:239–246

Shen Y, Rattan V, Sultana C, Kalra VK (1996) Cigarette smoke condensate-induced adhesion molecule expression and transendothelial migration of monocytes. Am J Physiol 270: H1624–H1633

Sheps DS, Herbst MC, Hinderliter AL, Adams KF, Ekelund LG, O'Neil JJ, Goldstein GM, Bromberg PA, Dalton JL, Ballenger MN et al (1990) Production of arrhythmias by elevated carboxyhemoglobin in patients with coronary artery disease. Ann Intern Med 113:343–351

Smith CJ, Fischer TH (2001) Particulate and vapor phase constituents of cigarette mainstream smoke and risk of myocardial infarction. Atherosclerosis 158:257–267

Sorensen LT, Nielsen HB, Kharazmi A, Gottrup F (2004) Effect of smoking and abstention on oxidative burst and reactivity of neutrophils and monocytes. Surgery 136:1047–1053

Stuehr DJ, Wei CC, Santolini J, Wang Z, Aoyagi M, Getzoff ED (2004) Radical reactions of nitric oxide synthases. Biochem Soc Symp(71):39–49

Stupack DG, Cheresh DA (2004) Integrins and angiogenesis. Curr Top Dev Biol 64:207–238

Sumida H, Watanabe H, Kugiyama K, Ohgushi M, Matsumura T, Yasue H (1998) Does passive smoking impair endothelium-dependent coronary artery dilation in women? J Am Coll Cardiol 31:811–815

Szabo C, Day BJ, Salzman AL (1996) Evaluation of the relative contribution of nitric oxide and peroxynitrite to the suppression of mitochondrial respiration in immunostimulated macrophages using a manganese mesoporphyrin superoxide dismutase mimetic and peroxynitrite scavenger. FEBS Lett 381:82–86

Takajo Y, Ikeda H, Haramaki N, Murohara T, Imaizumi T (2001) Augmented oxidative stress of platelets in chronic smokers. Mechanisms of impaired platelet-derived nitric oxide bioactivity and augmented platelet aggregability. J Am Coll Cardiol 38:1320–1327

Ting HH, Timimi FK, Boles KS, Creager SJ, Ganz P, Creager MA (1996) Vitamin C improves endothelium-dependent vasodilation in patients with non-insulin-dependent diabetes mellitus. J Clin Invest 97:22–28

Totti N III, McCusker KT, Campbell EJ, Griffin GL, Senior RM (1984) Nicotine is chemotactic for neutrophils and enhances neutrophil responsiveness to chemotactic peptides. Science 223:169–171

Tracy RP, Psaty BM, Macy E, Bovill EG, Cushman M, Cornell ES, Kuller LH (1997) Lifetime smoking exposure affects the association of C-reactive protein with cardiovascular disease risk factors and subclinical disease in healthy elderly subjects. Arterioscler Thromb Vasc Biol 17:2167–2176

Treasure CB, Klein JL, Vita JA, Manoukian SV, Renwick GH, Selwyn AP, Ganz P, Alexander RW (1993) Hypertension and left ventricular hypertrophy are associated with impaired endothelium-mediated relaxation in human coronary resistance vessels. Circulation 87:86–93

Troost R, Schwedhelm E, Rojczyk S, Tsikas D, Frolich JC (2000) Nebivolol decreases systemic oxidative stress in healthy volunteers. Br J Clin Pharmacol 50:377–379

Tuut M, Hense HW (2001) Smoking, other risk factors and fibrinogen levels. evidence of effect modification. Ann Epidemiol 11:232–238

Tzemos N, Lim PO, Macdonald TM (2001) Nebivolol reverses endothelial dysfunction in essential hypertension: a randomized, double-blind, crossover study. Circulation 104:511–514

Ueda S, Matsuoka H, Miyazaki H, Usui M, Okuda S, Imaizumi T (2000) Tetrahydrobiopterin restores endothelial function in long-term smokers. J Am Coll Cardiol 35:71–75

Upston JM, Terentis AC, Stocker R (1999) Tocopherol-mediated peroxidation of lipoproteins: implications for vitamin E as a potential antiatherogenic supplement. FASEB J 13:977–994

Vasquez-Vivar J, Kalyanaraman B, Martasek P, Hogg N, Masters BS, Karoui H, Tordo P, Pritchard KA Jr (1998) Superoxide generation by endothelial nitric oxide synthase: the influence of cofactors. Proc Natl Acad Sci U S A 95:9220–9225

Vaziri ND, Ni Z, Oveisi F (1998) Upregulation of renal and vascular nitric oxide synthase in young spontaneously hypertensive rats. Hypertension 31:1248–1254

Vergnani L, Hatrik S, Ricci F, Passaro A, Manzoli N, Zuliani G, Brovkovych V, Fellin R, Malinski T (2000) Effect of native and oxidized low-density lipoprotein on endothelial nitric oxide and superoxide production: key role of L-arginine availability. Circulation 101:1261–1266

Verhaar MC, Stroes E, Rabelink TJ (2002) Folates and cardiovascular disease. Arterioscler Thromb Vasc Biol 22:6–13

Vita JA, Treasure CB, Nabel EG, McLenachan JM, Fish RD, Yeung AC, Vekshtein VI, Selwyn AP, Ganz P (1990) Coronary vasomotor response to acetylcholine relates to risk factors for coronary artery disease. Circulation 81:491–497

Vyssoulis GP, Marinakis AG, Aznaouridis KA, Karpanou EA, Arapogianni AN, Cokkinos DV, Stefanadis CI (2004) The impact of third-generation beta-blocker antihypertensive treatment on endothelial function and the prothrombotic state: effects of smoking. Am J Hypertens 17:582–589

Warnholtz A, Nickenig G, Schulz E, Macharzina R, Brasen JH, Skatchkov M, Heitzer T, Stasch JP, Griendling KK, Harrison DG et al (1999) Increased NADH-oxidase-mediated superoxide production in the early stages of atherosclerosis: evidence for involvement of the renin-angiotensin system. Circulation 99:2027–2033

Wassmann S, Laufs U, Muller K, Konkol C, Ahlbory K, Baumer AT, Linz W, Bohm M, Nickenig G (2002) Cellular antioxidant effects of atorvastatin in vitro and in vivo. Arterioscler Thromb Vasc Biol 22:300–305

Weber C, Erl W, Weber K, Weber PC (1996) Increased adhesiveness of isolated monocytes to endothelium is prevented by vitamin C intake in smokers. Circulation 93:1488–1492

White CR, Brock TA, Chang LY, Crapo J, Briscoe P, Ku D, Bradley WA, Gianturco SH, Gore J, Freeman BA et al (1994) Superoxide and peroxynitrite in atherosclerosis. Proc Natl Acad Sci U S A 91:1044–1048

Xia Y, Zweier JL (1997) Direct measurement of nitric oxide generation from nitric oxide synthase. Proc Natl Acad Sci U S A 94:12705–12710

Yamaguchi Y, Kagota S, Haginaka J, Kunitomo M (2000) Evidence of modified LDL in the plasma of hypercholesterolemic WHHL rabbits injected with aqueous extracts of cigarette smoke. Environ. Toxicol Pharmacol 8:255–260

Yamaguchi Y, Matsuno S, Kagota S, Haginaka J, Kunitomo M (2001) Oxidants in cigarette smoke extract modify low-density lipoprotein in the plasma and facilitate atherogenesis in the aorta of Watanabe heritable hyperlipidemic rabbits. Atherosclerosis 156:109–117

Yokode M, Kita T, Arai H, Kawai C, Narumiya S, Fujiwara M (1988) Cholesteryl ester accumulation in macrophages incubated with low density lipoprotein pretreated with cigarette smoke extract. Proc Natl Acad Sci U S A 85:2344–2348

Yong T, Zheng MQ, Linthicum DS (1997) Nicotine induces leukocyte rolling and adhesion in the cerebral microcirculation of the mouse. J Neuroimmunol 80:158–164

Yoshie Y, Ohshima H (1997) Synergistic induction of DNA strand breakage by cigarette tar and nitric oxide. Carcinogenesis 18:1359–1363

Zeiher AM, Schachinger V, Minners J (1995) Long-term cigarette smoking impairs endothelium-dependent coronary arterial vasodilator function. Circulation 92:1094–1100

Zou MH, Ullrich V (1996) Peroxynitrite formed by simultaneous generation of nitric oxide and superoxide selectively inhibits bovine aortic prostacyclin synthase. FEBS Lett 382:101–104

Zou MH, Shi C, Cohen RA (2002) Oxidation of the zinc-thiolate complex and uncoupling of endothelial nitric oxide synthase by peroxynitrite. J Clin Invest 109:817–826

Chapter 14

Nrf2: a Transcription Factor that Modifies Susceptibility to Cigarette Smoke-Induced Pulmonary Oxidative Stress and Emphysema

Shyam Biswal and Thomas W. Kensler

Contents

14.1	Introduction	366
14.2	Nrf2 as a Key Regulator of Antioxidative and Other Cytoprotective Genes	366
14.3	Emphysema Results from the Interplay of Oxidative Stress and Inflammation	367
14.4	Differences in Susceptibility to Cigarette Smoke-Induced COPD	369
14.5	Nrf2 as a Modifier Gene for Pulmonary Oxidative Stress, Inflammation, and Emphysema	369
14.5.1	Nrf2 Protects against Emphysema	370
14.5.2	Nrf2 Protects against Cigarette Smoke Pulmonary Oxidative Stress and Apoptosis	371
14.5.3	Nrf2 Protects against Pulmonary Inflammation	371
14.5.4	Activation of Nrf2 by Cigarette Smoke	372
14.5.5	Transcriptional Induction of Pulmonary Nrf2 Target Genes after Cigarette Smoke Induction	372
14.6	Conclusions	374
	References	375

14.1 Introduction

Pulmonary emphysema is a major manifestation of chronic obstructive pulmonary disease (COPD), which affects more than 16 million Americans (Blanchard 2003). COPD, which is caused primarily by cigarette smoking, is likely to become the third largest cause of death worldwide by 2020 (Viegi et al. 2001). Oxidative stress caused by chronic exposure of lungs to cigarette smoke contributes to the pathogenesis of emphysema and COPD. The capacity of the lungs to respond to this stress is an important determinant of their relative resistance or susceptibility to COPD. A battery of protective genes can be induced in a rapid and highly coordinated response to oxidants through activation of redox–sensitive transcription factors. The coordinated induction of these genes is fundamental to maintaining antioxidant and other cytoprotective functions against free radicals and electrophiles that arise from exposure to cigarette smoke. Multiple redox-sensitive transcription factors, such as activator protein 1, activator protein 2, nuclear factor kappa B (NF-κB), redox factor 1, signal transducer and activator of transcription, peroxisome proliferation activator receptor, p53, and aryl hydrocarbon receptor, are activated in lungs in response to oxidative stress. This chapter focuses on a relatively newly described basic leucine zipper transcription factor named nuclear factor erythroid 2-related factor 2 (Nrf2). Studies in knockout mice in particular are establishing Nrf2 as an important modifier of pulmonary oxidative stress, inflammation and emphysema.

14.2 Nrf2 as a Key Regulator of Antioxidative and Other Cytoprotective Genes

The capacity to detoxify environmental toxicants, such as may be found in tobacco smoke, is driven in part by the levels of expression of genes that enhance the conjugation and elimination of reactive intermediates by what have been classically termed phase II enzymes. A common regulatory element in the 5' flanking regions of many of these cytoprotective phase II genes has been defined and is termed the antioxidant-response element (ARE). A thorough characterization of the 5' upstream region of the murine NAD(P)H:quinone oxidoreductase (*nqo1*) gene has defined a 24-bp region spanning nucleotides –444 to –421 as the ARE consensus sequence (5'-gagTcA C aGTgAGt C ggCAaaatt-3') (Nioi et al. 2003). Several years ago, Nrf2 was recognized as the major transcription factor binding to AREs. As shown in Fig. 14.1, Nrf2 is an essential regulator of the coordinated expression of ARE-regulated genes. Nrf2 belongs to the cap 'n' collar (CNC) family of bZip transcription factors and primarily acts through formation of heterodimers with one of several small Maf proteins. Major insight into the contribution of Nrf2 in the regulation of phase II genes was provided by Itoh et al. (1997), who showed that disruption of *nrf2* in mice largely abrogated both the basal and inducible expression of prototypical phase II enzymes such as glutathione *S*-transferases (GSTs) and NQO1. As is discussed later in this chapter, genome-wide screening, using wild-type and *nrf2* knockout comparisons in several tissues, has now defined over 200 genes, composing a dynamic, highly coordinated, and diverse mammalian defense system against electrophilic and oxidative stresses. Indeed, *nrf2*-deficient mice are highly susceptible to environmental stresses in many forms because of the impaired expression of these cytoprotective genes.

An actin-binding cytoplasmic protein termed Keap1 represses the transcriptional activation of Nrf2-regluated genes (Itoh et al. 1999). Under basal conditions, Nrf2 is tethered to Keap1, which through interaction with components of ubiquitin ligase, leads to the degradation of Nrf2 by proteasomes (Itoh et al. 2003). Thus, transcription of Nrf2 target genes remains low. Conversely, expression of Nrf2 target genes is very high in *keap1*-disrupted mice (Wakabayashi et al. 2003). Following oxidative stress or exposure to pharmacological enzyme inducers, Nrf2 dissociates from Keap1, triggering the nuclear accumulation of Nrf2 and the transcriptional activation of its target genes (Chan et al. 2001; Cho et al. 2002; Kwak et al. 2002; Rangasamy et al. 2004). In this way, inducible expression of Nrf2-regulated genes can be targeted through the use of small molecules such as dithiolethiones and isothiocyanates (Kwak et al. 2002; Thimmulappa et al. 2002). Such agents are currently being evaluated for use in protection against carcinogenesis, neurodegenerative diseases, and other pathologies associated with inflammation and oxidative stress, including COPD. Keap1 is rich in cysteine residues, and it is currently thought that some of these sulfhydryl residues enable Keap1 to serve as a primary sensor molecule for oxidative stress and response to small molecule inducers (Dinkova-Kostova et al. 2002; Wakabayashi et al. 2004)

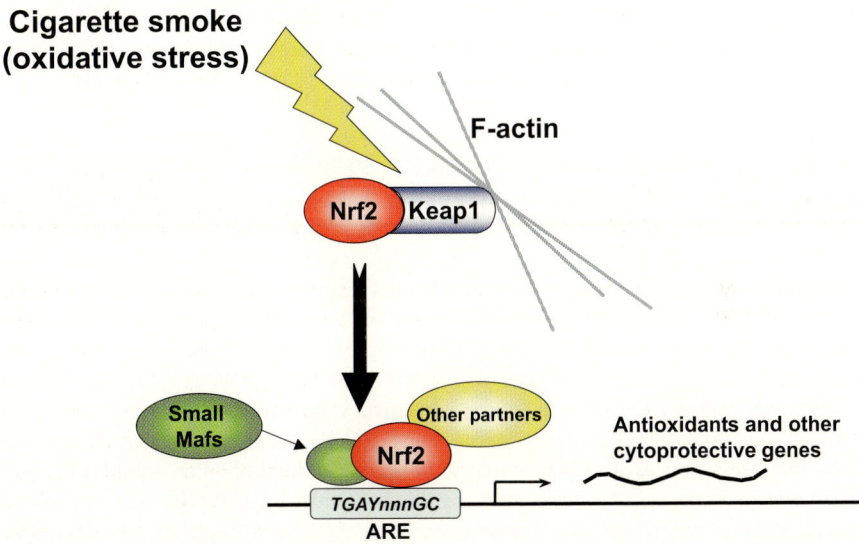

Fig. 14.1 Pathway for nuclear factor erythroid 2-related factor 2 (*Nrf2*)-mediated transcriptional regulation of antioxidant and cytoprotective genes following exposure to cigarette smoke

14.3 Emphysema Results from the Interplay of Oxidative Stress and Inflammation

Pulmonary emphysema is a complex disease characterized by abnormal inflammation, air space enlargement, and the loss of alveolar structures. Permanent destruction of peripheral air spaces distal to terminal bronchioles is the hallmark of emphysema (Hogg 2004). Imbalances in levels of expression of proteinases and antiproteinases as well as in levels of oxidants and antioxidants resulting from chronic insult with cigarette smoke contribute to the development of emphysema. There is accumulation of inflammatory cells such as macrophages and neutrophils in bronchioles and alveoli (Keatings et al. 1996). Greater numbers of neutrophils have been found in the bronchiolar lavage fluid (BALF) of COPD patients; however, there are relatively small increases in neutrophils in the lung parenchyma (Finkelstein et al. 1995). Neutrophils secrete serine proteases such as neutrophil elastase, cathepsin G, and matrix metalloproteinases (MMP)-8 and MMP-9. These and other proteases may cause alveolar destruction. Macrophages are the predominant inflammatory cells in the lower airways, and their number correlates with disease progression (Shapiro 1999). There is a several-fold increase in the number of macrophages in airways, lung parenchyma, and BALF of patients with COPD. Matrix metalloproteinases (specifically the macrophage elastase MMP-12) play a central role, as documented by the complete resistance of macrophage *mmp12* knockout mice to smoke induced-emphysema (Hautamaki et al. 1997). Mice defective in activation of latent transforming growth factor-β (TGF-β) develop emphysema because TGF-β suppresses the production of MMP-12 by macrophages and increases the tissue inhibitor of MMP (TIMP-1) (Morris et al. 2003). Moreover, pulmonary overexpression of interleukin 13 (IL-13) in transgenic mice results in MMP- and cathepsin-dependent emphysema (Zheng et al. 2000). More recently, MMP-12 has been shown to degrade α1-antitrypsin, and neutrophil elastase degrades TIMP-1. Thus, macrophages and neutrophils clearly alter the proteinase/antiproteinase balance (Shapiro et al. 2003). Neutrophil elastase is also involved in the conversion of proMMP-12 to active MMP-12 (Shapiro et al. 2003). Thus, crosstalk between neutrophils and macrophages enhances the inflammatory processes in mice following exposure to cigarette smoke.

The oxidative burden in the lungs of smokers has been estimated to be very high—10^{14} free radicals per puff (Church and Pryor 1985). The potent oxidants in cigarette smoke include superoxide anion (O_2^-), nitric oxide (NO·) and, through their interaction, the even more reactive peroxynitrite ($ONOO^-$) (Pryor and Stone 1993). Semiquinones and benzoquinones present in the cigarette tar along with superoxide radicals lead to production of reactive hydroxyl radicals (·OH) and hydrogen peroxide (H_2O_2) (Zang et al. 1995). Iron in the fluid of the epithelial lining and in tar causes production of ·OH by the Fenton reaction. Some of these reactive oxygen species cause lipid peroxidation, leading to destruction of membrane lipids (Rahman et al. 1996, 2002). Markers of oxidative stress (e.g., hydrogen peroxide and the end products of lipid peroxidation such as ethane, pentane, and 8-isoprostane) are elevated in the breath and serum of patients with COPD (Horvath et al. 2001). Oxidative stress also enhances inflammation and inactivates critical antiproteinase inhibitors such as α1-antitrypsin (Macnee and Rahman 2001). There is recent evidence that apoptosis of alveolar septal cells contributes to human emphysema (Yokohori et al. 2004) and is required for experimental emphysema caused by inhibition of the vascular endothelial growth factor (VEGF) receptor, a model where oxidative stress has been shown also to be involved (Tuder et al. 2003).

Evidence of the interplay between inflammation and oxidative stress in abetting lung destruction is highlighted by measures of significant release of reactive oxygen species from macrophages and neutrophils in smokers (Rahman and Macnee 1996; Rahman et al. 1996). The oxidants of cigarette smoke can activate alveolar macrophages to produce reactive oxygen species as well as several inflammatory mediators that attract neutrophils, macrophages, and other inflammatory cells into lungs. Inflammatory mediators such as interleukin-8 and tumor necrosis factor-α (TNF-α), whose levels are increased in BALF obtained from patients with COPD (Barnes 2000), are regulated by the proinflammatory redox-sensitive transcription factor NF-κB (Rahman et al. 2002, Rahman and Macnee 1998). Cigarette smoke has been shown to activate NF-κB in the lungs of mice (Churg et al. 2003). This activation leads to production of inflammatory mediators, such as macrophage chemoattractant protein 1 and macrophage inflammatory protein 2, which in turn attract macrophages and neutrophils, respectively. The initial increase in macrophages has been postulated to convert pro-TNF-α from macrophages to active TNF-α (Churg et al. 2003). TNF-α then activates endothelial cells with adhesion of neutrophils to the endothelial cells and subsequent entry of neutrophils into the lungs (Churg et al. 2003). Thus, the oxidant/antioxidant imbalance may crosstalk with NF-κB activation to aid in recruitment of inflammatory cells, thereby creating or exacerbating the proteinase/antiproteinase imbalance.

The net result of the interplay between oxidative stress and inflammation is increased release of proteases from activated inflammatory cells that then override the homeostatic control of antiproteinases and initiate the proteolysis of lungs. Further, the increased oxidant burden from the activated macrophages and neutrophils directly contribute to destruction of lung tissue by overwhelming the actions of protective antioxidants.

14.4 Differences in Susceptibility to Cigarette Smoke-Induced COPD

Only 10–20% of heavy cigarette smokers develop COPD (Fletcher and Peto 1977). Susceptibility to COPD is likely to be determined by multiple genes and their interaction with environmental factors. Twin studies examining lung function in monozygotic and dizygotic twins have indicated that 50–80% of variability in lung function has a genetic basis (Mcclearn et al. 1994, Redline et al. 1987, 1989). Modifier genes that regulate the oxidant/antioxidant and proteinase/antiproteinase balances and their interactions are candidates to contribute to susceptibility towards COPD in smokers. Other than congenital deficiencies of α1-antitypsin, which contribute to less than 1–2% of all COPD cases, the genes that determine susceptibility to emphysema are unknown (Sandford and Pare 2000; Sandford et al. 2001). Hence, it is important to elucidate genes and pathways that act as "risk modifiers" for emphysema. Recently, it has been shown that the development of emphysema in response to chronic cigarette smoke exposure in mice is strain dependent (Cavarra et al. 2001; Guerassimov et al. 2004). Factors that have emerged to play a role in susceptibility to emphysema in different mouse strains are α1-antitypsin and sensitivity to oxidants (Cavarra et al. 2001). The ICR strain has been shown to be resistant to cigarette smoke induced-emphysema, whereas the C57BL/6J and the DBA 2/J strains have been shown to be sensitive. These sensitive strains have significantly lower levels of antioxidant defenses. Thus, genetic factors, including Nrf2, that lead to lower antioxidant capacity of lungs may be determinants of susceptibility.

14.5 Nrf2 as a Modifier Gene for Pulmonary Oxidative Stress, Inflammation, and Emphysema

Numerous studies have demonstrated that the susceptibility of the lung to oxidative injury depends largely on the upregulation of protective antioxidant systems (Macnee

2001; Macnee and Rahman 2001). Critical host factors that protect the lungs against oxidative stress may either directly determine susceptibility to alveolar tissue destruction in emphysema or act as modifiers of risk by affecting the intensity of inflammation associated with chronic cigarette smoke inhalation. We have recently reported that disruption of the *nrf2* gene in a genetic background of (emphysema resistant) ICR mice led to early onset, severe emphysema with chronic exposure to cigarette smoke (Rangasamy et al. 2004). Emphysema in *nrf2*-deficient mice exposed to cigarette smoke for 6 months was associated with pronounced bronchoalveolar inflammation (mostly macrophages), enhanced oxidative stress, and apoptosis of alveolar septal cells (Rangasamy et al. 2004).

14.5.1 Nrf2 Protects against Emphysema

As assessed by computer-assisted morphometry, there was a dramatic increase in alveolar destruction in the lungs of *nrf2*-disrupted mice when compared to wild-type ICR mice after 6 months of exposure to cigarette smoke (Fig. 14.2). Both the alveolar diameter and mean linear intercept were significantly higher in smoke exposed *nrf2*-disrupted mice. Alveolar enlargement was detected in the lungs of *nrf2* knockout mice as early as after 3 months of exposure to smoke. The intrinsic resistance of *nrf2* wild-type ICR mice to cigarette smoke-induced pulmonary emphysema was evident from the modest increase (<10%) in the mean linear intercept and alveolar diameter, even after long-term exposure cigarette smoke. Thus, in this model, Nrf2 is critical for resistance to cigarette smoke-induced emphysema. It is noteworthy that *nrf2* knockout mice have also been shown to exhibit enhanced susceptibility to pulmonary damage from hyperoxia (Cho et al. 2002) and chemically induced lung injury (Chan and Kan 1999).

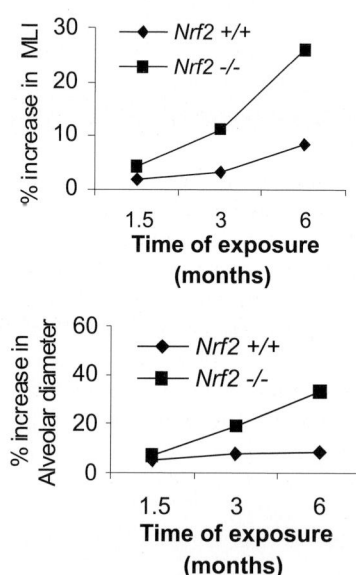

Fig. 14.2 Increased emphysema in nuclear factor erythroid 2-related factor 2 (*nrf2*)-deficient mice. The *nrf2*$^{+/+}$ and *nrf2*$^{-/-}$ mice (*n*=6) were exposed for 1.5–6 months of cigarette smoke. Alveolar diameter and mean linear intercept were measured by computed-assisted morphometry as described in Sect. 14.5.1

14.5.2 Nrf2 Protects against Cigarette Smoke Pulmonary Oxidative Stress and Apoptosis

Consistent with a central role for Nrf2 in the regulation of antioxidant defenses, levels of the oxidative DNA damage product 8-oxo-dG are markedly elevated in the lungs of *nrf2* knockout compared with wild-type mice, following chronic exposure to cigarette smoke. Chronic cigarette smoke also caused increased apoptosis of type II and endothelial cells in the lungs of *nrf2* knockout mice, as evidenced by terminal transferase dUTP nick end labeling (TUNEL) assay and caspase 3 immunostaining (Rangasamy et al. 2004). The presence of enhanced apoptosis in the lungs of *nrf2*-disrupted mice might be related to oxidative stress, inflammation, or excessive lung proteolysis. Oxidative stress and apoptosis are part of a mutually interactive feedback loop in VEGF receptor blockade-induced emphysema (Tuder et al. 2003). Furthermore, reactive oxygen and nitrogen species can modify and inactivate prosurvival cell signaling molecules and cause apoptosis. Inflammation and protease/antiprotease imbalance may also promote apoptosis by means of activated T lymphocytes, which are increased in COPD and seem to correlate with the degree of emphysema (Finkelstein et al. 1995; Majo et al. 2001) and unopposed leukocyte elastase, gelatinase, or collagenase activity. The relation of oxidative stress and apoptosis of lung cells with emphysema is emerging. Apoptosis is required for emphysema caused by VEGF receptor inhibition and is sufficient to cause emphysema (Kasahara et al. 2000; Tang et al. 2004; Tuder et al. 2003), as demonstrated in mice instilled intrabronchially with active caspase 3 (Aoshiba et al. 2003). Recent studies with lung samples derived from emphysema patients have indicated that there is increased apoptosis of alveolar cells (Yokohori et al. 2004). Our studies indicate that Nrf2 could be protecting against emphysema in part by decreasing oxidative stress and the resulting apoptosis of alveolar cells.

14.5.3 Nrf2 Protects against Pulmonary Inflammation

Proteinase/antiproteinase imbalance has been accepted as the most important factor leading to the destruction of the lung during emphysema. Prior and concomitant to airspace enlargement caused by exposure to cigarette smoke, there was increased infiltration of inflammatory cells, predominantly macrophages. These recruited macrophages may have contributed to the alveolar injury through the activity of their elastolytic enzymes, particularly MMP-12. A decrease in the activity and levels of antiproteases may follow the enhanced oxidative stress in our model, and thus contribute to protease/antiprotease imbalance. Studies with hyperoxia and bleomycin as stresses have also shown that Nrf2 protects against pulmonary inflammation. Even though the exact mechanism by which Nrf2 inhibits pulmonary inflammation remains unclear, at least in the cigarette smoke model, the net effect of the Nrf2-regulated pathway is to decrease oxidative stress in the lungs.

14.5.4 Activation of Nrf2 by Cigarette Smoke

Cigarette smoke contains several strong electrophiles such as acrolein, which has been shown to activate Nrf2 in lung cell lines in vitro (Tirumalai et al. 2002). In addition to electrophiles, free radicals and quinones found in smoke can activate Nrf2. Oxidative stresses can also activate several kinases in the lung, which may indirectly contribute to activation of Nrf2. Exposure of ICR mice to acute cigarette smoke (5 h) caused activation of Nrf2 in the lungs, as evident from a gel shift analysis showing increased binding of nuclear proteins to an oligonucleotide containing the ARE sequence (Rangasamy et al. 2004). Increased nuclear accumulation of Nrf2 is critical for the transcriptional activation of ARE-responsive genes. Understanding the targets of Nrf2 should provide insights into how this Keap1-Nrf2-ARE pathway confers protection against oxidative stress and inflammation, and hence, modifies host responses to chronic exposure to cigarette smoke.

14.5.5 Transcriptional Induction of Pulmonary Nrf2 Target Genes after Cigarette Smoke Induction

Comparison of global gene expression profiles in naïve and cigarette smoke-treated wild-type and *nrf2* knockout mice has greatly facilitated the identification of target genes that are directly or indirectly regulated by this transcription factor. Genes differentially expressed in wild-type compared to *nrf2* knockout mice can be assumed to be Nrf2-regulated. Using a microarray approach, we have recently reported that activation of Nrf2 in the lung in response to cigarette smoke leads to transcriptional induction of many different antioxidant and xenobiotic detoxication genes that can attenuate the formation or counteract the damage produced by a broad spectrum of reactive oxygen and reactive nitrogen species (Fig. 14.3) (Rangasamy et al. 2004).

Nrf2, in response to cigarette smoke, regulates genes involved in two major redox systems, the glutathione (GSH) and thioredoxin (Trx) systems. In response to activation of Nrf2 by cigarette smoke, the enzymes involved in GSH synthesis (γ-GCS catalytic and regulatory subunits), members of the GST family, glutathione reductase (GSR), glutathione peroxidases (GPx2, GPx3) and genes that constitute the thioredoxin system (*TrxR* and *Prx1*) were all induced in the lungs of *nrf2* wild-type mice. The members of these redox systems interact with various transducers and effector molecules to bring about antioxidant-specific responses. The regeneration of reduced Trx and GSH by TrxR and GSR, respectively, utilizes NADPH as a reducing equivalent generated by glucose-6-phosphate dehydrogenase (G6PDH) and phosphogluconate dehydrogenase (PGDH), both of which are also induced only in the lungs of wild-type mice. Prx1 and GPx reduce hydroperoxides by utilizing two electrons provided by Trx and GSH, respectively. In addition, GPx and peroxiredoxins have been shown to play a potential role in protection against peroxynitrite, the potent oxidant generated from the reaction of superoxide and nitrous oxide of cigarette smoke. The oxidized forms of GPx and peroxiredoxins are reduced back to their functional forms by Trx. These results suggest important interdependence between the thioredoxin and GSH redox systems and the NADPH generating system.

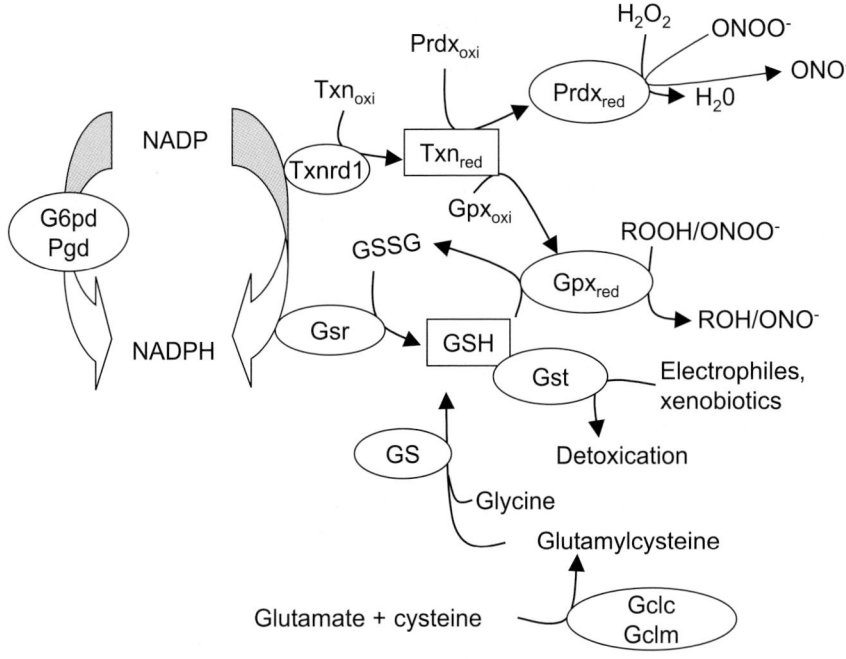

Fig. 14.3 Nuclear factor erythroid 2-related factor 2 (Nrf2)-regulated pulmonary antioxidant pathways

Several GSTs as well as UDP-glucuronosyl transferase (UGT) and NQO1 were selectively induced only in *nrf2* wild-type mice in response to cigarette smoke. Various isoforms of GSTs and UGTs play important roles in the detoxification of tobacco smoke carcinogens such as 4-(methylnitrosamino)-1-(3-pyridyl)-1-butanone, benzo[a]pyrene, and other polycyclic aromatic hydrocarbons that act as electrophiles and cause DNA damage and cytotoxicity. NQO1 blocks redox cycling of polyaromatic hydrocarbons and benzoquinones present in cigarette smoke, thereby reducing the levels of reactive oxygen species and, presumably, oxidative stress and its consequences such as formation of 8-oxo-dG. Various enzymes, including aldehyde dehydrogenase and aldo-keto reductase, which are involved in the detoxification of reactive aldehydes such as acetaldehyde and acrolein, were selectively induced in the lungs of cigarette smoke-exposed *nrf2* wild-type mice. Heme oxygenase 1 (HO-1), a critical enzyme involved in protection against oxidant-mediated cellular injury, as well as the iron sequestering protein, ferritin light chain 1, which prevents uncontrolled surges in the intracellular free concentration of the highly reactive, yet poorly soluble, ferric iron, were induced only in the lungs of cigarette smoke-exposed wild-type mice. Reduction of ferric ion by superoxide can generate reactive hydroxyl radicals via the Fenton reaction. Superoxide dismutase 3, the major extracellular antioxidant enzyme in the lung that attenuates reactive oxygen-mediated lung cell injury and inflammation, is also selectively upregulated in response to cigarette smoke. Other Nrf2-regulated genes included ubiquitin C, a protein involved in the degradation of oxidized proteins, the DNA damage repair protein GADD45G, and lung structural proteins, such as tropoelastin and procollagen type IV, alpha 2, and endomucin 1, sequestosome 1, MafF, and HIF-1α-related factor. One or more AREs in the upstream regions of most of these differentially expressed genes was located, indicating the likelihood of a direct role for Nrf2 in their transcriptional induction (Rangasamy et al. 2004).

14.6 Conclusions

Although oxidative stress, which originates directly from components of cigarette smoke and indirectly via infiltrating inflammatory cells, has been suspected to be involved in the etiopathogenesis of emphysema, there has been limited experimental evidence to support this hypothesis. Genetic manipulation of the Nrf2 pathway in mice has provided a model that indicates that oxidative stress because of cigarette smoke may be a central player in the development of emphysema. Oxidative stress regulates the intensity of alveolar inflammation, the extent of alveolar cell apoptosis, and ultimately, the rate of onset and severity of emphysema. There is now a clear experimental link between

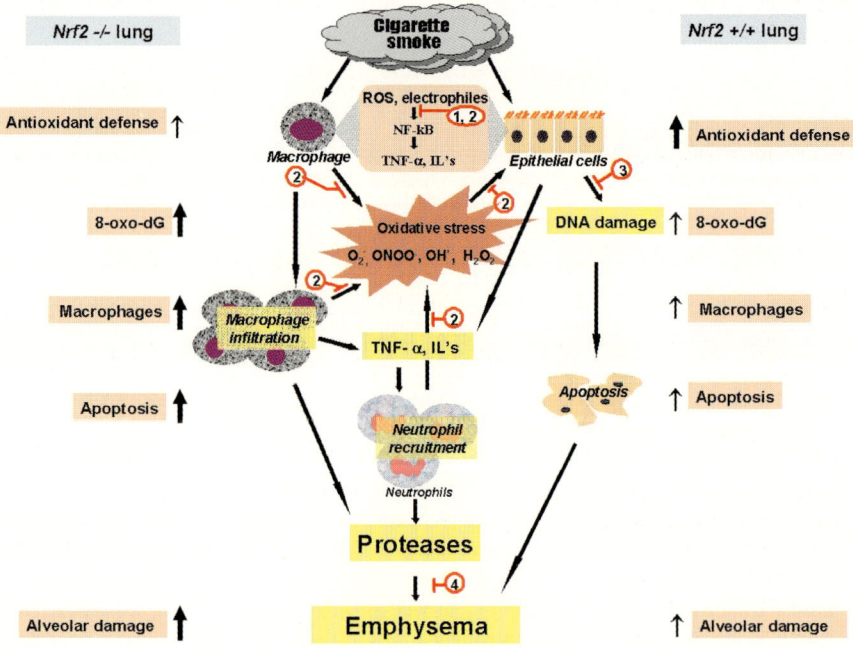

Fig. 14.4 Schematic indicating the increased susceptibility of lungs of nuclear factor erythroid 2-related factor 2 (*nrf2*)-deficient mice to emphysema and probable sites at which Nrf2 targets can block the progression of emphysema. *1* S-transferase (GST), UDP-glucuronosyl transferase (UGT), NAD(P)H: quinone oxidoreductase (NQO1), carboxyl esterase, aldo-keto reductase, antidiuretic hormone (ADH), aldehyde dehydrogenase (ALDH); *2* glutathione peroxidase (GPx), glutathione reductase (GSR), superoxide dismutase 3 (SOD3), pregnane X receptor reductase (PXR), thioredoxin reductase (TXR), glucose-6-phosphate dehydrogenase (G6PDH); *3* DNA damage repair protein GADD45; and *4* antioxidants may decrease inactivation of antiproteinases that inhibit proteases. ▲ High, ▼ Less *3*

excessive oxidative stress, increased apoptosis, inflammation, and worsened emphysema with the functional status of the Keap1-Nrf2-ARE signal transduction pathway. Nrf2 is activated in response to cigarette smoke in the lungs of ICR wild-type mice, leading to transcriptional induction of target genes that provides resistance against the development of emphysema. Conversely, a lack of a responsive Nrf2 pathway confers susceptibility to severe emphysema following exposure to cigarette smoke in the *nrf2* knockout counterpart of this model. As summarized in Fig. 14.4, Nrf2 is a critical transcription factor that determines susceptibility to lung inflammation, oxidative stress, and alveolar cell apoptosis caused by chronic exposure to cigarette smoke. The identification of Nrf2 as a determinant of susceptibility may have wide implications to tobacco smoke-related lung diseases and may serve as a target for interventions that seek to retard or block pulmonary diseases where oxidative stress and inflammation play important roles.

Acknowledgements

This work was supported by NIH grants HL081205 (S.B.), P50 CA58184 (S.B.), NIEHS center grant P30 ES 03819, The Maryland Cigarette Restitution Fund (S.B.) and Flight Attendant Medical Research Institute (S.B.); R01 CA94076 (T.W. K.). We thank Dr. Rajesh Thimmulappa for the schematics.

References

Aoshiba K, Yokohori N, Nagai A (2003) Alveolar wall apoptosis causes lung destruction and emphysematous changes. Am J Respir Cell Mol Biol 28:555–562
Barnes PJ (2000) Mechanisms in COPD: differences from asthma. Chest 117:S10–S14
Blanchard AR (2003) Treatment of acute exacerbations of COPD. Clin Cornerstone 5:28–36
Cavarra E, Bartalesi B, Lucattelli M, Fineschi S, Lunghi B, Gambelli F, Ortiz LA, Martorana PA, Lungarella G (2001) Effects of cigarette smoke in mice with different levels of alpha$_1$-proteinase inhibitor and sensitivity to oxidants. Am J Respir Crit Care Med 164:886–890
Chan K, Kan YW (1999) Nrf2 is essential for protection against acute pulmonary injury in mice. Proc Natl Acad Sci U S A 96:12731–12736
Chan K, Han XD, Kan YW (2001) An important function of Nrf2 in combating oxidative stress: detoxification of acetaminophen. Proc Natl Acad Sci U S A 98:4611–4616
Cho HY, Jedlicka AE, Reddy SP, Kensler TW, Yamamoto M, Zhang LY, Kleeberger SR (2002) Role of NRF2 in protection against hyperoxic lung injury in mice. Am J Respir Cell Mol Biol 26:175–182
Church DF, Pryor WA (1985) Free-radical chemistry of cigarette smoke and its toxicological implications. Environ Health Perspect 64:111–126
Churg A, Wang RD, Tai H, Wang X, Xie C, Dai J, Shapiro SD, Wright JL (2003) Macrophage metalloelastase mediates acute cigarette smoke-induced inflammation via tumor necrosis factor-alpha release. Am J Respir Crit Care Med 167:1083–1089
Dinkova-Kostova AT, Holtzclaw WD, Cole RN, Itoh K, Wakabayashi N, Katoh Y, Yamamoto M, Talalay P (2002) Direct evidence that sulfhydryl groups of Keap1 are the sensors regulating induction of phase 2 enzymes that protect against carcinogens and oxidants. Proc Natl Acad Sci U S A 99:11908–11913
Finkelstein R, Fraser RS, Ghezzo H, Cosio MG (1995) Alveolar inflammation and its relation to emphysema in smokers. Am J Respir Crit Care Med 152:1666–1672

Fletcher C, Peto R (1977) The natural history of chronic airflow obstruction. Br Med J 1:1645–1648

Guerassimov A, Hoshino Y, Takubo Y, Turcotte A, Yamamoto M, Ghezzo H, Triantafillopoulos A, Whittaker K, Hoidal JR, Cosio MG (2004) The development of emphysema in cigarette smoke-exposed mice is strain dependent. Am J Respir Crit Care Med 170:974–980

Hautamaki RD, Kobayashi DK, Senior RM, Shapiro SD (1997) Requirement for macrophage elastase for cigarette smoke-induced emphysema in mice. Science 277:2002–2004

Hogg JC (2004) Pathophysiology of airflow limitation in chronic obstructive pulmonary disease. Lancet 364:709–721

Horvath I, MacNee W, Kelly FJ, Dekhuijzen PN, Phillips M, Doring G, Choi AM, Yamaya M, Bach FH, Willis D, Donnelly LE, Chung KF, Barnes PJ (2001) "Haemoxygenase-1 induction and exhaled markers of oxidative stress in lung diseases," summary of the ERS Research Seminar in Budapest, Hungary, September, 1999. Eur Respir J 18:420–430

Itoh K, Chiba T, Takahashi S, Ishii T, Igarashi K, Katoh Y, Oyake T, Hayashi N, Satoh K, Hatayama I, Yamamoto M, Nabeshima Y (1997) An Nrf2/small Maf heterodimer mediates the induction of phase II detoxifying enzyme genes through antioxidant response elements. Biochem Biophys Res Commun 236:313–322

Itoh K, Wakabayashi N, Katoh Y, Ishii T, Igarashi K, Engel JD, Yamamoto M (1999) Keap1 represses nuclear activation of antioxidant responsive elements by Nrf2 through binding to the amino-terminal Neh2 domain. Genes Dev 13:76–86

Itoh K, Wakabayashi N, Katoh Y, Ishii T, O'Connor T, Yamamoto M (2003) Keap1 regulates both cytoplasmic-nuclear shuttling and degradation of Nrf2 in response to nucleophiles. Genes Cells 8:379–391

Kasahara Y, Tuder RM, Taraseviciene-Stewart L, Le Cras TD, Abman S, Hirth PK, Waltenberger J, Voelkel NF (2000) Inhibition of VEGF receptors causes lung cell apoptosis and emphysema. J Clin Invest 106:1311–1319

Keatings VM, Collins PD, Scott DM, Barnes PJ (1996) Differences in interleukin-8 and tumor necrosis factor-alpha in induced sputum from patients with chronic obstructive pulmonary disease or asthma. Am J Respir Crit Care Med 153:530–534

Kwak MK, Itoh K, Yamamoto M, Kensler TW (2002) Enhanced expression of the transcription factor Nrf2 by cancer chemopreventive agents: role of antioxidant response element-like sequences in the nrf2 promoter. Mol Cell Biol 22:2883–2892

MacNee W (2001) Oxidative stress and lung inflammation in airways disease. Eur J Pharmacol 429:195–207

MacNee W, Rahman I (2001) Is oxidative stress central to the pathogenesis of chronic obstructive pulmonary disease? Trends Mol Med 7:55–62

Majo J, Ghezzo H, Cosio MG (2001) Lymphocyte population and apoptosis in the lungs of smokers and their relation to emphysema. Eur Respir J 17:946–953

McClearn GE, Svartengren M, Pedersen NL, Heller DA, Plomin R (1994) Genetic and environmental influences on pulmonary function in aging Swedish twins. J Gerontol 49:264–268

Morris DG, Huang X, Kaminski N, Wang Y, Shapiro SD, Dolganov G, Glick A, Sheppard D (2003) Loss of integrin alpha,beta6-mediated TGF-beta activation causes Mmp12-dependent emphysema. Nature 422:169–173

Nioi P, McMahon M, Itoh K, Yamamoto M, Hayes JD (2003) Identification of a novel Nrf2-regulated antioxidant response element (ARE) in the mouse NAD(P)H:quinone oxidoreductase 1 gene: reassessment of the ARE consensus sequence. Biochem J 374:337–348

Pryor WA, Stone K (1993) Oxidants in cigarette smoke. Radicals, hydrogen peroxide, peroxynitrate, and peroxynitrite. Ann N Y Acad Sci 686:1–27; discussion 27–18

Rahman I, MacNee W (1996) Role of oxidants/antioxidants in smoking-induced lung diseases. Free Radic Biol Med 21:669–681

Rahman I, MacNee W (1998) Role of transcription factors in inflammatory lung diseases. Thorax 53:601–612

Rahman I, Gilmour PS, Jimenez LA, MacNee W (2002) Oxidative stress and TNF-alpha induce histone acetylation and NF-kappaB/AP-1 activation in alveolar epithelial cells: potential mechanism in gene transcription in lung inflammation. Mol Cell Biochem 234-235:239–248

Rahman I, Morrison D, Donaldson K, MacNee W (1996) Systemic oxidative stress in asthma, COPD, and smokers. Am J Respir Crit Care Med 154:1055–1060

Rahman I, van Schadewijk AA, Crowther AJ, Hiemstra PS, Stolk J, MacNee W, De Boer WI (2002) 4-Hydroxy-2-nonenal, a specific lipid peroxidation product, is elevated in lungs of patients with chronic obstructive pulmonary disease. Am J Respir Crit Care Med 166:490–495

Rangasamy T, Cho CY, Thimmulappa RK, Zhen L, Srisuma SS, Kensler TW, Yamamoto M, Petrache I, Tuder RM, Biswal S (2004) Genetic ablation of Nrf2 enhances susceptibility to cigarette smoke-induced emphysema in mice. J Clin Invest 114:1248–1259

Redline S, Tishler PV, Lewitter FI, Tager IB, Munoz A, Speizer FE (1987) Assessment of genetic and nongenetic influences on pulmonary function. A twin study. Am Rev Respir Dis 135:217–222

Redline S, Tishler PV, Rosner B, Lewitter FI, Vandenburgh M, Weiss ST, Speizer FE (1989) Genotypic and phenotypic similarities in pulmonary function among family members of adult monozygotic and dizygotic twins. Am J Epidemiol 129:827–836

Sandford AJ, Pare PD (2000) Genetic risk factors for chronic obstructive pulmonary disease. Clin Chest Med 21:633–643

Sandford AJ, Chagani T, Weir TD, Connett JE, Anthonisen NR, Pare PD (2001) Susceptibility genes for rapid decline of lung function in the lung health study. Am J Respir Crit Care Med 163:469–473

Shapiro SD (1999) The macrophage in chronic obstructive pulmonary disease. Am J Respir Crit Care Med 160:S29–S32

Shapiro SD, Goldstein NM, Houghton AM, Kobayashi DK, Kelley D, Belaaouaj A (2003) Neutrophil elastase contributes to cigarette smoke-induced emphysema in mice. Am J Pathol 163:2329–2335

Tang K, Rossiter HB, Wagner PD, Breen EC (2004) Lung-targeted VEGF inactivation leads to an emphysema phenotype in mice. J Appl Physiol 97:1559–1566; discussion 1549

Thimmulappa RK, Mai KH, Srisuma S, Kensler TW, Yamamoto M, Biswal S (2002) Identification of Nrf2-regulated genes induced by the chemopreventive agent sulforaphane by oligonucleotide microarray. Cancer Res 62:5196–5203

Tirumalai R, Rajesh Kumar T, Mai KH, Biswal S (2002) Acrolein causes transcriptional induction of phase II genes by activation of Nrf2 in human lung type II epithelial (A549) cells. Toxicol Lett 132:27–36

Tuder RM, Zhen L, Cho CY, Taraseviciene-Stewart L, Kasahara Y, Salvemini D, Voelkel NF, Flores SC (2003) Oxidative stress and apoptosis interact and cause emphysema due to vascular endothelial growth factor receptor blockade. Am J Respir Cell Mol Biol 29:88–97

Viegi G, Scognamiglio A, Baldacci S, Pistelli F, Carrozzi L (2001) Epidemiology of chronic obstructive pulmonary disease (COPD). Respiration 68:4–19

Wakabayashi N, Itoh K, Wakabayashi J, Motohashi H, Noda S, Takahashi S, Imakado S, Kotsuji T, Otsuka F, Roop DR, Harada T, Engel JD, Yamamoto M (2003) Keap1-null mutation leads to postnatal lethality due to constitutive Nrf2 activation. Nat Genet 35:202–204

Wakabayashi N, Dinkova-Kostova AT, Holtzclaw WD, Kang MI, Kobayashi A, Yamamoto M, Kensler TW, Talalay P (2004) Protection against electrophile and oxidant stress by induction of the phase 2 response: fate of cysteines of the Keap1 sensor modified by inducers. Proc Natl Acad Sci U S A 101:2040–2045

Yokohori N, Aoshiba K, Nagai A (2004) Increased levels of cell death and proliferation in alveolar wall cells in patients with pulmonary emphysema. Chest 125:626–632

Zang LY, Stone K, Pryor WA (1995) Detection of free radicals in aqueous extracts of cigarette tar by electron spin resonance. Free Radic Biol Med 19:161–167

Zheng T, Zhu Z, Wang Z, Homer RJ, Ma B, Riese RJ Jr, Chapman HA Jr, Shapiro SD, Elias JA (2000) Inducible targeting of IL-13 to the adult lung causes matrix metalloproteinase- and cathepsin-dependent emphysema. J Clin Invest 106:1081–109

Chapter 15

Tobacco Smoke and Skin Aging

Akimichi Morita

Contents

15.1	Epidemiological Study	380
15.2	Molecular Mechanisms of Tobacco Smoke-Induced Skin Aging	380
15.2.1	Effects of Tobacco Smoke on Skin Models In Vitro	381
15.2.3	Effect of Tobacco Smoke In Vivo	381
15.3.	Some Molecular Mechanisms and Protective Factors	382
15.4.	Conclusions	383
	References	383

15.1 Epidemiological Study

As early as 1971, Daniell (1971) found that tobacco smoking has a deleterious effect on the skin, and smoker's wrinkles are typical clinical features of smokers. A recent epidemiological study has clearly shown that tobacco smoking is one of the numerous factors contributing to premature skin aging, which is dependent on age, sex, pigmentation, sun exposure history, alcohol consumption, and other factors (Ernster et al. 1995; Frances 1998; Grady and Ernster 1992; Kadunce et al. 1991). In a further cross-section study, sun exposure, pack years of smoking history, and potential confounding variables were assessed by questionnaire. Facial wrinkles were quantified using the Daniell score. Logistic statistic analysis of the data revealed that age, pack year, and sun exposure independently contributed to facial wrinkle formation (Yin et al. 2001a). In this survey, age (OR = 7.5, 95% CI = 1.87–30.16), pack year (OR = 5.8, 95% CI = 1.72–19.87), and sun exposure (OR = 2.65, 95% CI = 1.0–7.0) were independently contributing to the facial wrinkles, as estimated by a logistic regression analysis model. Using silicone rubber replicas combined with computerized image processing, an objective measurement of skin's topography, the association between wrinkle formation and tobacco smoking was investigated. Sixty-three volunteers were enrolled by assessing their skin replicas and in an attempt to elucidate the association between tobacco smoking and wrinkles (Yin et al. 2001b). The replica analysis showed that the depth (R_z) and variance (R_v) of furrows (R_v) in subjects with smoking history ≥35 pack years were significantly higher than nonsmokers ($p<0.05$). The lines of furrows (R_l) in subjects with smoking history were significantly lower than nonsmokers ($p<0.05$) (Yin et al. 2000a; 2001b).

Tobacco smoking, which is regarded as another an important environmental factor, can potentially cause "tobacco wrinkles" (Daniell 1971), although chronic exposure of skin to ultraviolet (UV) radiation results in marked alterations in the structure and composition of the epidermis and dermis, i.e., photoaging (Fisher et al. 1999; Grether-Beck 1997; Wenk et al. 2001). In a recent study, tobacco smoking per se or when smoking combined with UV exposure were strong predictors of skin aging (Leung and Harvey 2002).

15.2 Molecular Mechanisms of Tobacco Smoke-Induced Skin Aging

Tobacco smoking probably exerts its deleterious effects on skin directly through its irritant components on the epidermis and indirectly on the dermis via the blood circulation (Frances 1998; Lofroth 1989). The decreased stratum corneum moisture of the face contributes to facial wrinkling because of the direct toxicity of the smoke. Pursing the lips during smoking with contraction of facial muscles and squinting because of the irritating of smoke may cause the formation of wrinkling around the mouth and in the crow's foot area (Smith and Fenske 1996). The changes in the dermis of macromolecular metabolism have been brought into focus as a major factor leading to skin aging (Uitto et al. 1989). Specifically, it has been demonstrated that accumulation of elastosis material is accompanied by degradation of matrix protein, which is mediated by matrix metalloproteinases (MMPs) in skin aging. The molecular alteration in the dermis includes the decrease of collagen synthesis, induction of MMPs, abnormal accumulation of elastic fibers, and proteoglycans (Fisher and Voorhees 1998; Shuster 2001; Yin et al. 2000b).

15.2.1 Effects of Tobacco Smoke on Skin Models In Vitro

The biosynthesis of new collagen was decreased significantly by tobacco smoke extracts in cultured skin fibroblasts (Yin et al. 2006). The studies also showed that the production of both procollagen types I and III, the precursors of collagen, were significantly decreased from the supernatant of cultured fibroblast treated with tobacco smoke extracts, using Western blot analysis (Yin et al. 2006). This result indicated that the final production of collagen secreted into the medium as reduced, regardless of the rate of collagen synthesis in the cell tested in ^{3}H-proline incorporation.

Although elastic fibers account for only 2–4% of extracellular matrix, these provide elasticity and resilience to normal skin. Tobacco smoke extracts induced the significant increase in tropoelastin mRNA in cultured skin fibroblasts. Accumulation of abnormal elastic material (termed solar elastosis) is the prominent histopathologic alterations in photoaged skin (Montagna et al. 1989; Tsuji 1987). Boyd et al. (1999) reported that tobacco smoking could facilitate smoke's elastosis of the subjects with an average of 42 pack years of tobacco smoking. In an in vitro study using cultured skin fibroblasts, tobacco smoke extracts induced elevation of tropoelastin. This might be attributed to premature skin aging.

The expressions of *MMP-1* and *MMP-3* mRNA, extracellular matrix (ECM)-associated members of the MMPs gene family, were induced in cultured skin fibroblast stimulated with tobacco smoke extracts in a dose-dependent manner (Yin et al. 2000b). These results support the concept that MMPs are primary mediators of connective tissue damage in skin exposed to tobacco smoke extracts and of the premature skin aging. In addition, expression of *TIMP-1* and *TIMP-3* remained unchanged (Yin et al. 2000b). By inducing the expressions of *MMP-1* and *MMP-3*, but not the induction of tissue inhibitor of MMPs, tobacco smoke extracts could alter their ratio in favor of the induction of MMPs and appears to result in a more degradative environment that produces loss of cutaneous collagen (Yin et al. 2000b). In addition, MMPs comprise a family of degradative enzymes, which are responsible for the degradation of extracellular matrix components such as native collagen, elastin fibers, and various proteoglycans. MMP-3 and MMP-7 may play a key role in the degradation of elastin and proteoglycans (Saarialho-Kere et al. 1999). MMP-7 was increased in fibroblasts induced by tobacco smoke extract.

15.2.3 Effect of Tobacco Smoke In Vivo

In a clinical study, significant higher levels of MMP-1 mRNA were observed in the buttock skin of smokers, compared with nonsmokers, using quantitative real-time PCR (Lahmann et al. 2001). The elevated enzyme should lead to the degradation of collagen, elastic fibers, and proteoglycans. Therefore, the observations in dermal connective tissue induced by the treatments of tobacco suggested an imbalance between the biosynthesis and degradation, with less repair capacity on the face of the ongoing degradation, which leads to loss of collagen and elastic fibers, manifesting clinically as aging appearance of skin.

Although staining of skin specimen and biochemical analysis of photodamaged skin demonstrated increased glycosaminoglycan content of sun-damaged skin, the underlying molecular pathogenesis remains unclear. Versican, the large chondroitin sulfate (CS) proteoglycan, has been identified in the dermis in association with elastic fibers, which contain a hyaluronic acid-binding domain. The core protein has been postulated to play a role in molecular interactions and specifically, to facilitate the binding of these macromolecules to other matrix components or cytokines such as transforming growth factor (TGF) (Fisher et al. 1989). Decorin, a small CS proteoglycan, has been shown to codistribute with collagen fibers and postulated to function in cell recognition, possible by connecting extracellular matrix components and cell surface glycoproteins (Zimmermann and Ruoslahti 1989). Targeted disruption of decorin synthesis in mice resulted in a significant reduction in the tensile strength of skin (Danielson et al. 1997). There was a decrease in the proportion of large chondroitin sulfate proteoglycan (versican) and a concomitant increase in the proportion of small dermatan sulfate proteoglycan (decorin) as a function of age as reported by Carrino et al. (2000). Ito et al. (2001) also observed that versican was stained strongly in young rats and faintly in old rats. On the other hand, decorin was faintly stained in the young rats and distinctly stained in the old rats. There were several reports concerning the changes of proteoglycans on photoaging, especially UVB irradiation (Bernstein et al. 1995; Margelin et al. 1993). The analysis of new synthesized proteoglycans showed a marked increase after UVB radiation in mice (Margelin et al. 1993). Versican and decorin immunostaining increased in photoaged tissue samples, accompanied by similar alterations in gene expression (Bernstein et al. 1995). Tobacco smoke extracts decreased both versican protein and mRNA levels in cultured akin fibroblasts. However, tobacco smoke extract exposure resulted in a significant increase of decorin. These results have a similar to those observed in photoaging.

15.3. Some Molecular Mechanisms and Protective Factors

Based on experimental evidence, a working model for UVA damage skin was proposed in which UV irradiation gene expression was mediated via the generation of singlet oxygen through a pathway involving activation of transcription factor AP-2 (Grether-Beck 1997). In order to define whether the reactive oxygen species (ROS) were involved in upregulation of MMPs induced by tobacco, sodium azide (NaN_3), L-ascorbic acid, and vitamin E, which are potent quenchers of singlet oxygen and other ROS, were employed. NaN_3, L-ascorbic acid, and vitamin E abrogated the induction of MMPs after exposure of fibroblast to tobacco smoke extract. Among the antioxidant reagents, L-ascorbic acid most obviously diminished the increase in MMP-1 expression level on exposure of fibroblasts to tobacco smoke extracts (Yin et al. 2000b). This points at that ROS were most probable responsible for the enhanced induction of MMPs by tobacco smoke extract.

The transforming growth factor-β1 (TGF-β1) is a multifunctional cytokine that regulates cell proliferation and differentiation, tissue remodeling, and repair (Massague 1998). TGF-β1 is a potent growth inhibitor in the epidermis, playing an important role in maintenance of tissue homeostasis. In the dermis, however, TGF-β1 acts as a positive growth factor, inducing the synthesis of extracellular matrix proteins. TGF-β signals through a heteromeric complex of type I/II TGF-β receptors, which initiate signal transduction (Kadin 1994; Piek 1999). A recent report showed that UV irradiation can cause downregulation of TGF-β type II receptor mRNA and protein, and induction of Smad7 mRNA and protein in human skin (Quan et al. 2001).

Tobacco smoke extracts induced the latent form TGF-β, not the active form, assayed by enzyme-linked immunosorbent assay (ELISA), in the supernatants of cultured skin fibroblasts (Yin et al. 2003). The induction of endogenous TGF-β1 from tobacco-exposed cells contributes to the intracellular defense capacity. Fibroblasts responses to TGF-β1 are mediated through its active form binding to the cell surface receptor. Tobacco smoke extracts blocked cellular responsiveness to TGF-β1 through the induction of nonfunctional latent form and downregulation of TGF-β1 receptor (Yin et al. 2003). Exogenous addition of TGF-β1 might be useful to stimulate the collagen production or to protect against the deleterious effects of tobacco smoke.

15.4. Conclusions

Tobacco smoke contains numerous compounds, with at least 3,800 constituents (Batsch et al. 1993). Just which constituents that contributed to the damage of connective tissue are still unclear. The tobacco-induced skin aging provides a tool for studying the effects of smoking. Also, detailed knowledge may provide a motivation to stop smoking, especially among those who are more concerned about their appearances than the potential internal damage associated with smoking.

References

Bartsch H, Malaveille C, Friesen M, Kadlubar FF, Vineis P (1993) Black (air-cured) and blond (flue-cured) tobacco cancer risk IV: molecular dosimetry studies implicate aromatic amines as bladder carcinogens. Eur J Cancer 29A:1199–1207

Bernstein EF, Fisher LW, Li K, LeBaron RG, Tan EM, Uitto J (1995) Differential expression of the versican and decorin genes in photoaged and sun-protected skin: comparison by immunohistochemical and northern analyses. Lab Invest 72662–669

Boyd AS, Stasko T, King LE Jr, Cameron GS, Pearse AD, Gaskell SA (1999) Cigarette smoking-associated elastotic changes in the skin. J Am Acad Dermatol 41:23–26

Carrino DA, Sorrell JM, Caplan AI (2000) Age-related changes in the proteoglycans of human skin. Arch Biochem Biophys 373:91–101

Daniell HW (1971) Smoker's wrinkles. A study in the epidemiology of "crow's feet." Ann Intern Med 75:873–880.

Danielson KG, Baribault H, Homes DF, Graham H, Kadler KE, Iozzo RV (1997) Targeted disruption of decorin leads to abnormal collagen fibril morphology and skin fragility. J Cell Biol 136:729–743

Ernster VL, Grady D, Miike R, Black D, Selby J, Kerlikowske K (1995) Facial wrinkling in men and women, by smoking status. Am J Public Health 85:78–82

Fisher GJ, Talwar HS, Lin J, Voorhees JJ (1999) Molecular mechanisms of photoaging in human skin in vivo and their prevention by all-*trans*-retinoic acid. Photochem Photobiol 69:154–157

Fisher GJ, Voorhees JJ (1998) Molecular mechanisms of photoaging and its prevention by retinoic acid: ultraviolet irradiation induces MAP kinase signal transduction cascades that induce Ap-1-regulated matrix metalloproteinases that degrade human skin in vivo. J Investig Dermatol Symp Proc 3:61–68

Fisher LW, Termine JD, Young MF (1989) Deduced protein sequence of bone small proteoglycan I (biglycan) shows homology with proteoglycan II (decorin) and several nonconnective tissue proteins in a variety of species. J Biol Chem 264:4571–4576

Frances C (1998) Smoker's wrinkles: epidemiological and pathogenic considerations. Clin Dermatol 16:565–570

Grady D, Ernster V (1992) Does cigarette smoking make you ugly and old? Am J Epidemiol 135:839–842

Grether-Beck S, Buettner R, Krutmann J (1997) Ultraviolet A radiation-induced expression of human genes: molecular and photobiological mechanisms. Biol Chem 378:1231–1236

Ito Y, Takeuchi J, Yamamoto K, Hashizume Y, Sato T, Tauchi H (2001) Age differences in immunohistochemical localizations of large proteoglycan, PG-M/versican, and small proteoglycan, decorin, in the dermis of rats. Exp Anim 50:159–166

Kadin ME, Cavaille-Coll MW, Gertz R, Massague J, Cheifetz S, George D (1994) Loss of receptors for transforming growth factor beta in human T-cell malignancies. Proc Natl Acad Sci U S A 91:6002–6006

Kadunce DP, Burr R, Gress R, Kanner R, Lyon JL, Zone JJ (1991) Cigarette smoking: risk factor for premature facial wrinkling. Ann Intern Med 114:840–844

Lahmann C, Bergemann J, Harrison G, Young AR (2001) Matrix metalloprotease-1 and skin ageing in smokers. Lancet 357:935–936

Leung W-C, Harvey I (2002) Is skin ageing in the elderly caused by sun exposure or smoking? Br J Dermatol 147:1187–1191

Lofroth G (1989) Environmental tobacco smoke: overview of chemical composition and genotoxic components. Mutat Res 222:73–80

Margelin D, Fourtanier A, Thevenin T, Medaisko C, Breton M, Picard J (1993) Alterations of proteoglycans in ultraviolet-irradiated skin. Photochem Photobiol 58:211–218

Massague J (1998) TGF-beta signal transduction. Annu Rev Biochem 67:753–791

Montagna W, Kirchner S, Carlisle K (1989) Histology of sun-damaged human skin. J Am Acad Dermatol 21:907–918

Piek E, Heldin CH, Ten Dijke P (1999) Specificity, diversity, and regulation in TGF-beta superfamily signaling. FASEB J 13:2105–2124

Quan T, He T, Voorhees JJ, Fisher GJ (2001) Ultraviolet irradiation blocks cellular responses to transforming growth factor-beta by down-regulating its type-II receptor and inducing Smad. J Biol Chem 276:26349–26356

Saarialho-Kere U, Kerkela E, Jeskanen L et al (2001) Accumulation of matrilysin (MMP-7) and macrophage metalloelastase (MMP-12) in actinic damage. J Invest Dermatol 113:664–672

Shuster S (2001) Smoking and wrinkling of the skin. Lancet 358:330

Smith JB, Fenske NA (1996) Cutaneous manifestations and consequences of smoking. J Am Acad Dermatol 34:717–732

Tsuji T (1989) Ultrastucture of deep wrinkles in the elderly. J Cutan Pathol 14:158–164

Uitto J, Fazio MJ, Olsen DR (1989) Molecular mechanisms of cutaneous aging. Age-associated connective tissue alterations in the dermis. J Am Acad Dermatol 21:614–622

Wenk J, Brenneisen P, Meewes C et al (2001) UV-induced oxidative stress and photoaging. Curr Probl Dermatol 29:83–94

Yin L, Morita A, Tsuji T (2000a) Tobacco smoking: a role of premature skin aging. Nagoya Med J 43:165–171

Yin L, Morita A, Tsuji T (2001b) Skin premature aging induced by tobacco smoking: the objective evidence of skin replica analysis. J Dermatol Sci 2001b; 27 Suppl 1:S26-31

Yin L, Morita A, Tsuji T (2001a) Skin aging induced by ultraviolet exposure and tobacco smoking: evidence from epidemiological and molecular studies. Photodermatol Photoimmunol Photomed 17:178–183

Yin L, Morita A, Tsuji T (2000b) Alterations of extracelluar matrix induced by tobacco smoke extract. Arch Dermatol Res 292:188–194

Yin L, Morita A, Tsuji T (2003) Tobacco smoke extract induces age-related changes due to the modulation of TGF-β, Exp Dermatol 12:51–56

Zimmermann DR, Ruoslahti E (1989) Multiple domains of the large fibroblast proteoglycan, versican. EMBO J 8:2975–2981

Chapter 16

Cigarette Smoke and Oxidative DNA Modification

Henrik E. Poulsen, Allan Weimann, and Barry B. Halliwell

Contents

16.1.	Introduction	388
16.2	Nature and Extent of Oxidative DNA Modifications in DNA	388
16.3	Urinary Excretion of Oxidatively Modified DNA Components	390
16.4	Analysis of Oxidative DNA Lesions	391
16.4.1	Specific Chemical Analysis	391
16.4.2	Nonspecific Analysis	392
16.4.2.1	The Comet Assay	392
16.4.2.2	Alkaline Elution	393
16.4.2.3	Immunological-Based Methods	393
16.5	Planning In Vivo Experiments to Investigate Oxidative DNA Lesions: Design Considerations	394
16.6	Some Aspects of DNA Repair of Oxidative Modifications	394
16.7	How Important Are Oxidative DNA Lesions for the Causal Relation between Cigarette Smoke and Development of Cancer and Other Diseases?	395
	References	396

16.1. Introduction

In this chapter, we give an overview of the nature of oxidative DNA modification, which factors are of importance for oxidation and repair of DNA, how to analyze the lesions and avoid pitfalls of oxidation, how to set up experiments, and how to interpret such experiments. We end up with an evaluation about the degree to which we can associate oxidative DNA modifications with cancer, particularly in relation to cigarette smoking.

In 1992, Leandersson and Tagesson (1992) showed that cigarette smoke increased DNA damage in cultured human lung cells, and at the same time our group showed that cigarette smoking induced increased DNA modification in humans (Loft et al. 1992), measured by urinary excretion of 8-hydroxy-2'-deoxyguanosine (8oxodG); this lesion is the most examined prototype of oxidative DNA modification. Later we showed that smoking cessation reduced DNA modification. Hiroshi Kasai's group (1997) showed that cigarette smoking induces an increase in 8-hydroxydeoxyguanosine in a central site of the lung. Taken together, these findings provide strong evidence that cigarette smoking induces oxidative stress to DNA in the form of increased oxidative base modification.

The area of oxidative DNA modification has particularly been promoted by the pioneers in this area: Hiroshi Kasai, who was the first to report the 8-hydroxy-2'-deoxyguanosine modification in 1984 (Kasai and Nishimura 1984), based on studies on mutagens in heated glucose, and Robert Floyd, who reported that this lesion could be measured by high-performance liquid chromatography (HPLC) with electrochemical detection (Floyd et al. 1986). In an excellent review in 1997, Hiroshi Kasai listed most of the reports about findings in different organs and diseases (Kasai 1997).

Bruce Ames promoted the relationship between oxidative DNA modification and aging, and also the relationship to the antioxidant intake (Ames 1989a, b; Ames et al. 1993), and hypothesized that micronutrient deficiency was a major cause of cancer (Ames 2001).

16.2 Nature and Extent of Oxidative DNA Modifications in DNA

The elucidation of the chemical nature of DNA oxidation was done by the pioneering work of Miral Dizdaroglu (Dizdaroglu 1985, 1991, 1993, 1994; Dizdaroglu and Bergtold 1986; Dizdaroglu et al. 2002) and Jean Cadet (Cadet and Treoule 1978; Cadet et al. 1986, 2003, 2005), preceded by the first report of the 8oxodG modification in 1984 (Kasai and Nishimura 1984).

Oxidation can modify DNA in several positions, in the purine/pyrimidine moiety as well as in the sugar moiety in almost any part of the molecule. After the initial oxidative modification, further rearrangements/changes can occur. For example, the initial modification of guanine can form the C8-OH radical of guanine, which can undergo ring opening, forming the Fapy (2,6-diamino-4-hydroxy-5-formamidopyrimidine) or forming the 8-oxo form dependent on the redox conditions in the reaction mixture or in cells. In total, the reported number of different possible modifications to DNA from oxidation is close to 100; however, only a few of these have been demonstrated in the in vivo situation (Cadet et al. 1997, 2003; Dizdaroglu 1991,1994; Guetens et al. 2002; Schram 1998).

With regard to oxidative modifications because of cigarette smoke, there are no reports of specific oxidative adducts, rather the reports unanimously indicate an increase in preexisting modifications. On the other hand, the literature is mainly focused on the 8oxodG lesion, so it is not known for certain if tobacco smoke gives a specific pattern of oxidation. The reported levels of 8oxodG in nuclear DNA vary over a vide range but may be about 1–10 per million dGs, as expected because 8oxodG is repaired very fast (Asami et al. 1996, 1997; Halliwell 2002; Spencer et al. 1996). In comparison, the levels of polycyclic aromatic hydrocarbon-derived adducts are about 1–10 per 100 million nucleotides (Farmer and Shuker 1999; Godschalk et al. 2002), i.e., about 100 times less frequent. However, as pointed out in an excellent review of smoking-related DNA adducts in a variety of human tissues (Phillips 2002), the half-life of polycyclic aromatic hydrocarbon-derived adducts in the lung is about 1–2 years. In animals exposed to oxidative stress the levels of, e.g., liver 8oxodG returns to normal values within 24 h (Deng et al. 1998), indicating an elimination half-life of some hours. In cellular systems, elimination half-lives of various types of oxidative damage range from minutes to hours. Some studies suggest that oxidized purines are eliminated faster than oxidized pyrimidines (Spencer et al. 1996); other investigators report the reverse (Jaruga and Dizdaroglu 1996). Injected 8oxodG is eliminated with at half-life of few hours into urine (Loft et al. 1995), and after smoking cessation, urinary excretion of 8oxodG decreases within weeks (Prieme et al. 1998a).

Exposure to environmental tobacco smoke in the workplace resulted in a 63% increase in white blood cell DNA 8oxodG levels. The same study included a nonrandomized and noncontrolled intervention showing that the high 8oxodG levels were mitigated by antioxidant supplementation (Howard et al. 1998b). In another study on occupational exposure of metal fume and residual oil fly ash, urinary excretion of 8oxodG was higher in nonsmokers than in smokers (Mukherjee et al. 2004) at the beginning of the work week, but after 2 days of work, the excretion rates were identical.

Taken together, it appears that oxidative lesions are much more frequent than polycyclic aromatic hydrocarbon (PAH)-derived adducts, i.e., with several orders of magnitude, and that the repair of the PAH adducts occurs with a much slower half-life. In this situation, it is very difficult to infer which of the adducts are most important for carcinogenesis, because all the adducts/modifications show mutagenic properties; rather, such information should rely on the predictive values of the lesions in prospective studies, e.g., case-control or cohort studies. Such studies are not presently published (reviewed by Halliwell 2002).

With the use of the Comet assay, a long list of studies has shown increased DNA modification in lymphocytes from smokers compared with nonsmokers (Einhaus et al. 1994; Holz et al. 1993; Lam et al. 2002; Park and Kang 2004; Piperakis et al. 1998; Poli et al. 1999; Welch et al. 1999; Zhu et al. 1999), in lung, stomach, and liver of mice exposed to cigarette smoke (Tsuda et al. 2000) and in oocyte-related cumulus cells (Sinko et al. 2005). On the other hand, there are also reports of no differences between smokers and nonsmokers (Hoffmann and Speit 2005; Speit et al. 2003; Wojewodzka et al. 1999), even after taking genetic polymorphisms in the glutathione S-transferase mu (*GSTM1*), cytochrome P450 1A1 (*CYP1A1*), xeroderma pigmentosum group D (*XPD*), X-ray repair cross complementing group 1 (*XRCC1*), and X-ray repair cross complementing group 3 (*XRCC3*) genes into account (Hoffmann et al. 2005). Regarding environmental tobacco smoke exposure, there are reports showing increased DNA strand breaks as measured by the Comet assay (Collier et al. 2005; Wolz et al. 2002).

Most animal studies have focused on target tissue of interest in relation to cigarette smoke-related cancers, whereas human studies mainly use peripheral lymphocytes as a surrogate tissue. However, one study focused on the DNA modification in placenta and found that 8oxodG increased in smokers as well as after exposure to environmental tobacco smoke (Daube et al. 1997). In mice exposed to acute side stream tobacco smoke, heart and lung levels of 8oxodG increased (Howard et al. 1998a). These findings indicate that cigarette smoke also leads to a more general oxidative stress that just to the DNA of the most directly exposed organ, i.e., the lungs.

16.3 Urinary Excretion of Oxidatively Modified DNA Components

Simple back-of-the-envelope calculation from an estimated average of 2,500 hits to bases in each cell's genome per 24 h gives the result that it would take 1 year to oxidize 1% of the genome if the lesions were not repaired (Poulsen et al. 1998), or about 50% at the age of 50. The excretion of such lesions into urine has been proposed to reflect the oxidative stress to DNA and its precursors (Poulsen et al. 2000, 2003).

In 1992, we showed that smokers excreted on average (big overlapping ranges) about 50% more 8oxodG than nonsmokers (Loft et al. 1992), and later we showed that smokers randomized to smoking cessation decreased their 8oxodG excretion as compared with smokers randomized to continued smoking (Loft et al. 1992; Prieme et al. 1998a). A subsequent study showed that smokers also excreted more of the corresponding base 8oxoG (Suzuki et al. 1995), a finding that could not be repeated in a later study (Harman et al. 2003), and the Poulsen laboratory did not find a difference in 8oxoG excretion between smokers and nonsmokers (unpublished observations). These finding are in agreement with the experimental findings that rats exposed to cigarette smoke for 30 days increased the content of 8oxodG and decreased glutathione levels in all tissues analyszd (Park et al. 1998) and that L-buthionine sulfoximine (BSO) treatment, which depletes glutathione levels, led to a further increase in liver and lung 8oxodG levels. Together with our findings, there is a clear indication that tobacco smoke induces oxidative stress in the lungs but also in other tissues, if not all tissues. In lung cancer patients, the 8oxodG antibody-based assay indicated higher excretion of 8oxodG (Erhola et al. 1997).

Also, urinary 5-(hydroxymethyl)uracil has been reported increased in smokers (Bianchini et al. 1998); however, only when given per excreted creatinine, and only an increase of about 10%. The corresponding nucleoside was also measured in this study, but levels were close to the detection limit. Interestingly, the urinary excretion of 5-(hydroxymethyl)uracil appears higher than other oxidative modifications such as 8oxodG and thymine glycol. A later study from the same group did not find a difference in 5-(hydroxymethyl)uracil excretion, but this time they found a 16% higher excretion of 8oxodG in smokers versus nonsmokers (Pourcelot et al. 1999). A more recent study measured three nucleic acid oxidation products (Harman et al. 2003). In a reasonably sized study, no difference between smokers, ex-smokers, and never smokers could be found with regard to excretion of 8oxodG and the corresponding base 8oxoG, whereas the 5-(hydroxymethyl)uracil was found increased just as in the study mentioned above, however, with a 55% increase. Interestingly, the excretion of the modified base 8oxoG did not differ between never smokers and smokers. In the Malmö Diet and Cancer Cohort (Wallstrom et al. 2003), plasma autoantibodies against 5-hydroxymethyl-2'-deoxy-uridine were higher in the smokers lacking glutathione S-transferase M1 activity and in the persons with high alcohol consumption. In urban bus drivers, the urinary 8oxodG excretion rate was higher than in rural bus drivers, regardless of exposure to environmental tobacco smoke and smoking (Loft et al. 1999).

16.4 Analysis of Oxidative DNA Lesions

The analysis of oxidative DNA lesions falls in two distinct categories, specific chemical analysis and unspecific analysis.

16.4.1 Specific Chemical Analysis

This type of analysis is based on a combination of chromatographic separation systems coupled with more or less specific detections systems. A very comprehensive and detailed review of the subject has been published recently (Guetens et al. 2002), and also several more selected reviews are available (Cadet et al. 2004; Cooke et al. 2003; Evans et al. 2004; Halliwell and Whiteman 2004; Jaruga et al. 2001; Loft and Poulsen 1999; Poulsen et al. 2000; Ravanat et al. 1999) including in the forthcoming fourth edition of *Free Radicals in Biology and Medicine, 2006*, by Halliwell and Gutteridge (Oxford University Press).

Choosing a system of analysis depends on a variety of factors. Is the system is to be used for determination of a single or several base oxidation products, and is it to be used to measure in tissue extracts or for urine determinations? Naturally, resources such a price and infrastructure have to be considered.

If a single lesion such as 8oxodG is to be measured in tissue extracts, the system of choice is HPLC with electrochemical detection. This is the most widely used system, and it provides a high sensitivity and specificity. From a cost point of view it is also the most favorable system, and it does not require the special skill that, e.g., mass spectrometry does. HPLC with electrochemical detection can also be used to measure 8-hydroxyadenine, 5-hydroxycytosine, 5-hydroxyuracil and the corresponding 2'-deoxyribonucleosides (Guetens et al. 2002). There are, however, very few reports on simultaneously measured modifications except from the lab of Miral Dizdaroglu by gas chromatography/mass spectrometry (GC/MS), and in human samples such reports are scarce.

If a single lesion such as 8oxodG is to be measured in urine, HPLC with electrochemical detection is also a choice. It should be noted, however, that urinary measurement is a tricky business and only few laboratories have been able to analyze large series of samples. Whereas analysis on tissue extracts is done by a relatively uncomplicated system, i.e., single column with straight or gradient elution, analysis of urine requires separation on a multicolumn system with reverse phase and cation exchange columns combined with selection of relevant fractions (Kasai 2003, 2005; Loft et al. 1993) or reverse phase combined with a proprietary carbon column (Bogdanov et al. 1999). Lin et al. (2004) have reported a GC/MS method that can be used for analysis of 8oxodG in urine.

When multiple lesions are to be measured, the prevailing method used is chromatography combined with MS. Initially, GC combined with MS was extensively used. For analysis of tissue extracts, derivatization at high temperature has been used to make the modified bases volatile and thereby suitable for GC. This can introduce artificial oxidation of nonmodified bases. Since nonmodified bases are in concentrations that are about a million times higher than the oxidized, even a minor artificial oxidation can produce erroneous results. For this reason GC with MS, if used, requires modifications of the derivatization process to reduce or eliminate such artifacts, or one can utilize the progress in the coupling between liquid chromatography (LC) and MS and thereby avoid such cumbersome procedures. It is also possible to use GC/MS if the samples are preseparated by liquid chromatography (Gackowski et al. 2003; Rozalski et al. 2004, 2005).

LC coupled with MS (LC-MS) (Dizdaroglu et al. 2001, 2002; Jaruga et al. 2001) or with tandem MS (LC-MS/MS) can be used to measure multiple oxidative modifications (Harman et al. 2003; Ravanat et al. 1998, 1999; Weimann et al. 2001, 2002), in urine as well as in tissue samples.

Whereas much emphasis has been put on the chromatography and detection systems, early investigations did not put much emphasis on the tissue sample preparation. In late 1997, a workshop was held in Scotland, where the problems in the analysis were discussed (Collins et al. 1997) and later compilation of reported values of 8oxodG showed a 5,000-fold range in nuclear estimates and a 60,000-fold range in mitochondrial DNA. It became clear subsequently that this was not correct and that a large part of the variation was because methodological problems and artificial oxidation. This prompted a group to set up a European Union Framework 5-sponsored project, where the problems were identified and a standard protocol for tissue sample preparation established (Collins et al. 2002a, b, 2004; Gedik and Collins 2004; Lunec 1998; Riis and European Standards Committee on Oxidative DNA damage [ESCODD] 2002. Also, US researchers took initiative to optimize the quality of assays for the 8oxodG modification (Huang et al. 2001).

It is beyond the scope of this chapter to detail the quality control and optimization of the analysis of 8oxodG, alone or together with other modifications. Caution should be taken when reading the scientific literature on this subject, because results might be because artifacts and poor methodology rather than to real biological events. Particularly, results where the levels are high should be regarded with skepticism, i.e., levels for 8oxodG that are substantially higher than the levels of 1–10 per million dGs found by ESCODD. This applies to analysis of tissue extract levels, i.e., nuclear or mitochondrial DNA extracts. In urine measurements, the level of dG (Weimann et al. 2002) is very low, and artificial oxidation is not a problem even if using GC (Lin et al. 2004).

16.4.2 Nonspecific Analysis

16.4.2.1 The Comet Assay

The most commonly used method is single-cell gel electrophoresis, or the Comet assay. This method uses single cells on a glass slide and is based on the charge on DNA subjected to an electrophoretic field followed by DNA staining. If there is a conformational change or strand breaks in the DNA, this part will move faster in the electrophoretic field than unmodified DNA. When conditions are adjusted properly, intact cells will appear as round, stained nuclei and with increasing DNA modification, the nucleus will shrink as the DNA migrates in the field and a comet-like picture will appear. There are several ways of expressing the results, but a method where, e.g., 100 cells are scored on a damage scale up to 5 and total cumulative scores for 100 cells as a semiquantitative measure of damage/modification gives reproducible results (Collins 2004; Collins et al. 2002b).

It is evident that strand breaks or conformational DNA changes do not equal oxidative damage, and consequently, the Comet assay cannot be taken as a specific marker for oxidative damage. In addition, the Comet assay may underestimate damage/modification if clustered, say, e.g., that all oxidation occurs on all guanosines in a segment of DNA. The method can be made more specific by the use of DNA repair enzymes that will nick DNA at sites with a certain modification, and measuring with and without incubation with such enzymes, e.g., 8-oxoguanine DNA *N*-glycosylase (hOGG1) (Collins 2005). But this assumes that these enzymes have access to all base lesions (unlikely in chromatin) and thus may tend to underestimate.

16.4.2.2 Alkaline Elution

Alkaline elution is a technique where DNA is eluted through filters. If DNA is fragmented, it will elute earlier because of small molecular size, compared with nonfragmented DNA. Such methodology has been applied to oxidative damage (Osterod et al. 2001; Pflaum et al. 1997), and the same argument about specificity as for the Comet assay can be done. We have only been able to find a single report relating to tobacco smoke and oxidative DNA modification using this method. Human lung cells exposed to smoke in buffered saline showed strand breaks that were abolished by catalase (Fielding et al. 1989; Mukherjee et al. 2004).

16.4.2.3 Immunological-Based Methods

Several commercial enzyme-linked immunosorbent assay (ELISA)-based assays have been marketed, and some investigators have produced similar assays. As of today there has not been an assay developed based on immunological methods that has shown sufficient specificity. Testing out an assay, Poulsen et al. found both lack of specificity and sensitivity (Prieme et al. 1996), and recently we tested a newer commercially available assay on different HPLC fractions of urine samples and found that several of the eluted fractions other than 8oxodG reacted in the ELISA kit (unpublished data). Comparison between an ELISA method and HPLC-electrochemical detection (ECD) showed that for quantification HPLC, clean up was necessary (Shimoi et al. 2002). Nevertheless, this paper has been quoted for a demonstration that there is agreement between the HPLC-ECD and ELISA measurements. We have doubt about what the ELISA kit measures besides 8oxdG. It has been suggested that oligonucleotides in urine containing 8oxodG are comeasured by ELISA; however, we demonstrated that such oligonucleotides do not exist in urine at measurable concentrations. We believe that it is very difficult to make an antibody that is sufficiently specific for detection of 8oxodG because of other unknown substances in urine. Consequently, data based on such ELISA methods should be interpreted with caution. Antibodies can be very useful for upconcentrating samples.

16.5 Planning In Vivo Experiments to Investigate Oxidative DNA Lesions: Design Considerations

According to the design used scientific evidence can be graded for quality (Concato et al. 2000) into five groups:
- Grade 1: Evidence obtained from at least one properly randomized, controlled trial
- Grade 2-1: Evidence obtained from well-designed controlled trials without randomization
- Grade 2-2: Evidence obtained from well-designed cohort or case–control analytical studies, preferably from more than one centre or research group
- Grade 2-3: Evidence obtained from multiple time series with or without the intervention. Dramatic results in uncontrolled experiments (such as the results of the introduction of penicillin treatment in the 1940s) could also be regarded as this type of evidence.
- Grade 3: Opinions of respected authorities, based on clinical experience; descriptive studies and case reports; or reports of expert committees

Taking starting point in the studies cited in Sects. 16.4.2.2 and 16.4.2.3, it is evident that the studies belong to grade 2-2 or lower. The only study with quality grade 1 is that of Prieme et al. (1998b), who used a design where smokers were randomized to continued smoking, later followed by a smoking cessation program, or immediately entering a smoking cessation program. This design is the ethically acceptable alternative to randomize nonsmokers to smoking or nonsmoking. Evidence from comparing cases and controls most often overestimates the effects (Kunz and Oxman 1998), and indeed, when we compare our cohort study (Loft et al. 1992) with the randomized intervention study (Prieme et al. 1998b), we find a 2- to 3-fold difference in the effect of smoking.

Although we have not performed a complete survey of studies on oxidative DNA markers and smoking with regard to quality, it is clear that most researchers use a design that is inferior regarding quality of design.

Regarding the total evidence available, however, it is quite clear, that the single grade 1 quality design and several grade 2-2 and grade 3 quality studies performed provides strong evidence that tobacco smoking induces oxidative modification to DNA

16.6 Some Aspects of DNA Repair of Oxidative Modifications

Whereas focus has been on the modification to DNA, it is becoming increasingly clear that DNA repair processes may have equal importance. Repair of oxidative modification in DNA is extensive, and individual differences in DNA repair are proposed to be important for development of cancer and premature aging (Hoeijmakers 2001a, b).

There are a large number of enzyme systems that can recognize oxidative DNA modifications and start a multistep process of repair that seems important for the modulation of oxidative mutagenesis and carcinogenesis (Nohmi et al. 2005).

The human homologue of the MutT protein (hMTH1) enzyme hydrolyses 8oxodGTP and prevent its incorporation into DNA. In lung cancer tissue, the activity of hMTH1 is lower than in normal lung tissue (Speina et al. 2005), and expression, i.e., mRNA levels, in lung cancer cells parallels cellular levels of 8oxodG (Kennedy et al. 1998).

hOGG1 is the initial step in recognition and incision of the 8oxodG lesion and in a case control study, the activity of hOGG1 was lower in peripheral lymphocytes from lung cancer patients than in those from controls (Paz-Elizur et al. 2003). hOGG1 shows a single nucleotide polymorphism (SNP), Ser326Cys, that gives relative risk (RR) of 5.8 in women and 2.0 in men for developing lung cancer in smokers with occupational exposure to smoky coal (Lan et al. 2004), as also observed inanother study where an odds ratio (OR) of 2.1 was found (Le Marchand et al. 2002). Lung tumors with loss of heterozygosity at loci associated with *hOGG1* and the glutathione peroxidase 1 (*GXP1*) genes had about double levels of 8oxodG in nuclear DNA (Hardie et al. 2000).

The xeroderma pigmentosa type a (XPA) protein is involved in nucleotide excision repair and a SNP A-G in the 5' non–coding region of the *XPA* gene and one or two G alleles is associated with a reduced lung cancer risk from smoking (Wu et al. 2003).

In a recent study where several polymorphisms was studied simultaneously, including the repair genes *XRCC1* (one polymorphism) and *ERCC2* (two polymorphisms), their interaction with smoking was studied, and the most striking finding was that the adjusted ORs for lung cancer of individuals carrying five or six variant alleles was 0.3, whereas it was 5.2 for the wild-type alleles/nonsmokers (Zhou et al. 2003).

The *XRCC1* has a SNP, Arg194Trp, and this allele also seems to lower the risk of lung cancer, RR 0.4 in cases with high serum retinol values (Ratnasinghe et al. 2003); however, a SNP, Arg399Gln, gave an OR of 1.4 for smokers developing bladder cancer (Kelsey et al. 2004).

DNA ligases also plays a role in DNA repair, but a SNP (A to C) in exon 6 of DNA ligase I (*LIG1*), seems not related to a changed risk of lung cancer (Shen et al. 2002).

16.7 How Important Are Oxidative DNA Lesions for the Causal Relation between Cigarette Smoke and Development of Cancer and Other Diseases?

The bulk of evidence indicates that tobacco smoking and exposure to environmental smoke lead to increased levels of oxidative modifications in DNA and to increased excretion of repair products into urine. As argued above, urinary excretion does not reflect repair but the total "stress-burden," i.e., the rate of oxidation of DNA and its precursors, and therefore smoking cessation reduces this oxidative stress to DNA. The lesions have been shown to be promutagenic, and it can therefore be concluded that tobacco smoking leads to increased promutagenic oxidative lesions in DNA, as discussed by Halliwell (2002).

The quality of the evidence is strong, and some of the studies demonstrating the oxidative stress to DNA in humans are of the highest grade of scientific evidence, as detailed above.

The subsequent question is: How important is this increased oxidative stress in the development of tobacco related diseases? In this aspect, oxidative DNA modification by mechanistic implications relates mostly to cancer development. Several facts are important to realize. (1) The oxidative DNA modifications are not specific for tobacco exposure; rather, tobacco smoke exposure increases preexisting oxidative modifications. (2) Tobacco smoke contains many chemicals that may modify DNA and form premutagenic lesions, or other types of disease-relevant DNA modifications. (3) The locations within

DNA of the oxidative modifications are not known, and location may be very important in disease processes. (4) The relative contribution of oxidative DNA modifications to the overall number of mutational events in DNA is not known, and the number of mutational spots in DNA from oxidative modification may represent a large or small fraction of other mutations/modifications and therefore also a minor or large contribution to disease. (5) Other endogenous and/or exogenous factors may be important for development of cancer.

Based on the data available as of today, it is clear that oxidative stress to DNA can be an important initial part of the pathogenesis of tobacco-related cancer development as well as in the later stages after malignant clones has been formed. Whereas there is a clear biological plausibility that oxidative stress could be important, it is important to make quantitative estimations of the importance of oxidative stress among all other biological possible mechanisms. One way of doing this is from trials or epidemiological studies where the relative risk of cancer risk from measures of, e.g., high or low oxidative stress to DNA are estimated; such studies are presently not available, but are under way. Even if such data reveal a low cancer risk from oxidative stress, this will not rule out its importance. It could very well be that oxidative stress to DNA in combination with other factors may be very important. Such factors could be DNA repair activity, inflammatory response, baseline DNA damage in nonsmokers, and so forth. Clearly, there is continued need for considering oxidative stress to DNA in the conquest for deciphering the mechanisms of tobacco-related diseases, particularly cancer.

References

Ames BN (1989a) Endogenous DNA damage as related to cancer and aging. Mutat Res 214:41–46
Ames BN (1989b) Endogenous oxidative DNA damage, aging, and cancer. Free Radic Res Commun 7:121–128
Ames BN (2001) DNA damage from micronutrient deficiencies is likely to be a major cause of cancer. Mutat Res 475:7–20
Ames BN, Shigenaga MK, Hagen TM (1993) Oxidants, antioxidants, and the degenerative diseases of aging. Proc Natl Acad Sci U S A 90:7915–7922
Asami S, Hirano T, Yamaguchi R, Tomioka Y, Itoh H, Kasai H (1996) Increase of a type of oxidative DNA damage, 8-hydroxyguanine, and its repair activity in human leukocytes by cigarette smoking. Cancer Res 56:2546–2549
Asami S, Manabe H, Miyake J, Tsurudome Y, Hirano T, Yamaguchi R, Itoh H, Kasai H (1997) Cigarette smoking induces an increase in oxidative DNA damage, 8-hydroxydeoxyguanosine, in a central site of the human lung. Carcinogenesis 18:1763–1766
Bianchini F, Donato F, Faure H, Ravanat JL, Hall J, Cadet J (1998) Urinary excretion of 5-(hydroxymethyl) uracil in healthy volunteers: effect of active and passive tobacco smoke. Int J Cancer 77:40–46
Bogdanov MB, Beal MF, McCabe DR, Griffin RM, Matson WR (1999) A carbon column-based liquid chromatography electrochemical approach to routine 8-hydroxy-2'-deoxyguanosine measurements in urine and other biologic matrices: a one-year evaluation of methods. Free Radic Biol Med 27:647–666
Cadet J, Bellon S, Douki T, Frelon S, Gasparutto D, Muller E, Pouget JP, Ravanat JL, Romieu A, Sauvaigo S (2004) Radiation-induced DNA damage: formation, measurement, and biochemical features. J Environ Pathol Toxicol Oncol 23:33–43

Cadet J, Berger M, Douki T, Ravanat JL (1997) Oxidative damage to DNA: formation, measurement, and biological significance. Rev Physiol Biochem Pharmacol 131:1–87

Cadet J, Berger M, Shaw A (1986) The radiation chemistry of the purine bases within DNA and related model compounds. Basic Life Sci 38:69–74

Cadet J, Douki T, Gasparutto D, Ravanat JL (2003) Oxidative damage to DNA: formation, measurement and biochemical features. Mutat Res 531:5–23

Cadet J, Sage E, Douki T (2005) Ultraviolet radiation-mediated damage to cellular DNA. Mutat Res 571:3–17

Cadet J, Treoule R (1978) Comparative study of oxidation of nucleic acid components by hydroxyl radicals, singlet oxygen and superoxide anion radicals. Photochem Photobiol 28:661–667

Collier AC, Dandge SD, Woodrow JE, Pritsos CA (2005) Differences in DNA-damage in non-smoking men and women exposed to environmental tobacco smoke (ETS). Toxicol Lett 158:10–19

Collins A, Cadet J, Epe B, Gedik C (1997) Problems in the measurement of 8-oxoguanine in human DNA. Report of a workshop, DNA oxidation, held in Aberdeen, UK, 19–21 January, 1997. Carcinogenesis 18:1833–1836

Collins A, Gedik C, Vaughan N, Wood S, White A, Dubois J, Duez P, Dehon G, Rees JF, Loft S, Moller P, Poulsen H, Riis B, Weimann A, Cadet J, Douki T, Ravanat JL, Sauvaigo S, Faure H, Morel I, Morin B, Epe B, Phoa N, Hartwig A, Pelzer A, Dolara P, Casalini C, Giovannelli L, Lodovici M, Olinski R, Bialkowski K, Foksinski M, Gackowski D, Durackova Z, Hlincikova L, Korytar P, Sivonova M, Dusinska M, Mislanova C, Vina J, Lloret A, Moller L, Hofer T, Nygren J, Gremaud E, Herbert K, Chauhan D, Kelly F, Dunster C, Lunec J, Cooke M, Evans M, Patel P, Podmore I, White A, Wild C, Hardie L, Olliver J, Smith E (2002a) Comparative analysis of baseline 8-oxo-7,8-dihydroguanine in mammalian cell DNA, by different methods in different laboratories: an approach to consensus. Carcinogenesis 23:2129–2133

Collins AR (2004) The comet assay for DNA damage and repair—principles, applications, and limitations. Mol Biotechnol 26:249–261

Collins AR (2005) Assays for oxidative stress and antioxidant status: applications to research into the biological effectiveness of polyphenols. Am J Clin Nutr 81:S261–S267

Collins AR, Cadet J, Moller L, Poulsen HE, Vina J (2004) Are we sure we know how to measure 8-oxo-7,8-dihydroguanine in DNA from human cells? Arch Biochem Biophys 423:57–65

Collins AR, Gedik C, Wood S, White A, Dubois J, Duez P, Rees JF, Legall R, Degand L, Loft S, Jensen A, Poulsen H, Weimann A, Jensen BR, Cadet J, Douki T, Ravanat JL, Faure H, Tripier M, Morel I, Sergent O, Cillard P, Morin B, Epe B, Phoa N, Hartwig A, Pelzer A, Dolara P, Casalini C, Guglielmi F, Luceri C, Kasai H, Kido R, Olinski R, Bialkowski K, Durackova Z, Hlincikova L, Korytar P, Dusinska M, Mislanova C, Vina J, Lloret A, Moller L, Hofer T, Gremaud E, Fay L, Stadler R, Eakins J, Pognan F, O'Brien J, Elliott R, Astley S, Bailley A, Herbert K, Chauhan D, Kelly F, Dunster C, Lunec J, Podmore I, Patel P, Johnson S, Evans M, White A, Tyrrell R, Gordon M, Wild C, Hardie L, Smith E (2002b) Inter-laboratory validation of procedures for measuring 8-oxo-7,8-dihydroguanine/8-oxo-7,8-dihydro-2'-deoxyguanosine in DNA. Free Radic Res 36:239–245

Concato J, Shah N, Horwitz RI (2000) Randomized, controlled trials, observational studies, and the hierarchy of research designs. N Engl J Med 342:1887–1892

Cooke MS, Evans MD, Dizdaroglu M, Lunec J (2003) Oxidative DNA damage: mechanisms, mutation, and disease. FASEB J 17:1195–1214

Daube H, Scherer G, Riedel K, Ruppert T, Tricker AR, Rosenbaum P, Adlkofer F (1997) DNA adducts in human placenta in relation to tobacco smoke exposure and plasma antioxidant status. J Cancer Res Clin Oncol 123:141–151

Deng XS, Tuo J, Poulsen HE, Loft S (1998) Prevention of oxidative DNA damage in rats by Brussels sprouts. Free Radic Res 28:323–333

Dizdaroglu M (1985) Formation of an 8-hydroxyguanine moiety in deoxyribonucleic acid on gamma-irradiation in aqueous solution. Biochemistry (Mosc) 24:4476–4481

Dizdaroglu M (1991) Chemical determination of free radical-induced damage to DNA. Free Radic Biol Med 10:225–242

Dizdaroglu M (1993) Chemistry of free radical damage to DNA and nucleoproteins. In: Halliwell B (ed) DNA and free radicals. Horwood, Chichester, pp 19–39

Dizdaroglu M (1994) Chemical determination of oxidative DNA damage by gas chromatography-mass spectrometry. Methods Enzymol 234:3–16

Dizdaroglu M, Bergtold DS (1986) Characterization of free radical-induced base damage in DNA at biological relevant levels. Anal Biochem 156:182–188

Dizdaroglu M, Jaruga P, Birincioglu M, Rodriguez H (2002) Free radical-induced damage to DNA: mechanisms and measurement. Free Radic Biol Med 32:1102–1115

Dizdaroglu M, Jaruga P, Rodriguez H (2001) Measurement of 8-hydroxy-2'-deoxyguanosine in DNA by high-performance liquid chromatography-mass spectrometry: comparison with measurement by gas chromatography-mass spectrometry. Nucleic Acids Res 29:E12

Einhaus M, Holz O, Meissner R, Krause T, Warncke K, Held I, Scherer G, Tricker AR, Adlkofer F, Rudiger HW (1994) Determination of DNA single-strand breaks in lymphocytes of smokers and nonsmokers exposed to environmental tobacco smoke using the nick translation assay. Clin Investig 72:930–936

Erhola M, Toyokuni S, Okada K, Tanaka T, Hiai H, Ochi H, Uchida K, Osawa T, Nieminen MM, Alho H, Kellokumpu-Lehtinen P (1997) Biomarker evidence of DNA oxidation in lung cancer patients: association of urinary 8-hydroxy-2'-deoxyguanosine excretion with radiotherapy, chemotherapy, and response to treatment. FEBS Lett 409:287–291

Evans MD, Dizdaroglu M, Cooke MS (2004) Oxidative DNA damage and disease: induction, repair and significance. Mutat Res 567:1–61

Farmer P, Shuker DEG (1999) What is significance of increases in background levels of carcinogen-derived protein and DNA adducts? Some considerations for incremental risk assessment. Mutat Res 424:275–286

Fielding S, Short C, Davies K, Wald N, Bridges BA, Waters R (1989) Studies on the ability of smoke from different types of cigarettes to induce DNA single-strand breaks in cultured human cells. Mutat Res 214:147–151

Floyd RA, Watson JJ, Wong PK, Altmiller DH, Rickard RC (1986) Hydroxyl free radical adduct of deoxyguanosine: sensitive detection and mechanisms of formation. Free Radic Res Commun 1:163–172

Gackowski D, Speina E, Zielinska M, Kowalewski J, Rozalski R, Siomek A, Paciorek T, Tudek B, Olinski R (2003) Products of oxidative DNA damage and repair as possible biomarkers of susceptibility to lung cancer. Cancer Res 63:4899–4902

Gedik CM, Collins A (2004) Establishing the background level of base oxidation in human lymphocyte DNA: results of an interlaboratory validation study. FASEB J 19:82–84

Godschalk R, Nair J, Van Schooten FJ, Risch A, Drings P, Kayser K, Dienemann H, Bartsch H (2002) Comparison of multiple DNA adduct types in tumor adjacent human lung tissue: effect of cigarette smoking. Carcinogenesis 23:2081–2086

Guetens G, De Boeck G, Highley M, van Oosterom AT, de Bruijn EA (2002) Oxidative DNA damage: Biological significance and methods of analysis. Crit Rev Clin Lab Sci 39:331–457

Halliwell B (2002) Effect of diet on cancer development: is oxidative DNA damage a biomarker? Free Radic Biol Med 32:968–974

Halliwell B, Whiteman M (2004) Measuring reactive species and oxidative damage in vivo and in cell culture: How should you do it and what do the results mean? Br J Pharmacol 142:231–255

Hardie LJ, Briggs JA, Davidson LA, Allan JM, King RF, Williams GI, Wild CP (2000) The effect of hOGG1 and glutathione peroxidase I genotypes and 3p chromosomal loss on 8-hydroxydeoxyguanosine levels in lung cancer. Carcinogenesis 21:167–172

Harman SM, Liang L, Tsitouras PD, Gucciardo F, Heward CB, Reaven PD, Ping W, Ahmed A, Cutler RG (2003) Urinary excretion of three nucleic acid oxidation adducts and isoprostane F-2 alpha measured by liquid chromatography mass spectrometry in smokers, ex-smokers, and nonsmokers. Free Radic Biol Med 35:1301–1309

Hoeijmakers JH (2001a) DNA repair mechanisms. Maturitas 38:17–22

Hoeijmakers JH (2001b) Genome maintenance mechanisms for preventing cancer. Nature 411:366–374

Hoffmann H, Speit G (2005) Assessment of DNA damage in peripheral blood of heavy smokers with the comet assay and the micronucleus test. Mutat Res 581:105–114

Hoffmann H, Isner C, Hogel J, Speit G (2005) Genetic polymorphisms and the effect of cigarette smoking in the comet assay. Mutagenesis 20:359–364

Holz O, Meissner R, Einhaus M, Koops F, Warncke K, Scherer G, Adlkofer F, Baumgartner E, Rudiger HW (1993) Detection of DNA single-strand breaks in lymphocytes of smokers. Int Arch Occup Environ Health 65:83–88

Howard DJ, Briggs LA, Pritsos CA (1998a) Oxidative DNA damage in mouse heart, liver, and lung tissue due to acute side-stream tobacco smoke exposure. Arch Biochem Biophys 352:293–297

Howard DJ, Ota RB, Briggs LA, Hampton M, Pritsos CA (1998b) Oxidative stress induced by environmental tobacco smoke in the workplace is mitigated by antioxidant supplementation. Cancer Epidemiol Biomarkers Prev 7:981–988

Huang X, Powell J, Mooney LA, Li CL, Frenkel K (2001) Importance of complete DNA digestion in minimizing variability of 8-oxo-dG analyses. Free Radic Biol Med 31:1341–1351

Jaruga P, Dizdaroglu M (1996) Repair of products of oxidative DNA base damage in human cells. Nucleic Acids Res 24:1389–1394

Jaruga P, Rodriguez H, Dizdaroglu M (2001) Measurement of 8-hydroxy-2'-deoxyadenosine in DNA by liquid chromatography/mass spectrometry. Free Radic Biol Med 31:336–344

Kasai H (1997) Analysis of a form of oxidative DNA damage, 8-hydroxy-2'-deoxyguanosine, as a marker of cellular oxidative stress during carcinogenesis. Mutat Res 387:147–163

Kasai H (2003) A new automated method to analyze urinary 8-hydroxydeoxyguanosine by a high-performance liquid chromatography-electrochemical detector system. J Radiat Res (Tokyo) 44:185–189

Kasai H, Nishimura S (1984) Hydroxylation of deoxyguanosine at the C-8 position by ascorbic acid and other reducing agents. Nucleic Acids Res 12:2137–2145

Kasai H, Svoboda P, Yamasaki S, Kawai K (2005) Simultaneous determination of 8-hydroxydeoyguanosine, a marker of oxidative stress, and creatinine, a standardization compound, in urine. Ind Health 43:333–336

Kelsey KT, Park H, Nelson HH, Karagas MR (2004) A population-based case-control study of the XRCC1 Arg399Gln polymorphism and susceptibility to bladder cancer. Cancer Epidemiol Biomarkers Prev 13:1337–1341

Kennedy CH, Cueto R, Belinsky SA, Lechner JF, Pryor WA (1998) Overexpression of hMTH1 mRNA: a molecular marker of oxidative stress in lung cancer cells. FEBS Lett 429:17–20

Kunz R, Oxman AD (1998) The unpredictability paradox: review of empirical comparisons of randomised and non-randomised clinical trials. BMJ 317:1185–1190

Lam TH, Zhu CQ, Jiang CQ (2002) Lymphocyte DNA damage in elevator manufacturing workers in Guangzhou, China. Mutat Res 515:147–157

Lan Q, Mumford JL, Shen M, DeMarini DM, Bonner MR, He X, Yeager M, Welch R, Chanock S, Tian L, Chapman RS, Zheng T, Keohavong P, Caporaso N, Rothman N (2004) Oxidative damage-related genes AKR1C3 and OGG1 modulate risks for lung cancer due to exposure to PAH-rich coal combustion emissions. Carcinogenesis 25:2177–2181

Le Marchand L, Donlon T, Lum-Jones A, Seifried A, Wilkens LR (2002) Association of the hOGG1 Ser326Cys polymorphism with lung cancer risk. Cancer Epidemiol Biomarkers Prev 11:409–412

Leanderson P, Tagesson C (1992) Cigarette smoke-induced DNA damage in cultured human lung-cells—role of hydroxyl radicals and endonuclease activation. Chem Biol Interact 81:197–208

Lin HS, Jenner AM, Ong CN, Huang SH, Whiteman M, Halliwell B (2004) A high-throughput and sensitive methodology for the quantification of urinary 8-hydroxy-2'-deoxyguanosine: measurement with gas chromatography-mass spectrometry after single solid-phase extraction. Biochem J 380:541–548

Loft S, Fischer-Nielsen A, Jeding IB, Vistisen K, Poulsen HE (1993) 8-Hydroxydeoxyguanosine as a urinary biomarker of oxidative DNA damage. J Toxicol Environ Health 40:391–404

Loft S, Larsen PN, Rasmussen A, Fischer-Nielsen A, Bondesen S, Kirkegaard P, Rasmussen LS, Ejlersen E, Tornøe K, Bergholdt R, Poulsen HE (1995) Oxidative DNA damage after transplantation of the liver and small intestine in pigs. Transplantation 59:16–20

Loft S, Poulsen HE (1999) Measurement of oxidative damage to DNA nucleobases in vivo. In: Dizdaroglu M, Karakaya A (eds) Advances in DNA damage and repair. Kluwer, New York, pp 267–279

Loft S, Poulsen HE, Vistisen K, Knudsen LE (1999) Increased urinary excretion of 8-oxo-2'-deoxyguanosine, a biomaker of oxidative DNA damage, in urban bus drivers. Mutat Res 441:11–19

Loft S, Vistisen K, Ewertz M, Tjonneland A, Overvad K, Poulsen HE (1992) Oxidative DNA damage estimated by 8-hydroxydeoxyguanosine excretion in humans: influence of smoking, gender and body mass index. Carcinogenesis 13:2241–2247

Lunec J (1998) ESCODD: European Standards Committee on Oxidative DNA damage. Free Radic Res 29:601–608

Mukherjee S, Palmer LJ, Kim JY, Aeschliman DB, Houk RS, Woodin MA, Christiani DC (2004) Smoking status and occupational exposure affects oxidative DNA injury in boilermakers exposed to metal fume and residual oil fly ash. Cancer Epidemiol Biomarkers Prev 13:454–460

Nohmi T, Kim SR, Yamada M (2005) Modulation of oxidative mutagenesis and carcinogenesis by polymorphic forms of human DNA repair enzymes. Mutat Res 591:60–73

Osterod M, Hollenbach S, Hengstler JG, Barnes DE, Lindahl T, Epe B (2001) Age-related and tissue-specific accumulation of oxidative DNA base damage in 7,8-dihydro-8-oxoguanine-DNA glycosylase (Ogg1) deficient mice. Carcinogenesis 22:1459–1463

Park E, Kang MH (2004) Smoking and high plasma triglyceride levels as risk factors for oxidative DNA damage in the Korean population. Ann Nutr Metab 48:36–42

Park EM, Park YM, Gwak YS (1998) Oxidative damage in tissues of rats exposed to cigarette smoke. Free Radic Biol Med 25:79–86

Paz-Elizur T, Krupsky M, Blumenstein S, Elinger D, Schechtman E, Livneh Z (2003) DNA repair activity for oxidative damage and risk of lung cancer. J Nat Can Inst 95:1312–1319

Pflaum M, Will O, Epe B (1997) Determination of steady-state levels of oxidative DNA base modifications in mammalian cells by means of repair endonucleases. Carcinogenesis 18:2225–2231

Phillips DH (2002) Smoking-related DNA and protein adducts in human tissues. Carcinogenesis 23:1979–2004

Piperakis SM, Visvardis EE, Sagnou M, Tassiou AM (1998) Effects of smoking and aging on oxidative DNA damage of human lymphocytes. Carcinogenesis 19:695–698

Poli P, Buschini A, Spaggiari A, Rizzoli V, Carlo-Stella C, Rossi C (1999) DNA damage by tobacco smoke and some antiblastic drugs evaluated using the Comet assay. Toxicol Lett 108:267–276

Poulsen HE, Loft S, Jensen BR, Sørensen M, Hoberg AM, Weimann A (2003) HPLC-ECD, HPLC-MS/MS (urinary biomarkers). In: Cutler RG, Rodriguez H (eds) Critical reviews of oxidative stress and aging: advances in basic science, diagnostics, and intervention, vol 1. World Scientific, Singapore, pp 233–256

Poulsen HE, Loft S, Weimann A (2000) Urinary measurement of 8-oxodG (8-oxo-2'-deoxyguanosine). In: Lunec J, Griffiths HR (eds) Measuring in vivo oxidative damage: a practical approach. Wiley, London, pp 69–80

Poulsen HE, Prieme H, Loft S (1998) Role of oxidative DNA damage in cancer initiation and promotion. Eur J Cancer Prev 7:9–16

Pourcelot S, Faure H, Firoozi F, Ducros V, Tripier M, Hee J, Cadet J, Favier A (1999) Urinary 8-oxo-7,8-dihydro-2'-deoxyguanosine and 5-(hydroxymethyl) uracil in smokers. Free Radic Res 30:173–180

Prieme H, Loft S, Cutler RG, Poulsen HE (1996) Measurement of oxidative DNA injury in humans: evaluation of a commercially available ELISA assay. In: Kumpulainen JT (ed) Natural antioxidants and food quality in atherosclerosis and cancer prevention. Royal Society of Chemistry, London, pp 78–82

Prieme H, Loft S, Klarlund M, Gronbaek K, Tonnesen P, Poulsen HE (1998a) Effect of smoking cessation on oxidative DNA modification estimated by 8-oxo-7,8-dihydro-2'-deoxyguanosine excretion. Carcinogenesis 19:347–351

Prieme H, Nyyssonen K, Gronbaek K, Klarlund M, Loft S, Tonnesen P, Salonen JT, Poulsen HE (1998b) Randomized controlled smoking cessation study: transient increase in plasma high density lipoprotein but no change in lipoprotein oxidation resistance. Scand J Clin Lab Invest 58:11–18

Ratnasinghe DL, Yao SX, Forman M, Oiao YL, Andersen MR, Giffen CA, Erozan Y, Tockman MS, Taylor PR (2003) Gene-environment interactions between the codon 194 polymorphism of *XRCC1* and antioxidants influence lung cancer risk. Anticancer Res 23:627–632

Ravanat J-L, Duretz B, Guilller A, Douki T, Cadet J (1998) Isotope dilution high performance liquid chromatography-electrospray tandem mass spectrometry assay for the measurement of 8-oxo-7,8-dihydro-2'-deoxyguanosine in biological samples. J Chromatogr B 715:349–356

Ravanat J-L, Guicherd P, Tuce Z, Cadet J (1999) Simultaneous determination of five oxidative DNA lesions in human urine. Chem Res Toxicol 12:802–808

Riis B, ESCODD (2002) Comparison of results from different laboratories in measuring 8-oxo-2'-deoxyguanosine in synthetic oligonucleotides. Free Radic Res 36:649–659

Rozalski R, Siomek A, Gackowski D, Foksinski M, Gran C, Klungland A, Olinski R (2004) Diet is not responsible for the presence of several oxidatively damaged DNA lesions in mouse urine. Free Radic Res 38:1201–1205

Rozalski R, Siomek A, Gackowski D, Foksinski M, Gran C, Klungland A, Olinski R (2005) Substantial decrease of urinary 8-oxo-7,8-dihydroguanine, a product of the base excision repair pathway, in DNA glycosylase defective mice. Int J Biochem Cell Biol 37:1331–1336

Schram KH (1998) Urinary nucleosides. Mass Spectrom Rev 17:131–251

Shen HB, Spitz MR, Qiao YW, Zheng YX, Hong WK, Wei QY (2002) Polymorphism of DNA ligase I and risk of lung cancer—a case-control analysis. Lung Cancer 36:243–247

Shimoi K, Kasai H, Yokota N, Toyokuni S, Kinae N (2002) Comparison between high-performance liquid chromatography and enzyme-linked immunosorbent assay for the determination of 8-hydroxy-2'-deoxyguanosine in human urine. Cancer Epidemiol Biomarkers Prev 11:767–770

Sinko I, Morocz M, Zadori J, Kokavszky K, Rasko I (2005) Effect of cigarette smoking on DNA damage of human cumulus cells analyzed by comet assay. Reprod Toxicol 20:65–71

Speina E, Arczewska KD, Gackowski D, Zielinska M, Siomek A, Kowalewski J, Olinski R, Tudek B, Kusmierek JT (2005) Contribution of hMTH1 to the maintenance of 8-oxoguanine levels in lung DNA of non-small-cell lung cancer patients. J Natl Cancer Inst 97:384–395

Speit G, Witton-Davies T, Heepchantree W, Trenz K, Hoffmann H (2003) Investigations on the effect of cigarette smoking in the comet assay. Mutat Res 542:33–42

Spencer JP, Jenner A, Aruoma OI, Cross CE, Wu R, Halliwell B (1996) Oxidative DNA damage in human respiratory tract epithelial cells. Time course in relation to DNA strand breakage. Biochem Biophys Res Commun 224:17–22

Suzuki J, Inoue Y, Suzuki S (1995) Changes in the urinary excretion level of 8-hydroxyguanine by exposure to reactive oxygen-generating substances. Free Radic Biol Med 18:431–436

Tsuda S, Matsusaka N, Ueno S, Susa N, Sasaki YF (2000) The influence of antioxidants on cigarette smoke-induced DNA single-strand breaks in mouse organs: a preliminary study with the alkaline single cell gel electrophoresis assay. Toxicol Sci 54:104–109

Wallstrom P, Frenkel K, Wirfalt E, Gullberg B, Karkoszka J, Seidegard J, Janzon L, Berglund G (2003) Antibodies against 5-hydroxymethyl-2'-deoxyuridine are associated with lifestyle factors and *GSTM1* genotype: a report from the Malmo Diet and Cancer cohort. Cancer Epidemiol Biomarkers Prev12:444–451

Weimann A, Belling D, Poulsen HE (2001) Measurement of 8-oxo-2-deoxyguanosine and 8-oxo-2-deoxyadenosine in DNA and human urine by high performance liquid chromatography-electrospray tandem mass spectrometry. Free Radic Biol Med 30:757–764

Weimann A, Belling D, Poulsen HE (2002) Quantification of 8-oxo-guanine and guanine as the nucleobase, nucleoside and deoxynucleoside forms in human urine by high-performance liquid chromatography-electrospray tandem mass spectrometry. Nucleic Acids Res 30:E7

Welch RW, Turley E, Sweetman SF, Kennedy G, Collins AR, Dunne A, Livingstone MB, McKenna PG, McKelvey-Martin VJ, Strain JJ (1999) Dietary antioxidant supplementation and DNA damage in smokers and nonsmokers. Nutr Cancer 34:167–172

Wojewodzka M, Kruszewski M, Iwanenko T, Collins AR, Szumiel I (1999) Lack of adverse effect of smoking habit on DNA strand breakage and base damage, as revealed by the alkaline comet assay. Mutat Res 440:19–25

Wolz L, Krause G, Scherer G, Aufderheide M, Mohr U (2002) In vitro genotoxicity assay of sidestream smoke using a human bronchial epithelial cell line. Food Chem Toxicol 40:845–850

Wu XF, Zhao H, Wei QY, Amos CI, Zhang K, Guo ZZ, Qiao YQ, Hong WK, Spitz MR (2003) XPA polymorphism associated with reduced lung cancer risk and a modulating effect on nucleotide excision repair capacity. Carcinogenesis 24:505–509

Zhou W, Liu G, Miller DP, Thurston SW, Xu LL, Wain JC, Lynch TJ, Su L, Christiani DC (2003) Polymorphisms in the DNA repair genes *XRCC1* and *ERCC2*, smoking, and lung cancer risk. Cancer Epidemiol Biomarkers Prev 12:359–365

Zhu CQ, Lam TH, Jiang CQ, Wei BX, Lou X, Liu WW, Lao XQ, Chen YH (1999) Lymphocyte DNA damage in cigarette factory workers measured by the Comet assay. Mutat Res 444:1–6

Index

2,6-diamino-4-hydroxy-5-
   formamidopyrimidine   388
3-nitrotyrosine   4
4-hydroxy-nonenal   54
4-hydroxynonenal   56, 58, 61, 65
5-(hydroxymethyl)uracil   390
5-hydroxycytosine   391
5-hydroxyuracil   391
8-hydroxy-2'-deoxyguanosine (8oxodG)   388
8-hydroxyadenine   391
α-lipoic acid   207
α1-antitrypsin   284
β-receptor blocker
 – nebivolol   355
γ-glutamylcysteine synthetase   79

A

acrolein   48, 50, 51, 52, 53, 56, 57,
   58, 59, 61, 62, 63, 65, 66
alcohol dehydrogenase   59
aldehyde dehydrogenases   59
aldo-keto reductase   59
aldose reductase   59
alkenal/one oxidoreductase   59
Angiotensin II   354
animal models   285
antioxidant   2, 280, 282, 283, 284, 353
AP-1   79
apoptosis   61, 62, 63, 78, 371
aryl hydrocarbon receptor   88
ascorbate free radical   240
ASK1   80
ATBC Study   203

B

benzo[a]pyrene   88
benzoquinone   10
biomarker of oxidative stress   3, 4
biomarkers   282
bronchoalveolar lavage fluid   282

C

c-fos   94
C/EBPβ   90
cadmium   77
CARET study   203
Carl Wilhelm Scheele   2
carotenoid   201
caspase   62, 64
catalyst   283
catechol   12, 16, 17, 20, 21, 23, 24, 31, 38, 88
cells   262
 – A549 cells   273
 – alveolar epithelial cells   262
 – alveolar macrophages   262
 – BEAS-2B cells   270
 – bronchial epithelial cells   262
 – CULTEX®   272
 – HFBE21   272
 – inlets   272
 – LA-4   271
 – lung tissue slices   264
 – NCI-H157 cells   271
 – THP-1 cells   270
 – tracheal explants   268
cell survival   78
ceramide   84

chronic obstructive pulmonary disease 366
cigarette smoke 366
– carbon monoxide 345
– gas phase 343
– polycyclic aromatic hydrocarbons 346
– tar 343
combustion 280
Comet assay 389, 392, 393
complex mixtures 262
– ambient air 262
– cigarette smoke 262
– diesel exhaust 262
COX-2 83
crotonaldehyde 48, 51, 52, 53, 56, 58
Cyp1A1 88

D

decorin 382
dehydroascorbic acid 239
device
– intracellular ATP 264
dietary guidelines 242
dietary intake 240
dietary intakes of antioxidants 238
DNA Repair 394

E

elastic fibers 381
electron spin resonance 3
emphysema 94, 283
endoplasmic reticulum 3
endothelial dysfunction 239
endpoint 263
– alkaline phosphatase 264
– cell proliferation 271
– DNA damage 265
– glutathione 263
– microporous membranes 265
– mitogen-activated protein kinase 272
– tumor necrosis factor-α [TNF-α] 264
– viability 271
eNOS 346
– uncoupling 346, 347

environmental tobacco smoke 207, 281, 389, 391
enzyme-linked immunosorbent assay 393
EPIC Study 201
epidemiological study 380
– cross-section study 380
– matrix metalloproteinases 380
– replica analysis 380
– ultraviolet 380
EPR 27, 29, 37
exposure 262
– air–liquid interface 266, 268
– catalase 267
– cell protein content 267
– diffusion barrier 263
– dynamic exposure 270
– GHS peroxidase (GPx) 267
– requirements 262
– superoxide dismutase (SOD) 267
exposure system 262
– biphasic cell culture system 268
– Millicell-CM system 270
– roller bottles 263
– rotating or rocking platforms 263

F

F2-isoprostanes 4, 200
fatigue 245
Fenton reaction 10, 12
First National Health and Nutrition Examination Survey Epidemiologic follow-up study 202
Fos 85
free radicals 281
fruit and vegetable 201

G

gas 263
– nitrogen dioxide (NO2) 263
– NO 263
– ozone 263
gas phase 77
genetically-engineered models 285
genetic engineering 285

gene transcription 284
gingival inflammation 245
glutahione (GSH) 53
glutaredoxin 78
glutathione 14, 390
glutathione peroxidase 1 395
glutathione peroxidases 372
glutathione S-transferase 59, 389, 390
GSH 54, 55
GSH S-transferases 55
GSH synthesis 372

H

heat shock proteins 95
heme oxygenase-1 79
HIF-1α 80
hMTH1 394
hOGG1 395
hydrogen peroxide 10
hydroquinone 9, 10, 13, 16, 17, 20, 21, 23, 24, 31, 33, 36, 38, 87
hydroxyl radical 2
hydroxynonenal 59
hypovitaminosis C 242

I

IL-8 87
imbalance 284
incidence 283
inflammation 282, 283, 284, 285, 286
inflammatory processes 280
inflammatory response 283

J

JNK 80

K

Keap1 367
Keap1-Nrf2-ARE pathway 372

L

l-buthionine sulfoximine 390
large prospective studies 238
lavage fluid 284
lipid peroxidation 200, 351
low-densitylipoprotein(LDL) 351

M

mainstream smoke 280, 281
malondialdehyde (MDA) 54, 204
matrix metalloproteinase 87
metals 11, 24
Michael addition 54, 64, 65
mitochondria 3
MMP-1 381
MMP-3 381
MMP-7 381
mucin 87
MutT 394

N

N-acetyl cysteine 78
nAChR 89
NAD(P)H:quinone oxidoreductase 1 79
NADPH 372
necrosis 95
neutrophil infiltration 284
NF-κB 60, 61, 64, 79, 369
nicotine 19, 77, 346
NO· 13, 14, 31, 38
NO2· 13
Nrf2 80
nuclear factor-kappaB (NF-κB) 56
nuclear factor-κB 284
nuclear factor erythroid 2-related factor 2 284
nuclear factor erythroid 2-related factor 2 (Nrf2) 366

O

oil fly ash 389
oxidant/antioxidant 369

oxidation 2
oxidative damage 3, 200, 393
oxidative stress 2, 3, 280, 282, 283, 284, 285, 286, 366, 389, 390
oxygen 280
ozone 280

P

p38 80
p53 80
pallid mouse 285
particulate phase 77
passive smokers 207
path length 281
peroxynitrite 14, 38, 82, 342
phase I 88
phase II 85
Physicians' Health Study 203
PKB/Akt 89
PKC 83
placenta 390
platelets 352
polycyclic aromatic hydrocarbon 389
proinflammatory mediators 286
prooxidant 2
proteinase/antiproteinase 369
protein carbonyl 52, 54
proteoglycans 381
proteolysis 286

R

radicals 9, 10, 12, 13, 26, 27, 29, 31, 33, 34, 35, 36
– carbon-centered 13, 27
– gas-phase 13, 31
– hydroxyl 10, 12, 36
– oxygen-centered 27
– semiquinone 9, 27, 31, 33, 34, 35, 36
– superoxide 9, 10, 13, 31, 36
– TPM 27, 29
RDA for vitamin C 241
reactive oxygen species 382
redox-sensitive transcription factors 366
Ref-1 80

S

scurvy 239
semiquinone 11, 36
side stream tobacco smoke 281, 390
single-cell gel electrophoresis 392
smoke 7, 13, 14, 15, 16, 18, 30, 32
– cytotoxicity 15, 31, 33
– electrophiles 15
– gas-phase 8, 13, 15
– mainstream 7
– metals 24
– particulate 14, 15, 18, 30
– particulate matter 8
– particulate phase 7
– sidestream 7
– TPM 16, 19, 24, 27, 29, 33
smoking machines 281
smoking system 271
– ADL/II 271
– VC10 273
sodium-dependent vitamin-C transporter 1 243
stroke 203
superoxide 9, 13, 14, 36, 37, 39, 342
surfactant 280
surrogate markers of disease 239
susceptible 284

T

tetrahydrobiopterin 248, 346
– BH4 deficiency 354
– BH4 depletion 348
thiobarbituric acid-reactive substances (TBARS) 204
thymine glycol 390
TIMP-1 381
TIMP-3 381
TNF-α 369
tobacco 6, 11, 16, 17, 20, 21
– carbohydrate 21, 23
– lignin 21, 23
– polyphenolic 27
– polyphenols 17, 23
tobacco-related aldehydes 77
– acetaldehyde 77

- acrolein 77
- crotonaldehyde 78
- formaldehyde 77

tobacco-specific nitrosamine 89
TPM 8, 19
transforming growth factor-β1 382
transgenic mouse model 285

V

versican 382
vitamin C 238
vitamin C deficiency 244
vitamin C intervention 243

X

xeroderma pigmentosa 395
xeroderma pigmentosum 389